Nuclear Medicine
Technology and Techniques

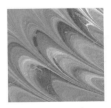

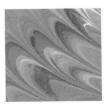

Nuclear Medicine
Technology and Techniques

Edited by

Donald R. Bernier, CNMT, FSNMTS
Clinical Instructor (Retired)
Nuclear Medicine Technology Program
School of Allied Health Professions
Saint Louis University
St. Louis, Missouri

Paul E. Christian, BS, CNMT, FSNMTS
Technical Director
Division of Nuclear Medicine
Department of Radiology
University of Utah Health Sciences Center
Salt Lake City, Utah

James K. Langan, CNMT, FSNMTS
Assistant Administrator
Department of Radiology
The Johns Hopkins Hospital
Baltimore, Maryland

Fourth Edition
with 420 illustrations

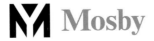

St. Louis   Baltimore   Boston   Carlsbad   Chicago   Naples   New York   Philadelphia   Portland
London   Madrid   Mexico City   Singapore   Sydney   Tokyo   Toronto   Wiesbaden

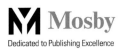
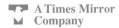

Publisher: Don E. Ladig
Senior Editor: Jeanne Rowland
Senior Developmental Editor: Lisa Potts
Developmental Editor: Sheryl Krato
Project Manager: John Rogers
Production Editor: Cheryl Abbott Bozzay
Designer: Yael Kats
Manufacturing Manager: Theresa Fuchs

Cover: The large background image is a whole-body scan using ^{111}In octreotide with normal radiopharmaceutical distribution in the liver, spleen, and kidneys. Two areas of radiopharmaceutical uptake in the chest are tumors.

   The smaller images are myocardial perfusion images. The polar map of myocardial perfusion (upper) shows decreased myocardial perfusion in the lower half of the heart, where the colors are less intense. The lower image is a three-dimensional display of myocardial perfusion also showing diminished perfusion as seen by darker colors in the lower portion of the heart.

Printed in the United States of America
Composition by The Clarinda Company
Printing/binding by Maple-Vail Book Manufacturing Group

Mosby–Year Book, Inc.
11830 Westline Industrial Drive
St. Louis, Missouri 63146

International Standard Book Number 0-8151-1991-7

97 98 99 00 / 9 8 7 6 5 4 3 2 1

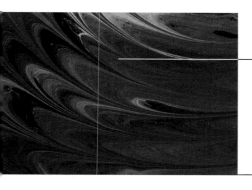

Contributors

Carolyn J. Anderson, PhD
Assistant Professor of Radiology
Division of Radiation Sciences
Mallinckrodt Institute of Radiology
Washington University School of Medicine
St. Louis, Missouri

Marcia Boyd, MS, CNMT
Director of Quality Management
Administration
Shelby County Government
Memphis, Tennessee

Paul H. Brown, PhD
Medical Physicist
Imaging Service
Veteran's Affairs Medical Center;
Associate Professor of Diagnostic Radiology
Diagnostic Radiology
Oregon Health Sciences University
Portland, Oregon

Julia W. Buchanan, BS
Research Associate
Department of Nuclear Medicine
The Johns Hopkins Medical Institutions
Baltimore, Maryland

Paul E. Christian, BS, CNMT, FSNMTS
Technical Director
Division of Nuclear Medicine
Department of Radiology
University of Utah Health Sciences Center
Salt Lake City, Utah

R. Edward Coleman, MD
Professor of Radiology
Vice Chairman
Department of Radiology
Duke University
Durham, North Carolina

James Conway, MD
Chief, Division of Nuclear Medicine
The Children's Memorial Hospital
Chicago, Illinois

Joanna B. Downer, MA
Division of Radiation Sciences
Mallinckrodt Institute of Radiology
Washington University School of Medicine
St. Louis, Missouri

†Robert L. Dressler, PhD
Professor of Chemistry
Department of Chemistry
Fort Hays State University
Hays, Kansas

Helen H. Drew, CNMT
Chief Technologist
Nuclear Medicine
The Johns Hopkins Medical Institutions
Baltimore, Maryland

Stanley J. Goldsmith, MD
Director, Nuclear Medicine
The New York Hospital Cornell Medical Center
New York, New York

L. Stephen Graham, PhD, FACR
Professor of Biomedical Physics
Department of Radiological Science
UCLA School of Medicine;
Medical Physicist
West Los Angeles VA Medical Center
Los Angeles, California

Landis K. Griffeth, MD, PhD
Chief of Nuclear Medicine
Baylor University Medical Center
Dallas, Texas

†Deceased.

Robert J. Gropler, MD
Associate Professor, Radiology and Medicine
Division of Nuclear Medicine
Mallinckrodt Institute of Radiology
Cardiovascular Division
Department of Internal Medicine
Washington University School of Medicine
St. Louis, Missouri

Jonathan Links, PhD
Associate Professor
Environmental Health Sciences and Radiology
Johns Hopkins University
Baltimore, Maryland

Leon S. Malmud, MD
Vice President of Health Sciences
Temple University Hospital
Philadelphia, Pennsylvania

Patricia McIntyre, MD (Retired)
Associate Professor of Medicine, Radiology,
    and Health Science
Radiology and Environmental Health Science
The Johns Hopkins Medical Institutions
Baltimore, Maryland

Marlene M. Moore, MS
Assistant Professor of Radiology
Medical Physicist
Department of Radiology
University of Vermont
Burlington, Vermont

David J. Phegley, BS, MBA, CNMT
Supervisor, Nuclear Medicine and PET Imaging
    Centers
Saint Louis University Hospital
St. Louis, Missouri

David Preston, MD
Professor of Radiology (Nuclear Medicine)
Director, Division of Nuclear Medicine
Department of Radiology
University of Kansas Medical Center
Kansas City, Kansas

Jay K. Rhine, BS, CNMT
Director, Nuclear Medicine Technology Program
The Johns Hopkins Medical Institutions
Baltimore, Maryland

Henry D. Royal, MD
Associate Director
Division of Nuclear Medicine
Mallinckrodt Institute of Radiology;
Professor of Radiology
Washington University School of Medicine
St. Louis, Missouri

Ursula Scheffel, ScD
Associate Professor
Radiology and Environmental Health Science
The Johns Hopkins Medical Institutions
Baltimore, Maryland

Sally Schwarz, MS, BCNP
Research Instructor in Radiology
Division of Nuclear Medicine
Mallinckrodt Institute of Radiology
Washington University School of Medicine
St. Louis, Missouri

Roger H. Secker-Walker, MB, FRCP
Professor of Medicine
College of Medicine
University of Vermont
Burlington, Vermont

Farrokh Dehdashti Shahrokh, MD
Assistant Professor of Radiology
Division of Nuclear Medicine
Mallinckrodt Institute of Radiology
Washington University School of Medicine
St. Louis, Missouri

Jay Spicer, MS
Assistant Professor of Diagnostic Radiology
    and Pharmacy
Director of Nuclear Pharmacy Service
Departments of Diagnostic Radiology and Pharmacy
University of Kansas Medical Center
Kansas City, Kansas

H. William Strauss, MD
Professor of Radiology
Chief, Division of Nuclear Medicine
Stanford Medical Center
Palo Alto, California

Kathy E. Thompson, BS, CNMT
Nuclear Medicine Technology Program Director
Allied Health Division
Baptist Memorial College of Health Sciences
Memphis, Tennessee

Richard A. Vitti, MD
Clinical Associate Professor
Department of Radiology
Pennsylvania Hospital
Philadelphia, Pennsylvania

Henry Wagner Jr., MD
Professor of Medicine
Radiology and Radiological Health Sciences
The Johns Hopkins Medical Institutions
Baltimore, Maryland

Susan Weiss, CNMT
Radiation Safety Officer
Department of Radiation Safety
The Children's Memorial Hospital
Chicago, Illinois

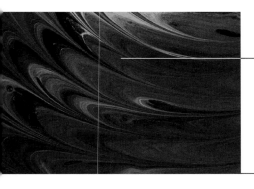

Foreword

Many textbooks fail to be published in a second edition. The popularity of the topic, the changes in medical practice or technology, and the energy of the authors are determinants of whether future editions are forthcoming. The first edition of *Nuclear Medicine Technology and Techniques* was published in 1981. Significant changes in nuclear medicine technology mandated that a second edition be published in 1989. The continuing popularity of this book led to a third edition in 1994. You now have before you the fourth edition, which places this textbook into the rarefied status of a "classic" textbook.

The editors have responded to the evident need for a timely continuing update of the technology of nuclear medicine. The second edition occurred after 8 years because of the significant advances in the field. The introduction of new techniques, especially that of cardiology, required additional revisions. The third edition followed after only 5 years and emphasized the technology of SPECT and PET imaging. This edition follows after only 3 years and represents further evidence of the continuing evolution of nuclear medicine technology. The editors have selected renowned authors with expertise in their field, who can convey their knowledge of the topic through the written word. The editors themselves are founding members and leaders within the Technologist Section of the Society of Nuclear Medicine and the Nuclear Medicine Technology Certification Board. They have served as editors or associate editors of the most important scientific journals devoted to nuclear medicine technology. Most importantly, they all have an abundance of experience as practicing nuclear medicine technologists, allowing them to recognize the important trends and developments in the field.

The success of a textbook can be recognized by its well-worn character, dog-eared pages, and underlining of passages, which are caused by frequent and continuous use. This textbook, which is used in our training program at The Children's Memorial Hospital, has these characteristics. It is not only utilized continuously by the nuclear medicine technology students in our training programs, but it is also used by our nuclear medicine residents and fellows.

It is said that the first edition of any book is the most desired by collectors, but the subsequent editions are the most valuable from a utility point of view. Being the fourth edition establishes this textbook as the "classic" in the field of nuclear medicine technology, and as such, it belongs in the laboratory of every practitioner of the discipline. Its up-to-date bibliography and images will serve not only as a reference for improving the quality of practice but also as the major resource for a quick and efficient method to find references for additional reading.

James J. Conway, MD

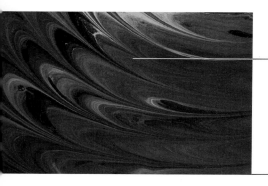

Preface

The fourth edition of *Nuclear Medicine Technology and Techniques* has been written to provide an update to the ever changing field of nuclear medicine. This new edition incorporates many exciting changes that have occurred in the last few years. The first section covers the fundamentals of mathematics, statistics, and physics, which are required as background information for other topics to build on. Chapters on instrumentation, computer science, laboratory techniques, radiochemistry and radiopharmacology, and radiation safety follow. A chapter devoted to each organ system includes sections on anatomy and physiology, followed by the radiopharmaceuticals that apply to the specific organ system. The specific procedure, techniques, and interpretation of these studies are then discussed.

To provide a truly comprehensive review for the technologist, we have added a new chapter on patient care. This chapter covers all of the fundamental aspects of patient mechanics, including obtaining vital signs, injection techniques, patient ethics, infection control, and universal precautions. Information on nonradioactive medications used in nuclear medicine is also included. In addition, a section on total quality improvement describes planning and process management to monitor and control patient outcomes.

Furthermore, we have added important information to the instrumentation and computer chapters to expand the aspects of SPECT imaging, reconstruction, and image filtering. Plus, the radiation safety chapter now includes detailed information on occupational radiation safety. This chapter has been significantly reorganized to present the material in a fresh and more understandable order.

In addition, information on new radiopharmaceuticals and their applications have been included to enhance the understanding of students and technologists in these areas. These discussions appear within the clinical chapters where individual clinical applications are most applicable. Material including the use of Sestamibi for parathyroid imaging as well as Somatostatin and Technegas have been added to the appropriate chapters. Procedures have been updated, where applicable, in the majority of the clinical chapters. In addition, the chapter on the endocrine system now covers the care of patients receiving thyroid therapy using ^{131}I. Furthermore, we have added information on pain management of bone cancer using ^{89}Sr to the skeletal system chapter.

Readers will also find that we have added learning objectives and outlines to each chapter. These two elements should add considerable teaching and educational value. In addition, we have liberally used tables and illustrations throughout to support concepts and to provide helpful examples. This edition is generously illustrated to demonstrate expected results of various studies. Furthermore, the glossary has been thoroughly updated so that definitions of specialized terminology can be found without consulting other sources.

The preparation of this fourth edition has required the efforts of many people. We appreciate the cooperation and work of Mosby. In particular, we would like to thank Lisa Potts and Jeanne Rowland for their understanding and patience during the writing and publication process. We are grateful for the hard work and efforts of our distinguished contributors who are the key to the content and educational value of this book. We sincerely appreciate their expertise in their respective areas, their long hours of preparation, and their dedication to the success of this fourth edition.

Donald R. Bernier
Paul E. Christian
James K. Langan

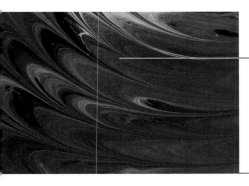

Contents

Nuclear Medicine
Technology and Techniques

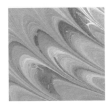

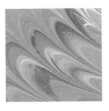

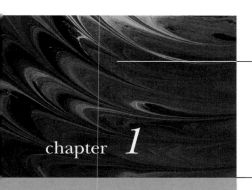

Paul H. Brown

chapter 1

Mathematics and Statistics

Objectives

Use scientific notation in performing algebraic operations.

Use the inverse square law to calculate the intensity of a radiation field at various distances.

Perform radioactive dilution calculations.

Define the units of radioactivity, radiation exposure, radiation absorbed dose, and radiation dose equivalent.

Perform calculations with logarithms and exponents using a calculator.

Discuss numeric accuracy, significant digits, and rounding.

Calculate quantities of radioactivity using the general form of the decay equation and decay factors.

Compute the concentration of Mo-99 in Tc-99m.

Compute effective half-life and biologic half-life.

Calculate intensity with half-value layers.

Diagram various types of graphs and graphing techniques.

Discuss curve fitting techniques.

Define mean, standard deviation, and coefficient of variation.

Discuss Gaussian and Poisson distributions.

State the formula for standard deviation, and perform calculations in the presence of background.

Explain the function of the chi-square test and interpretation of results.

Interpret the results of a chi-square test using a probability table.

Discuss the use and interpretation of *t*-tests.

Describe techniques for the interpretation used in medical decision making relative to the application of sensitivity, specificity, prevalence, and accuracy.

*N*uclear medicine technology occupies a unique position in the allied health sciences because of its strong dependence on quantitative, or mathematical, results. This chapter provides a sound basis for performing calculations that are typically required of nuclear medicine technologists. The emphasis here is on practical use, not on theoretical principles. Practical examples are provided, and the first of each type of calculation includes a discussion on the use of pocket calculators. This chapter reviews elementary algebra, graphing techniques, and statistical principles, always with an emphasis on practical applications. It is presumed that readers have a working knowledge of high school level mathematics. The more advanced reader may wish to skip to the

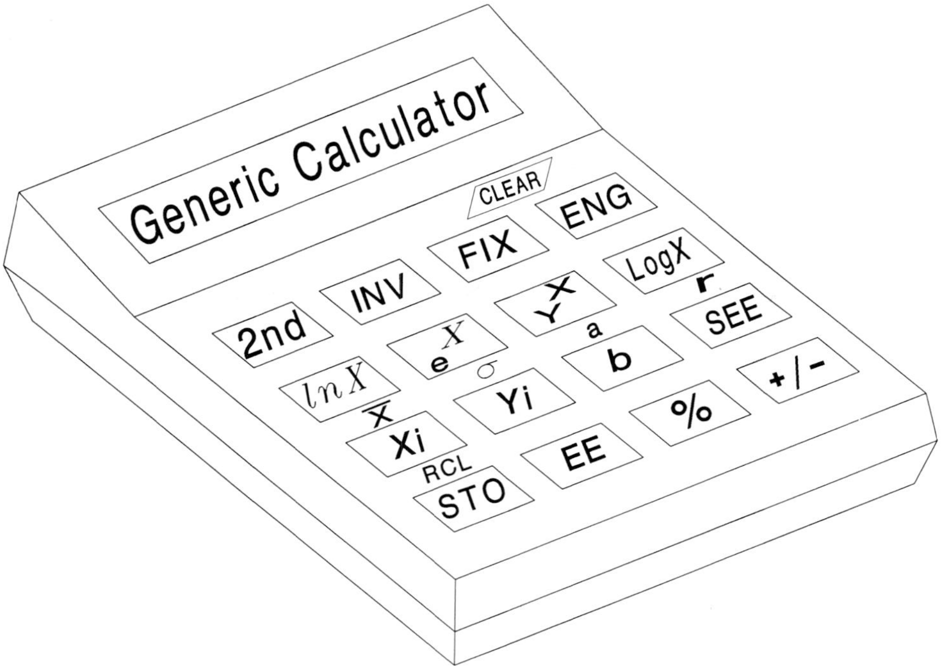

Figure 1-1 Generic scientific calculator demonstrating keys useful in nuclear medicine. The *2nd* key produces function above key, e.g., *2nd* and *Xi* produce mean of Xi values. The *INV* key produces functional inverse of key. For example, *INV* and *lnX* are e^x functions. Most calculators do not have an e^x key if they also offer *INV* and *lnX* keys. The *FIX* key sets number of decimal places to be displaced, e.g., *FIX* and 3 will display only three decimal places for all subsequent calculation. The *ENG* key causes the calculator to display results in scientific notation. *Xi* key is used to enter x values to calculate mean $\bar{x}$ and standard deviation σ. *Xi* and *Yi* keys are used to enter x and y values for least squares curve fit (linear regression) to produce straight line with intercept (a), slope (b), correlation (r), and standard error of estimate (SEE). $+/-$ key changes sign of number.

pertinent sections of this chapter. The reader who requires a more basic review of algebra may wish to consult another mathematics text.[4,8]

FUNDAMENTALS

Scientific Notation

Numbers in scientific calculations are often very small, such as 0.0015, or very large, such as 23,000. Scientific notation allows these numbers to be presented in a more convenient notation without cumbersome commas and zeros: 1.5×10^{-3} and 2.3×10^4. The exponent on the 10 specifies how many places the decimal point in the number is to be shifted to the left (for negative exponents) or shifted to the right (for positive exponents). Sometimes these numbers are alternatively represented as 1.5E − 3 and 2.3E + 4, a form found on pocket calculators or in printed tabular data (for example, in calculations of internal radiation dosimetry), where the superscript is cumbersome to print. Pocket calculators typically have an EE key (for **e**nter **e**xponent), which allows easy entry of data in scientific notation. For example, if it is desired to calculate

$$(1.5 \times 10^{-3}) \div (2.3 \times 10^4)$$

the procedure on the calculator would be as follows (refer to Figure 1-1):

1.5	enter value for numerator
EE	*enter exponent* key
±	*change sign* key to make the exponent negative
3	enter the value of the exponent
÷	division key
2.3	enter the value for denominator
EE	*enter exponent* key
4	enter the value of the exponent
=	*equals* key, causes calculation to proceed
6.5217391E-8	(see result in display)

This is precisely the same result as would be obtained by dividing 0.0015 by 23000 on the calculator.

It is often desirable to use numeric prefixes to represent very small or large numbers (Table 1-1). The value 6.52×10^{-8} g (or 6.52E-8 g) can be more conveniently represented by converting the exponent to one of the exponent values shown in Table 1-1, which are usually exponents divisible by 3 (such as 3, 6, 9 . . .).

Table 1-1	Numeric prefixes	
Abbreviation	**Prefix**	**Numeric value**
a	atto-	10^{-18}, one quintillionth
f	femto-	10^{-15}, one quadrillionth
p	pico-	10^{-12}, one trillionth
n	nano-	10^{-9}, one billionth
μ	micro-	10^{-6}, one millionth
m	milli-	10^{-3}, one thousandth
c	centi-	10^{-2}, one hundredth
d	deci-	10^{-1}, one tenth
dk	deka-	10^{1}, ten
h	hecto-	10^{2}, hundred
k	kilo-	10^{3}, thousand
M	mega-	10^{6}, million
G	giga-	10^{9}, billion
T	tera-	10^{12}, trillion
P	peta-	10^{15}, quadrillion
E	exa-	10^{18}, quintillion

Thus 6.52×10^{-8} g can be represented as 65.2×10^{-9} g, or in convenient shorthand form as 65.2 ng (nanograms), where the *nano-* stands for 10^{-9}. Notice that the decimal point in the number 6.52×10^{-8} can be shifted to the right by making the exponent smaller by 1 for each right shift of the decimal (e.g., $6.52 \times 10^{-8} = 65.2 \times 10^{-9}$), the object being to have an exponent that is divisible by 3 so that the numeric prefixes in Table 1-1 can be used. Similarly, a number like 2.3×10^{4} ct (or counts) can be expressed as 23.0×10^{3} ct, or 23k ct, the k denoting *kilo,* or thousand.

This type of notation is often used for units of radioactivity, which is measured in becquerels (Bq). A patient might be injected with 7.4×10^{8} Bq of radioactivity, which can be written 0.74×10^{9} Bq (the decimal point can be shifted *left* if the exponent is *increased* by 1 for each left shift). So the injected radioactivity could be conveniently represented as 0.74 GBq. Alternatively, the value 7.4×10^{8} Bq could be written 740.0×10^{6} Bq = 740 MBq (the decimal was shifted two places to the right so the exponent is decreased by 2). Choosing between the two forms is simply a matter of preference. Note that pocket calculators often have an engineering notation key, which controls the scientific notation exponents in the calculator display to always be a power of 3. For example, 7.4×10^{8} Bq will be displayed as 740E6 on the calculator, which the user understands to be the same as 740 MBq.

Fractions and Percentages

Fractions, such as ⅓, consist of a numerator (1) that is to be divided by a denominator (3). The value of a frac-

tion may also be expressed decimally, such as ¾ = 0.750 (a fraction that terminates in a zero digit), or ⅓ = 1.3333 . . . (a fraction that never terminates in a zero digit). The mathematical manipulation of fractions requires care as to the number of digits and placement of the decimal point. The safest way to handle mathematical manipulation of fractions is to simply use the power of the pocket calculator to perform calculations such as ⅓ + ¾ by first converting the fractions to decimals and then carrying out the other arithmetic.

$$\frac{1}{3} = 0.333$$
$$\frac{3}{4} = 2.250$$
$$\text{sum} = 2.583$$

As a general rule the arithmetic should maintain at least one more digit in each fraction than is necessary in the final result. For example, if it is desired to describe the area of a rectangle (area = width $\times$ length) to the nearest centimeter, then measurements of the width and length of the rectangle should be made to the nearest tenth of a centimeter. Use of the pocket calculator generally produces at least eight digits of accuracy, which is more than enough for nuclear medicine calculations.

Percentages are values expressed as a fraction of some whole, entire value: 75% of some number is the same as 0.75 multiplied by that number.

$$75\% \text{ of } 5 \text{ ml} = 0.75 \times 5 \text{ ml} = 3.75 \text{ ml}$$

Many pocket calculators have a % key, which makes it unnecessary to first convert the percentage to a decimal:

75	enter percent value
%	*percent* key
$\times$	*multiply* key
5	enter 5
=	(see display results of 3.75)

Percentages are often expressed as a percentage change between two values. For example, a patient may have had a kidney function test last month that showed a kidney clearance rate of 42 ml/min. The patient returns today and has a kidney clearance rate of 58 ml/min. The patient's kidney function has increased by 38% based on the following:

$$\% \text{ change} = [(\text{new value} - \text{old value})/\text{old value}]$$
$$\times 100$$
$$= [(58 - 42)/42] \times 100$$
$$= (16/42) \times 100$$
$$= 0.38 \times 100 = 38\%$$

Algebraic Equations and Ratios

Calculations in nuclear medicine often involve expressing a mathematical concept as a ratio. For example, an intensity setting of 240 on a display screen may produce a suitable image for a bar phantom with 500,000 cts in the acquisition. Now it is desired to change to 300,000 cts in the image. The intensity on the screen is known to change linearly with the intensity control setting. What intensity setting should be used for the new 300,000 ct image? This translates mathematically to:

$$\frac{x}{300k\ ct} = \frac{240\ intensity}{500k\ ct}$$

This is typical of numeric equations in nuclear medicine. First, it is necessary to translate a mathematical concept, expressed in words, into an algebraic equation. The equation generally contains several numbers and one unknown value; here the new intensity setting is the unknown value (x). The object is to solve for the unknown value by rearranging the terms in the equation. In this example the unknown intensity x can be isolated on one side of the equation by multiplying both sides of the equation by 300k ct. Remember, we can always do any math operation to both sides of an equation without changing the equality. Many students may have learned this technique as cross-multiplying to solve a proportion.

$$300k\ ct \times \frac{(x)}{300k\ ct} = 300k\ ct \times \frac{240\ intensity}{500k\ ct}$$

The 300k ct cancels in the left numerator and denominator, so

$$x = 300k\ ct \times \frac{240\ intensity}{500k\ ct} = 144\ intensity$$

Another frequently encountered problem relates to radioactivity concentrations in patient doses. For example, the morning elution of the ^{99}Mo-^{99m}Tc generator yields 943 mCi of ^{99m}Tc radioactivity in 20 ml of saline eluate. What volume should be withdrawn from the eluate vial into a patient syringe to immediately perform a 20 mCi patient scan?

$$\frac{x}{20\ mCi} = \frac{20\ ml}{943\ mCi}$$

$$x = 20\ mCi \times \frac{20\ ml}{943\ mCi} = 0.42\ ml$$

Inverse Square Law

The radiation exposure from a radioactive point source is governed by a mathematical relationship called the *inverse square law*. This states that the radiation exposure or intensity (I) at a distance (d) from a radioactive source is proportional to the inverse square of the

distance. This law holds for a point source (a source that is very small when compared to the large distances from the source involved) that emits radiation not absorbed in the distances involved. A syringe source of x rays or γ rays at a distance of 1 m or more in air would qualify as a point source. Air is only very weakly absorbing of x rays or γ rays in the energy ranges typically encountered in nuclear medicine. A syringe source for exposure to the hands does not qualify for the inverse square law, since the distance from the syringe to the hands is not large compared to the syringe dimensions. Similarly, the exposure from standing near patients does not follow the simple inverse square law. Mathematically the inverse square law states:

$$I \propto \frac{k}{d^2}$$

where k is a proportionality constant that depends on the type of radioactive source and its activity. This inverse square law results in the radiation intensity quadrupling if the distance from the source is halved, or the radiation intensity is decreased to one fourth its value if the distance is doubled. Changing the distance by a factor of 3 results in a factor of 9 change in intensity (9 times more intensity for a third the distance, or one ninth the intensity for 3 times the distance). This is usually stated in a form relating the old intensity (I_2) at some old distance (d_2) to a new intensity (I_1) at some new distance (d_1).

$$I_1(d_1)^2 = I_2(d_2)^2$$

The intensity of radiation is usually measured in units of roentgens (R) or milliroentgens (mR) per hour. For example, a technologist is working 2 m from a small vial of radioactivity that results in an intensity or exposure level of 2.5 mR/hr at this distance. If the technologist moves to a distance of 3 m from the source, what will be the new radiation intensity?

$$I_1 \times (3\ m)^2 = (2.5\ mR/hr) \times (2\ m)^2$$

or

$$I_1 = (2.5\ mR/hr) \times 2^2/3^2$$
$$I_1 = (2.5\ mR/hr) \times (4/9) = 1.1\ mR/hr$$

The technologist's radiation exposure is more than halved by his moving further from the source. Note that pocket calculators generally have an x^2 key, which facilitates the calculation:

2.5	enter intensity value
$\times$	*multiply* key
2	enter old distance value
x^2	*squaring* key
$\div$	*division* key
3	enter new distance value
x^2	*squaring* key
=	(see result of 1.1 in display)

In another example, a technologist is working 4 ft from a point source that results in an intensity of 0.62 mR/hr. Concerns of radiation safety suggest that the intensity should be maintained at no more than 0.25 mR/hr for a safe working environment. To what distance from the source should the technologist move to achieve an exposure level of 0.25 mR/hr?

$$0.25 \text{ mR/hr} \times (d_1)^2 = 0.62 \text{ mR/hr} \times (4 \text{ ft})^2$$

$$(d_1)^2 = \frac{(0.62 \text{ mR/hr}) \times (4 \text{ ft})^2}{0.25 \text{ mR/hr}}$$

$$(d_1)^2 = \frac{(0.62 \text{ mR/hr}) \times 16 \text{ ft}^2}{0.25 \text{ mR/hr}}$$

$$(d_1)^2 = 39.7 \text{ ft}^2$$

$$\sqrt{(d_1)^2} = \sqrt{39.7 \text{ ft}^2}$$

$$d_1 = \sqrt{39.7 \text{ ft}^2} = 6.3 \text{ ft}$$

Again, pocket calculators generally have a square root key ($\sqrt{}$), which facilitates calculation:

0.62	enter old intensity value
$\times$	*multiply* key
4	enter old distance value
x^2	*squaring* key
$\div$	*division* key
0.25	enter new intensity value
$=$	results of division
$\sqrt{}$	*square root* key (see result of 6.3 in display)

Notice that in solving this problem the left side of the equation contained $(d_1)^2$, but since we wanted to solve for d_1, we took the square root of both sides of the equation. The squaring function and the square root function canceled on the left side of the equation because $\sqrt{x^2} = x$. Functions that have this property are called inverse functions. The squaring function $(x)^2$ and the square root function ($\sqrt{}$) are inverse functions.

For example, say a dilute standard solution is made by diluting a 1 ml volume of some standard radioactivity up to a 500 ml volume. This dilute standard, which has a low enough radioactivity to be accurately counted in a well counter, is then counted, and 2 ml of the diluted standard yields 15,346 ct. How many counts were in the original 1 ml of the standard?

$$C_1 V_1 = C_2 V_2$$

$$C_1 \times 1 \text{ ml} = \left(\frac{15,346 \text{ ct}}{2 \text{ ml}}\right) \times 500 \text{ ml}$$

$$C_1 = 3,836,500 \text{ ct/ml}$$

Notice how the units are carefully included with each number.

The dilution principle can also be used to measure an unknown volume. For example, suppose a 2 ml sample of a standard solution produces 647,530 ct per minute (cpm) in a well counter. This standard sample is then injected intravenously into a patient, and a 2 ml sample of patient blood yields 2600 ct in 10 minutes (or 260 cpm). What is the patient's blood volume?

$$C_1 V_1 = C_2 V_2$$

$$\left(\frac{260 \text{ cpm}}{2 \text{ ml}}\right) \times V_1 = \left(\frac{647,530 \text{ cpm}}{2 \text{ ml}}\right) \times 2 \text{ ml}$$

$$V_1 = 4981 \text{ ml}$$

Often it is necessary to inject a patient with a more concentrated solution than can be accurately counted in a well counter to ensure an adequate measure of the patient blood counts, without undue statistical counting noise. In the previous example, for instance, the patient blood counts yielded only 260 cpm/2 ml, which would be subject to a large statistical uncertainty (as discussed below). It would therefore be necessary to obtain more blood counts. This requires increasing the activity in the standard source, which then becomes too concentrated to be accurately counted in the well counter. The problem is either that the standard is too strong or the patient sample is too weak because of the large dilution in the patient blood volume. The answer to the problem is to dilute a portion of the standard and count this diluted standard, while the full-strength undiluted standard can be injected into the patient. The standard can be diluted by adding 1 ml of it to a flask, which is then filled to 500 ml. The dilution factor is then 500. For example, a 2 ml sample of the 1:500 diluted standard in a well counter might yield 26,835 cpm. Then 5 ml of the undiluted standard is injected into the patient, producing blood plasma counts of 26,500 cpm in 2 ml of plasma. What is the plasma volume?

$$C_1 V_1 = C_2 V_2$$

$$\left(\frac{26,500 \text{ cpm}}{2 \text{ ml}}\right) \times V_1 = \left(500 \times \frac{26,835 \text{ cpm}}{2 \text{ ml}}\right) \times 5 \text{ ml}$$

$$V_1 = 2530 \text{ ml}$$

Notice here that the standard counts had to be multiplied by the dilution factor of 500 to obtain the true standard concentration, which was injected into the patient.

Units

When manipulating numbers, it is critical to always consider the units of the numbers involved. Forgetting to specify whether a patient was injected with 5 μCi or

5 mCi of iodine-131 radioactivity can have disastrous consequences. It is best to develop a habit of writing down the units for all the numbers in question.

Units are agreed upon standard quantities of measurement. They are generally composed of some combination of the three fundamental divisions of mass, length, and time. These are the properties that can be measured in our physical or biologic world. From these fundamental units we can derive other units, such as speed in meters per second (m/sec), centimeters per second (cm/sec), or feet per second (ft/sec). These three units of speed are derived from the three different measurement systems that arose about 50 years ago: the meter-kilogram-second, or mks, system of units; the centimeter-gram-second, or cgs, system of units; and the foot-pound-second system of units. Also commonly encountered are energy units of 1 joule (1 kg $\times$ m^2/sec^2) in the mks system and 1 erg (1 g $\times$ cm^2/sec^2) of energy in the cgs system. Table 1-2 lists units frequently encountered in nuclear medicine. In 1977 the situation of having three existing unit systems was simplified when a worldwide Système International d'Unités (SI) was developed. Although the intent of SI units was simplification, both the old units and SI units seem to be in use. In SI an attempt was made to name each unit after a person and to avoid any numeric factors in the definition of the new unit. For example, the old temperature scale of centigrade was replaced by Celsius (named after a person), and the old unit of radioactivity, the curie (3.7 $\times$ 10^{10} disintegrations per second [dps]), was replaced in SI units by the becquerel (1 dps), which has no complicating numeric factor in the definition. The reader should be familiar with both the old units and the SI units shown in Table 1-2. It is often necessary to convert between various systems for consistency in applying mathematics equations. Most common is the necessity to convert between the old units and SI units for radioactivity, radiation exposure, absorbed dose, and dose equivalent. For example, what is the activity in becquerels for 20 mCi of a radionu-

clide? This can be calculated from the conversion factor in Table 1-2 as follows:

$$\text{Activity in Bq} = 20 \text{ mCi} \times \left(10^{-3} \frac{\text{Ci}}{\text{mCi}}\right) \times$$
$$\left(3.7 \times 10^{10} \frac{\text{Bq}}{\text{Ci}}\right)$$
$$= 20 \times 10^{-3} \times 3.7 \times 10^{10} \text{ Bq}$$
$$= 7.4 \times 10^8 \text{ Bq} = 740 \times 10^6 \text{ Bq}$$
$$= 740 \text{ MBq (or 0.74 GBq)}$$

So 20 mCi is the same activity as 740 MBq. Notice how all the units except Bq canceled between numerator and denominator in the conversion. Use of the *enter exponent* key on the pocket calculator will facilitate such calculations.

Similarly, it might be desired to convert a radiation absorbed dose of 5 rad into the new SI units of grays (Gy):

$$\text{Absorbed dose} = 5 \text{ rad} \times \frac{1 \text{ Gy}}{100 \text{ rad}} = 0.05 \text{ Gy} = 5 \text{ cGy}$$

So 5 rad is the same absorbed dose as 5 cGy.

To convert dose equivalent in the new SI units of 1 cSv into the old unit of rem:

$$\text{Dose equivalent} = 1 \text{ cSv} \times 10^{-2} \frac{\text{Sv}}{\text{cSv}} \times \frac{100 \text{ rem}}{\text{Sv}}$$
$$= 1 \text{ rem}$$

So 1 cSv is the same dose equivalent as 1 rem. Again, notice that all the units except the final desired value cancel in numerator and denominator.

Use of the radioactive decay equations discussed below often requires converting between different time units. Suppose it was necessary to convert the time difference between 10:45 AM and 1:20 PM into units of days. The time difference is 155 minutes, which can be converted to days:

Table 1-2	Units		
Measured property	**Old unit**	**New SI unit**	**Conversion factor**
Radioactivity	curie (Ci) = 3.7 $\times$ 10^{10} dps	becquerel (Bq) = 1 dps	1 Ci = 3.7 $\times$ 10^{10} Bq
			1 Bq = 2.7 $\times$ 10^{-11} Ci
Radiation exposure	roentgen (R) = 2.58 $\times$ 10^{-4} C/kg	coulomb/kg (C/kg)	1 R = 2.58 $\times$ 10^{-4} C/kg
			1 C/kg = 3.88 $\times$ 10^3 R
Radiation absorbed dose	rad = 100 erg/g	gray (Gy) = 1 J/kg	1 rad = 0.01 Gy
			1 Gy = 100 rad
Radiation dose equivalent	rem = QF $\times$ rad	sievert (Sv) = QF $\times$ Gy	1 rem = 0.01 Sv
			1 Sv = 100 rem

QF = quality factor.

$$155 \text{ min} \times \frac{1 \text{ hr}}{60 \text{ min}} \times \frac{1 \text{ day}}{24 \text{ hr}} = 0.108 \text{ day}$$

The process of converting such units consists of repeatedly multiplying by a conversion factor of 1 (expressed as a fraction, such as 1 hr/60 min) until the desired final unit result is obtained. For example, to convert the speed of light (3×10^{10} cm/sec) into a speed measured in furlongs (⅛ mi) per fortnight (14 d):

$$\frac{3 \times 10^{10} \text{ cm}}{\text{sec}}$$

$$\times \frac{\left(\dfrac{1 \text{ in}}{2.54 \text{ cm}}\right) \times \left(\dfrac{1 \text{ ft}}{12 \text{ in}}\right) \times \left(\dfrac{1 \text{ mi}}{5280 \text{ ft}}\right) \times \left(\dfrac{8 \text{ furlong}}{\text{mi}}\right)}{\left(\dfrac{1 \text{ min}}{60 \text{ sec}}\right) \times \left(\dfrac{1 \text{ hr}}{60 \text{ min}}\right) \times \left(\dfrac{1 \text{ day}}{24 \text{ hr}}\right) \times \left(\dfrac{1 \text{ fortnight}}{14 \text{ days}}\right)}$$

$$= \frac{(3 \times 10^{10}) \times \left(\dfrac{1}{2.54}\right) \times \left(\dfrac{1}{12}\right) \times \left(\dfrac{1}{5280}\right) \times (8) \text{ furlong}}{\left(\dfrac{1}{60}\right) \times \left(\dfrac{1}{60}\right) \times \left(\dfrac{1}{24}\right) \times \left(\dfrac{1}{14}\right) \text{ fortnight}}$$

$$= \frac{1.49 \times 10^{6}}{8.27 \times 10^{-7}} \frac{\text{furlong}}{\text{fortnight}}$$

$$= 1.8 \times 10^{12} \text{ furlong/fortnight}$$

The conversion factors in the numerator convert centimeters to furlongs, and the conversion factors in the denominator convert seconds to fortnights. Completion of this otherwise silly problem on the calculator provides useful practice in unit conversion and calculator manipulation. Notice how the units in juxtaposed conversion factors always cancel between numerator and denominator until only the final desired units remain.

Lengthy calculations such as this one may best be handled on the calculator by first calculating the numerical value of the numerator and denominator separately. Calculate for the numerator with the following progression of keys:

3
EE
10
÷
2.54
÷
12
÷
5280
×
8
=   (see result 1.4912909E6 for numerator)

Calculate for the denominator with the following progression of keys:

1
÷
60
÷
60
÷
24
÷
14
=   (see result 0.0000008)
EE   put calculator in scientific notation
       (see result 8.2671958E-7)

Notice that the calculator had to be placed in scientific notation for the denominator to observe more than one significant figure in the display. Calculators from various manufacturers might function differently. The calculation is then completed by dividing the numerator by the denominator to obtain the final answer of 1.8×10^{12} furlongs/fortnight. Most scientific calculators have memory locations; you can temporarily store the numerator result in one memory location, with the denominator result stored in another. Then the memory locations can easily be recalled to divide numerator by denominator without having to enter the intermediate results by hand.

Exponent Laws and Logarithms

This section expands the algebra of exponents and logarithms. In general, exponent notation is set up as follows:

$$\text{base}^{\text{exponent}} = \text{number}$$

For example:

$$10^4 = 10,000$$

The exponent notation of 10^4 means the same as 10 multiplied 4 times:

$$10^4 = 10 \times 10 \times 10 \times 10 = 10,000$$

Generally, we are confronted with exponential calculations involving raising a base of 10, 2, or e to some power. Base 2 problems often arise in computer considerations where it might be required to calculate:

$$2^8 = 2 \times 2 \times 2 \times 2 \times 2 \times 2 \times 2 \times 2 = 256$$

Scientific pocket calculators generally have a Y^x key, meaning raise the base Y to the power x, which facilitates this type of calculation. To find 2^8 using the calculator:

2   enter base value Y
Y^x *exponentiation* key
8   enter exponent value x
=   (see result 256 in display)

A special case arises when the exponent is zero. By mathematics definition any number (except zero) raised to the zero power is equal to 1:

$$B^0 = 1$$
$$10^0 = 1$$
$$2^0 = 1$$

Negative exponents provide a convenient form for representing small numbers:

$$10^{-4} = \frac{1}{10^4} = 0.0001$$

Notice that this shows how a number in exponent notation can be moved from numerator to denominator simply by changing the sign of the exponent:

$$2^8 = \frac{1}{2^{-8}} = 256$$

The algebra of exponents in equations follows certain rules. *Multiplication:* add the exponents.

$$B^x \times B^y = B^{x+y}$$
$$10^2 \times 10^3 = 10^5$$
$$10^4 \times 10^{-5} = 10^{-1}$$

To find the area of a rectangle multiply width times height:

$$\text{area} = 20 \text{ cm} \times 30 \text{ cm} = 600 \text{ cm}^2$$

Notice how this follows the rule for multiplying exponents:

$$\text{cm}^1 \times \text{cm}^1 = \text{cm}^2$$

Division: subtract the exponents.

$$\frac{B^x}{B^y} = B^{x-y}$$

$$\frac{10^2}{10^3} = 10^{2-3} = 10^{-1}$$

$$\frac{10^4}{10^{-5}} = 10^{4-(-5)} = 10^9$$

$$\frac{2^3}{2^3} = 2^0 = 1$$

A practical problem might involve calculation of the *mass* attenuation coefficient μ_m, which is defined by the quotient of the *linear* attenuation coefficient μ (in units of cm^{-1} or $1/\text{cm}$) divided by the density ρ (in units of g/cm^3) for some substance, such as human soft tissues. For example:

if $\mu = 0.12 \; 1/\text{cm}$ and $\rho = 3.4 \; \text{g/cm}^3$, then

$$\mu_m = \frac{0.12 \; 1/\text{cm}}{3.4 \; \text{g/cm}^3}$$

The difficulty here is how to evaluate the units. First eliminate denominator units within each term of the equation, i.e., write $1/\text{cm}$ as cm^{-1} and g/cm^3 as $\text{g} \times \text{cm}^{-3}$, according to the rule discussed above for moving from denominator to numerator by changing sign of the exponent. Then:

$$\mu_m = \frac{0.12 \text{ cm}^{-1}}{3.4 \text{ g} \times \text{cm}^{-3}}$$

Now follow the rule above for division of exponents with cm dimensions:

$$\mu_m = \frac{0.12 \text{ cm}^{-1-(-3)}}{3.4 \text{ g}} = \frac{0.12 \text{ cm}^2}{3.4 \text{ g}} = 0.035 \; \frac{\text{cm}^2}{\text{g}}$$

Or the units of μ_m might be written as $\mu_m = 0.035$ $\text{cm}^2 \times \text{g}^{-1}$.

Another example is hertz (Hz), the measure of frequency expressed as the number of waves or cycles per second. For example, if 3 waves pass by a certain point in space in 1 sec, then the frequency (ν) is given by:

$$\nu = 3 \; 1/\text{sec, or } 3 \text{ sec}^{-1}, \text{ or } 3 \text{ Hz}$$

Taking the root of a number is the inverse of raising to a power. A special case is the square root $\left(\sqrt{} \right)$ of a positive number *x*, which is defined by:

$$\sqrt{x} \times \sqrt{x} = x$$
$$\sqrt{9} \times \sqrt{9} = 3 \times 3 = 9$$

Note that finding the square root is the same as raising a number to the ½ power: $\sqrt{x} = x^{1/2}$. As mentioned previously, the square root and squaring operation are inverses of each other, since:

$$\sqrt{(x^2)} = x$$
$$(\sqrt{x})^2 = x$$

Whether the squaring or the square root is performed first, the inverse function always cancels the other operation and simply returns the number *x*. Other roots can be calculated as the nth root of a number, which is written as $\sqrt[n]{x}$. For example, $\sqrt[3]{64} = 4$, because $4 \times 4 \times 4 = 64$. Some pocket calculators have a root key, such as $\sqrt[x]{y}$. Or the calculator might have an inverse (INV) key (see Figure 1-1), which is pressed before pressing another function to get the inverse of that function. For example, to calculate $\sqrt[3]{64}$ on the calculator:

64	enter value y to find cube root
INV and Y^x	or root key $\sqrt[x]{y}$, which is $\text{INV} - Y^x$
3	enter root value x
=	(see display of result, 4)

The base e ($= 2.718 \ldots$) is an irrational number called *Euler's number,* named after Swiss mathematician and physicist Leonhard Euler (1707-1783). Calculations involving e pervade our mathematical, physical, and biological world: radioactive decay, absorption of radiation, growth of bacteria, and radiation damage to cells. Scientific pocket calculators often have a special e^x key that is used for calculations. Many calculators require the user to invoke the e^x function by virtue of the fact that the e^x function and the natural logarithm function (ln x) are inverse of each other. This means that ln $(e^x) = x$, and $e^{(\ln x)} = x$. For example, a radioactive decay problem might require the following calculation:

$$e^{-0.693} \times 4.5/6.0 = e^{-0.51975} = 0.59$$

This can be performed on the pocket calculator as follows:

0.693	enter value
+/−	*change sign* key
x	multiply
4.5	enter value
÷	
6	enter value
=	(see result of division)
INV and ln x	or e^x key
	(see result, 0.59)

Logarithms provide another convenient system of notation that can make mathematical problems easier to solve. In nuclear medicine logarithms can be used to linearize certain graphs (change a curved line into a straight line), to solve problems in radioactive decay or radiation absorption, and to provide a graphic axis scale capable of utilizing a wide range of numeric values. The pocket calculator quickly computes logarithms so the reader need become familiar only with their algebraic properties. The logarithm ($\log_b$ x) of a number (x) is the value to which the base (b) must be raised to equal the number:

$$x = b^{\log_b x}$$

For example, for base 10 logarithms the $\log_{10} 1000 = 3$, because $1000 = 10^3$. Note that the expression $\log_{10} 1000$ is read as "the base ten log of 1000." Some examples follow:

$$\log_{10} 0.01 = -2$$
$$\log_{10} 0.1 \ = -1$$
$$\log_{10} 1 \ \ \ = 0$$
$$\log_{10} 10 \ \ = 1$$
$$\log_{10} 100 = 2$$
$$\log_{10} 10^n = n$$

If a $\log_b$ x is written without any value specified for the base (as log x) then base 10 is understood.

The blackness of a nuclear medicine image on a piece of photographic film is measured by the optical density (OD) of the film, which is defined by shining a beam of light through the film:

$$OD = \log (100\%/\% \text{ transmitted through film})$$

The human eye can generally distinguish optical densities in the 0.25 to 2.25 range; below 0.25 is too dim to be seen and above 2.25 is too black. The OD corresponds to the percentage of light transmitted through the film.

% **light transmitted through film**	**OD**
100	$\log \dfrac{100}{100} = 0$
10	$\log \dfrac{100}{10} = 1$
1	$\log \dfrac{100}{1} = 2$
0.1	$\log \dfrac{100}{0.1} = 3$

Logarithms have certain algebraic properties that can simplify mathematical calculations.

Multiplication: $\log xy = \log x + \log y$

Division: $\log x/y = \log x - \log y$

Exponents: $\log x^n = n \times \log x$

The other frequently encountered base for logarithms is the base e, or the natural logarithm, which is denoted by the special symbol

$$\ln x = \log_e x$$

Pocket calculators usually have an ln x key, which allows easy calculation. The major use of natural logarithms in nuclear medicine is to solve problems in radioactive decay and radiation absorption, such as the time of decay (t) in the following equation:

$$0.25 = e^{-0.693 \times t/6 \text{ hr}}$$

The difficulty here is to solve for *t* by removing it from within the exponent. To eliminate a function (like e^x) we can use the inverse function on both sides of the equation:

$$\ln 0.25 = \ln e^{-0.693 \times t/6 \text{ hr}}$$

Using the rule for log of exponents:

$$\ln 0.25 = \left(\frac{-0.693 \times t}{6 \text{ hr}} \right) \times \ln e$$

And now using ln e = 1:

$$\ln 0.25 = \frac{-0.693 \times t}{6 \text{ hr}}$$

Notice that the minus sign and units are carefully retained. Simply rearranging algebraically to solve for *t* then results in:

$$t = \frac{-6 \text{ hr} \times \ln 0.25}{0.693}$$

$$= \frac{-6 \text{ hr} \times (-1.386)}{0.693} = +12 \text{ hr}$$

The minus from the original equation times the negative value of ln 0.25 results in a + sign.

Numeric Accuracy: Significance and Rounding

The accuracy of mathematical calculations is governed by three concepts: significant *figures, rounding,* and significant *decimal places.* Significant figures refers to the number of digits required to preserve the mathematical accuracy in a number.

Numeric accuracy rule 1. For a number with no leading or trailing zeros, the number of significant figures is the number of digits.

Number	Number of significant figures
3	1
3.45	3

Numeric accuracy rule 2. For a number with leading zeros, the leading zeros are not significant.

Number	Number of significant figures
0.0015	2
−0.0463	3

Notice that expressing a number like 0.0015 in scientific notation as 1.5×10^{-3} eliminates the leading zeros and therefore eliminates the need for rule 2!

Numeric accuracy rule 3. Trailing zeros in a number should be retained only if they are significant, which depends on the context of the problem. Thus a problem may state that a drug costs $37; the cost has two significant figures. Or the problem may state that the drug costs $37.00, which is interpreted as being accurate in both dollars and cents; it has four significant figures. A length measured as 4 cm has one significant figure; the length was measured to the nearest centimeter. But a length measured as 4.0 cm has two significant figures; the length was measured more accurately to the nearest millimeter.

Numeric accuracy rule 4. The accuracy of the result in multiplication or division is such that the product or quotient has the number of significant figures equal to that of the term with the smaller number of significant figures.

For example, $2 \times 2.54 = 5$; the correct answer has only one significant figure, since the 2 in the calculation has only one significant figure. But $2.00 \times 2.54 = 5.08$; the result has three significant figures because we presume that the trailing zeros in the 2.00 are significant. In another example:

$$\frac{0.061}{12.34} = 0.0049$$

or

$$\frac{6.1 \times 10^{-2}}{12.34} = 4.9 \times 10^{-3}$$

The result has only two significant figures. Note that a calculator display might show 0.0049433 or 4.9432739E-3, but the proper answer to record as a result is 0.0049 or 4.9E-3, with only two significant figures.

It is necessary to properly round off the result from the calculator before recording the result. For example:

$$\frac{0.061}{1.233} = 0.0494728 = 0.049$$

whereas

$$\frac{0.061}{1.232} = 0.0495130 = 0.050$$

Both answers have two significant figures, but the results are different because of rounding. The mechanics of rounding off a number consist of carrying the mathematical calculations to several more digits than are needed in the final answer. Then the final result is rounded off by the following rules.

Numeric accuracy rule 5. If the right-most digits, beyond the significant figures in the final result, are less than . . . 5000, then simply drop the right-most digits. As an example, consider $0.061/1.233 = 0.0494728$, which must be rounded to two significant figures (because 0.061 has two significant figures). The right-most digits are . . . 4728, which is less than . . . 5000, so the 0.049 is the correct rounded-off final answer.

Numeric accuracy rule 6. If the right-most digits, beyond the significant figures, are greater than . . . 5000, then increase the least significant figure by 1. As an example, consider $0.061/1.232 = 0.0495130$, which again must be rounded to two significant figures (because of the 0.061). The right-most digits are . . . 5130, which is greater than . . .5000, so the final answer needs to be rounded up by one least significant digit $(0.049 + 0.001)$. The final answer is 0.050, rounded off correctly to two significant figures.

Numeric accuracy rule 7. It may sometimes be necessary to round off a number when the right-most digit is exactly 5. The rule here is to round down the number if the digit to the left of the 5 is even, and round up the number if the digit to the left of the 5 is odd. For example: 2.45 is 2.4, rounded to two significant figures; 1.5 is 2, rounded to one significant figure. This rounding scheme for numbers that end in 5 is arbitrary and results in averaging out rounding errors when a large number of calculations are performed.

Numeric accuracy rule 8. For addition and subtraction the final result has the same number of significant *decimal places* (rather than significant figures) as the number in the problem with the least number of significant decimal places. For example:

$$0.123 + 3.42 = 3.54 \text{ (two significant decimal places)}$$
$$0.1 + 3.42 = 3.5 \text{ (one significant decimal place)}$$
$$1 + 3.42 = 4 \text{ (0 significant decimal places)}$$

Sometimes addition and rounding must be employed simultaneously, as in $0.125 + 3.42 = 3.547$, which should properly be rounded to 3.55 with only two significant decimal places, since the 3.42 has only two significant decimal places.

Scientific pocket calculators often have a key for fixing the number of decimal places to be used in a calculation. The calculator also does the rounding off, simplifying such calculations.

Calculators

Examples throughout this chapter have emphasized the use of the pocket scientific calculator. These scientific calculators are available from many manufacturers and should offer, as a minimum, the *ln x* and e^x functions. Often these options are presented via a combination of an *ln x* and an inverse key as discussed in examples above. Figure 1-1 shows a typical calculator keyboard that would be useful in nuclear medicine. Generally, for just a few dollars more, a calculator will also offer very useful statistical functions, such as mean, standard deviation, and linear regression (or least squares curve fitting). Mastering the pocket calculator will greatly speed the results of many common nuclear medicine tests. Calculation of the variability in a nuclear counting system via chi-square test, for example, can be conveniently derived from the standard deviation function on the pocket calculator.

A programmable calculator allows the user to store the instructions for frequently performed functions in the calculator memory or on a magnetic media program card of some sort that is inserted into the calculator. This would allow the user to program a function such as

$$GFR = a[1 - e^{-b(c-d)}]$$

into the calculator. Simply entering *a*, *b*, *c*, and *d* would produce the answer for *GFR*. Other options for calculating such results include using a programming language such as BASIC, FORTRAN, or C, which is generally available on imaging computers or on PC-type computers within the nuclear medicine department. Either way—pocket calculator or other computer—the user must master some programming language to extend the range of the calculator to user-defined calculations. The simplest way is to buy a scientific calculator with built-in functions so that user-developed programs are unnecessary.

PRACTICAL APPLICATIONS

Radioactive Decay

Nuclei that have an unstable balance of neutrons and protons will spontaneously undergo radioactive decay to a more stable nuclear configuration. The number of radioactive nuclei that decay per unit time interval defines the radioactivity, which is measured in curies or becquerels (see Table 1-2). A radioactivity level as follows

$$1 \text{ mCi} = \left(1 \times 10^{-3} \frac{\text{Ci}}{\text{mCi}}\right) \times \left(3.7 \times 10^{10} \frac{\text{dps}}{\text{Ci}}\right)$$
$$= 3.7 \times 10^7 \text{ dps}$$

means that there are 3.7×10^7 dps (disintegrations per second) arising from the sample of radioactive material. The equation that defines the decay of the activity (A) over time (t) arises from a differential equation, which states that the number of atoms decaying per second is proportional to the number of atoms present. If we double the number of atoms in a sample of radioactive material, then the number of atoms decaying per second is also doubled. Solving the differential equation yields the radioactive decay law:

$$A = A_0 e^{-\lambda t}$$

where

$$A = \text{activity at time t}$$
$$A_0 = \text{activity at starting time}$$
$$\lambda = \text{decay constant}$$
$$t = \text{time}$$

The decay constant λ is the fraction of atoms that decay per (small) time interval and has units of 1 over time (e.g., 1/hr) or inverse time (hr^{-1}). The decay constant for ^{99m}Tc, for example, is 0.1153 hr^{-1}, which means that a fraction of *about* 0.115 (or 11.5%) of the ^{99m}Tc atoms decay per hour.

Note carefully that the verbal *interpretation* of the decay constant λ as the fraction that decays per some time interval is an *approximation* that holds only when the time period being considered leads to a very small fractional decay. It is incorrect, for example, to conclude that $\lambda = 0.115 \text{ hr}^{-1}$ means that in 6 hours a fraction of 6×0.115 or 69% of the atoms decay (it's really 50%). Even saying 11.5% decay per hour is only approximate (it's really 10.9%). It is advisable to simply use λ for the exact mathematical calculations using the radioactive decay equation and avoid using the inaccurate verbal interpretation as fractional decay.

The typical radioactive decay calculation required in nuclear medicine will specify three of the four variables (A, A_0, λ, t) in the decay equation, requiring that the fourth unknown variable be solved for. For example, a radiopharmacy delivers a 20.0 mCi dose of ^{99m}Tc ($\lambda = 0.115$ hr^{-1}) to the nuclear medicine department at 8 AM. What amount of radioactivity would be injected into the patient for an 11 AM nuclear medicine scan?

$A_0 = 20.0$ mCi, $\lambda = 0.115$ hr^{-1}, and $t = 3.00$ hr
$A = A_0 e^{-\lambda t}$
$A = 20.0$ mCi $\times e^{-(0.115\,\text{hr}-1) \times (3.00\,\text{hr})}$
$A = 20.0$ mCi $\times e^{-0.345}$
$A = 14.2$ mCi

To solve this problem on the pocket calculator, it is best to first evaluate the exponential expression and then multiply by 20.

0.115	enter λ value
+/−	*change sign* key to make negative
×	*multiply* key
3	enter t value
=	do the multiplication
INV − ln x	or e^x key
×	*multiply* key
20	enter A_0 value
=	(see result 14.2 in display)

The radioactive decay law is often expressed in an algebraic form involving the half-life ($t_{1/2}$), rather than the decay constant λ. The $t_{1/2}$, which depends on the radioactive material involved, is that time at which the activity is decreased to half its original value. The radioactive decay law may alternatively be expressed as:

$$A = A_0 e^{-0.693 \times (t/t_{1/2})}$$

The factor 0.693 is actually ln 2, which is commonly written with three significant figures. Each half-life of radioactive decay causes the activity level to drop by 50%. Following is a time line for radioactivity remaining:

Activity remaining	= 100% →	50% →	25% →	12.5%. . .
At time	= 0	$t_{1/2}$	$2t_{1/2}$	$3t_{1/2}$ . . .

(see Figure 1-3 for a graph of the radioactive decay law as a function of time for ^{99m}Tc with $t_{1/2} = 6$ hr).

Since both forms of the radioactive decay law are valid:

$$A = A_0 e^{-\lambda t} = A_0 e^{-(0.693) \times (t/t_{1/2})} = A_0 e^{-(0.693/t_{1/2}) \times t}$$

We can see that there is a relationship between λ and $t_{1/2}$ given by

$$\lambda = \frac{0.693}{t_{1/2}}$$

The λ and $t_{1/2}$ are inversely proportional to each other: a large λ means a small $t_{1/2}$ and vice versa. Whether to use one form of the radioactive decay law or the other is simply a matter of convenience. Given λ, we can easily calculate $t_{1/2}$ (and vice versa). For example, given that the decay constant λ for ^{99m}Tc is 0.1153 hr^{-1}, what is the $t_{1/2}$?

$$t_{1/2} = \frac{0.693}{\lambda} = \frac{0.693}{0.1153\,\text{hr}^{-1}} = 6.01\,\text{hr}$$

Careful attention to the units is necessary to avoid errors. To make the units clearer this might be restated as:

$$t_{1/2} = \frac{0.693}{0.1153\,\dfrac{1}{\text{hr}}}$$

To get the units of $\dfrac{1}{\text{hr}}$ out of the denominator, multiply both numerator and denominator by units of hours (essentially multiply by 1):

$$t_{1/2} = \frac{0.693}{0.1153\,\dfrac{1}{\text{hr}}}\,\dfrac{\text{hr}}{\text{hr}}$$

The $\dfrac{1}{\text{hr}}$ and the hr cancel in the denominator, leaving

$$t_{1/2} = \frac{0.693}{0.1153}\,\text{hr}$$

Here again the common radioactivity problem will be to solve for one of the four variables (A, A_0, t, $t_{1/2}$) when the problem specifies three of them. For example:

On Monday at 8 AM a sample of ^{131}I ($t_{1/2} = 8.04$ days) is calibrated for radioactivity of 10 μCi. What radioactivity will be given to the patient if the dose is administered on the following Friday at 2 PM?

Given: $A_0 = 10\,\mu$Ci, $t =$ Mon 8 AM → Fri 2 PM,
$t_{1/2} = 8.04$ days
Solve for: $A = A_0 e^{-(0.693) \times (t/t_{1/2})}$

Here a digression to discuss units is necessary. Remember the good practice of always writing down the units associated with every number. Any problem involving the e^x function must have a dimensionless number for the value of x. So it is absolutely necessary that identical units be used for both t and $t_{1/2}$. Then the units cancel in the numerator and denominator of $t/t_{1/2}$, making the calculation independent of the units chosen to measure time. In this problem the time of decay (Mon 8 AM → Fri 2 PM) is 102 hours. But we have already calculated $t_{1/2}$ in days. It would be correct to express the time of decay t as 4.25 days (rather than 102 hr) with the $t_{1/2}$ also in days, or it would be correct to express the $t_{1/2}$ as 193 hr (rather than 8.04 days), with the t also in hours.

$$A = 10 \ \mu Ci \times e^{-0.693} \times (4.25 \ days/8.04 \ days)$$

or

$$A = 10 \ \mu Ci \times e^{-0.693 \times (102 \ hr/193 \ hr)}$$
$$A = 10 \ \mu Ci \times e^{-0.366} = 6.93 \ \mu Ci$$

A quick check of the results of the calculator's answer is also useful, based on the $100\% \rightarrow 50\% \rightarrow 25\% \rightarrow$ . . . time line for each half-life. In this example the decay time of 4.25 days is less than one $t_{1/2}$ (8.04 days), so we know the answer should be between 100% and 50% of the initial 10 μCi activity. The calculator result of 6.93 μCi agrees with our mental check. Inadvertent calculator usage errors can be prevented with these mental checks.

A radionuclide is often calibrated for some activity level on a Friday, but it might have been administered to the patient on the previous Monday. This type of radioactivity problem can be calculated by using negative time values for times that precede the time of A_0 calibration. For example, a radionuclide with a 2-day half-life can be calibrated for Friday at noon to be 3 mCi. What activity level is present on the preceding Monday at noon?

Given: $A_0 = 3$ mCi
  $t = -96$ hr (4 days, $t_{1/2} = 2$ days)
Find: $A = A_0 e^{0.693 \times (t/t_{1/2})}$
  $A = 3 \ mCi \times e^{-0.693 \times (-4 \ days/2 \ days)}$
  $A = 3 \ mCi \times e^{+1.386}$ (notice ($-$) times ($-$) is ($+$))
  $A = 12$ mCi

This result is easy to check mentally since the time difference is exactly 2 half-lives; the answer should be that Monday noon has four times the activity of Friday noon, in agreement with our calculator result.

Sometimes a problem concerns only the fraction of remaining radioactivity (A/A_0), rather than with the actual remaining activity in mCi. For example, what fraction of radioactivity is left at a time equal to 3 half-lives? Here we are given $t = 3 \ t_{1/2}$ and asked to find A/A_0. The radioactive decay law can be algebraically rearranged (dividing both sides of the decay equation by A_0) as:

$$A/A_0 = e^{-0.693 \times (t/t_{1/2})}$$
$$A/A_0 = e^{-(0.693) \times (3t_{1/2}/t_{1/2})}$$
$$A/A_0 = e^{-0.693 \times 3}$$

$$A/A_0 = e^{-2.079}$$
$$A/A_0 = 0.125$$

A quick mental check confirms the result: in 3 half-lives the radioactivity should decay $100\% \rightarrow 50\% \rightarrow 25\% \rightarrow 12.5\%$.

Remember that the radioactive decay equation always refers to the remaining activity, which is the same as 100% less the decayed activity. It is important to determine whether the problem is stating the radioactivity remaining (which the decay equation predicts) or the radioactivity that has decayed (which some problems may require). For example, the previous problem showed that only 12.5% of the original radioactivity remains after 3 half-lives. This problem could also state that 87.5% of the radioactivity decays away in 3 half-lives.

Radioactive decay problems can also require you to solve for the t or $t_{1/2}$ value in the radioactive decay law. These values are contained in the decay law as part of the exponent function, so the exponent must be removed. An example might be to calculate the time necessary for 99.9% of a sample of ^{99m}Tc to decay away. Remember that the decay law works with the remaining radioactivity.

Given: $A/A_0 = 0.1\% = 0.001$
  $t_{1/2} = 6.01$ hr
Solve for t: $A/A_0 = e^{-(0.693) \times (t/t_{1/2})}$
  $0.001 = e^{-0.693 \times (t/6.01 \ hr)}$

Taking the natural logarithm of both sides and using $\ln (e^x) = x$, yields:

$$\ln (0.001) = -0.693 \times t/6.01 \ hr$$

Now the t value is out of the exponent and the equation can be simply rearranged algebraically:

$$t = -6.01 \ hr \times \ln (0.001)/0.693$$

Notice how the minus sign and the units are carried correctly. Now using $\ln (0.001) = -6.908$ yields:

$$t = -6.01 \ hr \times (-6.908/0.693) = 59.9 \ hr$$

The two minus signs are multiplied and cancel each other. About 60 hr (which is about 10 half-lives) is necessary for the radioactivity of ^{99m}Tc to decay to 1/1000 of its original value. For a radionuclide such as ^{131}I it is still true that 10 half-lives cause decay to 1/1000 of the original activity, but for ^{131}I ten half-lives is 10×8.04 days = 80.4 days.

As another example, an experiment finds that a sample of radioactivity decays to 30% of its original value in 5 hr. What is the $t_{1/2}$?

$$A/A_0 = e^{-0.693 \times (t/t_{1/2})}$$
$$0.30 = e^{-0.693 \times (5hr/t_{1/2})}$$
$$\ln (0.30) = -0.693 \times (5hr/t_{1/2})$$
$$-1.204 = -0.693 \times (5hr/t_{1/2})$$

so

$$t_{1/2} = -0.693 \times \frac{5 \text{ hr}}{-1.204} = 2.9 \text{ hr}$$

Do the mental check. Does this seem a reasonable answer? If 2.9 hr is the correct $t_{1/2}$, then a decay time of 5 hr is not quite 2 half-lives. So the expected answer is that 5 hr of decay with a 2.9-hr $t_{1/2}$ should leave slightly more than 25% of the radioactivity remaining. The problem has sensible results: 30% remaining at time just less than 2 half-lives.

In most practical problems it is necessary to combine radioactive decay calculations with concentration-volume problems. Usually the nuclear medicine department obtains its radioactivity from a ^{99}Mo-^{99m}Tc generator via an early morning elution of the generator. This eluate decays throughout the day, resulting in a changing concentration (in mCi/ml). For example, say a generator is eluted at 7 AM, yielding 900 mCi in 20 ml of eluate solution. What volume should be withdrawn from the eluate vial into a syringe to perform a 15 mCi scan at 2 PM? First calculate the radioactivity remaining in the eluate vial at 2 PM:

$$A = 900 \text{ mCi} \times e^{-0.693 \times (7 \text{ hr}/6.01 \text{ hr})} = 402 \text{ mCi}$$

(A quick mental check confirms the reasonableness of this answer; slightly less than 50% remaining at a time slightly greater than $t_{1/2}$.) The concentration (radioactivity per volume) in the eluate vial is then 402 mCi/20 ml at 2 PM. The volume needed to be withdrawn into the syringe for a 15 mCi dose at 2 PM can be calculated from the equation activity = concentration $\times$ volume.

$$A = C \times V$$

$$15 \text{ mCi} = \left(\frac{402 \text{ mCi}}{20 \text{ ml}} \right) \times V$$

$$15 \text{ mCi} = \left(\frac{20.1 \text{ mCi}}{\text{ml}} \right) \times V$$

so

$$V = \frac{15 \text{ mCi}}{\left(20.1 \dfrac{\text{mCi}}{\text{ml}} \right)} = 0.75 \text{ ml}$$

^{99}Mo-^{99m}Tc Radionuclide Generators

Another common problem for radioactive decay is to calculate the ratio of ^{99}Mo ($t_{1/2}$ = 65.9 hr) activity to ^{99m}Tc activity in generator eluate. The problem is that some ^{99}Mo is also eluted out along with the ^{99m}Tc in the morning elution. The ^{99}Mo is a radionuclide impurity that is limited by the current regulatory agencies to be less the 0.15 μCi ^{99}Mo per mCi ^{99m}Tc for injection into a patient. Consider a generator that is eluted

at 7 AM and yields an eluate vial containing 30 μCi ^{99}Mo along with 250 mCi ^{99m}Tc. Can this eluate be used for a brain scan at the elution time of 7 AM? Calculate the ratio of ^{99}Mo to ^{99m}Tc activity at 7 AM as:

$$\frac{^{99}\text{Mo}}{^{99m}\text{Tc}} = \frac{30 \ \mu\text{Ci} \ ^{99}\text{Mo}}{250 \ \text{mCi} \ ^{99m}\text{Tc}} = 0.12 \ \frac{\mu\text{Ci} \ ^{99}\text{Mo}}{\text{mCi} \ ^{99m}\text{Tc}}$$

This eluate is less than the regulatory limit (0.15) and may be used. Could this same eluate be used 6 hr later to prepare a lung scan? Now the ratio of activities at 1 PM is:

$$\frac{^{99}\text{Mo}}{^{99m}\text{Tc}} = \frac{30 \ \mu\text{Ci} \times e^{-0.693 \times (6 \text{ hr}/65.9 \text{ hr})}}{250 \ \text{mCi} \times e^{-(0.693) \times (6 \text{ hr}/6.01 \text{ hr})}}$$

$$= \frac{30 \ \mu\text{Ci} \times 0.939}{250 \ \text{mCi} \times 0.500} = \frac{28.17 \ \mu\text{Ci} \ ^{99}\text{Mo}}{125 \ \text{mCi} \ ^{99m}\text{Tc}}$$

$$= \frac{0.23 \ \mu\text{Ci} \ ^{99}\text{Mo}}{\text{mCi} \ ^{99m}\text{Tc}}$$

This eluate cannot be used, since the ^{99}Mo/^{99m}Tc ratio is greater than the 0.15 regulatory limit. The ^{99}Mo has not changed very much in the 6 hr since generator elution, but the ^{99m}Tc has halved, resulting in a large increase in the ^{99}Mo/^{99m}Tc ratio.

The mathematics of this type of radionuclide generator are governed by the laws of radioactivity,[5] relating radionuclides denoted as a parent-daughter-granddaughter- . . . decay chain. The parent radionuclide ^{99}Mo decays to the daughter ^{99m}Tc, which in turn decays to the granddaughter ^{99}Tc, and the decay chain continues. Without dealing with the exponential algebra for this type of decay, it is possible to easily calculate the ^{99m}Tc radioactivity expected to be eluted from the generator by knowing three values:

1. The activity of ^{99}Mo in the generator, which is given by the manufacturer's calibration date and the decay law for ^{99}Mo ($t_{1/2}$ = 65.9 hr)
2. The time since the last elution of the generator, which is commonly 24 hr for daily elutions
3. The ratio of ^{99m}Tc to ^{99}Mo in the generator, which depends on the time since the last elution (^{99m}Tc to ^{99}Mo ratios are shown in Table 1-3 as a function of the time since last elution)

For example, a generator is delivered on Saturday and calibrated by the manufacturer for the following Monday at 6 PM to contain 2 Ci of ^{99}Mo. The generator is eluted daily (Monday-Friday) at 7 AM. What activity of ^{99m}Tc is available in the generator at 7 AM on Tuesday? The required data are:

1. ^{99}Mo activity Tuesday 7 AM, 13 hr after calibration time.

$$A = 2 \text{ Ci} \times e^{-0.693 \times (13 \text{ hr}/65.9 \text{ hr})}$$
$$= 1744 \text{ mCi of } ^{99}\text{Mo in the generator,}$$
$$\text{Tuesday 7 AM}$$

Table 1-3	Generator ^{99m}Tc/^{99}Mo activity ratio
Time since last elution (hr)	**^{99m}Tc/^{99}Mo**
1	0.094
2	0.18
3	0.25
4	0.32
5	0.39
6	0.44
7	0.49
8	0.54
10	0.61
12	0.68
14	0.73
16	0.78
18	0.80
20	0.83
22	0.85
24	0.87
26	0.88
30	0.91
∞	0.95

From Lamson M, Hotte CD, Ice RE: Practical generator kinetics, *J Nucl Med Technol* 4:21, 1976.

2. Time since last elution is 24 hr, since the generator is eluted daily.
3. From Table 1-3, the ^{99m}Tc/^{99}Mo ratio is 0.87 for 24 hr since last elution.

So

$$\text{Activity } ^{99m}\text{Tc} = 0.87 \times \text{Activity } ^{99}\text{Mo}$$
$$= 0.87 \times 1744 \text{ mCi}$$
$$= 1518 \text{ mCi}$$

Depending on the quality of the generator, only a percentage of this 1518 mCi of ^{99m}Tc will appear in the eluate. This is known as the elution efficiency of the generator. If the elution efficiency is 95%, then the ^{99m}Tc found in the Tuesday morning eluate would be calculated as 0.95×1518 mCi = 1442 mCi. This is available for patient studies.

In most clinical applications the nuclear medicine gamma camera measures the radioactive counts over an organ of interest in the patient's body. Typically the patient organ excretes the radiopharmaceutical with some biologic half-life t_B, while the radioactivity also decays physically with a physical half-life, denoted t_P. The biologic half-life is an indicator of the physiologic fate of the radiopharmaceutical. The counts observed by the gamma camera follow an exponential decay law based on the effective half-life t_E, where

$$\frac{1}{t_E} = \frac{1}{t_P} + \frac{1}{t_B}$$

or

$$t_E = \frac{t_P \times t_B}{(t_P + t_B)}$$

For example, if the liver excretes a ^{99m}Tc radiopharmaceutical with $t_B = 3$ hr, then the gamma camera over the liver would observe an effective half-life:

$$t_E = \frac{6 \text{ hr} \times 3 \text{ hr}}{(6 \text{ hr} + 3 \text{ hr})} = 2 \text{ hr}$$

The effective half-life is always less than or equal to the smaller of t_P or t_B.

Attenuation of Radiation

The calculation of the intensity (I) of x-ray or γ-ray photons transmitted through some thickness *(x)* of absorbing material follows exactly the same algebra as the equations of radioactive decay. Figure 1-2 shows a beam of monoenergetic x-ray or γ-ray photons striking a thickness of absorbing material. Monoenergetic means that the photons all have the same energy, such as a beam of photons from a ^{99m}Tc radionuclide source that emits photons of energy 140 keV. The initial intensity (number of photons per second) entering the absorbing material is called I_0. The material attenuates, or absorbs, some fraction of the photons, and the photon beam emerges with a transmitted (i.e., not absorbed) intensity I. The intensity of the transmitted radiation is given by:

$$I = I_0 e^{-\mu x}$$

where μ is the linear attenuation coefficient, or the fraction of the beam absorbed in some (very small) thickness x. The linear attenuation coefficient μ is the analog of the decay constant λ in radioactive decay. The linear attenuation coefficient μ depends on the type of absorbing material and the energy of the photons. A large μ value means a strongly absorbing material. For ^{99m}Tc γ-rays the μ value in lead is about 23 cm^{-1}, whereas the μ in water is only 0.15 cm^{-1}. Lead is a much more strongly absorbing material than water.

A typical calculation deals with the fraction I/I_0 transmitted through a thickness x. For example, what percent of 140 keV photons are transmitted through 10 cm of water ($\mu = 0.15$ cm^{-1})?

$$I/I_0 = e^{-\mu x}$$
$$I/I_0 = e^{-0.15 \text{ cm}^{-1} \times 10 \text{ cm}}$$
$$I/I_0 = e^{-1.5} = 0.22, \text{ or } 22\%$$

Since 22% are transmitted, we can also say that 78% are absorbed in 10 cm of water.

Consider a problem that asks what fraction of ^{131}I photons at energy 364 keV is transmitted through ½

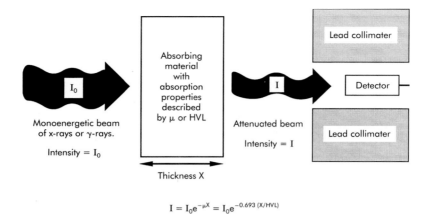

$$I = I_0 e^{-\mu X} = I_0 e^{-0.693\,(X/HVL)}$$

Figure 1-2 Attenuation of radiation in an absorbing medium.

in of lead ($\mu = 2.2$ cm^{-1} at 364 keV). Your inclination might be to calculate as follows:

$$I/I_0 = e^{-\mu x}$$

but

$$I/I_0 \neq e^{-2.2\ \text{cm}^{-1} \times 0.5\ \text{in.}}$$

The calculation is incorrect because the units in the exponent do not cancel each other. There must be a dimensionless number in the exponent to make the result independent of the units used to describe μ and x. We can use any units we choose, so long as the units of μ and x are inverse of each other. It is easiest to look up the μ values, from published tables, and then convert the thickness x to the corresponding units, rather than convert the units of μ to correspond with those of x. For this problem convert $x = 0.5$ in to 1.27 cm to obtain:

$$I/I_0 = e^{-2.2\ \text{cm}^{-1} \times 1.27\ \text{cm}} = 0.061$$

So 0.5 in of lead transmits only 6.1% of a beam of 364 keV photons from ^{131}I. This also means that the lead absorbs 93.9% of the photons. The linear attenuation coefficient suffers from the same problem as λ: it is difficult to conceptualize. It is therefore common to follow the method used in radioactive decay and define a *half-value layer (HVL)* as that thickness of material which absorbs 50% of the photons. The HVL is the analog of $t_{1/2}$ in radioactive decay. One HVL transmits 50% of the photons, two HVLs transmit 25% of the original beam, etc. The absorption line looks like the following:

Photon
  intensity = $\to 100\% \to 50\% \to 25\% \to 12.5\% \to \ldots$
Thickness =   0   1 HVL 2 HVL   3 HVL

The equation of photon attenuation then can be expressed as:

$$I = I_0 e^{-\mu x} = I_0 e^{-0.693 \times (x/HVL)}$$

And there is a relationship between μ and HVL given by: $\mu = 0.693/HVL$.

If you know the HVL or μ value, it is a straightforward calculation to find the other and use whichever attenuation equation is most convenient. As an example, what percent of 140 keV photons from ^{99m}Tc is attenuated by 10 cm of water? The HVL for 140 photons in water is 4.6 cm.

$$I/I_0 = e^{-0.693 \times (x/HVL)}$$
$$I/I_0 = e^{-0.693 \times (10\ \text{cm}/4.6\ \text{cm})}$$
$$I/I_0 = 0.22,\ \text{or } 22\%$$

Remember the units of x and HVL must be the same, and remember that this equation calculates the *transmitted* intensity. A fraction (0.22) of the photons is transmitted. This is precisely the same result that was obtained previously in this section using the attenuation equation with μ. The problem, however, asks what fraction is *attenuated* by the water, so $1 - 0.22 = 0.78$ is the attenuated fraction; 10 cm of water absorbs 78% of the photons emitted by ^{99m}Tc. This type of calculation can be carried out easily on the pocket scientific calculator.

0.693	enter value
$+/-$	change sign key
$\times$	*multiply* key
10	enter thickness value
$\div$	*divide* key
4.6	enter HVL value
$=$	(see result of division)
INV and ln x	or e^x key
	(see result 0.22)

Here again a quick mental check of the calculator result is very useful. The thickness here (10 cm) is just slightly more than 2 HVLs (since HVL = 4.6 cm), so the attenuation answer should be just slightly less than 25%.

Another problem might require solving the attenuation equation for either x or the HVL, both of which are contained in the exponent in the attenuation equation. Just as in radioactive decay (where we needed to solve for t or $t_{1/2}$) we can eliminate the exponent with the natural logarithm as the inverse function of e^x.

$$I/I_0 = e^{-\mu x} = e^{-0.693 \times (x/HVL)}$$

or

$$\ln (I/I_0) = -\mu x = -0.693 \times (x/HVL)$$

For example, if 10 cm is known to transmit 22% of the photon beam, what is the HVL?

$$\ln (0.22) = -0.693 \times (10 \text{ cm}/HVL)$$

so

$$HVL = \frac{-0.693 \times 10 \text{ cm}}{\ln (0.22)}$$

$$= \frac{0.693 \times 10 \text{ cm}}{-1.51} = 4.6 \text{ cm}$$

Note how the minus signs cancel and how the units are carefully carried. To calculate the HVL on the pocket calculator:

0.693	enter value
+/−	*change sign* key
×	*multiply* key
10	enter x value
÷	*divide* key
0.22	enter fraction value
ln x	*natural logarithm* key
=	(see result display 4.6 cm)

One further nuance occurs for attenuation of photons. The μ value, or the corresponding HVL value, for any material also depends on the physical density ρ (g/cm^3): the HVL in water vapor is different from the HVL in liquid water, is different from the HVL in ice, etc. This makes calculations using the μ or HVL values somewhat difficult, since the μ values are usually tabulated only for the common physical state of the material in question (e.g., for liquid water). To circumvent this problem, a new parameter is defined as the *mass attenuation coefficient* μ_m (cm^2/g) $= \mu/\rho$. The mass attenuation coefficient is *independent* of the physical density of the absorber and is therefore easily tabulated. The transmission of photons can then be expressed in one of three equivalent forms:

$$I/I_0 = e^{-\mu x}$$
$$I/I_0 = e^{-0.693 \times (x/HVL)}$$
$$I/I_0 = e^{-\rho \mu_m x}$$

Calculation of a result using the more easily tabulated value of mass attenuation coefficient also requires looking up the density (ρ) of the absorbing material.

It should also be noted that these equations for the transmitted fraction of photons apply only to a situation known as "good" geometry, or narrow beam geometry, meaning that a very thin pencil-like beam of photons enters the absorber and is detected by a small collimated detector. Scattered photons (photons not

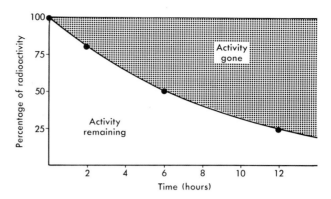

Figure 1-3 Linear plot of radioactive decay for $t_{1/2} = 6$ hr.

traveling in a straight line between the origin of the photon and the detector) are excluded by the good geometry. In most practical applications, such as photons arising in the patient's heart and being detected by a gamma camera, the geometry is broad beam. The photons can leave the patient's heart and move toward the thyroid, for example, then scatter in the thyroid and travel toward the gamma camera to be detected as a photon apparently arising from the thyroid. The scattered photons increase the apparent transmission through the patient's body, and the equation is typically modified by a multiplicative buildup factor B, with $B \geq 1$. Buildup factors are dependent on the absorbing material, on the energy of the photon, and on the geometry. A heavy, large patient has a buildup factor greater than that of a thin patient. So, in broad beam geometry:

$$I/I_0 = Be^{-\mu x}$$

Specification of the buildup factor, or some other correction for scatter (such as arbitrarily using a smaller μ value), may be necessary for accurate quantitation of photons originating inside a patient.

Graphs

The modern technologic world can often inundate us with data. Graphs provide a practical, highly visual way to convey large amounts of information. They can also be used to predict one variable based on another. The most common type of graph utilizes a linear set of x and y axes in the familiar Cartesian coordinate system. Figure 1-3 shows a graph or plot of the remaining radioactivity level versus time from a sample of radioactive material with $t_{1/2} = 6$ hr. The x axis (or abscissa) shows the time of each data point (for 0, 2, 6, and 12 hr), and the y axis (or ordinate) shows the activity in millicuries for each data point. One variable is often considered to depend on another independent variable. The independent variable is generally plotted on the x axis, with the dependent variable on the y axis. In Figure 1-3 time is considered the independent variable on the x axis, and activity level is considered the dependent variable on the y axis.

Mathematically, activity *(y)* is a function of time, or y = f(t). The data points in Figure 1-3 are called discrete data points because a measurement of activity was taken at four discrete, individual data points (0, 2, 6, and 12 hr). Graphs of discrete data points may or may not, at the user's discretion, show them joined by smooth curves or a connect-the-dots type of straight line. Our knowledge of the decay process suggests a smooth curve should best represent radioactive decay. On the other hand, a graph of the number of monthly kidney scans might be graphed as discrete data points joined in a connect-the-dots fashion, since there is no reason to imply a smoother curve.

Figure 1-3 shows a continuous curve of activity versus time for the radioactive decay equation:

$$A = A_0 e^{-\lambda t}$$

The $t_{1/2}$ for the data in Figure 1-3 is 6 hr, since the radioactivity drops 100%, 50%, and 25% in 0, 6, and 12 hr, respectively. If the natural logarithm is taken on both sides of the equation, the curve in Figure 1-3 will simplify into the straight line shown in Figure 1-4 because:

$$\ln A = \ln A_0 e^{-\lambda t}$$
$$\ln A = \ln A_0 + \ln e^{-\lambda t}$$
$$\ln A = \ln A_0 - \lambda t$$

or

$$y = a + bt$$

This is the equation of a straight line with y-intercept a = $\ln A_0$, and slope b = $-\lambda$. This is an important practical result: the logarithm of radioactive decay data plotted versus time is a straight line graph with negative slope equal to the decay constant. Note that the logarithmic plot of activity still shows the activity dropping by 50% every 6 hr.

A brief review of the graphic interpretation of straight line data seems pertinent. A straight line graph of *y* versus *x* is represented by the general formula:

$$y = a + bx$$

The y-intercept, which is the value of y at x = 0, is represented by *a*. The slope, which represents the "steepness" of the line, is represented by *b*. Figure 1-5 shows a straight line graph with b = 0.5 as the slope. The slope is calculated from any two arbitrary points on the line as:

$$\text{Slope} = \frac{\Delta y}{\Delta x} = \frac{y_2 - y_1}{x_2 - x_1}$$

In Figure 1-5 the slope is calculated from the points $(x_1, y_1) = (0, 5)$ and $(x_2, y_2) = (10, 10)$.

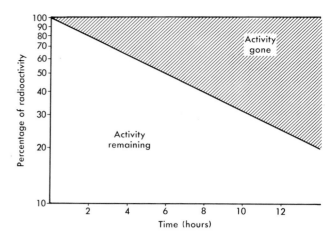

Figure 1-4   Semilog plot of radioactivity for $t_{1/2} = 6$ hr. y axis is logarithmic.

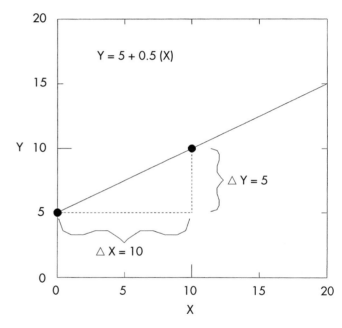

Figure 1-5   Straight line graph with slope = 0.5 and intercept = 5.

$$\text{Slope} = \frac{10 - 5}{10 - 0} = 0.5$$

For a straight line graph it does not matter which two points on the line are chosen to calculate the slope; the same answer will be obtained. In Figure 1-5 the y-intercept a = 5 because the value of y is 5 at x = 0. So the equation of the straight line in Figure 1-5 is given by:

$$y = 5 + 0.5x$$

Given any *x* value, the equation can be used to calculate the *y* value. The sign of the slope merely reflects whether the curve slopes upward (a positive slope) or downward (a negative slope). Straight line curves are generally used in nuclear medicine to prove a direct or linear relationship between two variables or to predict some y variable based on the value of the x variable. Mathematical relationships or curves that are nonlinear, such as radioactivity versus time, are often transformed by a mathematical operation to make the graph a straight line. For exponential curves, such as radioactive decay, taking the natural logarithm of the activity transforms the data into a straight line. The straight line form might be preferred because subsequent interpretation or calculations are simplified. The use of logarithms as a process to transform curvilinear data into straight lines is so common that a special type of graph paper is often used to simplify the process (Figure 1-6). Semilogarithmic graph paper has axes with divisions that are proportional to the logarithm of the y axis, so the y values are simply plotted at the appropriate point without the necessity of calculating the logarithm of the y axis data. Semilogarithmic graph paper is available with a varying number of cycles, or powers of 10, on the y axis. Figure 1-6 shows two-cycle graph paper, which can accommodate y values that span a range of no more than 10^2. The user simply relabels the numeric values on the y axis to correspond to the range of the data involved. For example, the y values could range from 0.23 to 7.9, with the y axis labeled with 0.1 at the bottom, 1.0 in the middle, and 10.0 at the top. Or the data might fall into the range of 200 to 8000, with the cycles labeled from 100 through 1000 to 10,000.

Measurement of Effective Half-life

A typical procedure with nuclear medicine data is to calculate the effective $t_{1/2}$ of excretion from some organ in the body. As an example, consider a patient who is given a meal of radioactive food to determine the $t_{1/2}$ of emptying of the stomach. The radioactivity counts emanating from the stomach are plotted on semilogarithmic graph paper (Figure 1-7). The $t_{1/2}$ of excretion can be determined by drawing a freehand straight line through the data points. Each data point is contaminated with statistical and systematic noise, or uncertainty, in the actual y value. So the straight line will probably not pass exactly through all, if any, of the data points. Use of this method to determine $t_{1/2}$ relies on the data points being reasonably well represented as a straight line on a semilogarithmic plot. Often the data appear more and more like a straight line at later time values, so these values are used to estimate the straight line fit. After the straight line is drawn, the $t_{1/2}$ can be determined as the interval needed for the straight line to decrease by a factor of ½. Just pick any convenient starting value for y, then read off the graph the time needed to reach y/2. In Figure 1-7 the estimated best fit straight line has a y-intercept (or Y_0) of 7800 ct, and the line falls to 3900 ct ($Y_0/2$) in 12.5 min. So $t_{1/2} = 12.5$ min.

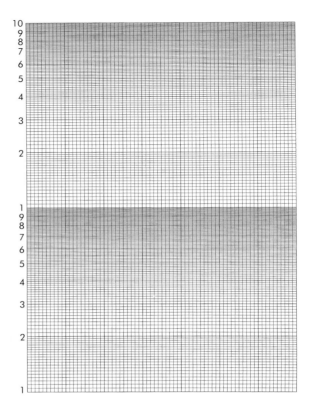

Figure 1-6 Two-cycle semilog graph paper.

In some cases the data never decrease by a factor of ½ over the time of the experiment, but it is still desired to calculate the $t_{1/2}$. In this case the proper calculation (remembering radioactive decay follows the equation $\ln Y = \ln Y_0 - \lambda t$) is to find the slope, which is equal to $-\lambda$, the negative decay constant, based on the counts (y) and time (t) of any two points on the straight line.

$$-\lambda = \frac{\ln (y_2) - \ln (y_1)}{t_2 - t_1}$$

Then the $t_{1/2}$ is calculated from the $t_{1/2} = 0.693/\lambda$. Note that the equation for the decay constant slope requires calculation of the natural logarithm of the count values in the numerator. The logarithm need not be calculated to *plot* the data (because of the convenience of semilogarithmic graph paper), but calculation of the slope *does* require calculation of the logarithm of any two arbitrary points on the straight line. Suppose that the data were acquired through only 10 minutes and that it was desired to still calculate $t_{1/2}$, although the data do not decrease to $Y_0/2$ in only 10 min. Using two points on the estimated best fit straight line (0, 7800) and (10, 4400) the decay constant is calculated as follows:

$$-\lambda = \frac{\ln (4400) - \ln (7800)}{10 - 0 \text{ min}} = \frac{-0.573}{10 \text{ min}}$$

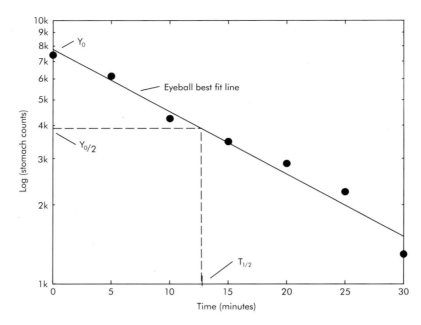

Figure 1-7 Measurement of effective $t_{1/2} = 12.5$ minutes in the stomach by visual estimate of best fit line on semilog plot.

So

$$\lambda = 0.0573 \text{ min}^{-1}$$

Then $t_{1/2} = 0.693/\lambda$ is calculated as 12.1 min, in close agreement with the graphic method above, which estimated $t_{1/2} = 12.5$ min.

Note that many nuclear medicine procedures yield graphs of counts versus time that do not follow a simple straight line on semilogarithmic plots. There might be several half-lives or several organs might be excreting a radiopharmaceutical from the body. It is then not correct to calculate a single $t_{1/2}$ from any data that do not appear to follow a straight line. Analysis of multiple half-life data requires other methods, such as curve stripping and nonlinear least squares.

Least Squares Curve Fitting

The technique of visually estimating the best fit straight line is fraught with inaccuracy and imprecision, since each observer's perspective is unique. This could result in different values for the $t_{1/2}$ (which is based on the straight line) or in different values for predicting a y value at any x value using the straight line fit to the data. A more mathematically precise method to fit the straight line to the data is the method of least squares, or linear regression.[1] In this technique a set of n data values at the points (x_i, y_i), where $i = 1 \rightarrow n$, is graphed and fitted with a mathematically exact technique. There is no imprecision; every observer who utilizes this method will obtain the exact same answer. This type of calculation is generally performed to show a linear relationship between two variables or to predict some y variable based on measurement of some x variable.

Figure 1-8 shows data for x, y values from an experiment involving measurement of cardiac ejection fraction *(EF)* by two different techniques: a previously used method and the new method (which involves some change in experimental technique). Do these data show that the old method and the new method yield identical results? Or, given some value for ejection fraction by the old method (an x value), what would be the predicted results for ejection fraction by the new method (a y value)? The least squares method, or linear regression, calculates the best fit values for y-intercept *(a)* and slope *(b)* in the best fit straight line: $y = a + bx$. The intercept and slope parameters define a straight line as discussed above. The least squares method uses a calculation for *a* and *b* that minimizes the square of the distance in the y direction between the best fit straight line and the data points. Use of a scientific pocket calculator can greatly speed calculations. Indeed, for any reasonably large number of data points a calculator or computer is the only practical way to do least squares curve fitting. Typically, a calculator requires the user to enter the first x value and press some key (such as *Xi* in Figure 1-1), telling the calculator this is x_i; then enter the corresponding first y value and tell the calculator this is Y_i (with the Y_i key, see Figure 1-1); then enter $X_2, Y_2, \ldots$, until all n data points have been entered. Then display the intercept and slope. Use of a computer is even simpler: the user enters x,y values in a spreadsheet format and instructs the computer to plot the data and the regression line. Almost all popular spreadsheet and graphics software packages offer regression analysis (i.e., the program will calculate and plot the best fit line).

Calculation of the regression line by hand is tedious but not really complicated. The first step is the calcu-

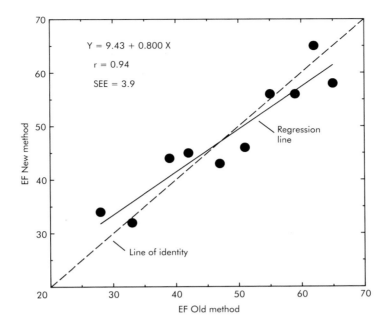

Figure 1-8 Regression analysis or least squares best fit curve to compare old and new method for calculating ejection fraction *(EF)*.

lation of four sums based on the (x,y) data values. Then some simple multiplication and division produce the intercept and slope as follows. First calculate the sums, using the data for Figure 1-8 as shown in Table 1-4:

$$\Sigma x = x_1 + x_2 + \ldots + x_n$$
$$= 47 + 62 + \ldots + 51 = 481$$
$$\Sigma y = y_1 + y_2 + \ldots + y_n$$
$$= 43 + 65 + \ldots + 46 = 479$$
$$\Sigma xy = x_1y_1 + x_2y_2 + \ldots + x_ny_n$$
$$= 47(43) + 62(65) + \ldots + 51(46) = 24165$$
$$\Sigma x^2 = x_1^2 + x_2^2 + \ldots + x_n^2$$
$$= 47^2 + 62^2 + \ldots + 51^2 = 24543$$

Then the intercept and slope are calculated as:

$$a = \frac{\Sigma x^2 + \Sigma y - \Sigma x \times \Sigma xy}{n \times \Sigma x^2 - \Sigma x + \Sigma x}$$

$$a = \frac{24543(479) - 481(24165)}{10(24543) - 481(481)} = 9.43$$

and

$$b = \frac{n \times \Sigma xy - \Sigma x \times \Sigma y}{n \times \Sigma x^2 - \Sigma x \times \Sigma x}$$

$$b = \frac{10(24165) - 481(479)}{10(24543) - 481(481)} = 0.800$$

The best fit line is then given by:

$$y = 9.43 + 0.80 \times x$$

Now this line is drawn onto the graph of y versus x by calculating two points at the endpoints of the regression line and then joining these points with a straight

Table 1-4	Linear regression: comparison of two methods for calculation of ejection fraction*	
Old method: x (%)	**New method: y (%)**
47	43
62	65
39	44
33	32
55	56
42	45
59	56
65	58
28	34
51	46

*y = 9.43 + 0.800 x; r = 0.94; standard error of the estimate (SEE) = 3.9.

line. At x = 20 the best fit line value of y is 9.43 + 0.80(20) = 25; and at x = 70 the best fit line value of y is 9.43 + 0.8(70) = 65. The regression line has been drawn in Figure 1-8. Also shown in Figure 1-8 is the line of identity, which is the line with zero y-intercept and slope equal 1, defined by y = x. The line of identity is frequently drawn on regression graphs when the same parameter, here the ejection fraction, is being plotted on both the x and y axes. The line of identity facilitates an evaluation of whether the two methods (the x axis and y axis) are predicting the same result for ejection fraction. If the two methods produce the same value for ejection fraction, then the regression line should be the same as the line of identity. The line of identity is not a useful concept if the particular experiment being considered does not have identical parameters on the x and y axes. A regression of blood pressure versus age, for example, would not utilize the line of identity.

So what does the regression equation predict in Figure 1-8? The old and new method do not predict the same ejection fraction, since the predicted regression line does not coincide with the line of identity. For any given old method result (the x value), the regression equation or graph can be used to predict what the new method would yield for an ejection fraction result. This prediction of a y value, based on some measured x value, is the goal of regression analysis. Figure 1-8 shows that the new method produces results greater than the old method for ejection fractions below about 47 by the old method, since the regression line is above the line of identity. The new method underestimates the ejection fraction, compared with the old method, for ejection fractions greater than 47 by the old method.

Figure 1-8 also lists the value of goodness of fit parameters, which help determine whether it is reasonable that the data points are truly represented by a straight line. The linear correlation coefficient r is calculated from the sums used to find the intercept and slope, along with one additional sum from the data points (Σy^2):

$$r = \frac{n \times \Sigma xy - \Sigma x \times \Sigma y}{(n \times \Sigma x^2 - \Sigma x \times \Sigma x)^{1/2} \times (n \times \Sigma y^2 - \Sigma y \times \Sigma y)^{1/2}}$$

The sign of the correlation coefficient is merely the same as the sign of the slope. A correlation $r = 1$ is a perfect fit, with the straight line passing exactly through each data point. The closer r is to 1, the more highly correlated the x and y data are.

There is always a chance, or *probability (P)*, for data that are truly not linearly related to each other to randomly appear in a fairly linear fashion. Correlation values less than 1 must be evaluated from statistical tables of probability (Table 1-5). If the correlation value for the *n* data points shows a *P* value of less than 0.05 from the statistical tables, then the data are said to be linearly correlated. Figure 1-8 shows $r = 0.94$ for n = 10 data points, which from Table 1-5 has $P < 0.001$, so the data are highly linearly correlated. If the r value was 0.632 or less (the $P = 0.05$ value for n = 10 from Table 1-5), then the data are not shown to be linearly correlated and it would not be prudent to suggest a straight line fit to the data. A statistically significant correlation (meaning $P < 0.05$) merely implies a linear relationship between the x and y variables. This linear correlation or relationship does not necessarily imply that x causes y.[3] A graph, for instance, of number of babies (y) versus number of stork nests (x) would probably show a high correlation. But this does not mean storks

Table 1-5 Linear correlation coefficient r at a probability P

Number of data points	Probability (P)				
	0.10	0.05*	0.01	0.005	0.001
5	0.805	0.878	0.959	0.974	0.991
10	0.549	0.632	0.765	0.805	0.872
15	0.441	0.514	0.641	0.683	0.760
20	0.378	0.444	0.561	0.602	0.679
30	0.306	0.361	0.463	0.499	0.570

*Minimum value of correlation coefficient for significant correlation is in this column. Larger r values are more highly correlated.

bring babies. More likely both x and y depend on some other variable, such as the number of people in the house: people make babies, people live in houses, storks build nests on these houses.

The other goodness of fit parameter shown in Figure 1-8 is the standard error of the estimate (SEE) (sometimes denoted S_{yx}) defined as follows:

$$SEE = [\Sigma (y - a - bx)^2 / (n - 2)]^{1/2}$$

The SEE is the root mean square average deviation in the y direction of a data point from the regression line, i.e., how far away the average data point is from the regression line in the y direction. In Figure 1-8 SEE = 3.9, so the average data point is about 4 units on the y axis from the regression line. Another interpretation of SEE might be that the old and new ejection fraction methods disagree, on average, by 4. A line that passes exactly through each data point produces $r = 1$ and SEE = 0, for a perfect fit. The SEE grows larger as the data points fall farther from the regression line. There is no easy way to state a P value for whether the SEE is small enough or not small enough to say the fit is statistically acceptable.

Least squares curve fitting could also be used to improve the precision of measurement of effective $t_{1/2}$ of data such as that shown in Figure 1-7. The calculation merely requires using the time as x values, and the ln (counts) as the y values in the regression equations. The best fit line has a slope that is the decay constant λ, and the half-life is then $t_{1/2} = 0.693/\lambda$. This least squares fit eliminates the imprecision of estimated best fit lines.

There are several other caveats regarding least squares curve fitting. The linear correlation coefficient r describes only the degree of *linear* relationship between x and y. There may in fact be some exact nonlinear relationship between x and y that yields a nonsignificant linear correlation. Data generated from the relationship $y = x^2$ (x = −2, −1, 0, 1, and 2 with corresponding y = 4, 1, 0, 1, and 4) would produce the straight line fit $y = 0.0 + 2 \times x$, with $r = 0$. There is in

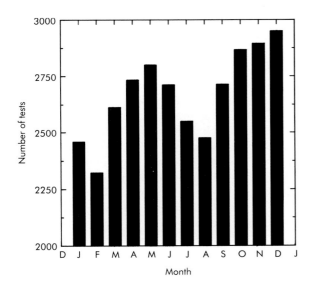

Figure 1-9   Histogram showing monthly variation in number of tests.

fact an exact relationship between X and Y, but it is not linear.

The least squares best fit line intercept and slope values have ± standard error uncertainties according to formulas available in the literature.[3] This results in a range of possible best fit lines. There is actually a statistical uncertainty in the predicted y value for any x value. These uncertainties in the predicted line can be used, for example, to ascertain whether the predicted regression line is really different from the line of identity. Or the x and y values can be tested for difference using *t*-tests, as discussed below.

Other Graphs

Another graph useful in nuclear medicine is a histogram, which is used to display a single list of numbers, such as number of tests per month (Figure 1-9). Note that the y axis is displayed with a minimum value of 2000, rather than 0, to accentuate month-to-month differences. Another type of graph is the pie chart, which is typically used to present some whole object broken down into its component parts. The width of each slice of the pie is proportional to each component's percentage share.

STATISTICS

Mean and Standard Deviation

Statistical analysis in nuclear medicine allows us to consider such things as how confident we are of the accuracy of some measurement, or how confident we are that a patient's test value is different from a normal result. Two concepts that emerge frequently in statistical

considerations are *precision* and *accuracy*. Precision refers to the spread, or range, of data values obtained when some parameter is measured many times or measured in many patients. A small precision means that there is little variation in the data values. Accuracy, on the other hand, refers to how close the results are to the true, or "gold standard," result. Suppose that the length of 96-in board is measured twice, obtaining results of 94 in and 98 in. These data could be called accurate because the average (or mean) value of the two yields the correct answer of 96 in. The large range of the data (94 to 98 in), however, would be considered not nearly precise enough for any practical construction measurements. Another person might measure the length of the board and obtain 96.25 and 96.50/in. These results are more precise (smaller range of data), but less accurate (the average is 96.37/in), than the previous measurement. A good measurement is both accurate and precise, but there is no necessarily fixed relationship between accuracy and precision in any experiment. Statistical parameters, such as the mean and standard deviation, allow quantitation of the concepts of accuracy and precision.

Suppose that some parameter x is measured n times. Then the mean of the n values of the parameters x is defined by the symbol $\bar{x}$:

$$\bar{x} = \frac{\Sigma x}{n}$$

The symbol Σx means the sum of all the measurements of x.

Suppose that a patient has four measurements of serum thyroxine (T_4, a thyroid hormone) given by: 9.5, 9.0, 9.2, and 8.7 $\mu g/dl$. The mean value x is:

$$\bar{x} = \frac{(9.5 + 9.0 + 9.2 + 8.7)}{4} = 9.1 \ \mu g/dl$$

If the true answer for the serum T_4 was known, then the mean value $x = 9.1 \ \mu g/dl$ could be compared to the true value to discuss the accuracy of the test. The *standard deviation*, a measure of the precision of the data, is given by the symbol σ, defined as:

$$\sigma = [\Sigma (x - x)^2 / (n - 1)]^{1/2}$$

Recall that an exponent of ½ means the same as the square root ($\sqrt{}$). The standard deviation is a measure of the deviation or spread of the data points from the mean value. For the thyroid T_4 data above:

$$\sigma = \{[(9.5 - 9.1)^2 + (9.0 - 9.1)^2 + (9.2 - 9.1)^2 + (8.7 - 9.1)^2]/(4 - 1)\}^{1/2}$$
$$\sigma = [(0.16 + 0.01 + 0.01 + 0.16)/3]^{1/2}$$
$$\sigma = (0.34/3)^{1/2} = 0.1133^{1/2} = 0.3366$$
$$\sigma = 0.3 \ \mu g/dl, \text{ correctly rounded to one significant decimal place}$$

The standard deviation is frequently expressed in a format of the mean value $\pm \sigma$, so this patient has a T_4 test result of 9.1 ± 0.3 $\mu g/dl$. A large σ value indicates data with a large range and therefore poor precision.

Sometimes it is more useful to express standard deviation as a percentage of the mean value, which is frequently called the percent standard deviation, or *coefficient of variation* (CV):

$$CV = \left(\frac{\sigma}{\overline{x}}\right) \times 100$$

For the thyroid function data above:

$$CV = \left(\frac{0.3367}{9.10}\right) \times 100 = 3.7\%$$

The CV merely shows how big the standard deviation is when compared with the mean value. For example, consider two separate experimental measurements of the length of an object. Both experiments produce the same standard deviation of 2 cm, but the two objects have different mean lengths of 2 m and 2 km. So one experiment has a CV of (2 cm/200 cm) $\times$ 100, or 1%, whereas the other experiment has a CV of (2 cm/200,000 cm) $\times$ 100, or 0.001%. The standard deviations of the two experiments are the same, but the CVs are vastly different, showing a much better precision in the second experiment (CV = 0.001%) than in the first experiment (CV = 1%).

As another example consider two different blueberry farms. Suppose farm A has blueberries of diameter 6 ± 7 mm and farm B has blueberries of diameter 9 ± 2 mm. Which farm would you rather have blueberries from? It depends on what you want. Farm A has a wider range of blueberry diameters. Indeed, some farm A blueberries must be quite small or very large to produce such a large 7 mm standard deviation, but the average blueberry is only 6 mm at Farm A. Farm B has blueberries that are bigger (9 mm) on the average, but the standard deviation for Farm B is smaller, so there are very few really big (or small) blueberries at Farm B.

The scientific pocket calculator generally has keys for calculation of mean and standard deviation. The user keys in the first data value and then pushes the key that tells the calculator this is x_1. Then the second data value is entered and the Xi key is pushed, telling the calculator this is x_2, etc. up to x_n. Then display the mean $\overline{x}$ and σ (sometimes denoted σ_{n-1}). Some calculators figure the variance, which is just σ^2. Most PC-type computers offer various spreadsheet, graphic, or statistical software that calculates the mean and standard deviation for columns of data values.

Further calculations with statistics require consideration of the *theoretical distribution* of the data values. We may know that a sample of blueberries produces diameters of 9 ± 2 mm. But suppose we want to know how many blueberries there are with diameters greater than 11 mm or what the probability is of getting a blueberry bigger than 13 mm. (The distribution refers to a theoretical measurement of *all* the blueberries of Farm A or of the T_4 values in *all* patients, etc.) The distribution is a theoretical graph of how many blueberries there are with which diameters or of how many patients there are with a certain value of T_4. What is usually measured in an experiment is not the theoretical distribution but rather *a sample* of data values (say 20 blueberries or 10 patients) that is part of the whole distribution. Two types of theoretical distributions of data values are important in nuclear medicine: the *Gaussian distribution* and the *Poisson distribution*. Many measurable quantities can be described by a Gaussian distribution, whereas the only thing of interest to nuclear medicine that follows a Poisson distribution is counting statistics.

Gaussian Distributions

The Gaussian distribution is also called the *bell-shaped distribution* and the *normal distribution*.[3] The theoretical equations for the Gaussian distribution need not concern us. In general, measurements of some parameter might be expected to follow a Gaussian distribution if a reasonably large sample is taken from a very large distribution, where the parameter being measured is expected to vary randomly. For example, the diameters of blueberries in a 1-gallon sample would be expected to follow a Gaussian distribution. The measurement of the decay counts of a sample of several thousand radioactive atoms (sampled from the distribution of about 10^{23} atoms in a small piece of radioactive material) would also be expected to follow a Gaussian distribution. Student scores on an examination might follow a Gaussian distribution. Saying that something follows a Gaussian distribution means that if the number of times a certain value occurs is plotted on the y axis, versus the value (say blueberry diameter or number of counts) on the x axis, then a graph such as Figure 1-10 is obtained. Analysis reveals that a Gaussian distribution has 68% of all results within the range $\overline{x} \pm 1\sigma$, 95% of all results within $\overline{x} \pm 2\sigma$, and 99% within $\overline{x} \pm 3\sigma$. (The actual values are 68.3%, 95.4%, and 99.7%.) Figure 1-10 shows this distribution. So, returning to the sample of blueberries, if $\overline{x} = 9$ mm and $\sigma = 2$ mm, then if all the blueberries in the bucket are examined, we would expect the following:

68% within 7-11 mm	$(\overline{x} \pm 1\sigma)$
95% within 5-13 mm	$(\overline{x} \pm 2\sigma)$
99% within 3-15 mm	$(\overline{x} \pm 3\sigma)$

The chance of getting a blueberry less than 5 mm or greater than 13 mm is only 5%. This is called *the area in the tails* (the ends) of the distribution. Since 95% are

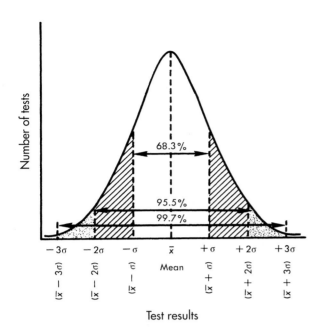

Figure 1-10 Gaussian distribution for test results can be expected to show distribution in large population where test value is expected to vary randomly. Note that 68% of all test results are within the mean ±1 standard deviation ($\bar{x} \pm 1\sigma$), 95% of all test results are in the range of $\bar{x} \pm 2\tilde{\sigma}$, etc.

within $x \pm 2\sigma$, it must be that only 5% are beyond the range $x \pm 2\sigma$.

The properties of the Gaussian distribution are often used in quality control procedures and to determine normal ranges (i.e., within acceptable tolerances). A quality control procedure might measure some daily parameter to determine whether an instrument is working properly. If today's value is beyond the $x \pm 2\sigma$ value (based on previous measurements), then the instrument might be considered to be operating improperly because the probability of getting a result beyond $x \pm 2\sigma$ is only 5%. The appropriate probability value to be used for rejection depends also on the number of parameters or control values being measured.[2]

Gaussian analysis is also frequently employed in determination of the normal range in radioimmunoassay (RIA) by measuring some RIA test in a large number of normal subjects. The normal range is then often defined as the mean ± 2σ range from the measurements in these normal subjects. A special type of graph paper, called probability paper, can be used[6] to plot the distribution (number of subjects versus their test value) as a straight line if the data follow a Gaussian distribution. Not all clinical data will follow a Gaussian distribution, especially if the study subjects are from a patient population rather than from true volunteer subject normal controls. Probability paper allows the "abnormal" patient high and low test results to be removed from the determination of the mean and standard de-

viation, since they appear as long tails on the ends of the Gaussian distribution.[5] This type of quality control, or normal value range determination, uses the 95% confidence interval (the $x \pm 2\sigma$ range) as a conventionally accepted range. This means that there is a 1 in 20 (or 5%) chance that we will incorrectly reject a quality control test, or that there is a 5% chance that a normal subject would be incorrectly called abnormal. The preponderance of results, 19 out of 20 (95%), will be correctly classified.

Poisson Distributions and Counting Statistics

Counting statistics, meaning the number of counts expected from a sample, follow the Poisson distribution. In the Poisson distribution the standard deviation (σ_C) for any number of counts (C) is fixed at the square root of C:

$$\sigma_c = \sqrt{C}$$

This fixed definition of standard deviation does not exist in Gaussian distributions; essentially only counting statistics are Poisson. One farm could have a Gaussian distribution of blueberries of diameter (mean ± σ) 9 ± 2 mm, and another farm could have blueberries of diameter 9 ± 4 mm. Neither has $\sigma = \sqrt{9}$. Any combination of a mean value and a standard deviation is possible in Gaussian data, whereas Poisson counting statistics always have the standard deviation of the counts from a sample equal to the square root of the counts.

EXAMPLE: What is the standard deviation of a sample that produced 10,000 counts?

$$\sigma_c = \sqrt{10,000} = 100 \text{ counts}$$

EXAMPLE: What is the coefficient of variation of 10,000 counts?

$$CV = \left(\frac{\sigma_c}{C}\right) \times 100 = \left(\frac{100}{10,000}\right) \times 100 = 1\%$$

EXAMPLE: What is the σ and CV for 100 counts?

$$\sigma_c = \sqrt{100} = 10 \text{ counts}$$

$$CV = \left(\frac{\sqrt{100}}{100}\right) \times 100 = 10\%$$

These examples show that, as the number of counts increases from 100 to 10,000, the absolute magnitude of the standard deviation goes up (from 10 to 100 counts), but the percent standard deviation or CV goes down (from 10% to 1%). There is less relative variability in large count values.

Counting statistics, besides being Poisson, are also described by a Gaussian distribution so long as the number of counts is greater than about 30. So now, given some number of counts C, we automatically know the standard deviation and we also know that 68% of repeat measures of the sample will fall within $C \pm \sqrt{C}$, and 95% of repeat measures of the sample will fall within $C \pm 2\sqrt{C}$, and so on.

EXAMPLE: A sample with 10,000 counts. What is the 95% confidence interval for this sample?

$$95\% \text{ confidence} = C \pm 2\sigma_c = C \pm 2\sqrt{C}$$
$$= 10{,}000 \pm 2\sqrt{10{,}000}$$
$$= 10{,}000 \pm 200 \text{ counts}$$

So the 95% confidence interval is from 9800 to 10,200 counts. If this represents a sample of the counts actually emanating from radioactive material, we can say we are 95% sure that the true counts from this radioactive material are in the 9800 to 10,200 range (or we would expect that 95% of repeat measurements would be in the range 9800 to 10,200 counts). The number of counts actually emitted by a radioactive source varies from time to time, in a random fashion, according to both Poisson and Gaussian distributions. The variation in the number of counts is often referred to as *counting noise*.

Sometimes this type of problem is expressed by saying that 10,000 counts are needed to be 95% confident that the true count is within 2% of the measured value. The presence of two different percentage values can seem confusing. The 95% confidence interval on 10,000 counts is ± 200 counts, and this 200 counts represents 2% of 10,000 counts. The general formula expressing the number of counts needed to be $n\sigma$ sure that the true answer is within some percent (*p*) of the measured counts is given by:

$$C = \left[\frac{n}{\left(\dfrac{p}{100\%} \right)} \right]^2$$

In this formula n is replaced with a 1 for 68% confidence, with a 2 for 95% confidence, and with a 3 for 99% confidence.

EXAMPLE: How many counts are needed to be 95% sure that the true answer is within 1% of the measured value? Here n = 2 and p = 1%.

$$C = \left[\frac{2}{\left(\dfrac{1\%}{100\%} \right)} \right]^2 = \left[\frac{2}{.01} \right]^2 = 40{,}000 \text{ counts}$$

If this sample were recounted, then 95% of repeat measurements would be in the range 40,000 ± 2$\sqrt{40{,}000}$ or 40,000 ± 400, which represents a 1% uncertainty (400 is 1% of 40,000). Some radiation counters may have a preset count dial labeled as the percent error at the 95% confidence level, rather than a preset count dial actually labeled in number of counts. Setting such a preset count dial at 1% error would be the same as collecting 40,000 counts. Setting such a preset count dial at 5% would mean collecting 1600 counts, since

$$1600 = \left(\frac{2}{0.05} \right)^2$$

Some problems may deal with the count rate R that is obtained by counting a number of counts C in time T:

$$R = \frac{C}{T}$$

The standard deviation in the count rate is σ_R:

$$\sigma_R = \left(\frac{\sqrt{C}}{T} \right)$$

This presumes that there is no error in measurement of the time T. By using $C = RT$, the σ_R can be alternatively written as:

$$\sigma_R = \frac{\sqrt{(RT)}}{T} = \sqrt{\left(\frac{R}{T} \right)}$$

EXAMPLE: A sample shows 43,627 counts in 5 minutes. What are the count rate and standard deviation in the count rate?

$$R = \frac{43{,}627 \text{ counts}}{5 \text{ minutes}}$$
$$R = \frac{8725 \text{ counts}}{\text{min}} = 8725 \text{ cpm}$$
$$\sigma_R = \frac{(\sqrt{43{,}627})}{5} = 42 \text{ cpm}$$

So the count rate might be expressed as 8725 ± 42 cpm.

EXAMPLE: The count rate is 8765 cpm for a 2-minute count. What range of count rates would be predicted to occur in 68% of repeat measurements? This is simply asking what is the value of σ_R, because $1\sigma_R$ is the 68% confidence interval.

$$\sigma_R = \sqrt{(R/T)} = \sqrt{(8765/2)} = \sqrt{4382.5} = 66 \text{ cpm}$$

So if the experiment were repeated, we would predict that 68% of the repeat measurements would be in the range 8765 ± 66 cpm.

Background counts are a problem in most measurements of counts from a radioactive sample. Background arises from natural terrestrial and cosmic sources of radioactivity or from other nearby sources of radioactive material. The sample is usually counted in the presence of some background radiation, yielding a gross count for sample plus background, denoted by the letter C. Then the sample is removed from the counter and the background B is counted. The net, or true counts, which represents the sample only, is denoted by N and given by:

$$N = C - B$$

The standard deviation of the net counts is given by

$$\sigma_N = \sqrt{(C + B)}$$

This is an example of the rules for combinations of errors,[1] which states that for addition or subtraction, errors add in quadrature within the square root:

$$\sigma_N = \sqrt{(\sigma_C^2 + \sigma_B^2)}$$

And since $\sigma_C = \sqrt{C}$ and $\sigma_B = \sqrt{B}$, we obtain $\sigma_N = \sqrt{(C + B)}$.

> **EXAMPLE:** A sample is counted in the presence of background yielding C = 1600 counts. Then the background is counted alone, producing 900 counts. What are the true or net counts and standard deviation?
>
> $$N = C - B = 1600 - 900 = 700 \text{ counts}$$
> $$\sigma_N = \sqrt{(1600 + 900)} = \sqrt{2500} = 50 \text{ counts}$$

So the net counts can be expressed as 700 ± 50 counts. Note that the presence of background increases the statistical uncertainty in the results. If there were *no* background, the sample in this example would have produced $N = 700 \pm \sqrt{700} = 700 \pm 26$ counts.

Similar considerations can yield the rules for the net count rate:

$$R_N = R_C - R_B = C/T_C - B/T_B$$
$$\sigma_{R_N} = \sqrt{(\sigma_{R_C}^2 + \sigma_{R_B}^2)}$$
$$\sigma_{R_N} = \sqrt{(C/T_C^2 + B/T_B^2)}$$

or

$$\sigma_{R_N} = \sqrt{(R_C/T_C + R_B/T_B)}$$

Chi-Square Tests

Suppose we wish to test the reliability of operation of some counting instrument, as a quality control test, by confirming that the instrument always produces the same counts in a reliable fashion. How can we do this when we now know that the number of counts recorded will vary from measurement to measurement because of the statistical nature of radioactive decay? The answer is to count a sample a reasonable number of times (typically 10 repeat measurements are used) and then determine if the 10 different values show a suitable amount of variation.[7] Too little or too much variation in the repeat measurements indicates a counter that may not be functioning properly. The chi-square (χ^2) test indicates an acceptable range of variability in the repeat measurements. The mean $\overline{C}$ of the 10 measurements is determined ($\overline{C} = \Sigma C/n$), and χ^2 is calculated as:

$$\chi^2 = \frac{[\Sigma(C - \overline{C})^2]}{\overline{C}}$$

Table 1-6 shows the calculation of χ^2 for some counter, which yielded a value of 24.7 for χ^2. Is this an acceptable amount of variation between the 10 measurements? The definition of acceptable χ^2 is given by looking up the probability *(P)* of this χ^2 value for the n (here 10) repeated measures in Table 1-7. Too little variation is shown by a χ^2 smaller than the $P = 0.9$ value; an amount of variation exactly as expected from the statistical nature of the decay process would yield $P = 0.50$; and an unacceptably large χ^2 would be for a P value greater than 0.10:

If $0.90 > (P \text{ of } \chi^2) > 0.10$, detector is OK
$(P \text{ of } \chi^2) > 0.90$, too little variation
$(P \text{ of } \chi^2) < 0.10$, too much variation

In Table 1-6 $\chi^2 = 24.7$. In Table 1-7 this n = 10 measurement has a P value < 0.01, so this detector is *not* operating properly, the χ^2 is too large. The detector probably needs to be repaired. An acceptable χ^2 for 10 measurements would be in the range: $4.17 < \chi^2 < 14.7$,

Table 1-6	Calculation of chi-square		
Observation	**Counts (C)**	**Deviation (C − C̄)**	**Square (C − C̄)²**
1	10,324	144.7	20,938.1
2	10,285	105.7	11,172.5
3	9847	−332.3	110,423.3
4	10,168	−11.3	127.7
5	10,352	172.7	29,825.3
6	10,234	54.7	2,992.1
7	9986	−193.3	37,364.9
8	10,139	−40.3	1624.1
9	10,356	176.7	31,222.9
10	10,102	−77.3	5975.3
	$\Sigma = 101,793$	$\Sigma = 0$	$\Sigma = 251,666$

$\overline{C} = 10179.3$
$\chi^2 = \Sigma(C - \overline{C})^2/\overline{C}$
$\chi^2 = \dfrac{251,666}{10,179.3} = 24.7$
$SD = [\Sigma(C - \overline{C})^2/(n - 1)]^{1/2}$
$SD = (251,666/9)^{1/2} = 167.2$

| Table 1-7 | Chi-square value at probability P |

Number of sample measurements	Probability (P)						
	0.99	0.95	0.90†	0.50	0.10*	0.05	0.01
5	0.30	0.71	1.06	3.36	7.78	9.49	13.3
10	2.09	3.33	4.17	8.34	14.7	16.9	21.2
15	4.66	6.57	7.79	13.3	21.1	23.7	29.1
20	7.63	10.1	11.7	18.3	27.2	30.1	36.2

*Largest acceptable χ^2 is in this column.
†Smallest acceptable χ^2 is in this column.

since this is the $0.90 > P > 0.10$ range. Here again it is only common convention that fixes the $P = 0.90 - 0.10$ range as acceptable. Some laboratories might be willing to accept more variation or be willing to use $0.95 - 0.05$ as the acceptable P range.

Notice the similarities in statistical approach for calculating the linear correlation coefficient r and χ^2. Both are calculated from the data based on some equation, and then the P value of the r or χ^2 is determined to assess significance of the result. This is typical of most statistical tests: calculate a parameter and then look up the probability of this result.

Does the result for the data in Table 1-6 seem sensible, that the detector is showing too much variation? Consider that we know that a properly operating detector should have 68% (about 7 out of 10) of repeat measurements within the mean count $\pm \sqrt{\text{mean count}}$. So the deviation $C - \overline{C}$ in Table 1-6 should be less than 1σ, less than $\pm \sqrt{10179.3} = 101$ counts in 7 out of 10 measurements. Examination of Table 1-6 shows that only 4 of the measurements (instead of the expected 7) have deviations from the mean smaller than $\pm 1\sigma$ or within ± 101 counts. The detector is not working properly by this crude visual check, in agreement with the too large χ^2 value. Similar visual checks can be made to assess that only 1 out of 20 measurements should have deviations from the mean of more than $\pm 2 \times 101$ counts. In fact, Table 1-6 shows that one measure is a deviation of -333 counts (about 3σ) and another is almost 2σ (actually -193 counts). So about 2 out of 10 are beyond $\pm 2\sigma$ in contrast to predicted 1 out of 20 measurements with this much variation. The calculated P value of χ^2 will always agree with such common sense data checks.

Last, a word about calculating χ^2. Most scientific pocket calculators do not have a calculation function for χ^2. But most can calculate the standard deviation of the repeat count measurements, here denoted SD:

$$SD = \left[\frac{\Sigma(C - \overline{C})^2}{(n-1)} \right]^{1/2}$$

This can be algebraically solved for $\Sigma (C - \overline{C})^2$:

$$\Sigma(C - \overline{C})^2 = (n - 1) \times (SD)^2$$

This is simply the numerator of the definition of χ^2, so the definition of χ^2 can be written in terms of the mean and SD as:

$$\chi^2 = (n - 1) \times \frac{(SD)^2}{\overline{C}}$$

To calculate χ^2, therefore, the pocket calculator (or the PC computer spreadsheet, etc., program) is used as described previously to calculate the SD and the mean, which are then used in the above equation for χ^2. The data in Table 1-6 show SD = 167.2 with a mean $\overline{C} = 10179.3$, so:

$$\chi^2 = \frac{(10 - 1) \times (167.2)^2}{10179.3} = 24.7$$

The χ^2 statistic has other uses besides a test for stability of counters in nuclear medicine. Chi-square is commonly used in 2×2 contingency tables,[3] which could consider, for example, the number of persons who are well or ill, tabulated according to their sex. Or a categorization could be made of the number of persons with positive or negative imaging tests using gamma cameras from two different manufacturers. A χ^2 calculation would show whether the two gamma cameras find different or same numbers of positive/negative test results.

t-Tests

The t-test is used to test for differences between *mean* values.[3,7] This test is also commonly referred to as the Student t-test because the original proposal for this test was published by W.S. Gosset in 1908 using the pseudonym *Student*. There are two forms of the t-test: for independent samples and for paired samples.

For independent t-tests there are two independent groups of data. For example, some test result is measured in a group of n_1 ill patients and a group of n_2 well patients. The two groups are independent. There is no relationship or correlation between the two groups, typically because the groups represent different patients. The two groups have mean and standard deviations denoted by $\bar{x}_1$, SD_1, $\bar{x}_2$, and SD_2.

The t-test is a test of a null hypothesis that the mean values in the two groups are equal. The hypothesis being tested can be abbreviated $H_0: \bar{x}_1 = \bar{x}_2$. The null hypothesis is statistical nomenclature meaning that there is no difference. This test is called a two-tailed test, since either group could be equally expected to have the larger mean value. The calculation of the t-test requires no new calculation details from the data, merely means and standard deviations in the two groups. The t-test result is calculated as follows:

$$t = (\bar{x}_1 - \bar{x}_2 / \left\{ \frac{[(n_1 - 1) \times SD_1^2 + (n_2 - 1) \times SD_2^2] \times \left(\frac{1}{n_1} + \frac{1}{n_2}\right)}{n_1 + n_2 - 2} \right\}^{1/2}$$

The calculated t compared to tabulated values of the critical t-test (Table 1-8) with $n_1 + n_2 - 2$ degrees of freedom (v) at the 0.05 level:

If $t \leq t_{n1 + n2 - 2, \, 0.05}$—the study does not reject $H_0: \bar{x}_1 = \bar{x}_2$, and no difference is shown between the two groups.

If $t > t_{n1 + n2 - 2, \, 0.05}$—the hypothesis $H_0: \bar{x}_1 = \bar{x}_2$ is rejected, and a difference between the two groups is demonstrated.

> **EXAMPLE:** One group of $n_1 = 6$ patients is given a drug, and their thyroid T_4 levels (8.8, 8.7, 9.2, 8.6, 8.5, and 9.0) have $\bar{x}_1 = 8.80$ and $SD_1 = 0.26$. A second group of $n_2 = 5$ patients is given a placebo, and their T_4 results (8.3, 8.5, 8.2, 8.1, and 8.4) are $\bar{x}_2 = 8.3$ and $SD_2 = 0.16$. Is there a difference in T_4 levels between the two groups? Did the drug affect T_4 level?

$$t = (8.80 - 8.30) / \left\{ \frac{[(6 - 1) \times (0.26)^2 + (5 - 1) \times (0.16)^2] \times \left(\frac{1}{6} + \frac{1}{5}\right)}{(6 + 5 - 2)} \right\}^{1/2}$$

$$t = \frac{0.50}{\left\{ \frac{[0.4404] \times (0.3667)}{9} \right\}^{1/2}}$$

$$t = \frac{0.50}{0.01794^{1/2}} = 3.73$$

From Table 1-8 the critical t value at the 5% or 0.05 level with $n_1 + n_2 - 2 = 9$ degrees of freedom is $t_{9,0.05} = 2.26$. Since calculated t is greater than critical t, we conclude that there is a statistically significant difference between the drug group and the placebo

Degrees of freedom (v)	Probability (P)			
	0.10	0.05*	0.01	0.001
4	2.13	2.78	4.60	8.61
5	2.01	2.57	4.03	6.87
6	1.94	2.45	3.71	5.96
7	1.89	2.36	3.50	5.41
8	1.86	2.31	3.36	5.04
9	1.83	2.26	3.25	4.78
10	1.81	2.23	3.17	4.59
15	1.75	2.13	2.95	4.07
20	1.72	2.09	2.84	3.85
30	1.70	2.04	2.75	3.65
60	1.67	2.00	2.66	3.46
∞	1.64	1.96	2.58	3.29

Table 1-8 t-Test value at probability P

*Minimum value of t-test for significant difference is in this column. Larger t values imply a more significant difference.

group. The drug *did* make a difference. In fact, the statistical tables show the critical t statistic at the 1% level $t_{9,0.01} = 3.25$, so we are actually more than 99% confident that a difference exists between the drug group and the placebo group (since calculated t is greater than $t_{9,0.01}$). We can also say that there is less than a 1% likelihood that the difference between the drug and placebo groups is due to a chance occurrence, rather than due to the drug.

Most PC-type computer software packages (spreadsheets, graphics, statistics software) offer calculation capabilities of t-tests for which the user simply enters two columns of data values and selects an independent or paired t-test. The PC computer will then calculate the t-test result and the associated probability, sparing the user from any tedious calculations. In using such software it can be helpful to enter some test data, such as from the examples given here, to insure that the software produces the same t-test and probability value as in the examples given here. Alternatively, the t-test can be performed as in the example here, after first using the pocket calculator to calculate the means and standard deviations of the two groups as discussed above.

A special term, *standard error,* is used when referring to the variability in *mean* values. The standard error (SE) governs the variability of the *mean* value, whereas the standard deviation (SD) governs the variability of any one *individual* patient measurement. The results of an experiment to measure a mean value will usually be expressed as $x \pm SE$, rather than $x \pm SD$, although this is not universal practice and there can be confusion if the specification of SE or SD is not made clear. The SE is given by:

$$SE = SD/\sqrt{n}$$

The data in the *t*-test example above would most commonly be specified as mean ± standard error:

Drug group mean = 8.80 ± 0.11 μg/dl
Placebo group mean = 8.30 ± 0.07 μg/dl

Stating the data in this manner helps compare the means in the two groups. A graphic representation often shows the individual data values as dots on the graph, with a separate symbol for the mean. The mean symbol on the graph often includes ± standard error bars, drawn as vertical lines of length equal to 1 SE above and below the mean value. The *t*-test is essentially a measure of how far apart the mean values are, measured in terms of their standard errors.

There is a nuance of independent *t*-tests which states that, before an independent *t*-test for equality of the means can be used, it is first necessary to verify that the standard deviations from the two independent groups are sufficiently similar. An independent *t*-test is thus properly preceded by the F-test, which concerns the null hypothesis that $SD_1 = SD_2$ (or $H_0:SD_1 = SD_2$). The F-statistic is easily calculated:

$$F = \frac{(SD_1)^2}{(SD_2)^2}, \text{ with } SD_1 > SD_2$$

Either group can be identified as group 1, so long as the identification results in $SD_1 > SD_2$. The value of the calculated F-statistic has degrees of freedom (ν_1 and ν_2) denoted by $n_1 - 1$ and $n_2 - 1$ for the numerator and denominator, respectively. The calculated F-statistic is compared to tables (from any statistics book) of critical F values $F_{n1}-1, n2-1, 0.05$ at the 5% level. If the calculated F is less than or equal to $F_{n1}-1, n2-1, 0.05$, then it is permissible to proceed with a *t*-test for $H_0:\bar{x}_1 = \bar{x}_2$. If the calculated F is greater than $F_{n1} - 1, n2 - 1, 0.05$, then it is not proper to use a *t*-test on these data. It is unfortunately not uncommon in scientific literature to see a *t*-test performed without first checking the F-test for similar standard deviations. The example data above have $SD_1 = 0.26$ and $SD_2 = 0.16$, so the F-statistic is calculated as:

$$F = \frac{(0.26)^2}{(0.16)^2} = 2.64$$

From statistical tables the critical F value $F_{5,4,0.05} = 6.26$; so the calculated F value is less than the critical F value. This means that the standard deviations are sufficiently similar and we can proceed with the *t*-test for equality of means in the two groups.

A paired *t*-test is used for testing differences between two mean values when they are from the *same* patient. For example, a group of *n* patients could have their ventricular ejection fraction measured before (x_1) and after (x_2) taking some drug. The ejection fractions before and after drug administration are correlated; a patient with a large ejection fraction before drug admin-

istration could also be expected to have a large ejection fraction after drug administration. What matters in paired data is the difference $d = x_1 - x_2$ between any two values. The difference between the first and second measurement is tabulated in each patient to calculate the mean difference $\bar{d}$:

$$\bar{d} = \frac{\Sigma(x_1 - x_2)}{n}$$

The standard deviation of the difference SDD is defined as:

$$SDD = \left\{ \frac{\Sigma(d - \bar{d})^2}{(n - 1)} \right\}^{1/2}$$

Note that the algebraic sign, either + or −, of the difference *(d)* in each patient must be carefully used in calculating $\bar{d}$ and SDD. Then the paired *t*-test tests the null hypothesis that there is no mean difference between the first and second measurements, $H_0:\bar{d} = 0$, by comparing the calculated *t*-statistic, $t = \bar{d}/(SDD/\sqrt{n})$, to the critical *t* value at the 0.05 level with $n - 1$ degrees of freedom ($= t_{n-1,0.05}$). If $t \leq t_{n-1,0.05}$, no difference is shown between the two measurements. If $t > t_{n-1,0.05}$, there is a statistically significant difference between the first and second measurements. If the calculated *t* is just greater than the critical *t* with $n - 1$ degrees of freedom at the *P* confidence level (e.g., $P = 0.05, 0.01, 0.005, 0.001$, etc.), then we say that a difference is shown between the two measurements at the *P* confidence level.

Table 1-9 shows calculation of $\bar{d}$ and SDD for the old versus new ejection fraction data from Table 1-4. Note carefully how the algebraic sign (+ or −) of d and $d - \bar{d}$ as in Table 1-9. The null hypothesis being tested is $H_0:$old = new. The calculated $t = 0.14$ is much less than the critical *t* value ($t_{9,0.05} = 2.26$) from Table 1-8. So the conclusion is that there is no statistically significant difference between the old and new EF values. This is another way of saying that the regression line in Figure 1-8 is not statistically different from the line of identity.

Note that a *t*-test either fails to show a difference ($t \leq t$-critical) or does show a difference ($t > t$-critical). A *t*-test that fails to show a difference does *not* prove that the two mean values are equal[3], it merely indicates that the data are inadequate to prove a difference exists. A semantic nuance that may be encountered is that independent *t*-tests consider the difference between the means, whereas a paired *t*-test considers the mean of the differences.

If more than two mean values are involved, the simple *t*-test is not appropriate. For example, we might wish to know whether a difference exists between the means of a test value in four independent groups of patients ($H_0:\bar{x}_1 = \bar{x}_2 = \bar{x}_3 = \bar{x}_4$). This test requires a method called *analysis of variance (ANOVA)* to most powerfully find differences between the four groups. Alter-

Table 1-9	Paired *t*-test data			
EF old method	EF new method	Difference (d = old − new)	d − d̄	(d − d̄)²
47	43	4	3.8	14.44
62	65	−3	−3.2	10.24
39	44	−5	−5.2	27.04
33	32	1	0.8	0.64
55	56	−1	−1.2	1.44
42	45	−3	−3.2	10.24
59	56	3	2.8	7.84
65	58	7	6.8	46.24
28	34	−6	−6.2	38.44
51	46	5	4.8	23.04
		d̄ = 0.2		sum = 179.60

$$SDD = [\Sigma(d - \bar{d})^2/(n-1)]^{1/2}$$
$$= [179.6/(10-1)]^{1/2}$$
$$= [19.96]^{1/2} = 4.47$$
$$t_9 = \bar{d}/(SDD/\sqrt{n})$$
$$= 0.2/(4.47/\sqrt{10}) = 0.14$$

natively, but less powerfully for finding differences, the data can be tested for all pairs of differences with a *t*-test using the Bonferroni method, which requires lowering the significant P value from 0.05 to $0.05/n$, where n is the number of possible tests. For four groups of patients there are six possible *t*-tests: group 1 versus 2,3,4; group 2 versus 3,4; group 3 versus 4. So we could do all six *t*-tests and claim a significant difference only between pairs of mean values with a t value larger than the critical t value at the $0.05/6 = 0.0083$ P value.

Medical Decision Making

Medical decision making would not be necessary if medical tests always produced a result that correctly identified the patient as either ill or well. Unfortunately, because of the diversity of biologic response, possible statistical noise in data, and other technological deficiencies, a medical test often produces identical results for ill and well patients. So by some, often arbitrary, method we establish a test result normal range for well people and then say that results outside this normal range indicate illness.

For example, suppose we measure T_4 thyroid hormone in a group of well people and find the mean ±2 SD normal range is $4 - 12$ $\mu g/dl$. So we define any subsequent patient test as normal or euthyroid for T_4 of ≥4 to ≤12, and hyperthyroid for $T_4 > 12$. But isn't this a little foolish? A patient with $T_4 = 11.9$ is labeled well, whereas a patient with $T_4 = 12.1$ is labeled ill, even though the difference in the two values may be within the limit of accuracy of the test technique. This is because most test values indicate a continuum of results, not a yes or no answer, as in pregnancy. What about a patient image test that produces an image that looks

suspicious, not quite clearly normal, but not extremely abnormal? We can call the image test either positive (yes it shows a defect) or negative (no defect is shown). What are the consequences of being a lax image reader (who calls lots of positive studies), versus a strict image reader (who requires very strong abnormal image characteristics before calling an image positive)? These are some of the questions that medical decision making can consider.[6]

A test that finds a result for which the test was performed is called a positive test. A positive test for hyperthyroidism would be a $T_4 > 12$ $\mu g/dl$. A positive $^{201}T1$ imaging test would be a patient image with a cold defect in the heart. A positive ^{99m}Tc MDP bone scan would be a patient image with a hot spot in the bone. The test result might be low, high, cold, or hot, but it is positive for the condition being tested for.

A test that does not show the tested for result is called a negative test. A T_4 result in the euthyroid (normal) range would be a negative test for hyperthyroidism. A $^{201}T1$ heart scan with no defects in the heart image would be a negative scan for coronary artery disease. Note carefully that the positive or negative value refers to the test result; positive or negative is not defined by the patient's clinical condition.

The patient condition can be similarly categorized as either well or ill. This categorization must be obtained from some test *other than* the one being considered as the nuclear medicine test with positive or negative result. The patient condition is usually established as well or ill via some other medical test, called the gold standard test. A patient, for example, could have either a positive or a negative $^{201}T1$ test, and the true state of the patient as well or ill is usually established from some other clinical test, such as coronary angiography. An imaging phantom study could have an image result that is called either positive or negative, and the true gold standard result is the known fact about whether the phantom contains an imaging abnormality or defect. Some presentations of this subject material might use the terms normal and abnormal in lieu of well and ill.

Given these definitions, all of the following material relates to placing test results into one of four categories:

1. *True positive (TP):* persons with a positive test result who are truly ill.
2. *False positive (FP):* persons with a positive test result who are not ill.
3. *True negative (TN):* persons with a negative test result who are truly well.
4. *False negative (FN):* persons with a negative test result who are not well.

A woman with a positive pregnancy test who is actually pregnant is called a TP result. If the pregnancy test result was negative, but the woman is actually pregnant, then the result is an FN result. More typically, in nuclear medicine a decision is made to call an image test positive if the image shows some agreed upon defect. Then patients are categorized as TP, FP, TN, or

FN by combining their nuclear medicine image test result with that of some other gold standard clinical test. A patient with a negative ^{201}T1 imaging test (no abnormal defects on the image study) who is known to have coronary artery disease would be called an FN test result. A phantom study that calls the image positive, in an area of the phantom where a lesion definitely exists, would be a TP result.

Now consider the following test results. A study of imaging tests in 1000 patients produced the following data:

Test result

	(−)	(+)
Well	836 = TN	44 = FP
Ill	26 = FN	94 = TP

From these categorized data we can derive several other interesting parameters that define the usefulness of the test.

The *sensitivity*, or *true positive fraction (TPF)*, is the percentage or fraction of ill patients who have a positive test.

$$\text{Sensitivity} = \text{TPF} = \frac{TP}{(TP + FN)}$$

For the above data

$$\text{Sensitivity} = \frac{94}{(94 + 26)} = 78\%$$

meaning that the study found a positive test result in 78% of the ill people. Note the distinction between similar appearing symbols, TP and TPF.

The *specificity*, or *true negative fraction (TNF)*, is the percentage or fraction of well patients who have a negative test.

$$\text{Specificity} = \text{TNF} = \left(\frac{TN}{TN + FP}\right)$$

For the above data

$$\text{Specificity} = \left(\frac{836}{836 + 44}\right) = 95\%$$

meaning that the study found a negative test result in 95% of the well people. Again, note the distinction between similar appearing symbols, TN and TNF. (The decision on whether to use the term sensitivity or TPF, and specificity or TNF is purely arbitrary.) The above data show a sensitivity of 78%, less than the specificity of 95%, which means that this test does a better job at correctly diagnosing well people than it does at correctly diagnosing ill people.

The ideal medical test would have sensitivity and specificity both equal 100%. Unfortunately, medical data usually appear as in Figure 1-11, with an overlap between the test results for the well and ill patient populations. Which is more important, a high sensitivity (correctly finding ill people), or a high specificity (correctly finding well people)? The answer to this question is complex, often depending on the medical/economic/social consequences of the test. If the imaging test is intended to detect brain tumors that are known always to be fatal, but for which there is a simple medical cure with no side effects even in well people, then a high sensitivity might be preferred.

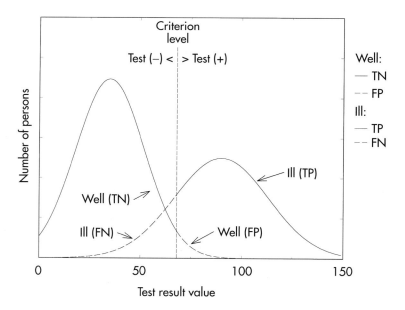

Figure 1-11   Distribution of test results for two groups: well (D−) and ill (D+). Test result is called negative or positive depending on whether it is below or above criterion level. Note that well and ill population overlap, creating well persons who are either TN or FP, and ill persons who are either TP or FN.

The consequences of misdiagnosing an ill person would be death, whereas the consequences of misdiagnosing a well person would be a harmless drug regimen. On the other hand, suppose the consequence of finding a positive result in an imaging scan was immediate total frontal lobotomy, which would prolong the patient's life by only a few months. Given the dire consequences of treatment, a high specificity would be preferred to avoid misdiagnosis in well patients.

Another factor that affects the most desirable sensitivity and specificity of a test is the prevalence of disease. The *prevalence* is the fraction or percentage of ill persons in the study population.

$$\text{Prevalence} = \frac{(TP + FN)}{(TP + FN + TN + FP)}$$

The above data had a prevalence of

$$\frac{(26 + 94)}{(26 + 94 + 836 + 44)} = 12\%$$

meaning that 12% of the study subjects were ill.

The prevalence is characteristic of the patient population; prevalence is not a characteristic of the test itself. Prevalence is shown graphically in Figure 1-11 by the area under the ill curve compared with the area under both the ill and well curves. The relative heights of the ill and well curves show the prevalence, which can vary from one hospital to another. If the prevalence is high, there are many sick people, and the optimum test may be one that gives priority to a high sensitivity at the expense of lowered specificity (we can more easily afford a few FP errors in the small number of well people). To the contrary, a screening test for some rare disease operates in a patient population with a low prevalence, where the optimum test may be one that gives priority to a high specificity at the expense of lowered sensitivity, to avoid a large number of FP results in the preponderance of well people.

A parameter that specifies the total number of correct answers, regardless of being ill or well, is the *accuracy* of the test.

$$\text{Accuracy} = \frac{(\text{Total number correct})}{(\text{Total number of persons})}$$

$$= \frac{(TN + TP)}{(TN + TP + FP + FN)}$$

The above data show an accuracy of

$$\frac{(836 + 94)}{(836 + 94 + 44 + 26)} = 93\%$$

meaning that the test correctly diagnosed 93% of all patients as ill or well. One problem is that the accuracy of a test depends strongly on the prevalence of disease for the same sensitivity and specificity of a test. This means that the accuracy between two hospitals can be very different for the same test because the prevalence at the two hospitals can be very different. Accuracy can be written specifically in terms of sensitivity, specificity, and prevalence as: Accuracy = Sensitivity × Prevalence + Specificity × (1 − Prevalence), where prevalence is expressed as a fraction, not a percent.

Using these several parameters for defining the goodness of a test, consider the following situation. A patient has a positive test result on some nuclear medicine study. We know this must be either a TP result in a truly ill person, or an FP result in a truly well person. The referring physician simply wants to know what is the probability of disease, given the positive test result? We can give the referring physician a wealth of parameters about the goodness of our *test:* the sensitivity = 78%, specificity = 95%, prevalence = 12%, accuracy = 93%. But these parameters do not answer the clinical question at hand—what is the chance that this patient with a positive test result is truly ill? We need a parameter that deals with the clinical usefulness of the test, not just goodness-of-the-test parameters such as sensitivity.

The *positive predictive value,* or *predictive value of a positive test* $P(D+ : T+)$ can be read as the conditional probability of having disease (D+), given a positive test result (T+). This is merely the fraction of persons with positive test results who are truly ill:

$$\frac{TP}{(TP + FP)}$$

For the above data

$$P(D+ : T+) = \frac{94}{(94 + 44)} = 68\%$$

meaning that the answer to the referring physician's question is that there is a 68% chance that the patient with the positive test result is truly ill. Of course this means that there is a 32% chance that the patient with this positive nuclear medicine test result is not ill. These considerations are a reflection of a mathematical concept called Bayes theorem, after Thomas Bayes (1702-1761), an English mathematician and theologian. It allows us to recalculate the probability of illness based on the new information of a positive test result. Before the nuclear medicine test, the chance that the patient had disease was simply the prevalence of 12%. But after a positive test, the probability of disease has jumped to 68%.

Conversely, the *negative predictive value,* or *predictive value of a negative test* $P(D- : T-)$ is the probability P of not having disease (D−), given a negative test result (T−), or the fraction of all persons with a negative test who are truly well: TN/(TN + FN).

For the above data $P(D- : T-) = 836/(836 + 26) = 97\%$, meaning that a patient with a negative nuclear medicine test result has a 97% chance of being truly well. Note Bayes theorem at work here. Before the nuclear medicine test, the patient had a (1-prevalence) or 88% chance of being well. After a negative nuclear medicine test the probability that the patient is truly well has jumped to 97%.

In all of the discussion so far we have not touched on how the patient's true condition, well or ill, is determined from some gold standard test. Calculation of all the parameters (such as TN, FP, sensitivity, specificity) requires that we know, from some other test, who is truly ill or well. So when evaluating the goodness of test results such as sensitivity, it is always necessary to ask what was used for the gold standard to define illness. Two hospitals may have vastly different parameters for sensitivity and specificity, not because of any difference in the nuclear medicine test result, but rather because the two hospitals define illness in different terms.

For example, an invasive procedure such as coronary angiography is often used as a gold standard to calculate the sensitivity and other parameters of nuclear medicine ^{201}Tl myocardial imaging. But there may be no commonly agreed on definition of illness in the gold standard test. One hospital might say that the test must show coronary arteries narrowed by only 40% for a diagnosis of illness, but a second hospital might say that a patient is not ill until the gold standard test shows more than 70% narrowing of the coronary arteries. This difference in gold standard will combine with the characteristics of the nuclear medicine test to produce different sensitivities and other parameters at the two hospitals.

When calculating sensitivity, for example, it is necessary to carefully define the test criterion level that characterizes a positive test. One hospital may say a positive test for hyperthyroidism is any $T_4 > 10.5$ μg/dl, whereas another hospital may say $T_4 > 12.5$ μg/dl is a positive test result. Different sensitivity values will result. In fact, when we receive information from the diagnostic test, we can operate with any criterion level we choose to define a positive test. A lax criterion level (e.g., calling a nuclear medicine study positive with just a hint of abnormality in the image) leads to high sensitivity and low specificity. If we want a high sensitivity, we can call all tests positive, resulting in sensitivity = 100%. Of course, there would then be no TN tests, so the specificity would be zero. Want a high specificity? Just call every test negative, resulting in specificity = 100%.

As the criterion level that defines a negative or positive test result is moved left or right in Figure 1-11, the sensitivity and specificity change accordingly. So sensitivity and specificity are not parameters fixed as constants in nature, or fixed by some inherent property of

a test, or fixed by an image reader's skill level. Rather, sensitivity and specificity depend on the gold standard used to define illness *and* on the criterion level that defines a positive test. In Figure 1-11, if we slide the criterion level to the right, so that it is stricter in calling a positive test result, the sensitivity decreases while specificity increases. Slide the criterion level to the left, so that it becomes more lax in defining a positive test, and the sensitivity improves while specificity worsens. To further guide our thinking in these matters we often plot a *receiver operating characteristic (ROC) curve,* which shows sensitivity and specificity as a function of the criterion level used to call a test positive.

An ROC curve[7] is shown in Figure 1-12. The y axis is the sensitivity, and the x axis is the specificity. Note that the x axis is inverted in the sense that it *decreases* left to right from 100% to 0% specificity. (An alternate labeling for the axes of an ROC curve will have TPF from 0 to 1 on the y axis and false positive fraction (FPF) = FP/(FP + TN) from 0 to 1 on the x axis.) The ideal point for a test result would be the upper left corner of the ROC curve in Figure 1-12, with sensitivity = 100% and specificity = 100%.

An ROC curve is a graphic representation of the effect of changing the criterion level, just as we moved the criterion level left or right in Figure 1-11. A wealth of information can be gleaned from an ROC curve concerning which sensitivity/specificity is the optimum operating point, i.e., what optimum criterion level should we use to call a test positive. There may be no definitive

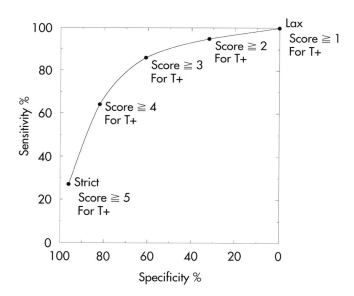

Figure 1-12 ROC curve showing sensitivity and specificity as function of minimum image score needed to call image positive. Note x axis for specificity reads left-to-right from 100 to 0. Lax reader might call any image with score ≥2 positive, with high sensitivity and low specificity. Strict reader would require high score to call image positive, resulting in low sensitivity and high specificity. Best test operates near upper left corner of ROC curve.

answers, but the ROC curve clearly shows the available options. The ROC curve is still dependent on prevalence and on the gold standard test to define illness. Suppose that a planar imaging study is reported in the literature with specificity = 61% and sensitivity = 86%. Another study in the literature reports a tomographic study with specificity = 82% and sensitivity = 64%. Which is the better test, planar or tomographic?

We cannot say which test is better *unless both* sensitivity and specificity are improved in one of the tests. In fact, these data could represent the same test results; the difference could simply be due to a changed criterion level for calling a test result positive. The hospital with the planar data could be calling a test result positive with a lower degree of image abnormality, leading to improved sensitivity but worsened specificity. We cannot clearly say which test is better without seeing the entire ROC curve for both the planar and tomographic data.

To form an ROC curve from any data we simply tabulate the TP, FN, TN, and FP results to calculate sensitivity and specificity for each criterion level that defines an abnormal test. For an in vitro T_4 blood test we just calculate sensitivity and specificity using different criterion levels for an abnormal test, e.g., for $T_4 > 0$, for $T_4 > 1$, for $T_4 > 2$, etc. Then a plot of sensitivity versus specificity at the various criterion levels yields the ROC curve. Image data are more difficult, since there is not always a quantifiable numeric result for imaging studies. So a rating scale is sometimes employed to score an image from 1-5 as follows:

Image score	Meaning
1	Definitely normal image
2	Probably normal image
3	Possibly abnormal image
4	Probably abnormal image
5	Definitely abnormal image

Suppose we had an imaging study with 50 patients. From some other gold standard test we know which patients are truly ill or well: 28 are well and 22 are ill. A reader scores each image as above. The sensitivity and specificity can be calculated from the TN, FP, FN, and TP results for each criterion level as follows:

A positive test is a score $\geq$	TN	FP	FN	TP	Specificity (%)	Sensitivity (%)
1 (lax)	0	28	0	22	0	100
2	9	19	1	21	32	95
3	17	11	3	19	61	86
4	23	5	8	14	82	64
5 (strict)	27	1	16	6	96	27

Figure 1-12 is an ROC curve for these data. The planar and tomographic results above *could* represent just two different operating points on this single ROC curve. The planar test could have been called abnormal for an image score $\geq$ 3, whereas the tomographic data may have been called a positive test only for a stricter image score $\geq$ 4. Alternatively, there could be a difference in ROC curves for the planar and tomographic results, but this could be ascertained only from seeing the entire ROC curve for both studies.

A medical test cannot be judged solely on sensitivity and specificity, since these parameters are a strong function of the definition of the test criterion level used to call a test positive. The ideal operating point on the ROC curve could be at the upper left corner, with sensitivity = 100% and specificity = 100%. In general, the test that is closest to this ideal is the better test, so the best operating point (at what score to call a test positive) may be the one that results in an operating point closest to the upper left corner of the ROC curve. Or, as discussed previously, considerations of prevalence of disease and consequences of diagnosis may suggest favoring sensitivity over specificity, or vice versa.

REFERENCES

1. Bevington PR: *Data reduction and error analysis for the physical sciences*, New York, 1969, McGraw-Hill.
2. Cembrowski GS, Carey RN: *Laboratory quality management*, Chicago, 1989, ASCP Press.
3. Colton T: *Statistics in medicine*, Boston, 1975, Little, Brown.
4. Highers MP, Forrester RA: *Mathematics for the allied health professions*, Norwalk, 1984, Appleton & Lange.
5. Martin HF, Gudzinowicz BJ, Fanger H: *Normal values in clinical chemistry: a guide to statistical analysis of laboratory data*, New York, 1975, Marcel Dekker.
6. Metz CE: Basic principles of ROC analysis, *Semin Nucl Med* 8:283-298, 1978.
7. Sorenson JA, Phelps ME: *Physics in nuclear medicine*, ed 2, Orlando, 1987, Grune & Stratton.
8. Stefani SS, Hubbard LB: *Mathematics for technologists in radiology, nuclear medicine, and radiation therapy*, St. Louis, 1979, Mosby.

SUGGESTED READINGS

Lamson M, Hotte CE, Ice RE: Practical generator kinetics, *J Nucl Med Technol* 4:21-27, 1976.

chapter 2

Paul E. Christian

Physics of Nuclear Medicine

Objectives

Describe the properties of electromagnetic radiation.

Describe the structure of the atom and its components and their properties.

Explain the structure of the chart of the nuclides, and define the line of stability.

State the relationship of mass and energy in Einstein's equation.

Write the correct form of radionuclide notation.

List the nuclear families, and state their characteristics.

Name and describe the primary forms of radioactive decay.

Diagram the schematics of the various radioactive decay processes.

Define decay constant.

Use the general form of the radioactive decay equation to calculate precalibration and postcalibration quantities of radioactivity.

List the radioactive units, and define curie and becquerel.

Write the equations for average half-life and effective half-life, and calculate effective and biologic half-lives.

Describe the interactions of charged particles with matter.

Discuss the processes of excitation and ionization.

Explain annihilation and the resultant products.

Describe the photoelectric effect, and explain the processes.

Describe Compton scattering, and explain the resultant products of this process.

Describe pair production, and explain the resultant products of this process.

Discuss the production of characteristic x rays.

Describe the process of the production Auger electrons.

Write the general form of the attenuation equation for gamma photons.

Calculate the reduction of gamma radiation using the general attenuation equation.

State the relationship between the linear attenuation coefficient and half-value layer.

*P*hysics is the study of both matter and energy and the properties, forces, and interactions that influence the behavior of matter. Nuclear medicine applies the principles of physics to all aspects of radioactive decay, to the interaction of radiation and matter, and to the detection and measurement of properties and quantity of radiation and radiation protection. A basic understanding of these principles is critical to the use of radioactive materials and radiation-detecting instrumentation.

ELECTROMAGNETIC RADIATION

Heat waves, radio waves, infrared light, visible light, ultraviolet light, and x rays and gamma rays are all forms of electromagnetic radiation (Figure 2-1). They differ only in frequency and wavelength. Longer wavelength, lower frequency waves (heat and radio) have less energy than the shorter wavelength, higher frequency waves (visible light, x and gamma rays). The wave properties of light were first shown by Christian Huygens in 1678 in his experiments with the separation of light into the color spectrum. The particulate characteristics of light were not appreciated until the experiments and research of Einstein, Planck, and Milliken in the early 1900s. Although electromagnetic energy has no mass, at very high frequencies it behaves more like a particle, whereas at lower frequencies it behaves more like a wave. The best way to think of electromagnetic radiation is as a wave packet called a photon. Photons are chargeless bundles of energy that travel in a vacuum at the velocity of light, *c*, which is 3×10^{10} cm/sec^{-1} or 186,000 miles/sec^{-1}.

The wave nature of electromagnetic radiation is symbolized by the Greek letter *lambda*, λ. Note that the Greek lambda used to refer to electromagnetic radiation should not be mistaken for the radioactive decay constant, discussed later. Electromagnetic waves, as their name indicates, consist of fluctuating fields of electric and magnetic energy. Figure 2-2 shows the pattern of the wave cycle. Since light travels at a constant velocity, the oscillating electromagnetic field wavelength and frequency are related by the equation:

$$c = \lambda v$$

where λ is the wavelength, v is the frequency, and c is the velocity of light. The time for one wave period, or cycle, is measured in cycles per second, called hertz. The relationship of the electromagnetic wave frequency to the energy was described by Planck as:

$$E = hf$$

Where f represents the frequency of the electromagnetic wave and h is Planck's constant, 6.625×10^{-27} erg.s/cycles. This equation can be manipulated to relate to energy and wavelength as:

$$E = \frac{12.4}{\lambda}$$

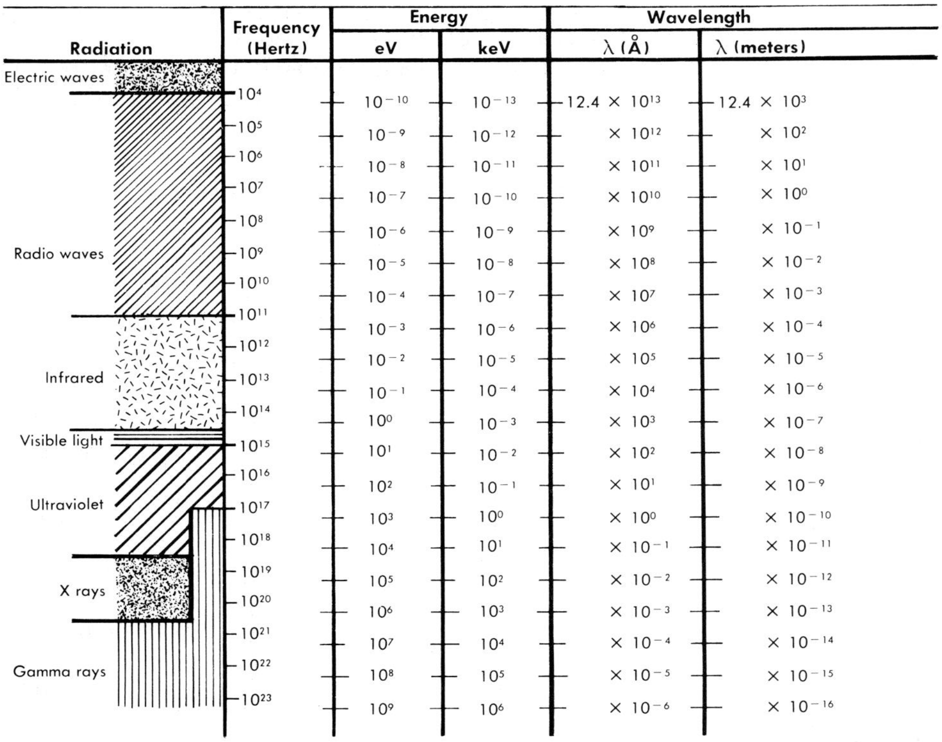

Radiation	Frequency (Hertz)	Energy eV	Energy keV	Wavelength λ (Å)	Wavelength λ (meters)
Electric waves	10^4	10^{-10}	10^{-13}	12.4×10^{13}	12.4×10^3
	10^5	10^{-9}	10^{-12}	$\times 10^{12}$	$\times 10^2$
	10^6	10^{-8}	10^{-11}	$\times 10^{11}$	$\times 10^1$
	10^7	10^{-7}	10^{-10}	$\times 10^{10}$	$\times 10^0$
	10^8	10^{-6}	10^{-9}	$\times 10^9$	$\times 10^{-1}$
Radio waves	10^9	10^{-5}	10^{-8}	$\times 10^8$	$\times 10^{-2}$
	10^{10}	10^{-4}	10^{-7}	$\times 10^7$	$\times 10^{-3}$
	10^{11}	10^{-3}	10^{-6}	$\times 10^6$	$\times 10^{-4}$
	10^{12}	10^{-2}	10^{-5}	$\times 10^5$	$\times 10^{-5}$
Infrared	10^{13}	10^{-1}	10^{-4}	$\times 10^4$	$\times 10^{-6}$
	10^{14}	10^0	10^{-3}	$\times 10^3$	$\times 10^{-7}$
Visible light	10^{15}	10^1	10^{-2}	$\times 10^2$	$\times 10^{-8}$
	10^{16}	10^2	10^{-1}	$\times 10^1$	$\times 10^{-9}$
Ultraviolet	10^{17}	10^3	10^0	$\times 10^0$	$\times 10^{-10}$
	10^{18}	10^4	10^1	$\times 10^{-1}$	$\times 10^{-11}$
X rays	10^{19}	10^5	10^2	$\times 10^{-2}$	$\times 10^{-12}$
	10^{20}	10^6	10^3	$\times 10^{-3}$	$\times 10^{-13}$
	10^{21}	10^7	10^4	$\times 10^{-4}$	$\times 10^{-14}$
Gamma rays	10^{22}	10^8	10^5	$\times 10^{-5}$	$\times 10^{-15}$
	10^{23}	10^9	10^6	$\times 10^{-6}$	$\times 10^{-16}$

Figure 2-1   Electromagnetic spectrum.

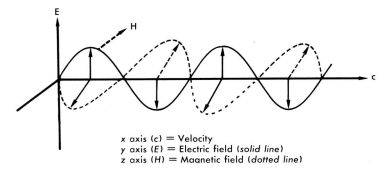

x axis (c) = Velocity
y axis (E) = Electric field (*solid line*)
z axis (H) = Magnetic field (*dotted line*)

Figure 2-2   Component energy fields of electromagnetic wave.

This equation expresses the energy in electron volts (eV) to the wavelength measured in angstroms (10^{-8} cm). The relationship indicates that very short wavelength photons have high energy, and vice versa.

ATOMS AND MOLECULES

Matter is anything that occupies space and has mass. Ancient Greek philosophers theorized that all matter was composed of small indivisible pieces, which they called atoms. An atom is the smallest quantity of an element (e.g., hydrogen, carbon, oxygen) that retains all of the chemical properties of that element. Atoms cannot be broken into smaller particles without losing their chemical properties. They are classified by their characteristics of weight, number of subparticles, and chemical properties. Two or more atoms may combine to form a molecule. A molecule is the smallest particle of a chemical compound that retains all of the chemical characteristics of that compound. Molecules can have as few as two or many hundreds of atoms; therefore tens of thousands of different chemical compounds can be created by changing the number of atoms or the configuration of atoms within the molecule.

The atom is made up of two basic parts, the nucleus and the orbital electrons. A simple representation of an atom is a structure similar to a miniature solar system (Figure 2-3). This elementary model of an atom divides the atom into two portions: nuclear (in the center) and extranuclear (the surrounding area). There are three principal types of subatomic particles that compose an atom—protons, neutrons, and electrons. The nucleus is composed of two types of these particles—protons and neutrons; hence protons and neutrons are called *nucleons*. The nucleus is a cluster of these particles and gives the atom most of its mass.

The extranuclear region of the atom is the area outside the nucleus and is mostly empty space with electrons that orbit the nucleus like planets revolving around the sun. This region of the atom, especially the outermost electrons, is responsible for all chemical interactions with other atoms, as well as being the area

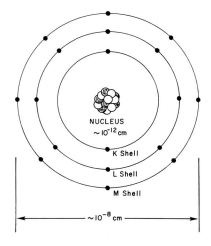

Figure 2-3   Bohr's atomic model with central nucleus surrounded by extranuclear region.

in which most of the interactions of radiation and matter occur.

In 1960 the International Unions of Pure and Applied Physics and Chemistry set the standard substance physical scale to the carbon 12 (^{12}C) atom, whose mass is defined to be exactly 12.00000 atomic mass units (amu). All other atomic and particle weights are measured from the ^{12}C atom.

Basic discussions of the composition of atoms are limited to the fundamental particles: electrons that orbit the nucleus and the particles in the nucleus; protons and neutrons. Particle physics describes several families that hold many dozens of subatomic particles. For example, protons and neutrons are in the family called hadrons, electrons and neutrinos are in a family of "light" mass particles called leptons, and photons are in a group called bosons.

In 1964 Murray Gell-Mann and George Zweig proposed that the hundreds of particles known at that time could be composed of combinations of three simpler fundamental particles that they called "quarks" (Figure 2-4). Experiments since that time have shown that there are actually six quarks that compose subatomic particles.

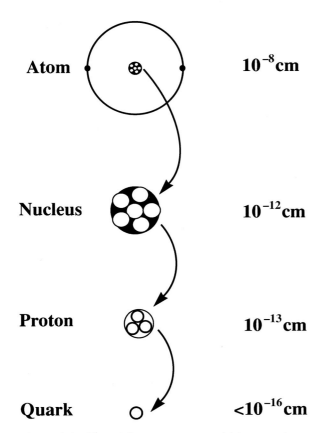

Atom	10^{-8} cm
Nucleus	10^{-12} cm
Proton	10^{-13} cm
Quark	$<10^{-16}$ cm

Figure 2-4 Size of the components within an atom.

Fortunately, for our purposes we can describe the composition of the atom and the processes of radioactive decay using the most common particles.

Electrons

Electrons are the smallest of the subatomic particles and are found in the extranuclear region of the atom. Electrons are also called negatrons and are given the symbol e or e^-. They have one negative unit of charge (1.6×10^{-19} coulombs) and a small mass of 9.1×10^{-28} g, or 0.000549 amu and travel at about one tenth the velocity of light. Since they carry a negative charge, they are deflected by electric or magnetic fields. Their mass allows them to have kinetic energy that is proportional to the square of their velocity. Electrons are held in their orbits around the nucleus by binding energy, which in conjunction with their motion and centrifugal force keeps them from being attracted into the positively charged nucleus. In an electrically neutral atom there are an equal number of protons and electrons.

Protons

Protons are found within the nucleus of an atom and are symbolized by the letter p or p^+. They have one positive unit of charge, which is equal but opposite to the charge of the electron. The protons within the nucleus provide its positive charge. The proton has a mass of 1.67×10^{-24} g, or 1.00759 amu, which is 1835 times that of an electron. The total number of protons is the atomic number, symbolized by the letter Z, and defines the element: for example, one proton is hydrogen, two protons is helium, three protons is lithium.

Neutrons

A neutral particle within the nucleus of the atom had been theorized by Rutherford in 1920, but neutrons were not experimentally found until 1932 by Chadwick. Neutrons are slightly heavier than protons, have no electric charge, and have a mass of 1.00898 amu. For simplification, the mass of a neutron and a proton are considered to be the same—1 amu. Neutrons are symbolized by the letter n.

For our purposes we can consider that a neutron is a combination of a proton and an electron. Neutrons are unstable particles and break down into the simpler more stable particles of a proton, an electron (beta-minus particle), and a neutrino. This instability of the neutron is the source of one type of radioactive decay. The decay process and the resultant particles are discussed later.

ATOMIC STRUCTURE

The model of the atom described by Neils Bohr in 1913 is one of the most easily understood representations. This miniature solar system has mostly empty space with the electrons in orbit around a small central nucleus. Three subatomic particles are used in this model. The electrons occupy specific orbits, or shells, around the center nucleus. The electron shells are labeled K, L, M, N, O, P, and Q (see Figure 2-3), beginning with the innermost, the K shell. Specific amounts of energy hold each electron in its orbit. The innermost electrons are more tightly bound to the nucleus, and therefore more energy is required to remove them. Outer electrons are more loosely bound and require only smaller amounts of energy to be removed. Electrons can be removed from their orbits only by overcoming the *binding energy* for that shell. Binding energies are greatest for the innermost electrons, and the binding energy of specific electron shells is greater in heavier elements.

The electrons do not actually revolve around the nucleus in circular orbits in one plane; they move around the nucleus in a spherical pattern. Collectively, the electrons swarming about the nucleus form an electron cloud. Individually, the electrons change their distance from the nucleus and can even occasionally pass right through the nucleus.

Remember that the chemical properties of the atom are determined by the outermost electrons. The num-

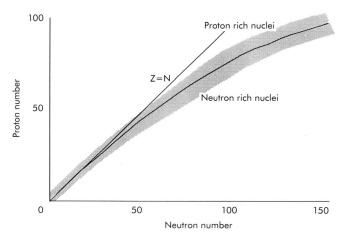

Figure 2-5   Neutron-proton ratio with line of nuclear stability.

ber of electrons that can occupy each orbit is limited. The formula $2n^2$ defines the number of atoms that can be contained in the major shells, where n is the shell number. For example, the K shell can contain only two electrons; the second shell can contain no more than eight; the third shell may contain 18; the fourth shell 32 electrons, etc. Each major shell is composed of several subshells.

The nucleus of an atom has an approximate diameter of 10^{-12} cm (see Figure 2-3) and is composed of a cluster of protons and neutrons. Most of the matter in the atom is located here; therefore the density of the nucleus is extremely high. Particles in the nucleus—protons and neutrons—are known as *nucleons*. The simplest atom, hydrogen, consists of one proton, no neutrons, and one orbital electron. The second element, helium, has a nucleus consisting of two protons, two neutrons, and two orbital electrons. More complex atoms have an increased number of protons and neutrons. In approximately the first 20 elements, there is a 1:1 ratio of neutrons to protons; however, elements with atomic numbers greater than 20 have more neutrons than protons to maintain nuclear stability. Very large atoms will have a neutron-to-proton ratio of 1.6:1 (Figure 2-5).

As with electrons in the extranuclear orbit structure of the atom, the protons and neutrons in the nucleus are bound there with a specific amount of energy. Stability of the nucleus is determined by the total binding energy of nucleons in addition to the number and configuration of the proton-neutron arrangement. Protons and neutrons tend to pair up, creating a more stable nucleus, depending on the neutron-to-proton ratio. Nucleons move about within the nucleus and occupy certain energy states. Some nuclei hold additional energy in a nearly stable, or metastable, state. The nucleus can emit this extra energy in a manner called an isomeric transition, with the emission of electromagnetic radiation (gamma ray).

MASS-ENERGY RELATIONSHIP

In Einstein's equation $E = mc^2$, c represents the velocity of light measured in centimeters per second, m is mass measured in grams, and E is energy measured in ergs. According to this equation, matter can be converted into energy and conversely, energy can create matter. This equation applies to a mass that is not moving and is therefore termed the *rest mass* of a particle of matter. When matter is converted to energy, the type of energy produced is of a form that is not imparted to or held by matter, such as heat or binding energy. Rather, it is pure energy— electromagnetic radiation.

The rest mass of an electron, 9.1×10^{-28} g, can be found by this equation to be equivalent to 0.511 MeV. Also, the rest mass of a proton can be found to be 931 MeV, and the rest mass of a neutron 939 MeV. This relationship is further defined in the discussions of radioactive decay and the interaction of radiation and matter.

Mass Defect

The relationship between mass and energy can be observed with the strong nuclear forces that exist in the nucleus. The sum of the masses of the nucleons in a ^{12}C atom is defined and measured as 12.00000 amu. However, the mass of a proton is 1.00759 amu; the mass of a neutron is 1.00898 amu; and the mass of an electron is 0.00054 amu. There are six protons, six neutrons, and six electrons in this atom, or a total mass of the individual particles of:

$$\begin{array}{r} 6 \times 1.00759 = 6.04554 \\ 6 \times 1.00898 = 6.05388 \\ \underline{6 \times 0.00054 = 0.00324} \\ 12.10266 \text{ amu} \end{array}$$

Since the carbon atom weighs 12.00000 amu, there is a difference of 0.10266 amu that has been converted into binding energy of the particles in the nucleus. The difference in mass of the constituent particles and the total mass is called the *mass defect*. This amount of mass converts to 95.62779 MeV of nuclear binding energy. Particles can be removed from the atom only by expending a force greater than the binding energy.

Nuclear Stability

The number of protons and neutrons that form all possible configurations of the nucleus are graphed in Figure 2-5. Any configuration of protons and neutrons forming an atom is called a *nuclide*. There are approximately 1500 nuclides, most of which are unstable and spontaneously release energy or subatomic particles in an attempt to reach a more stable state. This nuclear instability is the basis for the process we call *radioactive decay*. Approximately 280 of the nuclides are in a stable form, comprising only 83 elements. The remainder of

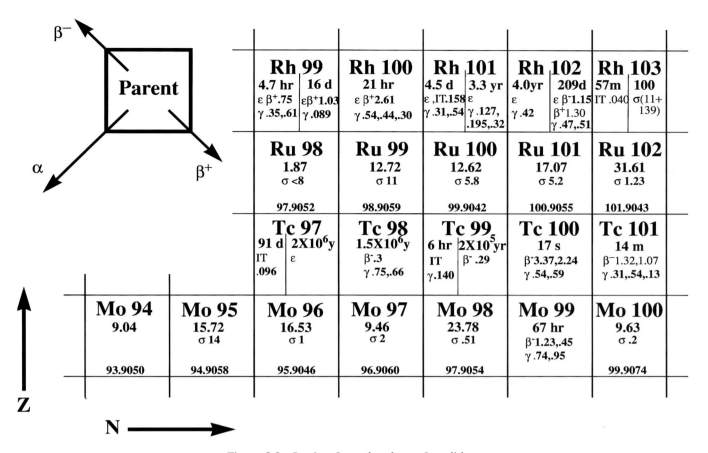

Figure 2-6 Section from the chart of nuclides.

the approximately 1500 nuclides are radioactive and are termed *radionuclides.*

The cause of nuclear instability stems from the energy configuration of the protons and neutrons in the nucleus. Although we might think of the structure of the nucleus being like a cluster of grapes, each nucleon has a certain energy state. For one specific radionuclide there is a specific release of particles and a specific amount of energy released by its unstable atoms in this decay process. For example, ^{131}I always decays by emitting beta-minus (β^-) particles and gamma rays of specific energies. From radioactive decay, each radionuclide has its own "fingerprint" of characteristic radiation.

In Figure 2-5 the approximately 280 stable nuclides follow along the center of the line of stability with radionuclide forms located on either side of this line. Radionuclides above the line of stability represent a region with a relative abundance of protons, termed *proton-rich* (or *neutron-poor*) *nuclei.* Radionuclides in this region achieve nuclear stability primarily by undergoing the decay processes of positron emission or electron capture. Radionuclides below the line of stability in the *neutron-rich* area undergo a radioactive decay process called *beta decay* in which a neutron becomes a pro-

ton followed by a release of a beta particle from the nucleus. The neutron-rich area can also be termed *proton-poor.*

Some radionuclei are in a metastable form. These radionuclides carry a slight amount of excess nuclear energy, which can be emitted as electromagnetic radiation to allow the atom to reach a more stable form.

The plotting of nuclides by their number of protons (vertical axis) and neutron number (horizontal axis) is the basis for the *chart of the nuclides* (Figure 2-6). This chart contains all possible nuclides, both stable and unstable radioactive forms. The chart is useful in identifying daughter decay products from a particular radionuclide or series of decays. Each nuclide is represented in a small square containing information such as the half-life, decay mechanism, and radiation type and energy.

NUCLEAR NOTATION AND NUCLEAR FAMILIES

There is a standard notation in the physical sciences for representing elements with a one- or two-letter chemical name symbol, taken primarily from the Greek names of the elements. The generalized symbol form appears as:

$$_{Z}^{A}X$$

where X is the chemical symbol; Z is the element's atomic number (number of protons); and A represents the atomic mass number of the atom (protons plus neutrons). Although the number of neutrons can be indicated as a trailing subscripted number, it is usually not written since it can be calculated by subtracting Z from A. As an example, carbon with 6 protons and 8 neutrons would be written as $_{6}^{14}C$. Since an atom with 6 protons will always be a carbon atom, there is a duplication of information by writing a 6 and C; therefore, by convention, it may be written simply as ^{14}C.

Although early scientists learned much about determining atomic weights and organizing the elements into the periodic chart, it was not immediately understood that there could be different atomic forms of the same element. The same element will always have a specific number of protons, as listed by the atomic number Z, and will have the same chemical properties; however, the number of neutrons can differ. The term *nuclide* refers to any configuration of the atom. The Greek terms *iso*, meaning same, and *topos*, meaning place, indicate the atoms have the same position on the periodic table of elements. The term *isotope*, although sometimes erroneously used interchangeably with nuclide, actually defines a specific element with different forms of that element, each containing different numbers of neutrons. ^{97}Tc, ^{98}Tc, ^{99}Tc, ^{100}Tc, and ^{101}Tc are all isotopes of element 43 (see Figure 2-6) and follow a horizontal line on the chart of the nuclides. Since the periodic chart of the elements is far too small to contain all of the different isotopes of each element, the chart of the nuclides is commonly used to list the 1500 isotopes of all the elements. Because the chart is laid out in a pattern following the line of stability listed by the number of protons and neutrons (see Figure 2-5), it is relatively simple to identify the isotopes. Isotopes for each element are found as a horizontal line, since the number of neutrons is plotted horizontally.

Additional families of nuclei are isotones, isobars, and isomers. Isotones are atoms of different elements that have the same number of neutrons, but varying numbers of protons. The following are isotones: $_{42}^{98}Mo$, $_{43}^{99}Tc$, $_{44}^{100}Ru$, and $_{45}^{101}Rh$, all having 56 neutrons and forming a vertical line on the chart of the nuclides (see Figure 2-6). Isobars are nuclides that have equal weights, or the same mass number (protons plus neutrons). Examples of isobars are ^{99}Rh, ^{99}Ru, ^{99}Tc, and ^{99}Mo; they are found on a 45-degree angle in Figure 2-6.

Isomers are atoms that have identical physical attributes as far as the number of protons, neutrons, and electrons; however, they contain a different amount of nuclear energy. Isomeric forms of an atom are identified by putting an m after the mass number A. The m means the atom is currently in a metastable form and will emit gamma radiation from the nucleus to achieve the more stable energy configuration. The most commonly used radionuclide in nuclear medicine is an isomer—^{99m}Tc. Technetium 99 (^{99}Tc) is a more stable form with a half-life of 2.13×10^{5} years. Other isomers that have been used in nuclear medicine are ^{113m}In and ^{87m}Sr.

The isotones are found in vertical columns on the chart, since the number of protons is represented on a vertical axis. Isobars are found on a 45-degree angle running from the lower right to upper left. Isomers are designated by a vertical line within the square for a specific radionuclide.

Another format for diagraming nuclide information is presented with a hexagonal box for each nuclide, as in Figure 2-7 (the Trilinear Chart), where vertically adjacent neighbors are isobars. Oblique neighbors from upper left to lower right represent isotones, and obliquely adjacent neighbors from lower left to upper right represent isotopes. Isomers are identified with a vertical line through the hexagon. Within each hexagon is a box that identifies the element symbol, atomic number, and mass number. As an example of the information contained in this chart, ^{99}Mo and ^{99}Tc should be carefully examined. In Figure 2-7 molybdenum 99 has a physical half-life of 2.76 days and emits both beta and gamma radiation during radioactive decay. The energy in MeV is listed as 1.230 for beta decay (β^{-}), and gamma ray emissions are identified. Vertical downward arrows show that 92% of the time molybdenum decays to the isomeric form of ^{99m}Tc and 8% of the time to ^{99}Tc. The left side of the hexagon representing technetium shows that isomeric transition (discussed later) will occur 100% of the time ^{99m}Tc decays. Also indicated in the left side is the gamma energy of 0.140 MeV (or 140 keV). Technetium 99, as represented on the right half of the box, is radioactive, with a half-life of 2.13×10^{5} years. Decay is by beta radiation to its daughter product ruthenium 99, which is a stable element. Note that the ^{99m}Tc decays first to ^{99}Tc before its decay to stable ruthenium.

DECAY PROCESSES

Alpha Decay

Alpha particles (helium nuclei consisting of 2 protons and 2 neutrons) are radioactive decay products from radionuclides having large mass. Using standard nuclear notation, the parent element M with atomic number Z, and mass number A decays by alpha (α) emission as:

$$_{Z}^{A}M = _{Z-2}^{A-4}N + \alpha + \text{energy}$$

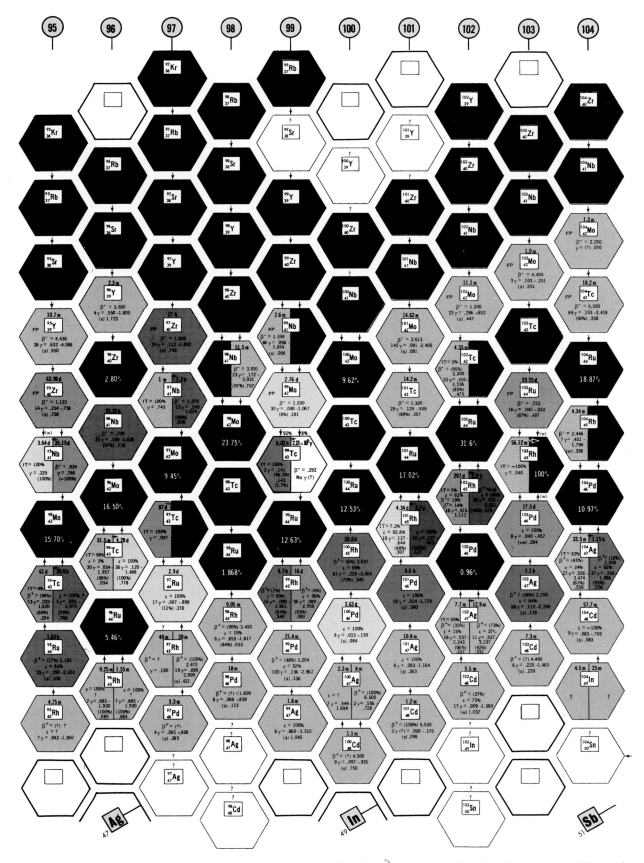

Figure 2-7 Trilinear chart of nuclides. *Black background,* Stable forms; *dark- to light-shaded areas,* instability. (Courtesy Mallinckrodt, Inc., St. Louis, 1979.)

to the daughter product symbolized by N. Since alpha particles have a +2 charge and a large mass of 4 amu, they are very damaging to biologic systems and therefore have no role in diagnostic nuclear medicine.

Beta Decay

The concept of a neutron being composed of a proton and electron is important in certain types of radioactive decay. A nucleus that is neutron rich becomes stable through the conversion of one of its neutrons by the reaction:

$$n = p + \beta^- + \bar{\nu} + energy$$

As a result, a proton and an electron (β^-) have been created from the neutron. The mass number of the new nuclei is the same as the parent nuclei, since the mass of a neutron and proton are virtually the same; however, a different element remains. The formation of a different element by a radioactive decay process is called *transmutation,* or *isobaric radioactive decay.* The β^- particle that has been created in the nucleus through this decay process is ejected. In this decay process an antineutrino ($\bar{\nu}$) is created and carries away part of the energy of this reaction. The laws of conservation of momentum and energy are accounted for by this particle. Neutrinos (ν) and antineutrinos have no electrical charge and a mass of almost zero. They travel at the velocity of light and are almost undetectable. The excess energy from the neutron is shared between the beta particle and antineutrino. This sharing of kinetic energy is not equal. Sometimes the electron receives more of the energy and the neutrino receives less, or vice versa. As a result, the energy of the beta particle varies in a continuous energy spectrum with some maximum energy (E_{max}) that was available from the nucleus (Figure 2-8). The nuclear decay process by this method is termed beta-minus (β^-) or simply beta decay. The parent element M with atomic number Z and mass number A decays by beta emission as

$$^A_Z M = ^{\ \ A}_{Z+1} N + \beta^- + \bar{\nu} + energy$$

The energy released by this process is shared as kinetic (motion) energy by the beta particle and the antineutrino. An example of a beta-emitting radionuclide used in nuclear medicine is ^{131}I, which decays as follows:

$$^{131}_{53} I = ^{131}_{54} Xe + \beta^- + \bar{\nu}$$

Positron (β^+) Decay and Electron Capture

A nucleus that is proton rich (neutron poor) reduces its proton surplus by two possible decay processes:

$$p = n + \beta^+ + \nu + energy \qquad (1)$$

or

$$p + e^- = n + \nu + energy \qquad (2)$$

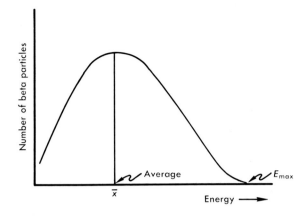

Figure 2-8 Generalized beta particle energy spectrum.

The first process is *positron decay,* and the second is termed *electron capture.*

Positron decay or emission (1) results when a proton is converted to a neutron, positron (β^+), neutrino, and energy. In nuclear notation the general form of positron decay is written as:

$$\beta^+ + e^- = \gamma(0.511\ MeV) + \gamma(0.511\ MeV)$$

An example of positron decay is:

$$^{18}_{9} F = ^{18}_{8} O + \beta^+ + \nu$$

An emitted positron loses kinetic energy through collision with surrounding matter, since it is then moving slowly enough to be attracted to an electron. The positron and negatron spiral in toward one another forming a temporary "positronium" atom for a brief instant before the two particles undergo annihilation. In the annihilation interaction the mass of each particle (positron and negatron) is converted into electromagnetic energy. The rest mass of each particle results in two 0.511 MeV photons. The two 0.511 MeV photons travel in opposite directions to conserve momentum (Figure 2-9).

Electron capture (2) occurs when an orbital electron travels in the proximity of the nucleus and is captured and combined with a proton to form a neutron. Remember from the cloud model of the atom that electrons can spend a very small amount of their time in the proximity of the nucleus. Electron capture is generalized as:

$$^A_Z M + e^- = ^{\ \ A}_{Z-1} N + \nu + energy$$

An example is the decay of ^{125}I:

$$^{125}_{53} I + e^- = ^{125}_{52} Te + \nu$$

Electrons involved in electron capture are usually those from the K or L shell. The probability for capture from another energy level is very unlikely. A result from electron capture is ionization of the atom with subsequent relocation of an outer shell electron to fill the vacancy created by the capture.

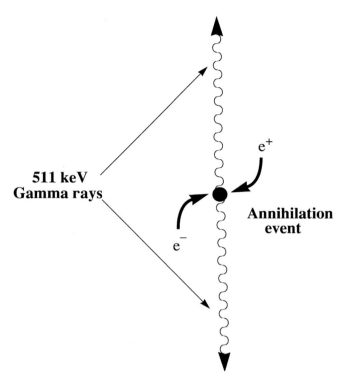

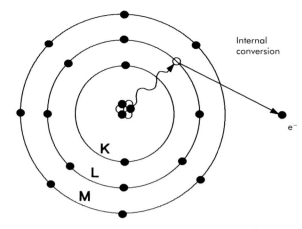

Figure 2-10 Internal conversion of L-shell electron. Energy transfer from nucleus ejecting orbital electron is alternative to gamma ray emission. Internal conversion electron will have kinetic energy equal to gamma ray energy minus binding energy.

Figure 2-9 Annihilation of a positron and negatron. The resultant pair of 0.511 MeV gamma rays travel 180 degrees apart.

Proton-rich nuclei can reach stability through either positron emission or electron capture. These are always competing processes; however, the configuration of the nuclei and a high energy content of some nuclei increase the probability of positron emission. If the energy content is less, then electron capture occurs. Some atoms can undergo either process with a certain probability.

A commonly used radionuclide in nuclear medicine, ^{67}Ga, undergoes electron capture. In addition to the changes that take place within the nucleus, characteristic x rays are emitted due to energy changes resulting from the electrons filling vacant positions.

Gamma Decay

Gamma ray emission represents a mechanism for an excited nucleus to release energy. The release of energy as a gamma ray (γ) may be as a part of another decay process, such as alpha or β^-. In addition, it is the process for releasing energy from a metastable nucleus.

Gamma ray emission usually occurs when there is greater than 100 keV of energy in the excited nucleus. It should be remembered that gamma rays and x rays are characteristically the same but are named based on their origin, gamma rays being emitted from the nucleus and x rays from the electron shells. The ideal radionuclides for nuclear medicine are those that emit only gamma rays without emitting particulate radiation. These radionuclides thereby provide gamma rays for imaging without increasing patient radiation exposure. With particulate radioactive decay the nucleus is most often left with additional energy, which is released promptly in the form of electromagnetic radiation.

When a metastable nucleus is present, there is a significant amount of time from any previous radioactive decay (such as from ^{99}Mo to ^{99m}Tc) before further release of energy. The release from the metastable state is termed an *isomeric transition*. In this transition the nucleus goes from a high-energy level to a lower energy level through emission of electromagnetic radiation (usually greater than 100 keV); this is sometimes termed *gamma decay*. The equation for an isomeric transition may be written as follows:

$$^A_Z M = ^A_Z M + \gamma$$

An example of an isomeric transition is:

$$^{99m}_{43}\text{Tc} = ^{99}_{43}\text{Tc} + \gamma$$

There is an alternative process to gamma ray emission in metastable nuclei. This process is termed *internal conversion* and is the transfer of energy from the nucleus to an orbital electron, which is then ejected from the atom (Figure 2-10). Internal conversion reactions usually involve electrons from the K shell but occasionally involve electrons from the L or M shell. In this process the ejected electron is called a *conversion electron*. This leaves an ionized atom, which follows normal processes of reshuffling its electrons, resulting in the release of characteristic x rays or Auger electrons.

Metastable nuclei are the most pure sources of gamma rays for nuclear medicine imaging. The isomeric forms for these medically important radionuclides require that they be generator produced within the nuclear medicine laboratory. Technetium-99m has become the most important radionuclide in nuclear medicine imaging.

SCHEMATICS OF RADIOACTIVE DECAY

The various decay processes of radionuclei can be represented diagrammatically to illustrate the relationship of individual processes that take place in radioactive disintegration. This diagram shows the relationship of the parent radionuclide to the daughter nuclide.

The diagrammatic representation of a decay scheme is based on representing the atomic number on the horizontal axis and energy of the nucleus on the vertical axis (Figure 2-11, *top*). The parent nucleus, being larger, contains more energy and is represented as a horizontal line at the top of the diagram. Through the process of radioactive decay the resulting daughter nucleus has less energy and is positioned lower on the diagram. Arrows are used to illustrate the emission of radiation. These arrows show the transition of the nucleus by alpha decay as a decrease in atomic number *(Z)*, shifting to the left, indicating the atomic number is decreased by 2 in the decay process. In β^- decay there is an increase in Z by 1, with a corresponding shift to the right. With positron decay and electron capture there is a decrease in Z by -1. Gamma emission is shown as a vertical down arrow, indicating the release of electromagnetic radiation and resulting only in a decrease in nuclear energy without a change in atomic number. The energy levels of the parent and daughter nuclei are represented as horizontal lines. The parent radionuclide, $_Z^A M$, is shown in general form as the decay process for β^- emission (Figure 2-12) to the daughter product $_{Z+1}^A M$. Two different diagonal arrows in this diagram represent two different energies of beta particle decay. In one case the longer diagonal line represents the emission of a beta particle going directly to the daughter nucleus without any additional energy release. This beta particle energy equals the difference between the parent and daughter energy levels. The shorter arrow represents release of a beta particle of lesser energy to an intermediate state with the prompt release of a gamma ray (vertical down arrow) to the daughter product. One individual atom of the parent radionuclide can release its energy in this beta decay by following either path; therefore one of two beta particles with different energies can be seen in this transition, and only those betas from the lower energy transition are accompanied by a gamma ray.

Figure 2-13 shows a simplified decay scheme for ^{131}I. The actual decay process for ^{131}I has several different beta energies, although only one is prominent (93%). With this beta particle is the gamma transition releasing 0.364 MeV. Figure 2-14 shows the decay scheme for ^{99}Mo followed by the transitions of ^{99m}Tc and ^{99}Tc to ^{99}Ru. Approximately 82% of the transition from ^{99}Mo

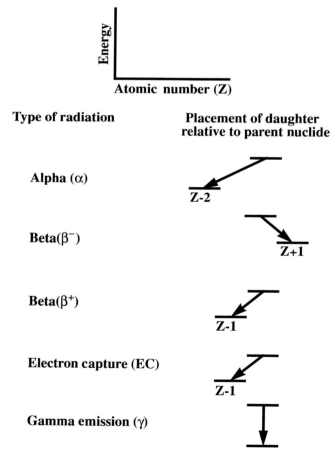

Type of radiation

Placement of daughter relative to parent nuclide

Alpha (α) Z-2

Beta(β⁻) Z+1

Beta(β⁺) Z-1

Electron capture (EC) Z-1

Gamma emission (γ)

Figure 2-11 Axes *(top)* show directions of increasing energy and atomic number in decay schemes. Directional placement of each daughter nucleus relative to parent in decay schemes.

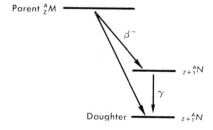

Figure 2-12 Hypothetical decay scheme representing beta particle emission.

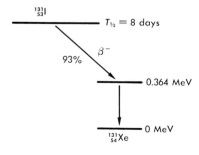

Figure 2-13 Generalized decay scheme for ^{131}I.

to ^{99m}Tc is by one particular beta energy. The radionuclide is then in the metastable form of ^{99m}Tc, which has a half-life of 6 hours. The isomeric transition of ^{99m}Tc is represented as a vertical line downward of a 0.140 MeV gamma ray to the daughter product ^{99}Tc. Technetium 99 has a long half-life (2.2×10^5 years) and by beta decay yields stable ^{99}Ru.

Figure 2-15 shows the decay process for ^{125}I, which is used in radioimmunoassay. The electron capture process is followed by an internal conversion process. The resulting daughter of tellurium, with the electron vacancy left by internal conversion, subsequently emits K-characteristic x rays.

The radioactive decay schemes shown in Figures 2-11, 2-13, 2-14, and 2-15 have been simplified. Some radionuclides can emit several different gamma ray energies, as illustrated in Table 2-1, for ^{67}Ga. Gallium 67 decays by electron capture to ^{67}Zn; the zinc nucleus then emits several energies of gamma photons. As indicated in Table 2-1 there is a gamma ray abundance percentage for each ^{67}Ga atom that decays. For every 100 atoms, approximately 38% emit gamma rays at 93.3 keV, etc. Decay schemes of this nature are helpful in identifying the most abundant peaks for selecting imaging windows. Two, three, or four peaks can be selected for imaging on some instruments. Certain decay schemes have more than one gamma ray emitted for each atom that decays. Figure 2-16 shows a radionuclide that yields more than one gamma ray for each

atom that disintegrates. Decay by beta 1 leaves the daughter nucleus with energy that will be released by gamma 1 and gamma 2. Decay of beta 2 is followed only by gamma 2.

Mathematics of Decay

Individual atoms undergo spontaneous transformations to release energy and form daughter nuclei. There is no way of predicting when that will occur for one specific atom. However, when a large number of atoms are present, a certain probability of radioactive decay is obtained and a mathematical average rate of decay can be determined. A sample that contains N radioactive atoms has on average a certain number of atoms decaying per unit time represented as $\Delta N/\Delta t$. This can be described mathematically as:

$$\frac{\Delta N}{\Delta t} = -\lambda N$$

where λ is the decay constant of the radionuclide. In this equation the minus sign indicates that $\Delta N/\Delta t$ is negative, or decreasing with time. The decay constant λ therefore represents a probability or average percent of atoms present that will decay in a certain time period. The units of λ are 1/time or time^{-1}. A value such as 0.10 hour^{-1} means that in each hour 10% of the at-

Table 2-1	Gallium 67 photon emissions	
Photons	**Abundance percentage**	**Mean energy (keV)**
Gamma 2	38	93.3
Gamma 3	21	184.6
Gamma 5	16	300.2
Gamma 6	4	393.5

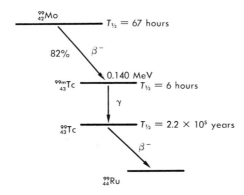

Figure 2-14 Generalized decay scheme for ^{99}Mo.

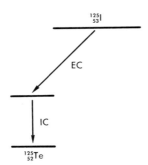

Figure 2-15 Generalized decay scheme for ^{125}I.

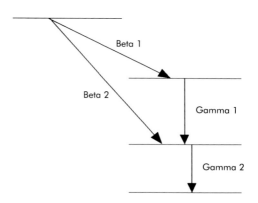

Figure 2-16 Decay by beta 1 is followed by emission of gamma 1 and gamma 2. Emission of higher energy beta 2 is followed only by single gamma emission, gamma 2. Some radionuclides yield several gamma rays for single disintegration.

oms undergo radioactive decay. Through calculus the above equation is manipulated to derive the number of atoms remaining at any specific time:*

$$N_t = N_0 e^{-\lambda t}$$

where N_t is the number of atoms that remain at any time t, and N_0 is the number of radioactive atoms at the original time zero.

The factor $e^{-\lambda t}$ represents the fraction of radioactive atoms that remain after time t and is called the *decay factor*. The e represents Euler's number, the base of natural logarithms (2.718); it has been raised to the power $-\lambda t$. The decay factor ($e^{-\lambda t}$) is an exponentially decreasing function with time and can be determined using a calculator (see Chapter 1). The decay factors for various time intervals can be calculated; decay factors for ^{99m}Tc are given in Table 2-2.

The number of radioactive atoms (N) is, by the above definition ($\Delta N/\Delta t = -\lambda N$), proportional to the radioactivity (A). This equation can therefore be written to apply to radioactivity. It is called the *general decay equation:*

$$A_t = A_0 e^{-\lambda t}$$

It is frequently difficult to work with the decay factor λ; it is much more practical to use another parameter $t_{1/2}$, known as *half-life*. The decay constant λ and $t_{1/2}$ are related by the equation:

$$\lambda = \frac{0.693}{t_{1/2}}$$

where 0.693 is the value of the natural logarithm of 2. This relationship can be derived from the general decay equation by inserting values for the initial activity (A_0) and the activity at the time t when the activity A_t is at 50% of the activity at time zero. The decay equation may be represented by substituting the relationship of half-life for decay constant and be written as:

$$A_t = A_0 e^{-0.693t/t_{1/2}}$$

where the decay factor (DF) equals the exponential portion of this equation:

$$DF = e^{-0.693t/t_{1/2}}$$

---

*Derivation of the general decay equation.

$$\frac{\Delta N}{\Delta t} = -\lambda N$$

$$\frac{dN}{dt} = -\lambda N$$

$$\frac{dN}{N} = -\lambda dt$$

$$\int \frac{1}{N} dN = -\int \lambda dt$$

$$\frac{N_i}{N_o} = e^{-\lambda t}$$

$$N_i = N_o e^{-\lambda t}$$

Table 2-2	Decay factors for ^{99m}Tc	
Hours	**Decay factor**	**Precalibration factor**
0	1.000	1.000
½	0.944	1.059
1	0.891	1.122
2	0.794	1.259
3	0.707	1.414
4	0.630	1.587
5	0.561	1.782
6	0.500	2.000
7	0.445	2.247
8	0.397	2.518
9	0.354	2.824
10	0.315	3.174
11	0.281	3.558
12	0.250	4.000

The fraction of elapsed time relative to the half-life can be generated and used for the determining decay factor for any radionuclide, sometimes called the *universal decay table*. The calculation of decay factors is reviewed in Chapter 1. Since the decay factor represents an exponential function, it can be plotted either linearly or semilogarithmically (Figure 2-17). When reviewing this graphic representation, it should be noted that the number of atoms remaining is 0.50 at one half-life. It should also be observed that the semilogarithmic plot (Figure 2-17, *bottom*) is represented as a straight line where the slope is determined by the decay constant.

RADIOACTIVITY UNITS

Radioactivity is quantitatively measured as the number of atoms that disintegrate per unit time. Two different units can be used to describe a quantity of radioactivity, the *curie* (Ci) and the *becquerel* (Bq). The curie was named in honor of Marie Curie, an early pioneer in the study of radioactivity. It is defined as the amount of radioactivity that decays at a rate of 3.7×10^{10} disintegrations per second (dps). This basic unit can be multiplied by standard mathematical scientific notation to yield larger and smaller multiples of the curie:

kilocurie (kCi) $= 10^3 \times$ Ci $= 3.7 \times 10^{13}$ dps
curie (Ci) $= 10^0 \times$ Ci $= 3.7 \times 10^{10}$ dps
millicurie (mCi) $= 10^{-3} \times$ Ci $= 3.7 \times 10^7$ dps
microcurie (μCi) $= 10^{-6} \times$ Ci $= 3.7 \times 10^4$ dps
nanocurie (nCi) $= 10^{-9} \times$ Ci $= 3.7 \times 10^1$ dps
picocurie (pCi) $= 10^{-12} \times$ Ci $= 3.7 \times 10^{-2}$ dps

The Systeme Internationale (SI) defines another unit of radioactivity, the becquerel (Bq). Henri Becque-

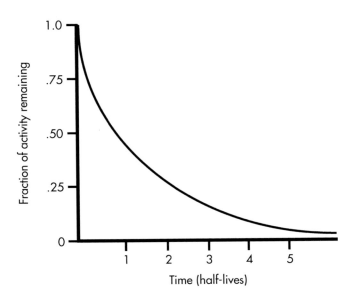

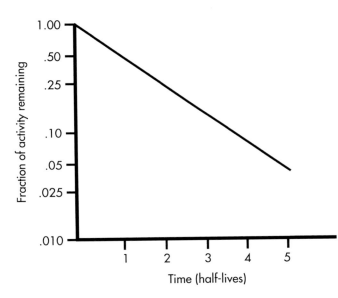

Figure 2-17 Fraction of radioactivity remaining (decay constant) as function of time is shown for a linear plot *(top)* and a semilogarithmic graph *(bottom)*. Slope of semilogarithmic straight line is determined by decay constant.

rel was the first person to identify radioactivity in 1894. One becquerel is the amount of radioactivity contained in a sample that decays at a rate of 1 dps. Since this unit is very small, nuclear medicine terminology uses multiples of the becquerel such as kilobecquerels (kBq) and megabecquerels (MBq).

Since most radioactivity in nuclear medicine is administered in doses of millicuries, or megabecquerels, it is important to understand rapid methods of converting between these two units of measure. The number of millicuries can be multiplied by 37 MBq/mCi to convert to the number of megabecquerels. For example, 20 mCi × 37 MBq/mCi = 740 MBq. Conversely, the number of megabecquerels can be converted to milli-

curies by dividing by 37 MBq/mCi, for example, 111 MBq/(37 MBq/mCi) = 3 mCi.

The quantities of radioactivity administered to most patients are on the order of several millicuries (several hundred MBq). The total radioactivity contained in a ^{99}Mo-^{99m}Tc radionuclide generator is on the order of 1 Ci (many tens of thousands of MBq). The quantity of radioactivity contained in patient specimens or assayed in a scintillation well counter is on the order of nanocuries to microcuries (kilobecquerels).

Decay Calculations

Decay factors (DFs) other than those in decay tables (see Table 2-2) for ^{99m}Tc can be found by multiplying together those that correspond to the decay interval. For example, a 14-hour DF equals the 12-hour DF (0.250) times the 2-hour DF (0.794), or 0.198; or you could multiply the 7-hour DF (0.445) by itself to get 0.198, or any other combination.

Sometimes it is necessary to dispense or use a radiopharmaceutical prior to the calibration time. Precalibration DFs may be calculated from the inverse (1/DF) of the decay factor for the time interval. As an example, the precalibration decay factor for 2 hours equals 1/DF or 1/0.794 = 1.26.

EXAMPLE 1: A vial contains 10 mCi of ^{99m}Tc; how much radioactivity remains after 2 hours?

DF for 2 hours = 0.794
10 mCi × 0.794 = 7.94 mCi

How much radioactivity was present 5 hours before for 10 mCi?

Precalibration DF for 5 hours = 1.782
10 mCi × 1.782 = 17.82 mCi

How much of the 10 mCi remains after 36 hours?

DF for 12 hours is 0.250, which we apply three times.
10 mCi × 0.250 × 0.250 × 0.250 = 0.156 mCi

EXAMPLE 2: Using the general decay equation, calculate the activity of 5 mCi/ml of ^{201}Tl after 48 hr ($t_{1/2}$ = 73 hr).

$A_t = A_0 e^{-0.693t/t_{1/2}}$
$A_t = 5 mCi/(ml) \times e^{-0.693t/t_{1/2}}$
$A_t = 5 mCi/(ml) \times e^{-0.693 \times (48hr)/(73hr)}$
$A_t = 5 mCi/(ml) \times e^{-0.456}$
$A_t = 3.17 mCi/(ml)$

Average Half-life and Effective Half-life

Average half-life describes the average lifetime of an atom. Mathematically, the average half-life can be calculated as:

$$T_{ave} = 1.44 \times t_{1/2}$$

Although this term represents the average interval for which a group of atoms exists, it has no clinical use in patient dose calculations. The decay constant of a radionuclide represents the physical radioactive decay. It does not indicate the nature of biologic turnover. Since rates are additive, the biologic decay constant can be added to the physical decay constant to give the *effective* decay constant:

$$\lambda_{\text{eff}} = \lambda_{\text{b}} + \lambda_{\text{p}}$$

Since $\lambda = 0.693/t_{1/2}$, and dividing by 0.693 this equation can be represented in terms of the half-life:

$$\frac{1}{t_{\text{eff}}} = \frac{1}{t_{\text{b}}} + \frac{1}{t_{\text{p}}}$$

where t_{eff} is the *effective half-life* (Figure 2-18), t_{b} is the biologic half-life, and t_{p} is the physical half-life.

An example of effective half-life might be the determination of the disappearance of ^{99m}Tc-MAA from the lungs. Assume that the biologic half-life is 3 hours.

$$\frac{1}{t_{\text{eff}}} = \frac{1}{(3 \text{ hr})} + \frac{1}{(6 \text{ hr})}$$

The effective half-life (t_{eff}) in the lung is thus 2 hours.

INTERACTIONS

Interactions of Charged Particles With Matter

Electrically charged particles (alpha particles, electrons, and positrons) have a high probability of interacting with the matter through which they move. Their mass and electrical charges interact with the mass of

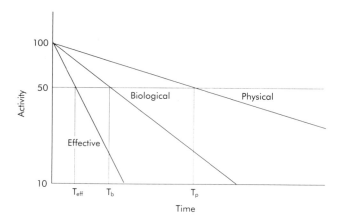

Figure 2-18   Semilogarithmic plot of physical (T_p) and biologic (T_b) half-life components of shorter effective half-life, T_{eff}.

the nucleus and electrical charges of atoms. In addition, the kinetic energy of these particles, along with the properties of the surrounding matter, determines how the particles will interact and how far these particles will travel. The density of matter, its atomic number, and its mass number influence the type and probability of these interactions.

Excitation and Ionization

Excitation is a process of absorbing small amounts of energy temporarily in the outer electron structure of an atom. Energy from a passing charged particle or from an interaction with electromagnetic radiation causes a short-lived or metastable excitement of an outer electron to a slightly higher energy level. The outer electron is not removed from the atom, and therefore no ionization occurs. Typically, excitation is very short-lived and the atom spontaneously gives up the extra energy in the form of electromagnetic radiation.

Ionization of an atom results from the collision of radiation with the electron structure of an atom. Ionization occurs only when there is sufficient energy of the radiation to completely remove an electron from its orbit. The energy must therefore be larger than the binding energy of the particular orbital electron. For example, if the binding energy of an electron were 54 keV and the incident energy were 78 keV, the electron would be ejected from the atom with 24 keV of kinetic energy. Ionization occurs in all forms of matter—solids, liquids, and gases.

Alpha Particles

An alpha particle (α) is the nucleus of a helium atom ($^4_2$He). Alpha particles are produced by radioactive decay in very large, unstable atoms. Their high mass and double-positive electrical charge give them a high ionizing potential in a short pathway in solids, liquids, or gases. They typically have energies between 3 and 8 MeV. Since it takes only about 34 eV to create one ion pair, the high energy of alpha particles along with their high mass and positive charge can create several hundred thousand ion pairs in only a fraction of a millimeter; this is devastating to biologic systems. Radionuclides that emit alpha particles have no use in nuclear medicine.

Beta Particles

The interaction of negatively charged beta particles in the proximity of the nucleus of an atom results in the attraction to the positively charged nucleus. As the beta particle is deflected and slowed in its path, there is a release of energy as x rays, called *bremsstrahlung radia-*

tion. These x rays are released in a continuous spectrum because of the variations in kinetic energy and path geometry of the beta particle. Bremsstrahlung interactions increase in probability with materials that have a high *Z* number. A beta particle emitting radionuclide, such as ^{32}P, should not be shielded by a high *Z* material such as lead. It is more appropriate to use a shielding material of low *Z*, such as plastic, since bremsstrahlung interactions are less likely to occur.

Annihilation

Positively and negatively charged electrons (positrons and negatrons) are antiparticles of one another. When positrons are produced in a decay process and are ejected from an atom, they have enough kinetic energy to travel a maximum of a few millimeters. The positron and an orbital electron from an atom are attracted due to their opposite charges, spiral in toward one another, and interact in a process called *annihilation.* The path distance required for a positron to find an electron for this interaction depends on the positron energy and number of electrons in the immediate area of the atom from which the positron was originally emitted. In the annihilation process the mass of the two particles is converted into energy according to Einstein's equation $E = mc^2$. The rest masses of the positron and negatron are identical (0.511 MeV), giving a total energy of 1.022 MeV. The mass of each particle is converted into a 0.511 MeV gamma ray (Figure 2-9). The gamma rays travel in opposite directions, 180 degrees from one another, to conform to the law of the conservation of momentum.

$$\beta^+ + e^- = \gamma(0.511 \text{ MeV}) + \gamma(0.511 \text{ MeV})$$

The detection of these two annihilation gamma rays is the foundation for positron emission tomography (PET) imaging.

PHOTONS

Electromagnetic radiation, or photons, is far more penetrating in matter than particulate types of radiation. There is no specific range for these photons, and their interaction with matter is based only on a probability of an interaction. In matter, photons may undergo scattering, might have no interaction with matter, or, since they are simply energy, might be completely absorbed and disappear. Although photons are more penetrating than particulate radiation, they demonstrate absorption, which diminishes exponentially with the distance traveled. For photons with energies associated with x rays and gamma rays, three types of interactions occur: photoelectric, Compton, and pair production (Table 2-3).

Photoelectric Effect

The photoelectric effect is an interaction that takes place between an incident photon and an inner orbital electron. For the photoelectric effect to occur, the energy of the incident photon must be greater than the binding energy of the orbital electron. In the photoelectric effect the photon energy is totally absorbed, with some of its energy used to break the bond of the electron in its shell and the remaining energy given to the electron in the form of motion or kinetic energy (Figure 2-19). Therefore a generalized relationship for this interaction can be written as:

Photon energy = Electron binding energy +
electron kinetic energy

The photoelectric effect usually occurs with electrons found in the K or L shell. Since an electron has been removed from the atom, there is no longer an electrically neutral balance between the number of protons and electrons; therefore the atom has been ionized with an inner shell vacancy created. In this interaction an ion pair has been formed—the positively charged atom and negatively charged photoelectron—which leaves the atom.

The electron vacancy can be filled (1) by another orbital electron dropping in to fill a vacancy with the subsequent emission of a characteristic x ray or (2) by an Auger electron (discussed later). The ejected photoelectron is no different from any other free electron in matter and is involved in other interactions, depending on its kinetic energy. The disappearance of the incident photon is important clinically because the energy has been absorbed completely by the patient.

The probability of a photoelectric interaction occur-

Table 2-3	Interactions between electromagnetic radiation and matter		
Interaction	**Interaction site**	**Energy range**	**Secondary effects**
Photoelectric	Inner electron shells	Several keV to 0.5 MeV	Photoelectrons, characteristic x rays
Compton	Outer electron shells	Several keV to several MeV	Compton electron, scattered photon
Pair production	Nuclear field	>1.02 MeV	Positron, electron, annihilation photons

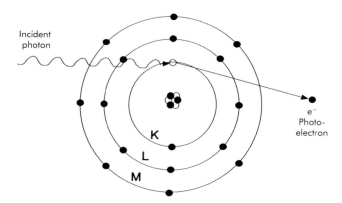

Figure 2-19 In photoelectric effect, incident photon is totally absorbed and transfers all of its energy to resultant photoelectron.

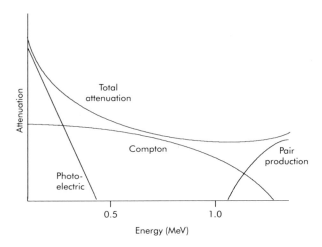

Figure 2-20 Interactions by photoelectric, Compton, and pair production combine to form attenuation coefficient. Probability of attenuation by photoelectric effect is dominant at low energy but decreases rapidly with increasing photon energy. Interactions through Compton scattering decrease more slowly and pair production becomes dominant above 1.02 MeV.

ring depends on the energy of the incident gamma ray and the atomic number of the material. Obviously, the photoelectric effect cannot occur unless the photon energy is above the binding energy. As a photon's energy increases, the probability for photoelectric interactions decreases (Figure 2-20). The probability of a photoelectric interaction increases dramatically with the atomic number, that is, photoelectric interactions are unlikely to occur in low Z materials such as water and tissue but are likely to occur in high Z materials such as the iodine in a sodium iodide crystal or in lead. The photoelectric effect is therefore the primary type of interaction for detecting gamma rays with nuclear medicine instruments. All of the gamma ray energy is given to the crystal material in a thallium-activated sodium iodide crystal. The photoelectric effect is therefore one of the most important interactions for nuclear medicine applications.

Compton Scattering

As its name implies, Compton scattering is an incomplete absorption of gamma rays or scattering of gamma radiation. The Compton effect involves an inelastic interaction of photons with outer orbital electrons. Like the photoelectric effect, there is the emission of an electron that is ejected from the atom; however, not all of the incident gamma ray energy is absorbed, and a scattered photon of lower energy and longer wavelength is emitted. Figure 2-21 illustrates the incident photon at a high energy with short wavelength and a scattered photon with lower energy and longer wavelength. The energy and wavelength of the scattered photon are always lower than those of the incident photon, and its energy also depends on the atomic number of the scattering material, the incident photon's energy, and the angle of scatter. The energy of the scattered photon is related to the angle of deflection.

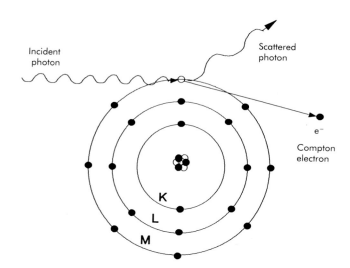

Figure 2-21 Compton scattering occurs in outer-shell electrons, with scattered photons having lower energy and longer wavelength. Ejection of Compton electron leaves ionized atom.

The minimum energy loss of the scattered photon will be at a shallow scatter angle and can be calculated using the relationship:

$$E_{min} = \frac{E_0}{(1 + 2E_0/0.511)}$$

where E_0 is the incident photon energy (in MeV). As an example, for a 0.140 MeV gamma ray, E_{min} equals 0.090 MeV, for 0.364 MeV E_{min} is 0.150 MeV.

The maximum energy E_{max}, or *backscatter energy,* will be at a scatter angle of 180 degrees and can be found from:

$$E_{max} = \frac{E_0{}^2}{(E_0 + 0.2555)}$$

This maximum scattered energy for a 0.140 MeV photon is 0.049 MeV and for a 0.364 MeV photon is 0.214 MeV. The maximum scatter energy identifies the sharp increase in scatter on the gamma ray spectrum, called the Compton edge.

The likelihood of Compton scatter is proportional to the atomic number, therefore there is more Compton scattering in high atomic number materials. Compton interactions are less likely to occur with higher energy photons (see Figure 2-20).

Pair Production

Pair production is an interaction produced when a photon with energy greater than 1.02 MeV passes near the high electric field of the nucleus. The strong electrical force brings about the energy-mass conversion. When the photon comes near the nucleus, it disappears totally and two particles of matter are created, an electron and positron, each possessing the mass equivalence of 0.511 MeV. For this interaction to occur, the initial photon must possess 1.02 MeV or more of energy. Any additional energy of the incident photon is converted into kinetic energy, which is given to the positron and negatron, thus conserving energy and momentum. The photon originally had zero charge and the offsetting positive and negative charges of the negatron and positron ensure that the net charge remains zero.

The fate of the negatron and positron are the same as if those particles were created by radioactive decay processes. The negatron interacts with surrounding atoms, possibly causing ionization and excitation. The positron loses some of its energy through interactions and ultimately undergoes annihilation with an orbital electron from an atom, producing a gamma ray pair with 0.511 MeV each. Figure 2-22 illustrates the pair production process.

Figure 2-20 shows the dominance of pair production interactions for very-high-energy photons. Note that there can be no pair production interactions below 1.02 MeV.

EXTRANUCLEAR ENERGY RELEASE

Three processes occur in the electron structure of the atom to release energy. These result in the creation of bremsstrahlung radiation, Auger electrons, and characteristic x rays.

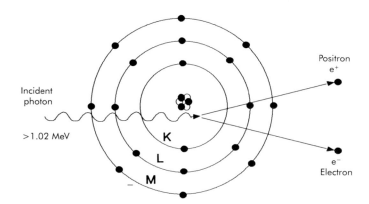

Figure 2-22 In pair production, photons with energy greater than 1.02 MeV may interact with strong forces near nucleus. Positron-electron pair is created with kinetic energy equal to excess above 1.02 MeV. Positron will undergo annihilation with electron.

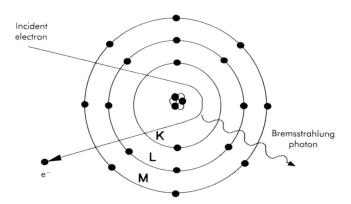

Figure 2-23 Deceleration of a charged particle passing near nucleus results in release of energy in the form of bremsstrahlung x rays.

Bremsstrahlung Radiation

Bremsstrahlung is a German word that simply means *braking radiation.* Bremsstrahlung is a process of the rapid deceleration of a charged particle as it comes under the intense electric field of the nucleus. The particle, electron or positron, has a very small mass in comparison with the nucleus. The rapidly moving particle is attracted to or repulsed from the nucleus and rapidly decelerated, and its direction changes. In this deflection and deceleration a significant loss of energy is emitted in the form of electromagnetic radiation in the x-ray region (Figure 2-23). In this type of interaction the conservation of energy and momentum must be maintained; therefore the energy of the incident charged particle is equal to the sum of the energy of the particle after deflection and the bremsstrahlung x ray.

The production of bremsstrahlung x rays can increase the total amount of radiation being produced and provide more hazard if thin lead shields are used. The production of bremsstrahlung radiation is not as significant in low atomic number materials, such as plastic; therefore it is better to shield pure beta-emitting radionuclides like ^{32}P with plastic shielding instead of thin lead.

Characteristic X Rays

The production of characteristic x rays occurs in atoms that have electron vacancies in their inner shell electron structure. In the process of filling these inner shells by electrons dropping in from outer orbits, there is a release of electromagnetic energy in the x-ray region (Figure 2-24). The characteristic x-ray energy is determined by the energy shell difference; electrons filling in the K shell are more energetic than those that fill an L shell because of the proximity to the nucleus and the higher binding energy.

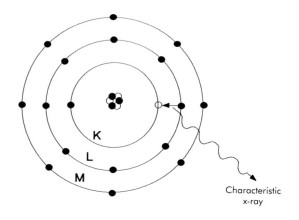

Figure 2-24 Characteristic x rays are produced when electron fills lower shell vacancy. Energy of x ray represents energy difference between two electron shells.

Auger Electrons

Characteristic x rays are produced in reducing excess energy when electrons fill vacancies in inner shells. An alternative to characteristic x rays is the Auger (pronounced *oh-zhay*) effect. In this interaction the surplus energy is given to another orbital electron, which is ejected (Figure 2-25). The ejected electron is called an Auger electron, and the atom is now left with two vacancies occurring in the electron structure. These vacancies are filled by additional electrons from outer orbits, which are also followed by the emission of characteristic x rays or secondary Auger electrons. The production of Auger electrons results in increased radiation exposure when these processes take place within the body tissue.

ATTENUATION AND TRANSMISSION OF PHOTONS

As discussed previously, gamma photons interact with matter through photoelectric, Compton, and pair production processes. These interactions combine into the linear attenuation coefficient, μ. The linear attenuation coefficient is the probability of attenuation per distance traveled through an absorber, therefore μ has the units of 1/distance (cm^{-1}). The general attenuation equation is:

$$I = I_0 e^{-\mu x}$$

where the initial intensity of radiation I_0 is reduced by the exponential function of the linear attenuation coefficient μ and distance traveled x, to give the reduced intensity of the radiation field I.

The linear attenuation coefficient μ is related to the half-value layer (HVL) of the material by:

$$\mu = \frac{0.693}{HVL}$$

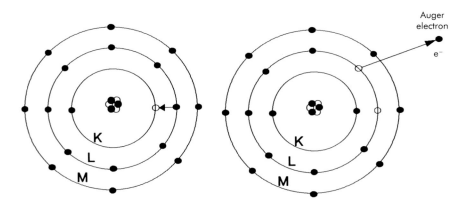

Figure 2-25 Alternative process to production of characteristic x rays is emission of Auger electron. As electron fills lower energy shell *(left)*, energy is transferred to release orbital electron. Atom *(right)* is left with two vacancies, which will be filled by outer orbital electrons with subsequent characteristic x rays or additional Auger electron production.

The HVL is the thickness of absorber necessary to diminish the intensity of the radiation to half its initial strength.

The general attenuation equation can be rewritten to incorporate the relationship to HVL as:

$$I = I_0 e^{-0.693x/HVL}$$

An example using these equations is the shielding of a source of ^{131}I with lead. The HVL for 364 keV gamma rays is 0.3 cm. The value of μ is then calculated to be 2.31 cm^{-1}. Assume that we have 0.9 cm of lead and an exposure rate of 5 mR/hr. Using the general attenuation equation we calculate:

$$I = 5(mR)/(hr)e^{-2.31 \times 0.9}$$
$$I = 5(mR)/(hr)e^{-2.079}$$
$$I = 5(mR)/(hr) \times 0.125$$
$$I = 0.625(mR)/(hr)$$

Since the thickness of the lead is 3 HVLs, an alternative method to more simply solve this problem is todivide the intensity of the radiation field by 2, three times, or:

$$\frac{([(5mR)/(hr)/2]/2)}{2} = 0.635(mR)/(hr)$$

The measure of attenuation can also be done with another parameter, the mass attenuation coefficient, μ_{mass}, which depends on the material's density. The units of this coefficient are cm^2/g. From the following, the relationship between these two attenuation coefficients is represented as:

$$\mu_{mass} = \frac{\mu_{linear}}{density}$$

Utilizing these attenuation relationships results in the following expression:

$$cm^2/g = \frac{cm^{-1}}{(g/cm^3)}$$

The mass attenuation coefficient can be broken down into its components for the processes of photoelectric, Compton, and pair production interactions.

chapter *3*

Instrumentation

Jonathan M. Links, L. Stephen Graham

Objectives

Describe the construction and operating principles of gas-filled detectors, including ionization chambers and Geiger-Mueller detectors.

Explain the operation of scintillation detectors and photomultiplier tubes.

Describe the mechanisms for performing spectrometry with a scintillation detector.

Diagram the differences between liquid scintillation counting systems and scintillation crystal systems.

Discuss count rate limitations of gas-filled and scintillation detectors relative to dead time, efficiency, geometry, and attenuation.

Diagram an Anger design of a scintillation camera system and explain the function of each component.

Diagram and discuss the properties of various camera collimators.

Discuss spatial resolution and sensitivity of the scintillation camera.

Diagram and describe the function of position logic circuitry for the scintillation camera.

Describe the operation of a pulse height analyzer for energy discrimination.

Explain how images are formed using photographic or digital systems.

Define SPECT and explain the principles behind emission computed tomography.

Describe the relative advantages of multiple detector SPECT cameras.

Describe the operation of positron imaging systems for dedicated PET tomography, PET imaging with SPECT, and coincidence imaging.

Describe quality control procedures required for survey instruments.

List the quality control procedures required for the dose calibrator and how each procedure is performed and results interpreted.

Explain quality control requirements for nonimaging scintillation detectors.

List and discuss quality control procedures required for the scintillation camera system, including SPECT.

Define NEMA standards and their application to nuclear medicine.

Define signal-to-noise ratio and its influence on data quality.

Nuclear medicine is a high-technology discipline. Accordingly, much more emphasis is placed on the design, manufacture, and use of its instruments than in some other fields. The equipment evolves out of a multidisciplinary approach, encompassing basic radiation physics, electronics, detector design, and computers. Although the nuclear medicine technologist does not need to become an expert in all of these fields, a basic knowledge of the principles behind the equipment is vital to maximizing a given imaging system's performance. The technologist is the key player, since he or she directly interacts with the equipment. A technologist needs an understanding of how nuclear instrumentation works far beyond knowing "which buttons to push."

This chapter emphasizes the principles of radiation detection, image formation, and tomography. A knowledge of basic mathematics and radiation physics is assumed. References to specific vendors or equipment are specifically avoided; the same general principles apply to all modern nuclear medicine imaging systems.

RADIATION DETECTION

There are two main types of detectors used in nuclear medicine: gas-filled detectors and scintillators. *Gas-filled detectors* are typically used in nonimaging instruments, whereas *scintillators* form the basis of most imaging instruments.

Gas-Filled Detectors

The basic approach of a gas-filled detector is quite simple: radiation is sensed by detecting the ionization of gas molecules produced by deposition of energy during radiation's passage through the gas-filled detector. In essence, a gas-filled detector is a container of gas with two electrodes, one positive (the anode) and one negative (the cathode). When ionizing radiation produces ion pairs in the gas, the resulting free electrons are attracted to the anode and the positively charged gas molecule ions are attracted to the cathode. (An *ion pair* is the positively charged gas molecule ion and the free electron that came from it.) This bulk movement of charge produces an electrical signal from the detector. Commonly used gases include helium, neon, argon, hydrogen, and air. Gases that have a high affinity for electrons, such as oxygen or halogens, are not used, since these would compete with the anode for the free electrons.

Types. There are three main types of gas-filled detectors: ionization chambers, proportional counters, and Geiger-Mueller detectors. Although in practice many factors determine which type a given detector represents, in theory the type is given by the value of the applied voltage across the electrodes in the detector. The curve that relates the applied voltage to the signal from a gas-filled detector is shown in Figure 3-1. The y axis is labeled *number of ion pairs collected per event*. An event refers to one alpha, beta, x ray, or gamma ray passing through the detector and depositing energy in the gas (in the process of ionizing gas molecules). Because the electrodes have a voltage across them, the free electrons are attracted to the anode and the gas molecule ions are attracted to the cathode. This movement of charge produces an electrical signal across the electrodes, whose size is proportional to the numbers of electrons and gas ions (i.e., ion pairs) collected at the electrodes. In general, a gas-filled detector gives one electrical pulse for every alpha, beta, x ray, or gamma ray it detects, with the *size of the pulse* determined by the number of ion pairs collected at the electrodes. The curve in Figure 3-1 is divided into six regions: recombination, ionization, proportional, limited proportional, Geiger-Mueller, and continuous discharge. These divisions imply different operational modes for a gas-filled detector.

When the applied voltage across the electrodes is very low, the gas ions and electrons feel very little attraction toward their respective electrodes. Even though many ion pairs may have been created in the gas by ionizing radiation, these gas ions and electrons are more apt to *recombine* with each other than to be separated and collected at the electrodes. There is reduced signal from a gas-filled detector in the recombination region of operation, thus detectors are not operated with voltages in this region.

If the applied voltage is increased to 100-400 V, the electrodes apply sufficient force to overcome the mutual attraction of the gas molecule ions and free electrons for each other. Thus all of the ion pairs produced by deposition of energy in the detector are collected. This means that the size of each pulse in this *ionization region* of operation is directly related to the amount of energy deposited in the gas by the ionization event. If the gas is air, ionization chambers can directly measure *exposure* in roentgens.

When the applied voltage is increased to 400-800 V,

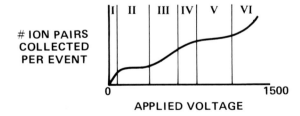

Figure 3-1 Relationship between applied voltage and number of ion pairs collected per event in a gas-filled detector. Curve is divided into six regions. *I,* Recombination; *II,* ionization; *III,* proportional; *IV,* limited proportional; *V,* Geiger-Mueller; *VI,* continuous or spontaneous discharge.

the free electrons gain a significant amount of kinetic energy on their way to the anode. The larger the voltage on the anode, the greater the electrons' acceleration and increase in kinetic energy. These electrons now have sufficient energy to cause ionization themselves. As they make their way to the anode, they produce more ion pairs. Most of this additional ionization occurs near the anode, because by this point the electrons have gained the most kinetic energy. Some of these secondary electrons also gain enough kinetic energy to cause further ionization. The end result is that many more ion pairs are collected than were initially produced in the gas by the incoming ionizing radiation. However, the final number of ions pairs collected is still *proportional* to the initial number produced. Thus the size of a pulse from a proportional counter is proportional to the energy deposited in the detector; the size is a factor of 100 to 10,000 times the size from an ionization chamber (depending on the particular counter) for the same energy deposited because of this *gas amplification.*

As the voltage across the electrodes is increased above about 800 V, free electrons from initial ionization events gain sufficient kinetic energy to ionize a significant fraction of the gas molecules in the detector. In this *limited proportional region* the detector is approaching its saturation point, such that the number of ion pairs collected (and thus pulse size) is not strictly proportional to energy deposited; detectors are not generally operated in this region.

If the applied voltage is increased to 1000-1500 V, the free electrons from initial ionization events gain enough kinetic energy to produce an *avalanche* of ionization, resulting in as complete an ionization of the gas in the detector as possible; this can be thought of as the *saturation point.* In this situation the number of ion pairs collected is independent of the initial number formed. Thus the size of the pulse from a detector operating in this *Geiger-Mueller region* is independent of the energy deposited by the ionizing radiation; every event yields the same large size pulse. It is interesting to note that the actual number of gas molecules ionized at saturation is still only a small fraction of the total number of molecules in the detector.

Figure 3-2 shows a characteristic curve for a Geiger-Mueller detector system, in which the observed pulse or count rate from a radioactive source is plotted as a function of applied voltage. Note that this curve has a different y axis than that in Figure 3-1. The y axis in Figure 3-1 refers to the size of a given pulse, whereas that in Figure 3-2 refers to the number of pulses per unit time. This curve has several features: *A,* starting voltage or threshold; *B,* knee; *C,* plateau region; and *D,* region of continuous discharge. This curve is used to characterize the voltage-response function of a particular Geiger-Mueller detector to select the appropriate operating voltage (usually about one-third of the way along the plateau).

Increases above about 1500 V can produce arcing between the electrodes; the actual voltage depends on several factors, including electrode separation distance. This spontaneous electrical discharge will create ion pairs in the same way that a bolt of lightning ionizes the air along its path. The electrical discharge is continuous. Operation in this region is not useful and is harmful to the detector.

Spontaneous discharge can also occur at lower voltages in Geiger-Mueller detectors if not prevented. X rays are released when positive gas molecule ions reach the cathode (the detector wall) and recombine with electrons from the wall. These x rays can produce ionization, leading to another avalanche and the generation of a pulse. This effect will continue indefinitely once started unless it is *quenched.* Quenching is accomplished by using a small concentration of a second polyatomic or halogen quenching gas. The energy released by recombination of the positive ions and electrons is absorbed by the quench gas, causing dissociation. Halogen quenched detectors have a long life, because the halogen molecules, typically Br_2 or Cl_2, recombine after dissociation. Quenching is not required in ionization chambers or proportional counters because the applied voltage is not high enough to cause sufficient gas amplification for the very low-energy x rays to produce a detectable pulse.

A complete detection system consists of the gas-filled detector itself, a high-voltage power supply, a preamplifier (used to shape the pulses by narrowing their width to increase count rate capability), an amplifier (used to linearly increase the size of the pulses), and a read-out device, consisting of either a scaler (used to actually count the pulses) and a timer (used to control the duration of counting) or a ratemeter. Since it is possible for noise to arise in the electronics that count the pulses, a discriminator is used to eliminate the noise pulses, which are typically of lower amplitude. This discriminator, which is located in the preamplifier or am-

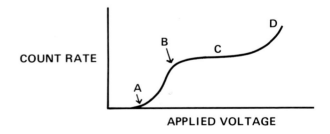

Figure 3-2 Characteristic curve for a Geiger-Mueller detector, showing relationship between applied voltage and observed count rate from a radioactive source. *A,* Starting voltage or threshold; *B,* knee; *C,* plateau region; *D,* region of continuous or spontaneous discharge.

plifier, is an electronic threshold that only allows pulses above a certain size to pass on to be counted. The presence of this discriminator produces the threshold seen in Figure 3-2; without it, counts would be observed at a very low applied voltage.

Uses. Gas-filled detectors are most commonly used in nuclear medicine as dose calibrators and survey meters. A *dose calibrator* is used to determine the radioactivity in a test tube, vial, or syringe (Figure 3-3). Dose calibrators are based on ionization chambers filled with a known volume of air; as such, they directly measure exposure rate. This direct measure of exposure rate can be converted into a measure of the amount of radioactivity present. Exposure is based on the production of a known number of ion pairs in a known volume of air. In a dose calibrator, measured exposure rate is converted to activity by

$$A = E\ d^2/G$$

where *A* is the activity of the source, *E* is the measured exposure rate, *d* is the distance between the source and the detector, and *G* is the specific gamma ray constant. This gamma ray constant expresses the ability of a given amount of activity of a radionuclide to ionize air molecules. This constant is based on the type, number, and energies of emissions from a given radionuclide and is thus different for each radionuclide. Dose calibrators thus have a selector switch or dial that selects the appropriate constant for that radionuclide, so that actual activity can be displayed on the calibrator's read-out.

The second application of gas-filled detectors is as a *survey meter* (Figure 3-4). These are used to locate a source of radioactivity and to assess the amount of radioactivity present or the exposure rate from the source. When the location of a radioactive source is not known, Geiger-Mueller detectors are frequently used. These typically read out in units of counts/min and thus indicate the relative amount of radioactivity present. They are the most sensitive gas-filled detector for this purpose. When the location of the source is known, an ionization chamber may be used to directly assess exposure rate in mR/hr. This is particularly useful in estimating the exposure risk from patients, syringes, and packages. Some manufacturers produce Geiger-Mueller detectors that also read out in units of mR/hr. These should be used with caution for measurement of exposure rate, since the calibration is very energy dependent.

It is very important to consider the materials used in constructing gas-filled detectors, for their characteristics and thickness will determine what radiations can penetrate the detector housing and interact in the gas. For example, *thin end-window* Geiger-Mueller detectors have one end of extremely thin mica, which allows counting of low-energy alphas and betas. Side-window Geiger-Mueller detectors, on the other hand, have windows that are typically ten times as thick and are only useful for higher energy betas and electromagnetic radiation.

If a detector read-out is in units of counts/time or exposure/time, it is called a *ratemeter*. Such a meter responds to changes in activity. The speed with which the meter responds is determined by the meter's *time con-*

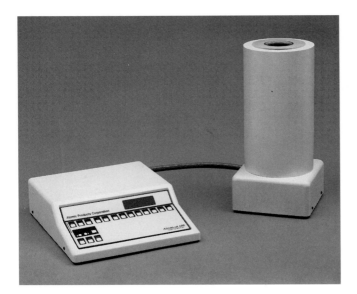

Figure 3-3 Dose calibrator used to assay amount of radioactivity in a syringe. System is based on a calibrated ionization chamber. (Courtesy Biodex Medical Systems, Shirley, New York.)

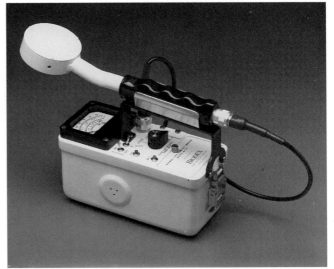

Figure 3-4 Survey instrument used to detect location and relative amount of radioactivity. System is usually based on a Geiger-Mueller counter. (Courtesy Biodex Medical Systems, Shirley, New York.)

stant. A long time constant means that the ratemeter responds sluggishly. If the activity rapidly changes, the meter's reading will lag behind. If the time constant is short, the meter will rapidly respond to changes, even if only due to the statistical nature of radioactive decay rather than to a true change in activity. The choice of a time constant reflects a compromise between the ability to detect true changes in activity and smoothing the rapid meter fluctuations due to statistical variation.

Scintillation Detectors

The most commonly used detector in nuclear medicine is the scintillation detector. This type of detector is based on the property of certain crystals to emit light photons *(scintillate)* after deposition of energy in the crystal by ionizing radiation. To understand how these inorganic scintillators work, the band theory of solids must be considered. In this theory the outer electrons have energy levels that lie in a *valence band.* Above the valence band is a band of electron energy levels called the *conduction band.* The region of energies between the valence and conduction bands is called the *forbidden gap* and represents electron energies that do not exist in a pure crystal. In the crystal's ground energy state, the valence band is completely filled with electrons and the conduction band is empty. If energy is imparted to the crystal, electrons may be raised from the valence band to the conduction band. Because this results in an energetically unstable state, the electrons fall back to the valence band, giving off energy (as electromagnetic radiation) in the process. This electromagnetic radiation represents the difference in energy between the valence band and the conduction band and is usually in the visible light range. In a typical scintillator the light photons have wavelengths from about 350-500 nm. The number of photons emitted is proportional to the energy deposited.

The most commonly used scintillation crystal in nuclear medicine is sodium iodide. This crystal absorbs moisture from the air; it is hygroscopic and is therefore hermetically sealed in an aluminum can. Because the aluminum absorbs alphas and betas, sodium iodide detectors are generally used only for detection of x and gamma rays. Interactions of x or gamma rays will not cause a crystal of pure sodium iodide to fluoresce at room temperature. However, if impurity atoms (usually thallium) are incorporated into the crystal, *luminescence centers* are created in the forbidden gap. Electrons excited during interaction of ionizing radiation are trapped in these centers. As the electrons return to the valence band, light is released in the crystal. In most thallium-activated sodium iodide crystals, about 20-30 light photons are released for each keV of energy absorbed.

The light photons are converted to an electrical sig-

nal through the use of a *photomultiplier tube,* which is optically coupled to the crystal. The photomultiplier tube is a vacuum tube with a large potential voltage distributed across a series of intermediate electrodes, called *dynodes.* The light photons leave the transparent crystal and impinge upon the photosensitive surface *(photocathode)* of the photomultiplier tube. The photocathode is an extremely thin layer of an alloy such as cesium and antimony, or cesium, antimony, sodium, and potassium (in a typical bialkali photomultiplier tube). For every 3-5 light photons incident upon the photocathode, one electron is released by the photoelectric effect. The photoelectrons are accelerated to the first dynode, which is positively charged and positioned a short distance from the photocathode. For each electron reaching the first dynode, 3-4 electrons are released. The second dynode has a higher voltage than the first; thus the liberated electrons are accelerated to it. Each of these electrons in turn liberates 3-4 electrons from this second dynode. This process is repeated at 10-14 successive dynodes in the photomultiplier tube, and 10^6-10^8 electrons reach the tube's anode for each electron liberated from the photocathode. Electrons collected by the anode are directed into a preamplifier circuit, which forms and shapes a pulse that is then further amplified by a linear amplifier from a few millivolts to a few volts. A complete scintillation counting system is shown in Figure 3-5.

Spectrometry

Measurement principles. The size or *height* of each pulse from the photomultiplier tube is proportional to the energy deposited in the crystal by ionizing radiation. As with gas-filled detectors, the number of pulses coming from the detector per unit time is related to the activity of the source. Scintillation spectrometry, or *pulse height analysis,* refers to the use of a scintillation counting system to obtain an energy spectrum from a radioactive source (Figure 3-6). This energy spectrum is simply a histogram of pulse height (which is propor-

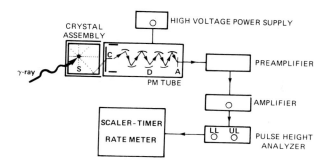

Figure 3-5 Scintillation spectrometry system. *S,* Scintillation event; *C,* photocathode; *D,* dynode; *A,* anode; *LL,* lower level discriminator; *UL,* upper level discriminator.

tional to the energy deposited in the crystal) on the x axis versus the number of pulses with a given pulse height on the y axis. This spectrum is a function of the energies of the x or gamma rays emitted by the source and the interactions of these radiations in the crystal. This spectrum has two main features: a broad range of energies called the *Compton plateau,* and a peak at the highest pulse heights or energies, called the *photopeak.* The broad plateau represents Compton scatter interactions in the crystal. The right-most limit of this plateau, called the *Compton edge,* represents Compton interactions in which the incoming x ray or gamma ray is backscattered 180 degrees in the crystal, thus depositing the maximum energy possible in a Compton interaction. The photopeak represents x rays or gamma rays that come directly from the source and deposit all of their energy in either a single photoelectric interaction or one or more Compton interactions followed by a photoelectric interaction. Because an x or gamma ray cannot lose all its energy in a single Compton scatter event, there is a separation between the Compton plateau and the photopeak. A typical pulse height spectrum (for ^{99m}Tc) is shown in Figure 3-6.

In an ideal detector the photopeak would be a single vertical line at the pulse height representing the energy of the emitted x ray or gamma ray. In reality the statistical nature of the light emission and the finite energy resolution of a pulse height analyzer smears out this line, producing a bell-shaped photopeak. In nuclear medicine imaging the general term *resolution* can be thought of as the ability of a system to accurately depict two separate events in space, time, or energy as separate. Resolution can also be thought of as the amount by which a system smears out a single event in space, time, or energy. These two ways of looking at resolution are, of course, related, because the less smearing a system produces, the closer in space, time, or energy two events can be and still be distinguished as being separate. The worse the energy resolution of

a pulse height analyzer, the broader the photopeak. Energy resolution can be quantified as the *full width at half maximum* (FWHM) of the photopeak (Figure 3-7). This is measured by first determining the counts at the peak of the photopeak and locating the points on either side of the peak where the counts are half of the peak counts. The width of the photopeak in pulse height units is obtained by subtracting the lower pulse height from the upper. Finally, this width is divided by the pulse height (energy) at the apex of the photopeak (and multiplied by 100) to yield an energy resolution measurement in percent.

$$\text{\% energy resolution} = (\text{FWHM/photopeak center}) \times 100$$

The smaller the number, the better the energy resolution; typical scintillation systems average 7%-9% for ^{137}Cs; typical camera systems average 8%-12% for ^{99m}Tc. It is important to note that the time resolution of the scintillation system also plays a role in energy resolution, in that two scintillation events that occur within the system's time resolution will produce a single, summed pulse of larger size. Such pulses can contribute to an apparent widening of the photopeak.

To calibrate a pulse height analyzer to establish the quantitative relationship between energy deposited and pulse height (e.g., 1 pulse height unit = 1 keV), either the applied voltage across the photomultiplier tube or the amplification in the electronics is adjusted until the photopeak from a known energy source falls at the desired pulse height. Changing the applied voltage across the photomultiplier tube changes the size of pulses coming out of the detector by changing the amplification in the tube. If the voltage across each dynode is increased, electrons liberated from the previous dynode gain more kinetic energy. Upon striking the next dynode, a larger number of electrons are liberated. This leads to a larger signal from the photomultiplier tube. Changing the amplification in the electronics directly changes the size of each pulse. In any event, there is a linear proportionality between pulse height and energy; calibrating the analyzer at one energy usually calibrates it for all energies. However, some systems are not perfectly linear. This is especially true at very low energies such as those of the photons from I-125.

Uses. Spectrometry systems are generally used to determine which radionuclides (and their amounts) are present in a mixed sample or to determine how much activity of a known radionuclide is present in a sample. To assay the amount of radioactivity in a test tube, a *well counter* is commonly used (Figure 3-8). This counter consists of a cylindrical lead-shielded sodium iodide detector 1-3 inches in diameter, containing a hole passing

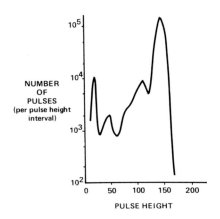

Figure 3-6 Pulse height spectrum of ^{99m}Tc.

through the lead and partway through the crystal, which permits the insertion of a test tube containing the radioactive sample. Because the crystal surrounds the test tube on all sides except the top, the counting geometry is very close to optimum. To count radioactivity in a patient, a *probe system* is often used (Figure 3-9). The probe consists of a sodium iodide crystal with a collimator attached to its front. This collimator is a piece of lead with a large hole in it (Figure 3-10). Its purpose is to limit the *field of view* of the crystal, so that the probe only detects activity from a defined volume in space in front of it. A major application of these probe systems is in thyroid uptake studies, in which the amount of orally ingested radioiodine that accumulates in the thyroid is determined. This requires the use of a *flat-field collimator*. This collimator provides relatively uniform detection sensitivity across the region of the thyroid, while excluding most radioactivity outside the neck from the probe's field of view.

Pulse height analyzers are very important in well-counters and probes in two ways. First, they can be used to determine which radionuclides are present in a sample by analysis of the pulse height spectrum. For example, a small sample of the liquid solution that is eluted from the chemical ion exchange column of a radionuclide generator system can be counted in a well counter. The pulse height spectrum from the counter will be a composite of the desired radionuclide's spectrum and spectra from any radioactive impurities in the eluate. Since each radionuclide has a characteristic pulse height spectrum, inspection of the composite spectrum will reveal the presence of impurities, as additional photopeaks on the observed spectrum and their amounts will be indicated by the heights of the peaks relative to the desired radionuclide's photopeak.

The second application of pulse height analyzers is to count a preselected range of energies (Figure

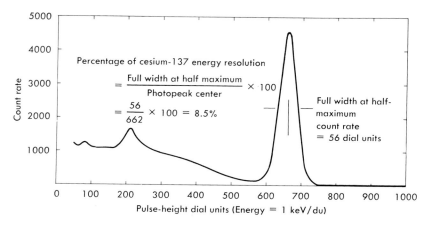

Figure 3-7 Cesium-137 energy spectrum and energy resolution. *du,* Dial or energy units. (From Rollo FD: *Nuclear medicine physics, instrumentation, and agents,* St. Louis, 1977, Mosby.)

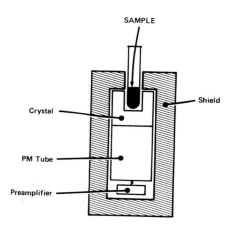

Figure 3-8 Arrangement of a standard well counter for assay of radioactivity. System is based on a crystal scintillator.

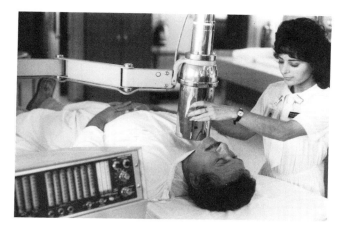

Figure 3-9 Probe system utilizing scintillation spectrometry, usually used for iodine or technetium thyroid-uptake studies.

3-11). This is accomplished through the use of a *pulse height window*. The pulse height window is a combination of a lower level discriminator and an upper level discriminator. The lower level discriminator only allows pulses above a certain size to pass and be counted, whereas the upper level discriminator allows only pulses below a certain size to pass and be counted. The combination of lower and upper level discriminators in an *anticoincidence circuit* permits the range of pulses between the lower and upper levels to pass and be counted. The importance of selecting a certain range of pulses, which represents a specific range of energies deposited in the crystal by x rays or gamma rays, is discussed later.

Liquid Scintillation Counting

One special spectrometry technique is liquid scintillation counting. This technique is used to assess the activity of small sources of beta emitters, such as tritium (^{3}H) or carbon 14. In liquid scintillation counting, the radioactive samples are dissolved in a liquid that scintillates, called a *cocktail*. This liquid scintillation cocktail is put into a vial and coupled to a photomultiplier tube.

Liquid scintillation cocktails are composed of three main ingredients: an organic solvent, a primary fluor, and a secondary fluor. The *solvent* is used to dissolve the small sample containing the radioactivity, which is usually biologic tissue. The solvent accounts for about 99% of the cocktail's volume. Because of this, most of the interactions of ionizing radiation with the cocktail are with solvent molecules, rather than directly with a scintillator. The *primary fluor* scintillates when energy is transferred to it from the solvent. The color of these scintillation photons from the primary fluor is generally not ideal for the photocathode of modern photomultiplier tubes, thus a *secondary fluor* (a so-called *waveshifter*) is usually used. This fluor produces a different color light from the primary fluor when energy is transferred to it from the primary fluor.

The pulses from liquid scintillation counting systems are very small, and electronic noise is thus a problem. Two techniques are used to reduce this noise. The first is to cool the entire counting system by putting it in a refrigerator. This reduces noise because stray electrical signals (the source of the noise) originate in the electronics as electrons that are "freed" from atoms by heat (this process is called *thermionic emission*). Reducing the temperature decreases thermionic emissions. The second technique to reduce noise is to use *coincidence counting*, in which two photomultiplier tubes view the vial from opposing sides. A special coincidence circuit determines if a pulse occurs at the same time in both tubes. When a flash of light occurs in the vial, both tubes will generate a pulse and the coincidence circuit will generate a pulse to be counted. Noise pulses will occur in only one photomultiplier tube/electronics stage at a time, thus no coincidence circuit pulse will be generated.

An additional problem in liquid scintillation counting is *quenching*, which refers to any undesirable reduction in light output from the scintillation cocktail. (This use of the term quenching should not be confused with its completely different meaning in Geiger-Mueller detectors.) There are three main types of quenching. Chemical quenching is caused by the presence of materials in the cocktail that interfere with the transfer of energy from the solvent to the fluor or from the primary fluor to the secondary fluor; oxygen is a common chemical quench agent. Color quenching is the result of any colored material in the cocktail that absorbs light

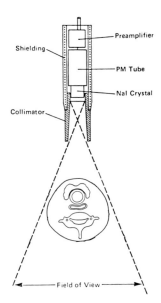

Figure 3-10 Flat-field collimator, which limits probe's field of view to region of interest—in this case, the neck.

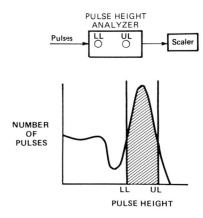

Figure 3-11 Use of pulse height window, defined by lower level and upper level discriminators, to select desired range of energies (usually photopeak energies, representing unscattered events).

from the primary or secondary fluor. Optical quenching is produced by condensation, fingerprints, or dirt on the vial.

Factors Affecting Count Rate

For both gas-filled and scintillation detectors, the size of each pulse (pulse height) is related to the energy deposited in the detector during the passage of a single ionizing particle or ray through the detector (except for detectors operated in the Geiger-Mueller region, where the pulses are always the same, large size), and the number of pulses produced per unit time (pulse rate) is proportional to the radioactivity of the source. Typically, pulses of certain sizes are counted, and these data are used to represent relative activity. In practice, the observed count rate from a detector is typically less than the actual disintegration or decay rate of the radioactive source.

Time. First, after the deposition of energy in the detector by an alpha, beta, x ray, or gamma ray, it takes a certain amount of time for the detector's response to occur (i.e., for the ions and electrons to travel to the electrodes in a gas-filled detector or for the light to be emitted in a scintillator). Figure 3-12 shows pulse size of a second event as a function of the time interval between two events for a gas-filled detector. During this time the detector is either not responsive or only partially responsive to the deposition of additional energy. The so-called *resolving time* represents how long it takes to "count" a given event. Thus for a nonparalyzable system its inverse yields the maximum count rate capability of the detector. For example, a typical counting system might have a resolving time of 4 μsec, resulting in a maximum count rate capability of 250,000 counts/sec.

The effects of timing can be separated into two types of situations: paralyzable and nonparalyzable systems (Figure 3-13). In a *nonparalyzable system,* as the activity increases, the count rate increases, until it reaches a maximum value given by the inverse of the resolving time. No matter how much the activity is further increased, the count rate will not increase. However, if the resolving time of the detector is known, comparison of its inverse with the observed count rate will indicate whether the detector is operating at an unacceptably high count rate. If so, the activity should be reduced until the count rate is at an acceptable level (i.e., below the maximum or plateau value). In a *paralyzable system,* as the activity increases, the count rate increases to a maximum value and then actually starts decreasing at higher activity levels. In this situation it is not possible to determine if the detector is operating on the ascending or descending portion of the curve. The ascending portion is, of course, where the detector should be operated. Accordingly, the user needs to know ahead of time what activity levels are reasonable to count with the detector. Alternatively, the user can count the activity, dilute it, and then recount the same size aliquot. If the observed count rate decreases after dilution, the detector was initially operating on the ascending portion of the curve (which is good); if it increases, the detector was on the descending portion (which is unacceptable).

Efficiency. The second factor is the *efficiency* of the detector itself. Not every alpha, beta, x, or gamma ray that passes through the detector will deposit energy in the detector material. If no energy is deposited, obviously no pulse will be generated. Gas-filled detectors can approach 100% efficiency for most alphas and betas that enter the detector but are only about 1% efficient for x rays and gamma rays, whereas sodium iodide scintillators are approximately 50% efficient for x rays and gamma rays.

Geometry. The third factor is called *geometry* and takes into account the inverse square law. The greater the distance between the source and the detector, the lower the observed count rate. The count rate is changed by

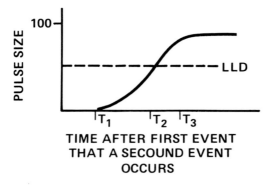

Figure 3-12 Timing characteristics of a detector system, showing relationship between the time after an event that a second event occurs and pulse size of the second event. T_1, Dead time; T_2, resolving time; T_3, recovery time; *LLD*, lower level discriminator setting.

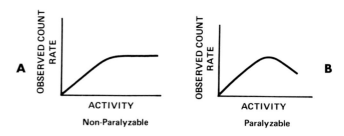

Figure 3-13 Effect of activity on observed count rate: **A,** Nonparalyzable system. **B,** Paralyzable system.

the square of the change in distance (e.g., if the distance is doubled, the count rate is reduced by a factor of four). Geometry also takes into account the front cross-sectional area of the detector. The larger the surface of the detector facing the source, the more radioactive emissions that will intersect the detector, and the higher the count rate. Efficiency and geometry are often combined into a single term called *sensitivity*. This term reflects the fraction of radioactive emissions from the source that is ultimately detected.

Attenuation. The fourth factor is attenuation of the radioactive emissions, either self-attenuation in the source itself or attenuation in the medium between the source and the detector. In either case, radioactive emissions from the source are "removed" from the beam before they can strike the detector, thus lowering the observed count rate.

Random decay. The preceding factors are deterministic in nature. One final factor is the random nature of radioactive decay itself. Radioactive decay is governed by Poisson statistics. In the Poisson distribution the mean and variance are equal. Thus the coefficient of variation decreases as the mean increases. In the case of nuclear medicine the "mean" is the total number of observed decays (i.e., the total acquired counts). The greater this number, the better the statistical precision

of the measurement. This statistical nature of decay is also the primary source of image noise.

ANGER SCINTILLATION CAMERAS

The Anger scintillation camera was invented by Hal Anger of Donner Laboratory, University of California at Berkeley, in the late 1950s. A picture of a modern scintillation camera is shown in Figure 3-14. It is the most commonly used imaging instrument in nuclear medicine today. The complete camera system consists of a lead collimator, a 10-25 in circular, square, or rectangular sodium iodide scintillation crystal, an array of photomultiplier tubes on the crystal, a positioning logic network, a pulse height analyzer, a scaler-timer, and a cathode ray tube (CRT) display, as shown in Figure 3-15.

Collimators

A *collimator* is typically a ½- to 2-in thick slab of lead the same dimensions as the scintillation crystal, with a geometric array of holes in it. (The pinhole collimator is the exception to this general description.) The lead in between each hole is called a *septum;* collectively the lead represents *septa.* The collimator provides an interface between the patient and scintillation crystal by only

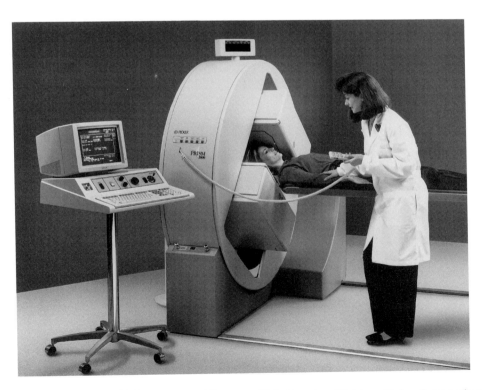

Figure 3-14   Dual detector Anger scintillation camera. (Courtesy Ohio Imaging Division, Picker International, Inc., Bedford Heights, Ohio.)

allowing those photons traveling in an appropriate direction (i.e., those that can pass through the holes without being absorbed in the lead) to interact with the crystal. Collimators thus discriminate based on direction of flight, not on whether the photons are scattered or not. There are several types of collimators used with Anger cameras: parallel-hole, converging, diverging, and pinhole, as shown in Figure 3-16.

Types. The most commonly used collimator is the *parallel-hole collimator,* which consists of an array of parallel holes, essentially perpendicular to the crystal face, and thus presents a real-size image to the crystal face. The resolution of a parallel-hole collimator is best at the collimator surface. The sensitivity is independent of the distance between the source and the collimator. Although this seems to contradict the inverse square law, it really does not (Figure 3-17). The field of view of each hole increases with increasing distance. This means that each hole "sees" a larger area at a greater distance from the collimator. Looking at it another way, more holes see the same source if it's farther away from the collimator. As a radioactive source is moved away from the face of the collimator, the count rate through each hole decreases due to the inverse square law. However, more and more holes see the source, and the total count rate remains constant. Since more holes see the source, its image is spread over a larger area of the crystal face (i.e., the image is progressively smeared out). Thus the resolution gets worse with increasing distance, as stated earlier.

Converging collimators have an array of tapered holes

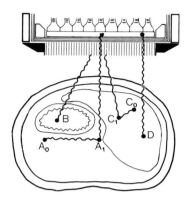

Figure 3-15 Side view showing arrangement of collimator, crystal, and photomultiplier tubes in an Anger camera. Photon A_0 scatters in the patient, resulting in photon A_1, which is detected in the crystal; photon B is absorbed by collimator; photon C_0 scatters in the patient, resulting in photon C_1, which is absorbed by collimator; photon D does not scatter and is detected in the crystal. Collimators discriminate based on direction of flight, not on scattered versus nonscattered photons.

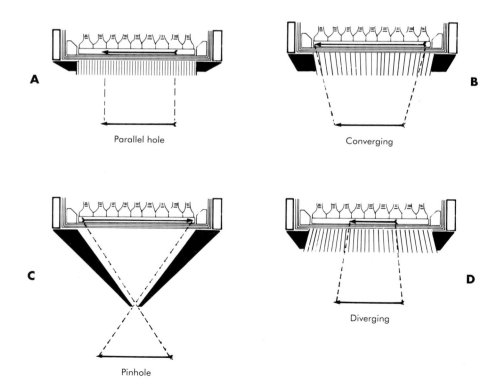

Figure 3-16 Four types of collimators for Anger cameras. Note how arrows are perceived by the crystal. **A,** Parallel hole; arrow is seen as actual size pointing to the left. **B,** Converging; arrow is magnified on crystal surface with point to the left. **C,** Pinhole; arrow is magnified on the crystal surface. Mirror image results with arrow pointing right. **D,** Diverging; arrow is minified on crystal surface with point to the left.

that aim at a point at some distance in front of the collimator; this point is called the *focal point*. The image that is presented to the crystal is a magnified version of the real object. Converging collimators have their best resolution at the surface of the collimator. The sensitivity of a converging collimator slowly increases as the source is moved from the collimator face back to the *focal plane* (the plane parallel to the collimator face that passes through the focal point) and then decreases.

Diverging collimators are essentially upside-down converging collimators. They have an array of tapered holes that diverge from a hypothetical focal point behind the crystal. The image presented to the crystal face is a minified image of the real object. Since converging and diverging collimators are simply flipped versions of each other, some collimators may have an insert that can be flipped either way, in effect producing two collimators in one. This combination collimator is sometimes called a *div/con collimator*.

Pinhole collimators are thick conical collimators with a single 2-5 mm hole in the bottom center. As a source is moved away from the surface of a pinhole collimator, the camera image gets smaller. However, the camera image is magnified (i.e., larger than real size) from the collimator face to a distance equal to the length of the collimator and is then progressively minified at larger distances.

Other types of collimators have more specialized functions. A *single-axis diverging collimator* is used for whole body scanning when the transverse field of view of the camera is smaller than the patient's width. This collimator has diverging holes in the transverse direction but has parallel holes in the axial direction. A *fan-beam collimator* is a combination of a parallel-hole collimator (along one axis) and a converging collimator (along the other axis). It is used in some tomographic studies. An *astigmatic collimator* is a converging collimator with unequal convergence behavior along the two axes. It is also used in some tomographic studies.

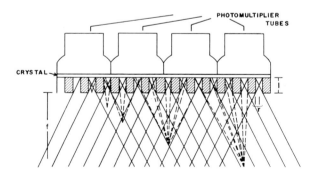

Figure 3-17 Relationship between each hole's field of view and distance from collimator face. (From Boyd CM, Dalrymple GV: *Basic principles of nuclear medicine,* St. Louis, 1974, Mosby.)

Spatial Resolution and Sensitivity

As stated earlier, *spatial resolution* can be defined in terms of the amount by which a system smears out the image of a very small point source or a very thin line source of radioactivity. A profile of the counts along a line through the point source image (which is called the *point spread function*) or through the line source image (perpendicular to the line, which is called the *line spread function*) is generated, usually with computer-aided analysis. Resolution is quantified as the FWHM of the point or line spread function and is generally expressed in millimeters. This measurement of spatial resolution is directly analogous to the measurement of energy resolution as the FWHM of the photopeak of a pulse height spectrum. In practice, the FWHM in millimeters will be nearly identical to the minimum distance by which two point sources must be separated in space to be distinguished as separate in an image. *Sensitivity,* on the other hand, is the overall ability of the system to detect the radioactive emissions from the source. The higher the sensitivity, the greater the fraction of the emissions that are detected. In practical terms, a higher sensitivity system detects more x or gamma rays when viewing the same radioactive source. In practice, there is always a trade-off between resolution and sensitivity. The simple relationship between spatial resolution and sensitivity for a pinhole collimator makes the point: the smaller the pinhole, the better the resolution and the worse the sensitivity, and vice versa for a larger pinhole.

Because of this trade-off, a collimator is not completely specified by its type. For multihole collimators, sensitivity can be increased (at the expense of resolution) by increasing the size or shortening the length of each hole. This reduces the amount of lead in the path of the x or gamma rays, so that a larger fraction can interact in the crystal. Resolution can be increased by using many more, smaller holes or by making the collimator longer, thus increasing the hole length. This reduces the sensitivity because of a net increase in the amount of lead in the collimator. *General all purpose* (GAP) collimators represent a compromise between high resolution and high sensitivity.

These relationships are illustrated in the following simplified equations for a parallel-hole collimator.

$$\text{Resolution} = \text{Diameter}\left(\frac{\text{Length} + \text{distance}}{\text{Length}}\right)$$

$$\text{Sensitivity} = \left(\frac{\text{Diameter}}{\text{Length}}\right)^2\left(\frac{\text{Diameter}}{\text{Diameter} + \text{thickness}}\right)^2$$

Resolution is the geometric resolution of the collimator (the smaller the number, the better), *diameter* is the diameter of each hole, *length* is the length of each hole, and *distance* is the distance between the face of the collimator and the patient or point in the organ of interest. Note that increasing hole diameter or distance increases the resolution value (i.e., makes it worse), whereas increasing hole length decreases the resolution value. *Sensitivity* is the geometric sensitivity of the collimator (the larger the number, the better), and *thickness* is septal thickness. Note that increasing hole diameter increases the sensitivity value (i.e., makes it better), whereas increasing septal thickness decreases the sensitivity value.

It is important to note that the geometric spatial resolution of a collimator is only one of several factors that influences the actual spatial resolution in an image. In planar imaging, instrinsic camera resolution, collimator resolution, scatter, and "patient resolution" effects caused by patient or organ movement all influence the actual resolution in the image. A simple way to estimate total resolution from intrinsic, collimator, scatter, and patient resolution is

$$R_T = \sqrt{R_I^2 + R_C^2 + R_S^2 + R_P^2}$$

Note that the total resolution cannot be any better (i.e., a smaller value) than the largest term in the equation. Thus changes in intrinsic resolution of less than 1 mm rarely, if ever, influence image resolution.

In general, there is an inverse relationship between spatial resolution and sensitivity. However, when using a converging collimator, an additional parameter must be considered. The magnification provided by such a collimator provides increased spatial resolution and sensitivity compared with a parallel-hole collimator with equivalent holes. This is because the part of the patient within the field of view is spread over a larger area of the crystal. Of course the actual field of view with a converging collimator is proportionately smaller than that with a parallel-hole collimator because of the magnification. The possible increase in spatial resolution and sensitivity with magnification is sometimes exploited in SPECT with fan beam collimators.

Collimators are currently either cast or fabricated from corrugated lead strips (the latter are termed *foil* collimators). In general, it is harder to produce fabricated foil collimators with uniform septal thickness. This led some users to automatically consider cast collimators superior to foil collimators. At present, with improved manufacturing technology, excellent foil and cast collimators are available. Originally the collimator holes were circular in cross section. This meant that the lead septa were thicker in some areas than they needed to be to ensure that the thinnest areas were thick enough to absorb the x rays or gamma rays. Recent cast or corrugated collimators have square, hexagonal, or triangular holes. With these collimators the septa are of uniform thickness around each hole. When compared with circular hole collimators, these newer collimator designs have better sensitivity for a given resolution (and better resolution for a given sensitivity).

Crystals

The properties of thallium-activated sodium iodide crystals as scintillation detectors have been described earlier. As with crystals used in scintillation spectrometry, those used in Anger cameras are extremely sensitive to moisture and are sealed in an aluminum housing. In addition, they are sensitive to temperature, especially rapid changes in temperature, which can produce cracking. The crystals used in Anger cameras vary from 7 to over 25 in in dimension. In the past, virtually all crystals were circular in cross section. At present, rectangular crystals are very popular, since these typically provide an increased field of view. Crystals are typically ¼-½ in thick, with ⅜ in the most common size. The thicker the crystal, the higher the probability that an incoming photon will interact, deposit its energy, and be detected. Thus the sensitivity of the camera is higher. However, the thicker the crystal, the poorer the spatial resolution due to the complex (geometric optics) interaction between the crystal, the photomultiplier tubes, and the light pipe that is generally used to optically couple the two. Crystals ¼ in thick have about 1 mm better intrinsic resolution than crystals ½ in thick. When counting low energy radionuclides such as ^{201}Tl, there is no difference in sensitivity. However, when counting ^{99m}Tc, crystals ¼ in thick have 15% less sensitivity than crystals ½ in thick. At higher energies the difference in sensitivity is even more significant. Crystals with a thickness of ⅜-½ in are required to efficiently detect gamma rays above 200 keV.

Positioning Logic

Anger cameras have an array of photomultiplier tubes optically coupled to the back of the scintillation crystal (Figure 3-18). The actual number of tubes is determined by the size and shape of both the crystal and each individual photomultiplier tube. In circular-field cameras the tubes are typically arrayed in a hexagonal

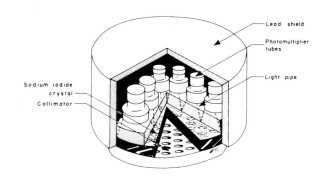

Figure 3-18 Arrangement of collimator, crystal, light pipe, photomultiplier tubes, and lead housing in an Anger camera. (From Boyd CM, Dalrymple GV: *Basic principles of nuclear medicine,* St. Louis, 1974, Mosby.)

geometric configuration in which the number of tubes follows a "6 n + 1" configuration. For example, early cameras had 7 or 19 photomultiplier tubes. At present, it is common for cameras to have 37, 55, or 61 tubes. In general, the more photomultiplier tubes, the better the spatial resolution and linearity. Early photomultiplier tubes had a round cross section. Current tubes often have a hexagonal cross section to cover more of the crystal area for more efficient detection of scintillation photons.

When a scintillation event occurs, each photomultiplier tube produces an output pulse. The amplitude of the pulse from a given photomultiplier tube is directly proportional to the amount of light (number of scintillation photons) its photocathode has received. Those photomultiplier tubes closest to the scintillation event produce the largest output pulses. If only that tube with the largest pulse were used for positioning, the spatial resolution of the camera would be equivalent to the cross-sectional size of each tube. By combining the pulses from each photomultiplier tube, a higher resolution x, y coordinate of the gamma ray location can be generated, based on a centroid (center-of-mass) approach. The general equation for a centroid is

$$x = \frac{\Sigma x_i T_i}{\Sigma T_i}$$

where x is the centroid, x_i is the location of the ith tube, and T_i is the ith tube's output pulse size. Note that the centroid is the weighted average of the tube locations, with the weighting factors determined by pulse size.

There are two ways in which the x and y centroids can be determined. In older, so-called *analog cameras*, an analog resistor network is used. A coordinate system is defined with the origin (0,0) at the center of the crystal (Figure 3-19). The network creates four signals: x^+, x^-, y^+, and y^-. All photomultiplier tubes whose output is above a preset threshold contribute to all four signals. The contribution of any photomultiplier tube to the four signal lines (representing the four coordinate directions) is inversely proportional to the square of its distance from the respective coordinate and is controlled (in a predetermined, fixed way) by the resistor network. The sum of these four signals, called the

z pulse, is proportional to the total energy deposited in the crystal by the photon interaction. The x coordinate of the interaction is given by

$$x = (x^+ - x^-)/z$$

Similarly, the y coordinate is given by:

$$y = (y^+ - y^-)/z$$

Compare these equations to the general equation for a centroid given above. Note the similarities—remember that x^+, x^-, y^+, and y^- are already weighted sums of voltages (with the resistors providing the weighting factors), and that z is the sum of all tubes.

In newer, so-called *digital cameras*, each photomultiplier tube's output is digitized with an analog-to-digital converter. The resulting digital signals are then used with a software-based positioning algorithm. In many cases this algorithm is simply a "digital version" of Anger positioning logic. In some cases more sophisticated algorithms are used. This highlights the theoretical advantage of a digital camera: the ability to more easily change and upgrade positioning algorithms. It should be noted, however, that the term "digital camera" does not have a universally accepted definition, and different vendors use the term to denote digitization of the signals at different stages. Although it is tempting to automatically consider a digital camera as superior to an analog camera, in practice, the functional performance, flexibility, and reliability of a camera determine its value. Thus excellent analog and digital cameras exist.

Energy Discrimination

The desired goal of the Anger camera is to create an image that portrays the distribution (i.e., sites and numbers of radioactive atoms) of radioactivity within the patient. Because the collimator only allows those photons traveling in predetermined directions to interact in the crystal, a line drawn from the scintillation event in the crystal through the nearest collimator hole is presumed to intersect the site of origin of the photon (i.e., the radioactive atom from which it originated) in the patient. If the photon has been scattered in the patient, a line drawn through its direction of flight will not intersect its site of origin, only the site of the Compton interaction. Thus photons scattered into the field of view could be falsely attributed to activity at the sites of Compton interactions in the patient. It is clearly not desirable to have these scattered photons contribute to the final image, since they significantly degrade resolution and contrast. It is important to note that a large percentage of photons striking the crystal have been scattered in the patient.

The z pulse is used by the pulse height analyzer to discriminate against these scattered photons. The pulse

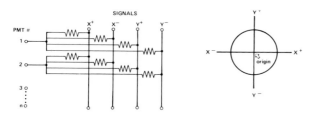

Figure 3-19 Coordinate system and resistor network for Anger positioning logic.

height analyzer is used to set a window around the photopeak. Because the window has a finite width, some scattered photons may still be accepted (those that are scattered through a small angle and thus retain most of their energy). For example, 140 keV photons can scatter by as much as 55 degrees and still be accepted by the often-used 20% window.

In practice, proper window setting is vital, since a window that is not centered around the photopeak (an offset window) can degrade field uniformity for many cameras (Figure 3-20). There is typically slightly better light collection efficiency directly under each photomultiplier tube. Thus events that occur under a tube tend to produce slightly larger z pulses, whereas those that occur between tubes tend to produce slightly smaller z pulses. If the manufacturer does not compensate for this effect, a pulse height window skewed to the "high side" of the photopeak will preferentially accept events occurring under tubes, producing a "hot-tube" pattern, whereas a window skewed to the "low side" will produce a "cold-tube" pattern. In practice, manufacturers of analog cameras frequently "tune" their cameras in a compensatory fashion to improve field uniformity. This has the effect of actually reversing the expected patterns with high-side and low-side peaking. Fortunately, newer cameras, with microprocessor-based correction circuitry (described later), generally maintain good uniformity even with offset pulse height windows. Such cameras may be purposely peaked to the high side of the photopeak to further reduce scatter by eliminating any Compton scattered photons that show up in the lower half of the photopeak (due to every camera's less than perfect energy resolution). Some cameras have two or three separate pulse height windows to simultaneously image the multiple emissions of some radionuclides (e.g., those from ^{67}Ga). In this way counts are

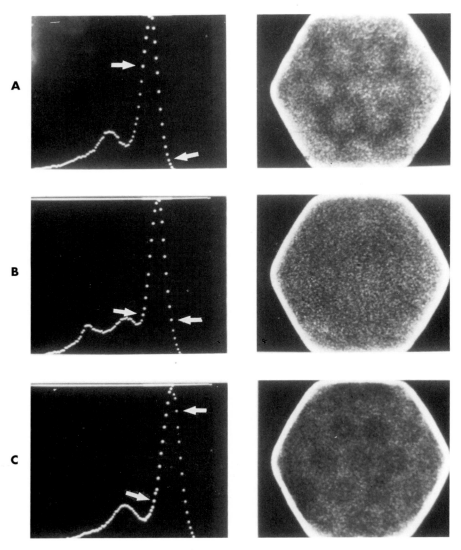

Figure 3-20 Effect of asymmetrically setting the pulse height window. **A,** Window set to high side of photopeak; **B,** window symmetrically positioned; **C,** window set to low side of photopeak.

acquired in a shorter time, as the multiple energy emissions are utilized.

The window can be set manually, or (in some cameras) automatically. Although *autopeaking* may be more accurate than manual peaking, automatic windows may be affected by the amount of Compton scatter present (which proportionately increases, for example, in larger patients) and generally perform poorly when multiple photopeaks are present.

Image Formation

There are two ways in which an image can be formed. In analog cameras, particularly older cameras, photographic images are directly formed during acquisition. Virtually all current analog and digital cameras form images via digital acquisition. In older analog cameras, the scaler-timer controls the on/off cycle of the camera. The camera may be set up to acquire an image for a predetermined time interval (preset time mode) until a predetermined amount of radioactivity has been detected (preset count mode) or until a certain number of counts/cm^2 has been reached (preset information density mode). In current cameras, acquisition is under computer control, although typically the same criteria as above are used to define the end of acquisition.

Photographic image formation. For each z pulse that passes through the pulse height analyzer, its associated x and y pulses are used to position a finely focused dot of light on the CRT face. A collection of these light dots over time produces the image. Since it takes time for a complete picture to be obtained, some sort of integrating medium must be used to record the image. The most frequently used media are various types of photographic film. A photographic camera is mounted on the CRT, and the shutter is left open during the entire image acquisition period. The film is developed, and an image of the distribution of radioactivity is obtained.

An alternative camera recording system is a multiformatter (Figure 3-21). The heart of a multiformatter is a very high-quality CRT. The signals going to the multiformatter can be reduced and repositioned in such a way that the image only occupies a portion of the CRT; thus it only exposes a corresponding portion of the photographic film. In this way, up to 80 images can be produced on a single piece of film. The usual practice is to have four, nine, or sixteen images on one piece of 8 × 10 inch film.

The proper use of film requires an understanding of the relationship between exposure and the appearance of the film. This relationship is characterized by the so-called *H and D curve* (after Heurter and Deerfield), which describes the film's response (optical density when developed) to a given amount of exposure (Figure 3-22). Since many nuclear medicine studies are displayed and stored on film, it is important to understand this relationship.

Optical density reflects how "dark" the film looks when held up to a light source. *Optical density* is given by

$$OD = -\log T$$

where T is *transmittance,* the fraction of light that passes through the film. The smaller the fraction, the higher the optical density and the darker the film appears. *Exposure* (on the x axis of the curve) can be taken to mean exposure to light. In Anger cameras this light comes

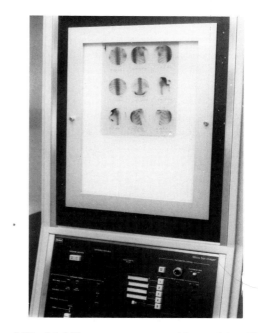

Figure 3-21 Multiformatter camera with resulting film displayed.

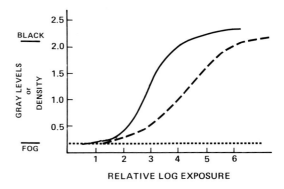

Figure 3-22 H and D curve, characterizing the response of a given film in terms of optical density, to a given amount of exposure. The film represented by the solid line is "faster" and has higher contrast than that represented by the dashed line, because a smaller exposure is required to produce the same optical density for the first film, and a smaller change in exposure produces a larger change in optical density. This means the faster film has higher contrast.

from the CRT. (In general diagnostic radiography, the light comes from the "screen" that is part of the film cassette.) In general, the term exposure represents the total amount of light, which is the product of the brightness of each individual flash of light and the total number of flashes at a given spot on the film. Note that the large middle range of the H and D curve is linear, indicating a linear proportionality between the logarithm of exposure and optical density. However, unusual things happen at the extremes of the curve. At the low end the optical density is not zero, even with no exposure. This baseline level of density is called *base fog* and in practical terms means that it is impossible to get perfectly transparent film. At the upper end the optical density reaches a plateau and does not increase with further exposure. It turns out that the human eye cannot distinguish between different "degrees of blackness"; all optical densities above 2.0 appear equally black. Furthermore, the ability of the eye to distinguish changes in the range 1.0-2.0 is less than its ability to distinguish changes in optical density below 1.0. Thus, the goal in producing an image from an Anger camera is to adjust the system so that the range of counts coming from the areas of interest within the patient produces optical densities on the film between 0.2 and (at most) 2.0. This is done by adjusting the exposure (e.g., adjusting the intensity of each flash of light) before the image is acquired.

Digital image formation. The x, y signals from an Anger camera are frequently entered directly into the computer in real time during image acquisition. As scintillation events occur within the crystal of the camera, corresponding x, y signals stream into the computer and are digitized with the computer's analog-to-digital converters (which in the past had 8-bit resolution but at present have as much as 12-bit resolution). These x, y signals are stored in one of two ways, based on the mode selected by the operator before acquisition begins. These two acquisition modes are *frame mode* and *list mode* (also called *serial mode*).

In frame mode acquisition a digital image of the data is built in computer memory as the x, y signals are received. In frame mode the camera face is represented by a matrix of pixels, each of which corresponds to a certain area of the camera face and is designated by a specific range of x, y signal values. When the computer receives an x, y signal from the camera, the pixel associated with that particular x, y signal value is increased by one count. When data acquisition is complete, images are immediately available for display.

In list mode acquisition the x, y signals are transferred directly to computer memory in the form of a list of x, y coordinates. In addition to the x, y signals, other types of data can be inserted in the list. Typically, time markers are inserted every 1-10 msec. Physiologic trigger marks, such as the occurrence of the R wave

from an ECG monitor of the patient's heart, can also be inserted. In list mode acquisition no matrices or images are formed within computer memory during acquisition. Although no images are produced immediately, list mode acquisition is useful because the x, y signals are permanently recorded in computer memory, allowing flexible control over subsequent formatting into digital matrices.

An extension of frame mode acquisition is *multiple-gated acquisition*. In this mode the data from the camera are distributed to a series of matrices in computer memory. A trigger signal (usually a physiologic trigger such as the R wave) controls the distribution of data among the matrices. Immediately after the trigger, data from the camera are placed in the first matrix for a fixed interval. When the interval has elapsed, data are then placed in the second matrix for the same interval. This process continues until the occurrence of a new trigger signal, at which time data distribution restarts at the first frame or until all the assigned matrices in computer memory are used, in which case no data are acquired until the occurrence of a new trigger signal. Multiple-gated acquisition is used to study a repetitive (cyclic) dynamic process. For example, in a cardiac-gated blood pool study, in which the circulating blood is labeled with radioactivity and the beating chambers of the heart examined, the data from the corresponding phases of many heartbeats are superimposed during acquisition, resulting in a series of images representing one "average" cardiac cycle. Typically, the cardiac cycle is divided into 16-64 frames, with each frame representing $\frac{1}{16}$-$\frac{1}{64}$ of the cycle.

Three different types of data sets can be produced from an acquisition. A single, static image can be produced by acquiring a single frame mode image or by ignoring the time markers and formatting list mode data into a single matrix. A dynamic study can be produced by acquiring a series of frame mode images over time or by formatting list mode data into a series of matrices with reference to the embedded time markers in the list. (These images may or may not represent equal intervals and may or may not be contiguous in time.) A cyclic-gated study can be produced by multiple-gated frame mode acquisition or by formatting list mode data into a series of images representing a single average cycle with reference to the embedded trigger markers in the list.

The most common matrix sizes used in nuclear medicine are 64 × 64, 128 × 128, and 256 × 256. The larger the matrix size, the better the digital spatial resolution in the image. The digital sampling requirements necessary to preserve the "optical" or "geometric" spatial resolution that the camera is capable of producing are given by the Nyquist theorem. This theorem states that to accurately portray a signal, the spatial sampling frequency must be twice the highest spatial frequency present in the signal. Thus pixel dimensions should be smaller than half the spatial resolution of the Anger camera. In practice, pixel dimensions range from 2-6 mm.

Multiple Crystal Cameras

Another type of scintillation camera currently in use is the multiple crystal camera. This type of camera was originally developed by Bender and Blau and called an *autofluoroscope*. In the original designs, small physically separate crystals were arranged in a matrix. Special light piping was used to couple the crystals to photomultiplier tubes. The light was arranged in such a way that each crystal was coupled to two photomultiplier tubes. One tube directly determined the x position and the other the y position, without the need for any Anger type of positioning logic (Figure 3-23). Thus the camera could handle very high count rates. Its spatial resolution was limited by the size and number of crystals used in the matrix.

In the current system (Scinticor) a single block of sodium iodide is divided into 400 "detector elements" in a 20 × 20 matrix, by partially cutting through the block. Photomultiplier tubes are directly coupled to the block, without any light pipes. The tubes are arranged in such a way that each scintillation event is seen by two tubes. The difference in signal from the two tubes is electronically coded to directly yield the specific crystal (i.e., x-y) location of the scintillation event. The system comes with a computer for camera operation, display, and processing of data.

The advantages of a multiple crystal camera over an Anger camera are that the multiple crystal camera can handle a higher count rate and the thicker crystal (e.g., 1½ in) is significantly more sensitive for higher energy photons. The main disadvantages are that the field of view is smaller than some large-field Anger cameras and the ultimate spatial resolution is not as good as state-of-the-art Anger cameras.

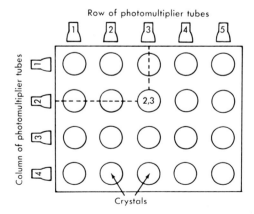

Figure 3-23 Arrangement of crystals and photomultiplier tubes in a multicrystal camera.

EMISSION COMPUTED TOMOGRAPHY

Tomography is the process of producing a picture of a section or slice through an object. In medical imaging, tomography is performed either by transmitting x rays through an object (as in transmission computed tomography, CT scanning), by measuring proton density (as in magnetic resonance imaging, MRI), or by tomographically determining the distribution of radioactivity in a patient (as in emission computed tomography).

Emission computed tomography (ECT), in its most general use, refers to the process of producing a picture of the distribution of radioactivity in a slice through the patient. The slice can be oriented orthogonal to the patient's long axis (a transaxial slice), parallel with the patient's long axis (coronal or sagittal slices), or at any arbitrary oblique angle to the long axis of the body. In the past, ECT utilized either limited angle tomography systems or true transaxial tomographic acquisition and reconstruction (as in CT). At present, only transaxial approaches are in widespread use; these include single photon emission computed tomography (SPECT) and positron emission tomography (PET).

Limited Angle Tomography

Limited angle tomography systems have been designed using multipinhole collimators, Fresnel zone plates, and rotating slant-hole collimators. The essence of limited angle tomography is that images of an object are obtained from a (limited) number of different angles. Of major importance (and in distinction to true transaxial tomography) is that the images are not orthogonal to each other and to the reconstructed slices. Typically, the images do not cover a full 360 degrees around the object. Each image contains information from a number of slices, but the data are different from image to image because of the difference in perspective. In some approaches (e.g., the seven-pinhole collimator system), each image is recognizable and has the appearance of a "conventional" planar image. In other systems (e.g., coded aperture tomography), the individual images are not recognizable as conventional images.

The tomographic reconstruction process involves a shifting and superimposition of original images in such a way that the data from the slice of interest are reinforced, whereas unwanted data are blurred. Although there certainly are differences among the various coded aperture techniques, the important point is that each reconstructed slice contains data from many slices.

The main advantage of limited angle tomographic techniques is simplicity, in that only a specialized collimator is needed, along with the appropriate computer program. The disadvantages include propagation of image data, such as abnormalities, to slices that actually do not contain them and the lack of a quantitative relationship between observed counts and actual radioactivity within the slice of interest. Limited angle tomographic systems were very popular several years ago but have largely been replaced by rotating Anger camera-based transaxial tomography.

Single Photon Emission Computed Tomography

Single photon emission computed tomography (SPECT) is generally used today to refer to true transaxial tomography with standard nuclear medicine radiopharmaceuticals (i.e., those that emit a single photon upon decay, as opposed to positron emitters, whose emissions ultimately result in two coincident annihilation photons). SPECT is performed with either specialized ring detector systems or rotating Anger cameras. The ring systems consist of an array of individual detectors (usually sodium iodide crystals) that surround the patient. These systems, which produce excellent tomograms, tend to be very expensive. By far the most popular method of doing SPECT is with a rotating Anger camera (usually with a large field of view detector) mounted on a special gantry that allows 360-degree rotation around the patient. The initial systems utilized a single Anger camera. At present, multidetector systems with two or three heads are common, since these provide increased sensitivity.

The essence of emission transaxial tomography is similar to that of CT: an object is viewed at a number of angles between 0 and 180 or 360 degrees around it. (Certain types of studies, such as myocardial perfusion studies, produce higher contrast when 180 degrees worth of data, from RAO to LPO, are used for reconstruction.) Images are acquired at many angles, each representing one *projection* of the object. In general, a parallel-hole collimator is used; thus the projections have parallel beam geometry. In some cases it is useful to magnify the image in-plane; this is particularly true when the organ of interest encompasses only a small fraction of the system's field of view. In such a situation a fan-beam collimator may be used. This collimator has holes that converge in the plane of the slice but are parallel from slice-to-slice. Projections from such collimators have fan-beam geometry.

Reconstruction. To reconstruct a slice through an object, each projection need only be a one-dimensional linear scan of the object. The use of an Anger camera, which produces two-dimensional images, therefore allows simultaneous acquisition of data for a number of contiguous transaxial slices. Note, however, that the data used to reconstruct a given slice come from only that slice.

Tomographic reconstruction of transaxial slices by filtered back-projection is the most common computer algorithm for tomography. From the computer's point of view, it does not matter if the data are from a transmission CT scanner, a rotating Anger camera SPECT system, or a PET scanner. The essence of the reconstruction is the smearing back *(back-projection)* into the reconstruction space of each projection, maintaining the correct angular offset (Figure 3-24).

Filtering. Simple back-projection results in a blurred image, with streaks emanating from areas of high activity. (This is called the star artifact.) This artifact can be eliminated by understanding the underlying mathematics of reconstruction, as was first done by Radon in 1917. The mathematical function describing the reconstruction process contains a *filter* that is used to modify each projection before back-projection. Conceptually, this filter produces negative side regions around hot ar-

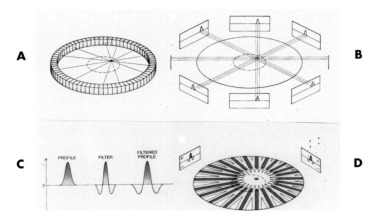

Figure 3-24   Reconstruction process. **A,** Arrangement of detection in positron tomography. **B,** So-called parallel detection geometry, from either reorganizing PET data or directly from Anger camera SPECT with parallel-hole collimation. **C,** Original projection data profile, shape of filter used to modify data, and resulting filtered profile to back-project. **D,** Back-projection process to reconstruct image. (From Ter-Pogossian M et al: *Sci Am* 243(4), 1980.)

eas in each projection. The negative side regions cancel out the positive streaks from other projections during a reconstruction.

Mathematically, a "perfect" filter exists, called the *ramp filter*. This filter progressively boosts the power of higher and higher *spatial frequencies*. Spatial frequencies are analogous to audio (temporal) frequencies. Audio frequencies are expressed in cycles/time; spatial frequencies are expressed in cycles/distance. High spatial frequencies are generated by the edges of organs and other structures in the patient and by image noise. Thus the ramp filter best preserves spatial resolution but also boosts noise significantly. In fact, the noise is no longer governed by Poisson statistics; rather, it is significantly worse. In practice, images are reconstructed with one of many different filters. These filters represent different trade-offs between noise reduction and spatial resolution (Figure 3-25). In general, the filters used in practice are a combination of the ramp filter with a "low-pass" or "smoothing" filter such as a Butterworth filter. The user must specify certain characteristics of the low-pass filter, including the "cutoff frequency" or "critical frequency." The lower this frequency, the poorer the spatial resolution and the greater the noise reduction (i.e., the more the "smoothing" action of the filter).

Two-dimensional prefiltering (followed by ramp filter reconstruction) is preferable to one-dimensional filtering during reconstruction (with the use of other than a simple ramp filter). With two-dimensional pre-

filtering, the spatial resolution in the data remains *isotropic* (uniform in all directions), whereas one-dimensional filtering produces a three-dimensional data set in which the transverse resolution is worse than the axial resolution. One-dimensional filtering thus produces coronal and sagittal images with horizontal smearing and oblique angle reorientations with nonuniform resolution. Contrast enhancing filters, such as the Wiener or Metz filter, are desirable at times.

Sometimes, projection data from adjacent slices are combined to reconstruct transverse slices that are more than 1 pixel thick. In general, even if ultimately the slices will be displayed with greater than 1 pixel thickness, it is preferable to reconstruct transverse slices 1 pixel thick to use as the input for coronal and sagittal image formation and for oblique angle reorientation. After the slices are reoriented, they may be added together if necessary. The use of slices 1 pixel thick for reorientation is superior to starting with thicker transverse slices, since interpolation artifacts are significantly diminished. Automated reorientation approaches are frequently helpful, since these reduce analysis variability, and particularly facilitate comparisons (both stress-to-rest and patient-to-database). In addition to reconstructing transaxial, coronal, sagittal, and oblique slices, it is often helpful to display the data in a "whole body" mode, particularly if the axial coverage is sufficient. This is often performed through a pseudo–three-dimensional volume rendering.

Multidetector SPECT. In an attempt to increase sensitivity, manufacturers are now producing multicamera SPECT systems. These systems incorporate two or three cameras to increase sensitivity. The increase in sensitivity depends on the acquisition arc, as illustrated in Table 3-1.

Optimizing acquisition. In many SPECT acquisitions the organs or structures of interest are at a significant distance from the collimator face (as much as 25-30 cm or more in some views). In an attempt to both increase resolution and (of greater importance) preserve good resolution with depth, the use of longer hole length collimation is desirable. Such collimators are typically labeled as "high-resolution" collimators; the corresponding loss in sensitivity is more than compensated for by the improved resolution at depth. The use of a multi-camera system greatly facilitates the use of high-resolution collimation, because the loss of sensitivity with the use of high-resolution collimators can be (at least partially) compensated for by the increase in sensitivity with the use of multiple detectors. Frequently, the increased sensitivity permits shorter imaging times, which reduces artifacts that might arise from patient motion or organ movement (e.g., so-called *upward creep* of the heart, a gradual upward movement of the heart during SPECT acquisition following a stress study).

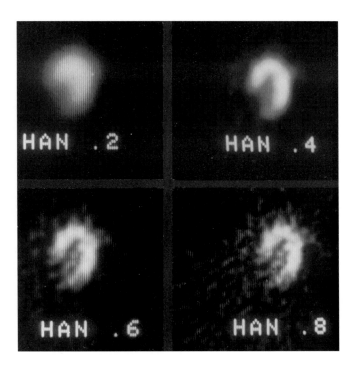

Figure 3-25 Effect of reconstruction of same raw projection data with four different filters.

Table 3-1

	360 Degree acquisition		180 Degree acquisition	
	Acq time	Rel sens	Acq time	Rel sens
Single	30	1	30	1
Double (heads at 180 degrees)	15	2	30	1
Double (heads at 90 degrees)	15	2	15	2
Triple	10	3	20	1.5

Shorter imaging times also reduce artifacts from tracer washout during acquisition.

It is important to preserve the "optical" or "geometric" resolution of the camera in the digital matrix. To do so, the "sampling" must be fine enough to not be the limiting factor. As stated above, according to the Nyquist sampling theorem, the linear pixel dimension must not be greater than half the resolution of the camera. For most practical situations, a pixel size less than about 6 mm is sufficient. It is also important that the angular sampling be adequate. If we assume that the angular sampling should be as fine as the linear sampling, the relationship between the two is given by

$$\text{Pixel size} = \frac{\text{Body diameter}}{\text{Number of pixels spanning body}}$$

$$\text{Angular step size} =$$
$$\frac{\pi \times \text{body diameter}}{\text{Number of projections in 360 degrees}}$$

For pixels to equal the angular step size, balance the following:

$$\frac{\text{Body diameter}}{\text{Number of pixels spanning body}} =$$

$$\frac{\pi \times \text{body diameter}}{\text{Number of projections in 360 degrees}}$$

Therefore the number of projections around 360 degrees should equal π times the number of pixels spanning the body. For example, if a 64×64 matrix is used to acquire SPECT projection data and the organ of interest fills about two thirds of the field of view, then 64 projections should be acquired over 180 degrees, and 128 over 360 degrees.

Studies have shown that Anger cameras must have significantly better performance for adequate SPECT than for adequate planar imaging. For example, nonuniformity must be reduced to less than 1%. This requires acquisition of a 30-120 million count flood for subsequent computer correction of nonuniformities. In older cameras, this correction had to be explicitly performed by the computer operator during the reconstruction process. In present systems, particularly those

with microprocessor-based real-time correction circuits, the correction maps themselves contain sufficient counts to obviate the need for a separate SPECT uniformity correction procedure, provided collimator defects are not present. The camera image must also be mechanically aligned within the computer matrix, or an axis-of-rotation correction should be made.

Positron Emission Tomography

One of the most exciting tomographic techniques is PET scanning. Positron emitting radionuclides are used with this technique. Recall that a positron is an antimatter electron, and consider a positron-emitting radiopharmaceutical distributed in a patient. As a positron is emitted, it travels several millimeters in tissue, depositing its kinetic energy. It then meets a free electron in the tissue, and mutual annihilation occurs. From conservation of energy, two 511 keV annihilation photons appear (511 keV is the energy equivalent to the rest mass of an electron or positron); from conservation of momentum, they are emitted 180 degrees back-to-back. We could use an Anger camera to individually detect these 511 keV annihilation photons. However, it makes more sense to surround the patient with a ring of detectors and electronically couple opposing detectors to simultaneously identify the pair of photons (Figure 3-26).

When two 511 keV annihilation photons are detected by opposing detectors in coincidence, we know that the annihilation event must have occurred along the line joining the two detectors. We thus know the direction of travel of the photons, without the need for a collimator. Conceptually, the raw PET scan data consist of a number of these *coincidence lines*. Reconstruction could simply be the drawing of these lines: they would cross and superimpose wherever there was activity in the patient. In practice, the data set is reorganized into projections, and filtered back-projection is used. In some PET scanners the difference in arrival times of the two photons is used to position the event along the coincidence line. In practice, time-of-flight spatial resolution is limited to several centimeters because of

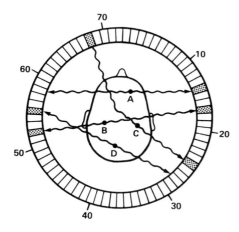

Figure 3-26 Geometry of PET detection system. Event *B* represents true coincidence detection, simultaneous detection of one gamma ray each from events *A* and *D* produces accidental coincidence detection, and event *C* represents scatter coincidence detection.

temporal resolution limitations (hundreds of psec); these limitations are due to both electronics and the decay time of the scintillation detectors used. (Decay time refers to the amount of time required for light to be emitted following deposition of energy in the crystal.) Thus, time-of-flight is used in combination with back-projection reconstruction. Even without time-of-flight, PET differs from SPECT in that the "electronic collimation" of coincidence counting reduces the need for conventional lead collimation, thus increasing sensitivity.

The excitement about PET is due to both the chemistry and physics inherent in positron tomography. The most commonly used radionuclides—^{11}C, ^{13}N, ^{15}O, and ^{18}F—are isotopes of elements that occur naturally in organic molecules. (Fluorine usually does not but is a bioisoteric substitute for a methane group.) Thus radiopharmaceutical synthesis is simplified, and the tracer principle (which mandates as small a change in the molecule to be traced as possible) is better satisfied. Indeed, useful PET radiopharmaceuticals are now available to measure in vivo such important physiologic and biochemical processes as blood flow, oxygen, glucose, and free fatty acid metabolism, amino acid transport, pH, and neuroreceptor densities. The short half-lives of the radionuclides (^{11}C, 20 min; ^{13}N, 10 min; ^{15}O, 2 min; and ^{18}F, 110 min) permit the acquisition of serial studies on the same day without background activity from prior injections interfering with the measurements. The physics of PET permits greater quantitative accuracy and precision. The use of small, high-density crystals improves spatial resolution (about 4 mm in the best commercial PET scanners). The lack of lead collimation to determine photon direction dramatically increases sensitivity. Finally, coincidence detection allows mathematically accurate attenuation correction.

Unfortunately, PET scanners generally cost over $2 million. They require more space, more electricity, and more air-conditioning than Anger cameras. Finally, although some generator systems exist (e.g., $^{68}Ge/^{68}Ga$), a cyclotron is required to produce ^{11}C, ^{13}N, and ^{15}O. Because of the short half-lives of these radionuclides, the cyclotron is generally on site. Cyclotrons cost a minimum of $1 million and are quite expensive to install and operate. At present, PET scanning is confined to 90 centers around the world.

Positron Tomography With Scintillation Camera Systems

In theory, positron-emitting radionuclides could be used in SPECT in two ways: collimated detection of one or both of the two photons in noncoincidence mode (i.e., by one or more collimated heads in a conventional SPECT system), or uncollimated coincidence detection of both photons by opposing detectors (i.e., by a dual-head, uncollimated 180-degree SPECT system). Each approach has its advantages and disadvantages.

511 keV collimators for SPECT. Most manufacturers have now developed 511 keV collimators. There are two main issues in the use of such collimators: (1) the design trade-offs between collimator resolution and sensitivity and (2) appropriate "tuning" and "correction" of the camera head's intrinsic spatially varying energy response, linearity, and uniformity.

With respect to the trade-off between resolution and sensitivity, the "optimum" design would be that which produces the highest image quality and accuracy in a given situation. For cardiac imaging with fluorodeoxyglucose (FDG), an abnormality is a *decrease* in FDG concentration compared with surrounding normal myocardium. Given the relatively large vascular territories involved, such abnormalities, like perfusion abnormalities, may commonly represent relatively large areas of myocardium. For tumor imaging with FDG, an abnormality is an *increase* in FDG concentration compared with surrounding normal tissues. These lesions may be very small in size (sub-cm). It is conceivable that the optimum collimator for FDG myocardial viability studies would require good sensitivity—even at the expense of resolution—to produce low noise images that depict a small reduction in FDG in a relatively large area, whereas the optimum collimator for FDG tumor detection/localization studies would require good sensitivity—even at the expense of resolution—to produce images with sufficiently low partial volume effects that small hot lesions are depicted with adequate quantitative recovery to be visible. The optimum design for these two applications may be significantly different.

One additional problem in 511 keV collimator design relates to the required septal thickness. Septal thickness depends on the minimum required path length for adequate attenuation. That is, the septa must be thick enough that photons traveling through them have a high probability of being absorbed. The μ for lead at 511 keV is 1.746 cm^{-1}. For comparison, the μ for lead at 140 keV is 21.43 cm^{-1}. Thus septal thickness for a given hole diameter and length must be significantly greater for 511 keV collimators than for 140 keV collimators.

For roughly equivalent resolution, low energy collimators have approximately three to four times the sensitivity of ultra–high-energy collimators. Accordingly, 511 keV collimators of comparable resolution yield about one fourth the counts for the same acquisition time. It is also of interest to note that the manufacturers have chosen long holes, which yield reasonable resolution at distances greater than 10 cm (i.e., good design for SPECT, rather than planar imaging). Because of the long holes, they are able to use larger diameters, which gain back some of the sensitivity. In spite of the difficulties in designing 511 keV collimators that are capable of producing images with adequate quality and accuracy, several important studies suggest that such an approach can provide useful clinical data.

511 keV coincidence imaging. As an alternative to the use of 511 keV collimators with "conventional" SPECT, dual-head SPECT systems may be used without collimators in a coincidence mode. The opposing cameras are electronically configured in coincidence, and the coincident detection of the two 511 keV annihilation photons is used to define a "coincidence line" that passes through the annihilation site. This annihilation site differs from the positron emission site by about 1 mm, which fundamentally limits the achievable resolution in coincidence imaging. However, the lack of collimation, coupled with high-speed electronics, permits spatial resolution only slightly worse than the intrinsic resolution of the camera (i.e., about 4-5 mm).

The lack of collimation also means that the sensitivity is quite high (at least a factor of 10^4 or higher per head than with collimation). However, since both photons must be detected, the effective sensitivity gain is about 100. Furthermore, since both photons must exit the body, the overall attenuation is actually greater than at 140 keV. Consequently, overall sensitivity is only about a factor of 10 higher. The count rate capability of the camera is not influenced by the presence or absence of a collimator; it thus remains the same in coincidence mode. Thus the activity in the field of view must be significantly decreased (e.g., to about 1 mCi) relative to "conventional" SPECT imaging to prevent operation of the heads in a paralyzable region.

This point is particularly important because only about 1% of the so-called singles counts at each head produce coincidence counts. Thus for a coincidence count rate of 10^3 counts/sec, the expected singles count rate is about 10^5 counts/sec. Thus to have a usefully high coincidence count rate, each camera's count rate capability must be exceptionally good (e.g., >500,000 counts/sec). To achieve this count rate capability, pulse shortening must be used. In addition, fewer photomultiplier tubes are allowed to contribute toward the positioning of each event. It is worth noting that such a system should not be called a "SPECT" system, since it deals with two photons, not "single photons."

Effects of Resolution, Scatter, and Attenuation in ECT

From a physics point of view, there are five major factors that affect the appearance of images and accurate quantification of absolute radioactivity in ECT. These include (1) attenuation of photons by tissue; (2) transaxial spatial resolution and effective slice thickness of the SPECT or PET scanner; (3) detection of scattered photons; (4) accidental counting of "random" (nonpaired) photons in coincidence, applicable only to PET; and (5) "noise" resulting from the random nature of radioactive decay. It is worth noting that these factors also affect planar imaging.

Resolution effects. All tomographic scanners have a limited ability to resolve small objects. The spatial resolution of a scanner can be thought of as that distance by which two small point sources of radioactivity must be separated to be distinguished as separate in the reconstructed image. Finite spatial resolution results in two important effects. First, the image is blurred, with the degree of blurring dependent on the spatial resolution. This blurring prevents the delineation of edges of larger structures and may not allow the visualization of smaller ones as distinct objects. Furthermore, neighboring areas are smeared and averaged together, reducing the measured value in the areas with greater radioactivity and increasing it in the areas with lesser radioactivity.

The second effect is more subtle. Finite spatial resolution produces an underestimation of radioactivity in small structures, with progressive underestimation as the structures get smaller. The effect is not eliminated until the object is approximately three times the resolution of the scanner. For example, the apparent radioactivity concentration in different portions of the myocardial wall will be influenced by myocardial wall thickness. Thinner regions of the myocardial wall will appear to have reduced radiotracer concentration. These effects, which also apply to the axial resolution (sometimes mistakenly called "slice thickness") of the scanner, are sometimes referred to as *partial volume effects*. Reduction of these effects requires improvement in spatial resolution, for example, through the use of higher resolution collimation and a filter with a higher frequency cut-off.

Scatter effects. The photons detected in SPECT and PET are electromagnetic radiation. As such, they may undergo two major types of interactions in the patient: photoelectric effect and Compton scattering. The photoelectric effect results in complete absorption of the photon, reducing the observed count rate, although scattered photons may still be detected. Large-angle scatter produces a low-level background "haze" in the image, which reduces contrast. Small-angle scatter influences apparent resolution. Approaches to reducing scatter effects include the use of narrower pulse height windows and subtraction of (estimated) scatter from the images. Both of these approaches reduce the net number of counts, and thus increase the noise. Large-angle scatter can be estimated through the use of a second "scatter" pulse height window or through the use of two or three windows around the photopeak (in which the scatter in the primary photopeak window is estimated by interpolation or extrapolation from the counts in the "accessory" windows). If a separate scatter correction is used, this must be taken into account when utilizing attenuation correction schemes.

Attenuation effects. Attenuation is produced through loss of photons by a combination of absorption (by photoelectric effect) and scatter (photons that Compton scatter in the patient and exit the field of view). Attenuation produces a gradual, progressive underestimation of radioactivity from the edge to the center of the body, by about a factor of five.

There are two main approaches to attenuation correction. In the first, attenuation is measured before the SPECT or PET scan begins by transmitting photons from a point, line, sheet, or ring source of single-photon or positron-emitting activity through the patient's body and relating this measurement to a second one without the patient. From these two measurements, the attenuation experienced by radioactivity at each point within the body can be determined.

The second approach to attenuation correction does not require any additional measurements. After the uncorrected image is reconstructed, the computer operator defines the body with either an ellipse or body-following outline. An average value for attenuation is then assumed for each point within this outline of the body. (This average value depends on both the tissues involved and the characteristics of the particular SPECT or PET scanner.) It is important to define the outline of the entire body, not just the organ of interest. Although this approach is easier than the transmission-based approach, it is not very accurate in the torso, where the attenuation coefficient varies significantly. Consequently, virtually all PET attenuation correction schemes in practice utilize a transmission

scan, and such approaches are becoming more popular in SPECT, particularly for cardiac SPECT.

QUALITY CONTROL

The interpretation of all diagnostic nuclear medicine procedures is based on the assumption that the performance of the system used for data acquisition, display, and analysis is reliable and accurate. To provide evidence that data of diagnostic quality are present, a standardized program of routine system performance assessment is essential. The quality control of nuclear instrumentation is the cornerstone of an effective overall nuclear medicine quality assurance program.

Quality control is the term used to refer to the routine assessment of instrument performance in nuclear medicine. Quality control, or "QC," is extremely important. It is first used to establish a baseline level of performance, which can be compared with the manufacturer's specifications and other units in the field. It is then used daily to monitor the continued performance of the instrument. Changes can be judged against both the baseline performance (relative assessment) and against standards or thresholds for action (absolute performance).

Survey Meter Quality Control

The survey meter is an essential part of a good radiation safety program. These meters are typically used to measure either exposure or count rate. Two types of survey instruments are commonly used in a clinical nuclear medicine unit. An ionization chamber (often referred to as a *cutie-pie*) is used in areas where high fluxes of x rays or gamma rays must be measured, and the Geiger-Mueller counter, because of its sensitivity, is used for low-level surveys. They both require annual calibration and daily constancy testing with long-lived radionuclide standards. Calibration techniques are the same for both types of instruments.

Accuracy. Survey instruments are calibrated before their first use, annually, and following repair. Calibration is performed at two different operating points on the instrument's read-out scale. The two points are approximately $1/3$ and $2/3$ of full scale. The standard used must be traceable within 5% accuracy to the National Institute of Standards and Technology (NIST, formerly known as the National Bureau of Standards). The same formula used to convert known exposure rate to activity can be rearranged to convert known activity to exposure rate:

$$E = AG/d^2$$

where E is the measured exposure rate, A is the activity of the source, d is the distance between the source and the detector, and G is the specific gamma ray constant. Readings are then made of the standard with the survey meter at those same distances. Each scale setting is calibrated over its entire range. The calculated points are plotted versus the measured readings (Figure 3-27). The line formed will allow one to determine the true exposure from the actual reading. Some users like to minify the graph and attach it to the survey meter so that the actual exposure rate can be easily ascertained while the instrument is being used. The indicated exposure rate should not differ from the calculated exposure rate by more than 20%. Many departments send their instruments to qualified laboratories for calibration if they do not wish to keep a standard source on hand.

It is extremely important to remember the differences between ionization chambers and Geiger-Mueller counters. Ionization chambers respond in proportion to the total energy deposited in the detector. Thus the output of an ionization chamber can be directly related to exposure rate, no matter what the energy of each incoming photon. On the other hand, Geiger-Mueller detectors produce pulses whose sizes are independent of energy deposited. Thus count rate may only be related to exposure rate if the energy of the radiation is known. Accordingly, the use of Geiger-Mueller counters to assess exposure is only possible if the photon energy used to calibrate the detector is the same as that of the source being measured.

Constancy. In addition to assessing accuracy, a reference source with a long half-life must be used to check the *constancy* of the survey meter's performance. The initial measurement of the source is made at the time of calibration and should be conspicuously noted on the instrument. The source is then counted with the same geometry each day the instrument is used, after a battery change, and after any maintenance. If the exposure rate (or count rate) is not within 10% of the expected results, the instrument should be recalibrated.

Dose Calibrator Quality Control

The accuracy of the dose of radiopharmaceutical given to patients depends on the performance of the dose calibrator. An acceptable quality control program for radionuclide dose calibrators consists of a series of procedures that measure its accuracy, linearity, geometry dependence, and constancy.

Accuracy. Instrument accuracy testing is performed at installation and annually thereafter. The accuracy of the dose calibrator is measured with at least two sealed reference standards whose activity is traceable to NIST. The instrument should be calibrated with standard sources of the radionuclide of interest whenever possible. When the use of short-lived nuclide standards is not possible, a long-lived standard of similar energy can be used, provided that the appropriate correction factors are employed. Several different radionuclides, such as ^{57}Co, ^{137}Cs, and ^{133}Ba, may be used. The activity shall be at least 50 μCi and preferably 200 μCi or more. At least one of the sources must have a principal photon energy between 100 keV and 500 keV.

By correcting the standards for decay, the exact activity is known for comparison with the amount indicated by the dose calibrator. The average of several net-activity measurements should be compared to the activity calculated for that particular standard. According to the Nuclear Regulatory Commission (NRC), if the measured activity is within 10% of the standard, the dose calibrator is functioning with acceptable accuracy. So-called agreement states (such as Maryland and California, which regulate activities themselves under an agreement with the NRC) may have different limits.

Constancy. Constancy is checked each day the instrument is used. After the accuracy of the dose calibrator has been determined, the constancy of its performance is monitored by daily testing with long-lived standards at each of the frequently used radionuclide settings. An activity control chart is established for each of the radionuclide settings (Figure 3-28). The average reading of the standard is obtained and plotted on semilogarithmic graph paper. The activity level of the standard is calculated, with use of the appropriate decay schedule, and plotted. These points are connected with a straight line, which indicates the decay of the stan-

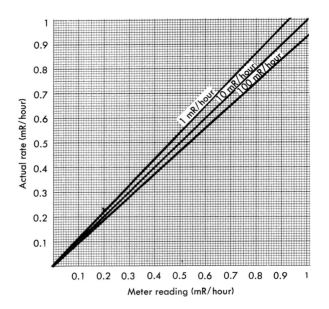

Figure 3-27 Survey meter calibration graph. Convert meter reading (abscissa) to actual dose rate by reading upward to intercept point and then across to ordinate. Multiple ranges may be plotted on the same graph.

dard. Two straight lines are drawn above and below the decay line, indicating the tolerance limits ($\pm 10\%$ for NRC-regulated states). Daily readings of the standard are plotted and should fall within the tolerance limit lines. If a reading repeatedly falls outside of the limits, the calibrator should be taken out of service until the problem is identified and corrected. Personal computer-based spreadsheets may easily be programmed to generate tables and graphs for this purpose.

Linearity. Instrument linearity is measured at installation and quarterly thereafter. The dose calibrator must function linearly over the range of its use between the highest dosage that will be administered to a patient and 20 μCi (for NRC-regulated states). There are several methods that may be used to determine the dose calibrator's response at different activity levels. A convenient method uses a vial of ^{99m}Tc that contains the desired amount of activity. The vial is assayed at frequent intervals, usually twice each day, over the appropriate range of activities. The observed activity versus time is plotted on semilogarithmic paper, and a best-fit straight line is drawn through the points. A point is chosen on the line where the accuracy of the measurement has been established by a reference standard and a straight line constructed with a slope equivalent to the half-life of ^{99m}Tc (6 hours). Compare this straight line to the line generated by the data from the observed counts. Any difference greater than 10% (again, for NRC-regulated states) indicates the need for repair or adjustment. Note that the use of radionuclides with a longer half-life than that for ^{99m}Tc would require a correspondingly longer measurement period.

An alternative method uses a set of calibrated lead attenuation sleeves to assess changes in linearity once the system's linearity has been established. It offers the advantage of shortening the time required to perform the test from days to minutes.

Geometric calibration. Geometric calibration is performed at installation and whenever a change is made in the type of vial or syringe used in radiopharmaceutical processing or the chamber is repaired. Changing the radionuclide sample volume or configuration can significantly affect the measurement of the sample's activity. To measure the effect of changing the volume of liquid within a vial, a 30 ml vial containing 1 mCi of ^{99m}Tc in a volume of 1 ml is used. This is assayed, and the volume is increased with water in steps of 1, 4, 8, 10, 15, 20, and 25 ml, with assays being taken at each step. The net activity at each volume is determined by subtraction of the background. One of the volumes should be selected as the standard, and the correction factor for each of the other volumes can be calculated as the ratio of the measured activity for the standard reference volume divided by the measured activity for each of the other volumes. These volume-specific multiplicative correction factors should be plotted against the volume on linear graph paper. Alternatively, the data may be put in tabular form. One can then calculate the true activity of a sample by taking the correction factor determined for that volume times the measured activity of the sample. This procedure should be used to determine the correction factors for various types and sizes of syringes, since significant changes in the measurement can occur when the radionuclide is assayed in different materials or the wall thickness of the container changes.

It is important to note that the sensitivity of a dose calibrator is affected by backscattering of photons by the shielding of the unit or other adjacent objects. An erroneous activity reading may be obtained if these variables are changed after calibration of the instrument.

The dose calibrator is a tool upon which all nuclear medicine departments rely heavily. Assurance that the indicated activity on the dose calibrator is close to the true amount is important for the proper dispensing of radiopharmaceuticals to the patients in technologists' care.

Quality Control of Nonimaging Scintillation Detectors

Scintillation probes are employed for external organ counting, and well detectors are used for sample counting. Their reliable performance is essential for accurate results in a variety of in vivo and in vitro studies.

Calibration. Calibration initially involves energy calibration, in which the relationship between pulse height units and energy is determined (and set). First, the pulse height spectrum is obtained for a long-lived radionuclide, usually ^{137}Cs, by selection of a narrow window width (e.g., 10 pulse height units) and then by obtaining a series of counts at each 10 pulse height unit increment of the spectrum until the principal photo-

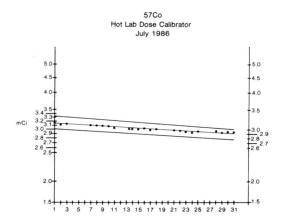

Figure 3-28 Typical count control chart used for measurement of dose calibrator constancy.

peak is passed or until the count rate approaches the background level. Plotting the resultant counts on linear graph paper will yield a pulse height spectrum. The pulse height position of the photopeak indicates the relationship between pulse height and energy. It is possible to adjust the amplifier gain or the high voltage across the photomultiplier tube to "move" the photopeak to a different pulse height position. It is frequently useful to move the photopeak to a pulse height position corresponding to photopeak energy (e.g., 662 pulse height units for the 662 keV photon from ^{137}Cs).

By measuring the FWHM of the ^{137}Cs photopeak, one may determine the percent energy resolution for that radionuclide (see Figure 3-7). Typical values for percent energy resolution should be less than 10%. Ordinarily, this procedure is performed by the manufacturer, and the values obtained are furnished with the instrument. It is prudent to repeat the procedure upon installation and annually thereafter.

Daily calibration should include counting a long-lived reference source at specified window and baseline settings while either the fine gain or the high voltage is adjusted. This procedure is referred to as *peaking*. In other words, a series of counts at various voltages or gain settings are made until the maximum count rate is determined. The voltage or gain setting that yields the maximum or peak counts is recorded in the daily calibration log. Background counts accumulated for a statistically sufficient interval are recorded as well. The number of counts obtained at the peak is plotted on a control chart. This control chart is merely a graph of the number of source counts plotted on the ordinate, with time (usually 1 year) represented on the abscissa. A line is drawn representing the estimate of the source counts over time. Parallel lines representing ±1, 2, and 3 standard deviations are drawn as well. If daily counts fall outside the +3 standard deviation limits repeatedly, the instrument most likely is malfunctioning.

Reproducibility. The ability of the instrument to reproducibly and reliably record and display events detected can be assessed by performing standard statistical fits of repetitive sample counts obtained using a radioactive source. The most prevalent statistical models used are the chi-square test, Poisson standard deviation, and Gaussian standard deviation. These statistical goodness-of-fit formulas should be performed on a minimum of 10 repetitive counts (observations), accumulating a statistically valid number of counts (greater than 10,000). It is sufficient to perform these tests initially when a program is begun or when a new instrument is placed in use. The data should be recorded and used for comparison at least twice per year and whenever the instrument is suspected of malfunctioning.

Reproducible sample geometry in multisample well counters is affected by the mechanical devices that po-

sition the sample in the well. There may be a combination of mechanical arms or elevators moving or lowering the sample into the well. Because of their mechanical design, the wearing of parts and belts or service adjustments may affect sample positioning and hence counting efficiency. This error may first appear as a decrease in the count rate of the long-lived standard used to monitor count rate stability and spectrometer calibration. As a result, it is not advisable to use the chi-square test for measurements made across samples that involve mechanical motion.

Calibration of Multicrystal Well Counters

The development of multicrystal gamma counters to increase the efficiency of counting large numbers of radioassay samples has introduced a special problem in assessing the balance or sensitivity of 10, 16, or 20 small sodium iodide crystals and their corresponding electronics. Discrepancies in the sensitivity of these multidetectors can drastically and insidiously affect the results of critically important tests. Most multicrystal systems employ a microprocessor-based program to assess the *balance* of detectors and often times match detector output by mathematically applying correction factors to counts from individual wells. The intrinsic balance of each well in these counters should be evaluated daily using a single long-lived standard of appropriate energy and count rate or a set of matched standards.

The actual measurement spread is determined by counting a source sequentially in all detectors for a minimum of 100,000 counts. The spread is defined by

$$\text{spread} = (\text{max} - \text{min})/\text{max} \times 100\%$$

where *max* and *min* are the maximum and minimum counts obtained from a set of detectors at any given count rate. The spread of absolute count rate should not exceed 3% at a counting rate not exceeding 10,000 counts/sec.

Scintillation Camera Quality Control

The performance of a scintillation camera system must be assessed each day of use to assure the acquisition of diagnostically reliable images. Performance can be affected by changes or failure of individual system components or subsystems and environmental conditions such as electrical power supply fluctuations, physical shock, temperature changes, humidity, dirt, and background radiation. Testing procedures that elucidate the presence of these performance-affecting variables must be utilized.

The most useful data to determine acceptability of camera performance reflect the parameters of field uniformity, spatial resolution, linearity, and sensitivity. These parameters must be measured at the time of installation to confirm specifications and provide the standard for all subsequent performance evaluations. These initial measurements are usually part of acceptance testing. It is also important to test the camera after service has been performed.

Uniformity. Perhaps the most basic measure of camera performance is *flood-field uniformity*. This is the ability of the camera to depict a uniform distribution of activity as uniform. It is assessed by "flooding" the camera with a uniform field of radiation and assessing the uniformity of the resulting image. In the past, field non-uniformity was thought to arise primarily from differences in sensitivity across the crystal face. To correct the nonuniformity, a uniform flood or sheet source of radioactivity was imaged and recorded in an electronic memory in the camera. Clinical images were corrected during acquisition by either adding counts to the image in areas where the flood had too few counts relative to the other areas, or by subtracting (i.e., purposely not recording) counts in areas with too many counts.

It is now well-known that the majority of the nonuniformity in a camera occurs as a result of *spatial distortion* (i.e., the mispositioning of events). To correct this distortion, references images are acquired and digital correction maps are generated and stored. Each map contains values that represent x,y correction shifts. Sophisticated microprocessor circuitry is used to reposition each count in real time during acquisition using these shifts. With many current cameras it is best to acquire correction maps with the same radionuclide as used for patient imaging. In some cameras several sets of corrections maps are stored on the computer, representing all the radionuclides used in the nuclear medicine department and the appropriate set chosen for a given patient study.

Variation in the position of a pulse from different areas of the camera within the pulse height window can also produce nonuniformities. This spatially dependent energy variation may also be corrected by microprocessor circuitry. The combination of energy variation and spatial distortion is responsible for loss of spatial resolution and imperfect linearity and uniformity. In present cameras, explicit uniformity correction is typically carried out with multiplicative factors, only after spatial distortion (and spatially dependent energy response) corrections.

Spatial resolution. Spatial resolution has been previously defined. A transmission phantom is commonly used to measure camera resolution. This type of phantom consists of some pattern in lead. The alternating patterns produce closely spaced areas of differing activity levels, which by definition allow for the analysis of resolution performance. The better the spatial resolution, the better the ability to detect small abnormalities manifested as different radionuclide concentra-

tions in clinical images. Since such phantom should only be used without a collimator to measure intrinsic performance, it is also useful at times to assess resolution with a point or line source. The spread of the point or line is indicative of the degree of blurring (loss of resolution) of the camera.

Linearity. Linearity deals with the ability to reproduce a linear activity source as linear in the image. A phantom with a linear arrangement of bars or holes is usually used. The image produced should look exactly like the phantom (i.e., straight lines should be reproduced as straight).

Approaches to Camera Quality Control

When embarking on a scintillation camera quality control program, a department must make several decisions regarding methods and apparatus to be used. There are three major decisions to be made: which radionuclides to use; whether to use intrinsic or extrinsic testing; and which phantoms to use.

The radionuclide used should be of a similar energy to (if not the same as) the radionuclide used most frequently for actual patient imaging. Because of the widespread use of ^{99m}Tc-labeled radiopharmaceuticals, the two most commonly used radionuclides are ^{99m}Tc itself and ^{57}Co. There are advantages and disadvantages for both radionuclides. ^{57}Co, with a principal gamma-ray energy of 122 keV, meets the criterion of a similar energy. The half-life of 271 days allows for longer use before replenishment or replacement and also facilitates daily sensitivity checks. A disadvantage is the relatively high cost compared with ^{99m}Tc. Another consideration is that the microprocessor-based correction maps may be appropriate for the ^{57}Co setting (122 keV) but not for the ^{99m}Tc setting (140 keV). (This is particularly possible if ^{57}Co was used to acquire the maps.) This could lead to a false sense of security when one sees acceptable ^{57}Co images, whereas the clinical images using ^{99m}Tc might be unacceptable. This would support the case for using ^{99m}Tc as a source, since it is the radionuclide used in the majority of nuclear medicine imaging procedures. Its availability makes cost an insignificant factor. The 6-hour half-life does necessitate daily replenishment.

Intrinsic testing (Figure 3-29, *A*) involves measuring the performance of the system without the collimator. A small volume or point source of the chosen radionuclide is positioned at a distance of five times the diameter of the camera's useful field of view to give a uniform radiation field across the crystal (Figure 3-30). Care must be taken to avoid contaminating or damaging the exposed crystal. The phenomenon known as *edge packing* is seen with some gamma cameras. This area of increased counts around the edge of the image must be masked for those scintillation cameras with

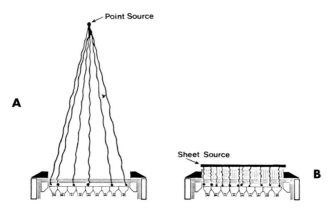

Figure 3-29 Schematic representation of (**A**) intrinsic and (**B**) extrinsic scintillation camera testing.

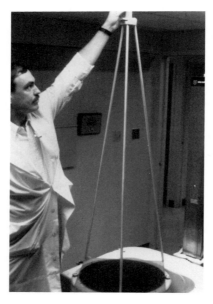

Figure 3-30 Tripod source receptacle used for intrinsic scintillation camera testing.

uniformity correction devices. The advantage of intrinsic testing is that a uniform radiation field is easily obtained using a small amount of radioactivity of the type used in clinical studies.

Extrinsic testing (Figure 3-29, *B*) allows evaluation of the total system, including the collimator. When a collimator is used during assessment, a planar source having a uniform radionuclide distribution is placed on the collimator. Two types of planar sources are in use: a Lucite sheet impregnated with ^{57}Co and a liquid-filled, flat plastic phantom. The solid sheet consists of an epoxy type of material with ^{57}Co dispersed uniformly throughout, ranging in size from 30-50 cm (Figure 3-31). The liquid-filled planar source (Figure 3-32), commonly called a *flood phantom*, is usually water filled, and radioactivity must be added. The phantom is a sealable, flat, thin-walled container usually made of Lucite.

It has a cavity that can be filled and then sealed. Thorough mixing of the radionuclide in the flood phantom is essential, since any nonuniformity in the distribution of radioactivity in the phantom could be interpreted as a camera malfunction. When this problem is suspected on a flood-field image, the phantom should be rotated 90 degrees and a second image should be obtained. A change in the pattern between images indicates a mixing problem in the phantom. Various examples are shown in Figure 3-33.

Analog cameras, not interfaced to computers, form photographic images in real time during acquisition. The use of exactly the same activity each day permits one to check the CRT intensity on such cameras. Figure 3-34 shows that a change in source strength greatly affects film density even though all imaging parameters including total counts were kept constant. This increased density at high count rates is due to two factors. When the electron gun in the CRT repeatedly strikes the same spot on the phosphor screen, the light output increases or it experiences pulse buildup. Also, the high rate of light deposition on the film causes a failure of the reciprocal nature of producing the film density. The effects of film exposure on uniformity and resolution images are illustrated in subsequent figures. In addition, maintenance of a reproducible source strength allows a quality control check on the sensitivity or counting efficiency of the system.

Quality Control Phantoms

Many transmission phantoms have been developed for resolution and linearity testing, with several gaining the widest acceptance. An ideal phantom allows the accurate, simultaneous acquisition of an image that evaluates the parameters of spatial resolution, linearity, and spatial distortion. Some controversy exists regarding the ideal phantom to be used in performing these checks. Two criteria must be met in selecting the phantom. First, the size and spacing of the holes or bars of the phantom selected should stress the maximum resolving capability of the instrument. Second, the same size pattern of holes or bars should be used to cover the entire camera field of view.

Three of the most widely used phantoms are pictured in Figure 3-35. The *parallel-line equal-space (PLES) phantom* consists of lead bars that have the same width and spacing and are embedded in Lucite. The bar width can be selected to match the lower limits of spatial resolution of the camera being evaluated. Two transmission images taken 90 degrees to each other provide the assessment of spatial resolution, linearity, and spatial distortion for the entire detector area.

The *orthogonal-hole (OH) phantom* consists of a sheet of lead in which rows and columns of equal-diameter holes are arranged at right angles to one another. Phantoms are available with hole diameters 0.64 cm (¼

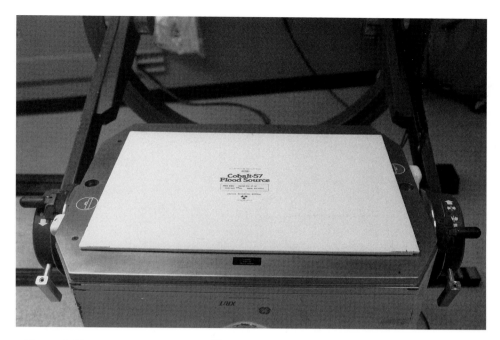

Figure 3-31 Planar disk source of ^{57}Co used for extrinsic scintillation camera testing.

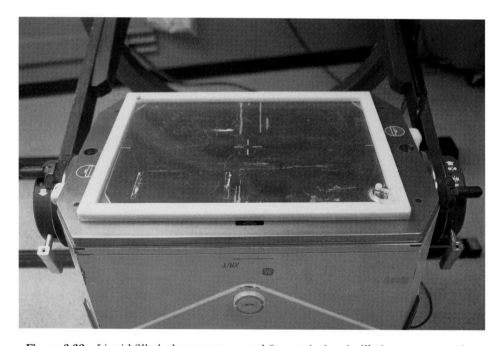

Figure 3-32 Liquid-filled planar source used for extrinsic scintillation camera testing.

in), 0.48 cm (³⁄₁₆ in), and 0.32 cm (⅛ in) spaced at intervals of 1 cm (½ in), 0.96 cm (⅜ in), and 0.64 cm (¼ in), respectively. A match of hole size to the lower limits of spatial resolution for the camera is important. A single image allows the assessment of spatial resolution, linearity, and spatial distortion for the entire detector area. The orthogonal and PLES phantoms are considered comparable for all the parameters being assessed.

Four different widths of bars and spaces are used in the *quadrant bar phantom*. The bars in the quadrants are arranged so that each set of bars is oriented 90 degrees from the set adjacent to it. The spaces and bars in each quadrant are equal. A higher resolution phantom going down to 2 mm bars is available for newer high-performance cameras. Measurement of the resolution of all detector regions requires imaging of the phantom in different positions, which is inconvenient. It

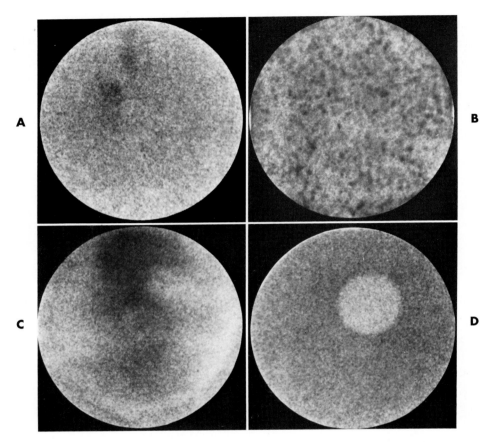

Figure 3-33 Complications arising from improper flood phantom preparation. **A,** Adherence of macroaggregated albumin particles to inner surface. **B,** Particulate formation within liquid. **C,** Incomplete mixing of radionuclide. **D,** Air bubble simulating a photomultiplier tube malfunction.

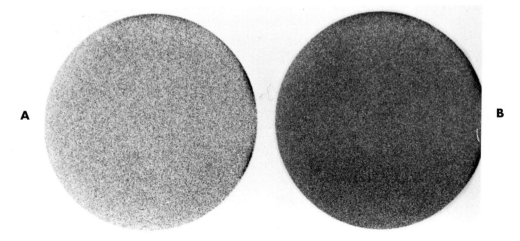

Figure 3-34 Effects of source activity on film density. Film density increases (**A** to **B**) when source activity is doubled. All other imaging parameters are kept constant.

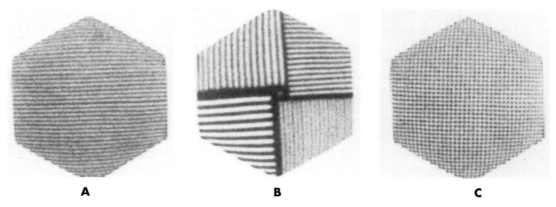

Figure 3-35 Transmission phantoms. **A,** Parallel-line equal-space (PLES) phantom. **B,** Four quadrant bar phantom. **C,** Smith orthogonal-hole phantom. (From Rollo FD: *Nuclear medicine physics, instrumentation, and agents,* St. Louis, 1977, Mosby.)

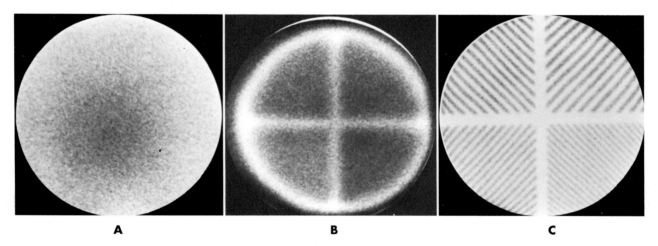

Figure 3-36 Source activity is important in assessing performance. Nonuniformity **(A)** and loss of resolution **(B)** occur when activity is too great. **C,** Resolution returns when activity is reduced to proper level.

should be noted that the effective resolution of the camera is about 1.7 times the smallest visible bars. The advantage of this phantom over the PLES and OH phantoms is that, because of the presence of four different bar size/spacing combinations, the same phantom can be used to assess cameras with a range of intrinsic resolutions.

Whatever source is used, the count rate should not exceed 20,000 counts/sec. At excessive counting rates, poor uniformity and spatial resolution arise because of counting losses and pulse pileup (Figure 3-36). It is also important to note that these transmission phantoms should only be used for intrinsic testing, without a collimator. Use of the phantom with a collimator can lead to moire type of artifacts because of the interference patterns produced by the combination of the transmission phantom pattern with the "pattern" of holes in the collimator. This is particularly a problem with poor-resolution and high-energy collimators; some are willing to use these transmission phantoms with a collimator as long as it's a high-resolution or ultra–high-

resolution design. It is also important to note that when acquiring transmission phantom images by computer, the digital acquisition matrix can act as a pattern. Thus these types of images should be acquired into a very large matrix (at least 256×256 and preferably 512×512).

Routine Camera Quality Control Procedures

Once intrinsic-versus-extrinsic testing, source considerations, and phantoms have been discussed and decisions have been made, a daily quality control program for scintillation cameras can be established. One of the keys to a reliable quality control program is the standardized performance of the quality control procedures. A number of steps dealing with camera system setup must be taken prior to any quality control imaging.

Photopeak settings. The correct energy window for the radionuclide being used must be selected, and the photopeak must be centered in the window. If peaking is performed manually, the setting should be recorded. A correct photopeak setting is absolutely essential for optimum camera performance. All the parameters being assessed for quality control are adversely affected if the system is off-peak. The clinical ramifications of incorrect photopeaking are seen in Figures 3-20 and 3-37.

Orientation controls. Image orientation must remain constant for quality control images, so the same detector area is always recorded in the same position on the image. This is important in the evaluation of gradual performance degradation in a particular detector area.

Intensity. Daily use of the same CRT intensity settings and image size to produce field uniformity images should result in a comparable daily image density. This ensures that established CRT intensities used for clinical studies remain valid. When the same CRT intensity does not reproduce the same image density daily, the most common causes are electronic drift, aging of the CRT, and changes in the film processor (if transparency film is used). The same image-recording devices used for patient studies are also used to record all the quality control images.

Uniformity. Use one of the following methods daily.

Extrinsic method. If the system's extrinsic uniformity is to be evaluated, a collimator is installed and a planar source, with a count rate that does not exceed 20,000 counts/sec, is centered over the detector. Covering the collimator surface with a plastic cover or enclosing the flood phantom in a plastic bag helps prevent collimator contamination.

1. Acquire a flood image that contains at least 3 million counts for a camera with a circular field of view and 5 million counts for a camera with a larger rectangular field of view.

2. If the camera has a microprocessor system for detector uniformity correction that can be turned off, daily flood-field images are acquired with and without microprocessor correction (Figure 3-38).
3. Evaluate and compare the image(s) with previous images for uniformity.
4. Record the data, photopeak setting, CRT intensity setting, total counts, and elapsed imaging time.
5. Place the image in the appropriate file.

Intrinsic method. If an intrinsic protocol has been adopted, the collimator must be removed. Extreme care must be taken to avoid physical shock and radionuclide contamination of the crystal. A collimator can be removed if contaminated, but crystal contamination can shut the camera down for days.

1. Place an appropriate size lead mask ring on the face of the detector if the gamma camera's edge packing is not masked.
2. Position a point source, with a count rate not exceeding 20,000 counts/sec, at a distance of at least fives times the diameter of the camera's useful field of view. The source can be positioned above or below the detector.
3. Acquire a flood image that contains at least 3 million counts for a camera with a circular field of view and 5 million counts for a camera with a larger rectangular field of view.
4. If the camera has a microprocessor system for detector uniformity correction that can be turned off, daily flood-field images are acquired with and without microprocessor correction if possible. Record the times taken to acquire both the corrected and uncorrected images, and note the difference.
5. Evaluate and compare the images with previous images for uniformity.

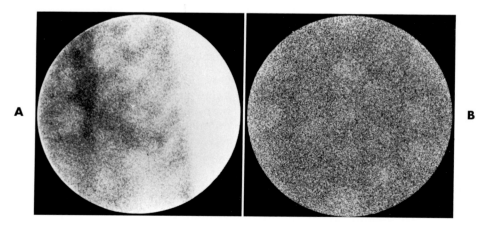

Figure 3-37 Improper photopeak selection. **A,** ^{99m}Tc pyrophosphate. **B,** ^{99m}Tc intrinsic flood-field images from camera peaked for ^{57}Co.

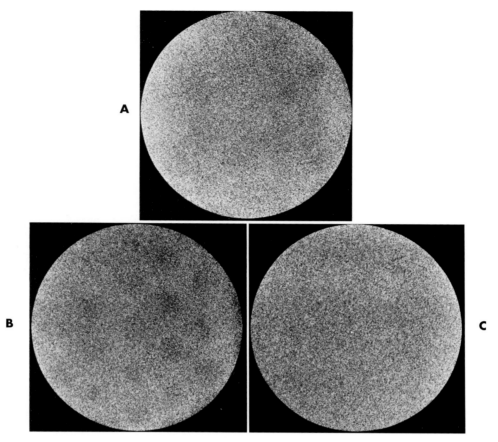

Figure 3-38 Detector performance without uniformity correction must also be assessed. **A,** Subtle nonuniformities. **B,** Increasing nonuniformity with time. **C,** Uniformity corrected flood of detector in **B.** Uniformity correction should not replace good detector calibration.

6. Record the date, photopeak setting, CRT intensity setting, total counts, and elapsed imaging time.
7. Place the images in the appropriate file.

Linearity and resolution. At a minimum, linearity and resolution should be checked weekly. An orthogonal-hole phantom is preferred, as long as the hole spacing is fine enough to "stress" present cameras. Other patterns may require multiple images of the phantom in different orientations for a complete evaluation of the system's performance.

1. Remove the collimator from the camera, and position the detector facing the ceiling.
2. Place the appropriate size lead mask ring on the face of the crystal if the cameras edge packing is not masked.
3. Position the transmission phantom on the detector housing.
   Note: Some cameras have transmission phantoms that may be attached like a collimator. In such a case the camera may be positioned facing downward or in any other convenient direction.

4. A point source of appropriate activity is positioned at a distance of five times the diameter of the camera's useful field of view. The count rate should not exceed 20,000 counts/sec.
5. Acquire an image that contains at least 3 million counts for a camera with a circular field of view and 5 million counts for a camera with a larger rectangular field of view.
6. Remove the point source before removing the phantom, particularly if the source is attached to the ceiling.
7. Evaluate and compare the image with previous images for linearity and intrinsic resolution.
8. Record the findings in the camera log, and place the image in the appropriate section of the logbook.

Collimators. The development of higher sensitivity and increased resolution low-energy collimators through the use of thinner septa and an increased number of holes has also produced the potential problem of physical damage or manufacturing defects, which can produce imaging artifacts (Figure 3-39).

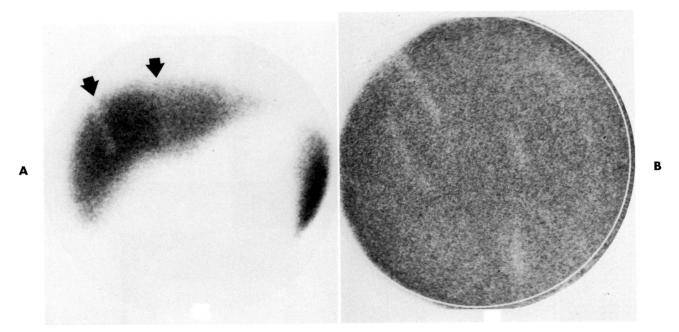

Figure 3-39 Anterior view (**A**) of liver with two photopenic areas suspected of being artifactual and (**B**) planar flood image demonstrating collimator damage as cause.

Checks for faulty or damaged collimators should be a part of a quality assurance program. These checks should include an initial check of all collimators plus subsequent checks at 12-month intervals. Each collimator should be evaluated by performing an extrinsic uniformity test in addition to a visual inspection for physical damage, dents, and separation of castings. The resultant images should be labeled with collimator name, date performed, total counts, time, and any pertinent comments. These images should be used in comparison for future evaluations.

Artifacts caused by the collimator can be confirmed by performing an extrinsic field uniformity image, then removing the collimator and rotating it 90 degrees or 180 degrees and reimaging (if possible). If the artifact position changes on the subsequent image, the collimator is the cause of the nonuniformity.

Photographic systems. Daily care and maintenance of the photographic system should be included as part of a quality assurance program. The CRT face and the lens and mirrors of the photographic camera system (when possible), including multiformatters, should be inspected and cleaned frequently. Dust and fingerprints on the mirrors and lens should be removed using professional lens paper. Do not use soap and water. The CRT face and protective cover can be cleaned with a lens cleaning solution. All surfaces should be checked for scratches and marks (Figure 3-40).

A suspected artifact in the photographic system can be confirmed or eliminated by the following procedure:

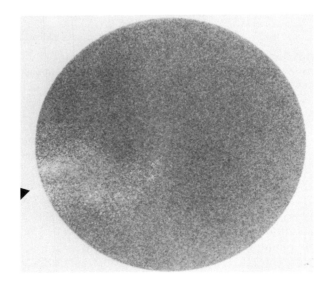

Figure 3-40 Cathode ray tube (CRT) artifact.

1. Obtain a flood-field image as described, noting the camera orientation, and observe where the suspected artifact is in the image.
2. Rotate the camera orientation 90 degrees and obtain another flood-field image.
3. Compare the two images: if the artifact did not change locations with a change in camera orientation, the artifact is on the CRT or photographic system; if the artifact moves with a corresponding change in orientation, the display system can be eliminated as a cause.

Streaking and other artifacts on Polaroid film can be caused by developer build-up on the rollers. These rollers should be cleaned daily using alcohol.

Multiple window spatial registration. Cameras that are equipped with multiple pulse height windows must be evaluated for spatial registration. Unless positional information (x and y signals) from each window is the same, images will be distorted. This distortion typically manifests as decreased spatial resolution compared with single window acquisition. Consequently, a practical approach to assessment of multiple window spatial registration is to compare single window to multiple window ^{67}Ga images of a quandrant bar phantom. To use this approach, the bar phantom must be adequately thick to attenuate the higher energy photons from ^{67}Ga.

Film Processor Quality Control

The processors used to develop nuclear medicine images require a program of maintenance and monitoring to assure that they function properly. A schedule should be established for cleaning, chemical change, temperature monitoring, and constancy of film development (density); this schedule should be strictly followed.

Computer Quality Control

The computer is an integral part of the imaging process for virtually all current scintillation cameras. Uniformity, linearity, resolution, dead time, and count rate response are all important parameters that must be monitored on a timely basis. A number of these quality control procedures are very similar to those used for the scintillation camera and can be performed at the same time.

Uniformity. The same method chosen for the scintillation camera is employed each day of use for uniformity. At a minimum, a 128×128 matrix is used to collect the computer image. Evaluate and compare the image(s) with previous images for uniformity. A count profile across the field of view may be generated to aid in evaluation of uniformity. Many present computer systems have the NEMA protocol for uniformity; this can be another useful aid in evaluation of uniformity. If uniformity can be quantified, it may be appropriate to establish actions levels. That is, if the integral uniformity is greater than x%, new corrections maps should be acquired or service should be requested.

Linearity and resolution. For weekly monitoring the orthogonal-hole phantom is used with the same technique described for scintillation camera linearity and resolution testing. The image is collected and displayed with the maximum digital resolution available (i.e., the

largest matrix size). Linearity is evaluated by assessing the straightness of the rows and columns. Spatial resolution is checked by evaluating the definition of the holes across the entire phantom image. Note that this test may produce erroneous results if too small a matrix (e.g., 64×64 or 128×128) is used.

Dead time determination. Follow this procedure yearly:

1. Prepare two sources of activity (approximately 300-500 μCi ^{99m}Tc); label one as source no. 1 and the other as no. 2. The activities of the sources must be within 10% of each other.
2. Remove the collimator, and place the lead masking ring on the detector.
3. Position the camera head to allow the sources to be placed approximately 1 m from the center of the detector.
4. Collect 1 min images in the camera (if analog) and the computer (64×64 matrix) of the individual sources and of the combined sources.
5. Calculate the dead time of the camera and the camera/computer system using the formula below

$$T = \frac{2R_{1,2}}{(R_1 + R_2)^2} \times \ln\left(\frac{R_1 + R_2}{R_{1,2}}\right)$$

where T is dead time in seconds, R_1 is counts/sec of source no. 1, R_2 is counts/sec of source no. 2, and $R_{1,2}$ is counts/sec of sources 1 and 2 combined.
6. Record these two values for comparison with subsequent monitoring measurements.
7. Identical counting conditions and nearly identical source activities must be employed each time the test is performed.

All of these tests are used to detect changes in performance over time. The results are usually interpreted in a subjective manner, and a decision is then made to determine if the system can be used for clinical studies.

SPECT System Quality Assurance

Adequate single photon emission computed tomography demands stringent quality assurance procedures. Field uniformity tolerances of $\pm5\%$, which are common for planar imaging, are not acceptable for SPECT imaging. Variations in uniformity of no greater than $\pm1\%$ are required. Additionally, alignment of the collimator crystal surface with the gantry axis of rotation as well as alignment of the computer image matrix and axis of rotation are critical.

Uniformity. Small changes in extrinsic camera uniformity may be misrepresented as different levels of activity or artifacts in reconstructed images (Figure 3-41).

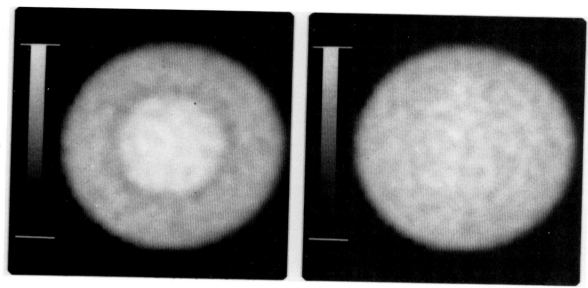

Figure 3-41   Slice through a water-filled cylinder containing a uniform distribution of ^{99m}Tc, reconstructed without *(left)* and with *(right)* compensation for nonuniformity in camera sensitivity. (From Greer K et al: *J Nucl Med Technol* 13:76-85, 1985.)

These artifacts typically take the form of alternating concentric hot and cold rings, which form a *bull's eye pattern.* Nonuniformities in multiple detector systems do not usually produce complete rings. SPECT imaging typically requires extrinsic uniformity variations which are less than 1%. This is particularly true for higher count SPECT studies, and perhaps less true for lower count (e.g., Tl-201 cardiac SPECT) studies. Extrinsic uniformity flood images (5 million counts, 64 × 64 matrix) should be acquired daily using clinical collimators. A uniform sheet source of ^{57}Co or ^{99m}Tc should be placed on the collimator, and the photopeak window should be properly set. Weekly, a 30-60 million count flood image using a 64 × 64 matrix should be acquired and analyzed for uniformity. If a 128 × 128 matrix is to be used clinically, at least 120 million counts will be required for adequate statistical precision. Updated high count flood images should be saved on the computer for performing uniformity correction. Different collimators and radionuclides may require separate uniformity correction matrices saved on the computer. Visual evaluation of high count flood images is not adequate for quality assurance of SPECT equipment. Quantitative computer programs are frequently required to evaluate the images to ensure less than ±1% extrinsic field variation.

^{57}Co sheet sources require no filling, since the radionuclide is impregnated into the plastic. However, not all commercially available ^{57}Co disk sources have the required uniformity to evaluate SPECT imaging systems. Furthermore, these sources might need to be replaced every 6-12 months to maintain reasonable count rates. Fillable liquid sheet sources can be used for long periods and may be filled with different radionuclides. Care must be used in ensuring uniform mixing of the

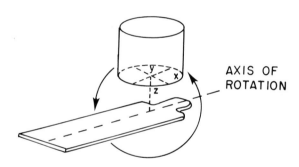

Figure 3-42   Camera x, y, and z coordinate system must be properly aligned with the axis of rotation of the SPECT gantry system. The camera y axis must be parallel to the axis of rotation for proper spatial registration on reconstructed images.

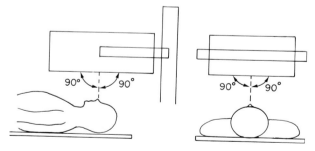

Figure 3-43   Camera head alignment must be perpendicular to the axis of rotation.

radionuclides with the liquid. Significant problems in filling or bulging with thin, fillable sheet sources may create artifacts in evaluating camera uniformity. A thick, water-filled phantom several centimeters thick may be used; however, care must be taken that no con-

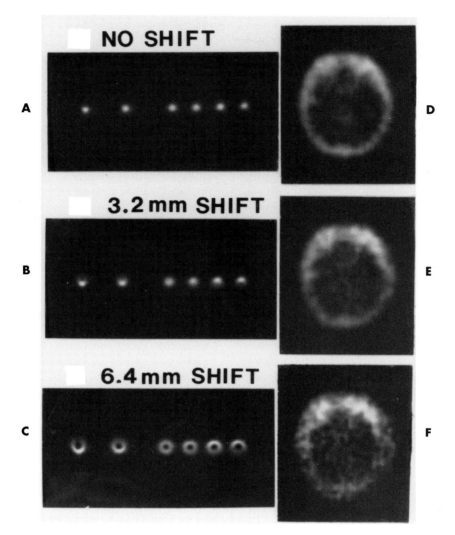

Figure 3-44 Top figures depict reconstructions for unaltered data from six line sources (**A**) and a slice from a brain scan (**D**). Centering error for **A** and **D** measured less than 1 mm. **B** and **E** show the effect of a 2-3 mm error in offset determination, accomplished by shifting the same projection data from **A** and **D** by one pixel (3.2 mm) prior to reconstruction. Note rapid deterioration of resolution and introduction of circular artifacts in **B** as compared to **A**. **C** and **F,** as in **B** and **E,** except data were shifted 6.2 mm from origin. (From Greer K et al: *J Nucl Med Technol* 13:76-85, 1985.)

tamination occurs when filling sources and that no leaks in the phantom occur.

SPECT system alignment. Proper x, y centering and gain adjustments are extremely important in SPECT imaging. The x and y gains of the computer image matrix should be evaluated in both directions using two point source markers separated by a known distance. The number of pixels between the two sources can be used to determine the dimension of a pixel. If the gains have drifted or are incorrectly set, they must be readjusted prior to any further SPECT imaging acquisitions.

The *axis of rotation* is an imaginary line that extends through the center of the camera gantry as a pencil would pass through a hole in a doughnut (Figure 3-42). As the camera moves in a circular orbit, the camera dis-

tance to this axis of rotation must not change; this requires that both the camera head and yoke rotation be carefully set to place the plane of the camera crystal parallel to the axis of rotation. Noncircular orbits may be implemented in several ways. In some approaches the camera head only moves in and out relative to the axis of rotation (i.e., the rotation radius changes). In this approach no additional alignment issues arise. In other approaches the gantry or bed may move in addition to the camera head, the effective axis of rotation changes from projection-to-projection, and additional alignment relationships (e.g., between gantry and bed) must be proper.

The computer image matrix must also be correctly aligned with the axis of rotation (Figure 3-43). Any misalignment in the acquired images, independent of the source of error, will cause blurring and a lack of resolution on the reconstructed images. Reconstruction of an image with an incorrect axis of rotation can create or mask lesions. The initial calibration of camera gains and offsets, necessary for correct planar imaging, provides a starting point for more sophisticated center-of-rotation corrections.

Center of rotation. Most SPECT systems should be able to maintain center of rotation alignment (Figure 3-44).Center-of-rotation evaluation is done to ensure that alignment exists between the mechanical and observed reference point. Proper camera alignment with the mechanical center of rotation must be checked weekly. Rotational image data are acquired of one or more point sources of ^{57}Co or ^{99m}Tc with a clinically used collimator and image matrix. A computer program is used to calculate the center of rotation, and the pixel value is recorded. Reconstructed transaxial images (see Figure 3-44) may show the point sources appearing too large or even having a cold center if the center of rotation is misaligned. Center-of-rotation shifts of 2-3 mm can significantly alter the quality of reconstructed transaxial slices. From center-of-rotation reconstructed data, the FWHM may be determined. Records of the center-of-rotation measurement (such as the correction shifts necessary) should be kept to evaluate any slight shift which may require service.

Phantom evaluations. At least monthly there should be a full system test using a phantom (Figure 3-45) that can evaluate system uniformity and resolution simultaneously. These tests should always be performed with the same amount of radioactivity, collimator, and other acquisition and processing parameters. Phantom studies frequently require the use of high amounts of activity in the phantom and long acquisition times exceed-

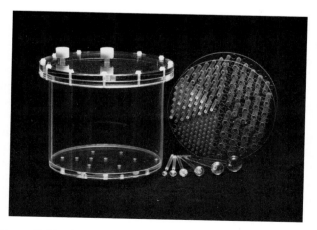

Figure 3-45 Commercially available SPECT phantom consisting of a cylinder with inserts to mimic hot or cold areas of activity. This may be used to measure complete system performance. (Courtesy Data Spectrum, Inc., Hillsborough, NC.)

ing techniques used in clinical studies. A simple large plastic bottle filled with a uniform concentration of ^{99m}Tc allows the reconstructed evaluation of transaxial slices for uniformity.

Resolution phantoms should have a variety of sizes of cold defects. Some resolution elements should be fairly easy to resolve, and some should exceed the resolution capabilities of the system. Having this variety of resolution elements allows the overall system to be pushed to its limit. Data acquisition with clinical parameters and subsequent reconstruction with a variety of filters will allow the user to optimally evaluate parameter selection to provide the most information.

Sinogram display. A extremely useful way of displaying SPECT quality control data is the sinogram. This image consists of the projection data for a given slice. Each row in the sinogram represents that one row of pixels in the projection corresponding to the slice of interest. Thus the horizontal direction in the sinogram corresponds to the linear horizontal direction in the projection data, and the vertical direction in the sinogram corresponds to projection angle.

Nonuniformities show up in the sinogram as straight vertical lines. Patient or organ motion or movement shows up as a "break" in the sinogram. Projections in which the organ moves out of the field of view produce sinograms with truncated activity.

National Electrical Manufacturers' Association (NEMA) Standards

NEMA consists of approximately 550 electrical manufacturing companies in the United States. One of its eight product divisions is the Diagnostic Imaging and Therapy Systems Division, with a section devoted to nuclear imaging. This section is made up of manufacturers of nuclear medicine equipment and includes all the major suppliers of scintillation cameras. This group has cooperatively formulated a set of standards that are used to measure the various performance characteristics of their products, including both planar imaging and SPECT performance.

After purchasing a scintillation camera, it is prudent to perform some type of acceptance test and not rely on the word of the installer that the system is working correctly. The usual quality assurance checks of uniformity, spatial resolution, and linearity should certainly be done. However, most nuclear medicine departments lack the expertise or equipment to measure all of the NEMA camera performance characteristics quoted by the manufacturer. For this reason, as well as the fact that there is a considerable dollar investment involved, it is wise to utilize the services of a consultant who has both the expertise and equipment to perform the NEMA measurements to ascertain that the system is performing as advertised.

MAXIMIZING IMAGE QUALITY

Image Quality and Signal-to-Noise Ratio

The goal of clinical nuclear medicine imaging is not to produce a "pretty picture" per se, but rather to aid diagnosis, prognosis, or treatment planning and monitoring. To do so, nuclear medicine images must be of high diagnostic and quantitative accuracy, depending on whether subjective visual interpretation or more objective quantitative analyses are used. In practice, the performance of a given instrument, technique, or study can only be judged in the light of rigorous assessment of diagnostic performance (by comparison with the results of "gold standard" tests or long-term follow-up) and quantitative accuracy (by comparison with the results of phantom studies and in vivo animal experiments). Subjective evaluation of "image quality," although frequently done in evaluations of new approaches, is of limited value in truly assessing the performance of an instrument or technique.

In general, the "quality" of an image can be described (quantitatively) by its *signal-to-noise* ratio (SNR). The signal-to-noise ratio directly affects diagnostic and quantitative accuracy. In essence, then, a major goal of nuclear medicine imaging equipment is to maximize the signal-to-noise ratio in an image.

The signal-to-noise ratio describes the relative "strength" of the desired information and the noise (e.g., due to the statistics of radioactive decay) in the image. As a simple example, consider a bone scan with hot lesions. The signal in this example is the difference between the lesions and the surrounding bone activity. Note that the signal is not the bone itself, but rather the contrast (or difference in image counts) between the lesions and the rest of the bone. As another example, consider a liver scan with cold lesions. Again, the signal is the contrast or difference between the lesions and the normal liver. For either the bone or liver scan, the only way the lesions can be detected is if their activity is sufficiently different than that of the surrounding areas. Contrast is often defined as

$$C = \frac{T - B}{T + B}$$

The greater the contrast between the lesions and the surrounding bone or liver, the greater the "signal" (Figure 3-46). In practice, this contrast is provided in the

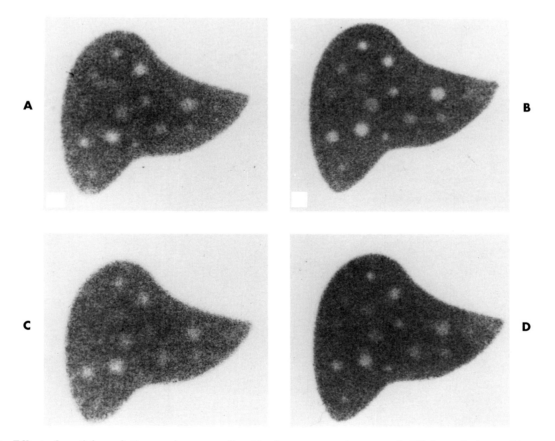

Figure 3-46 Effect of spatial resolution on image quality. Total counts are the same. **A,** High-resolution collimator with scattering material interposed. **B,** Same as **A** without scatter. **C,** Medium-energy collimator with scattering material interposed. **D,** Same as **C** without scatter. Note loss of contrast with lower resolution (medium energy) collimator and scatter.

patient by the radiotracer's distribution. The goal of the imaging system is to preserve this contrast in the image. Contrast is maintained by avoiding blurring, which smears counts from higher activity regions into lower activity regions (and vice versa), thus reducing image contrast. Thus spatial resolution and contrast are closely linked. This relationship is quantitatively described by the imaging system's *modulation transfer function* (MTF). Although the MTF is obtained from the Fourier transform of the point spread function (a measure of spatial resolution), it is actually the ratio of the contrast in the image to that in the object as a function of spatial frequency.

In addition, inclusion of scattered photons in the image reduces contrast (Figure 3-46). The imaging geometry of the system, along with its energy resolution, determines the amount of scatter present. It is important to note that the response of the imaging system to a point source of activity reflects both spatial resolution and scatter effects and can be used overall as an index of the ability of the system to preserve "signal."

The noise in this example is the statistical fluctuation within the lesions and within the surrounding bone or liver; this statistical fluctuation arises from the Poisson nature of radioactive decay. If there are few counts in the image, this fluctuation will be large, perhaps almost

as large as the true contrast between the lesions and the rest of the bone. In such a case the viewer would not be able to recognize the lesions as being "different" than the rest of the bone or liver (Figure 3-47).

For accurate quantification, many of the same factors that influence the image's signal-to-noise ratio are at play. Accuracy refers to the degree to which the average value (e.g., of radioactivity concentration) corresponds with the truth. An average value implies the existence of multiple measurements. By strict definition the values of these individual measurements can vary; if the average value agrees with the truth, the overall measurement is *accurate*. Accuracy is influenced by the spatial resolution of the imaging system—by its ability to accurately portray the correct contrast present in the patient. Accuracy is also affected by other factors, such as photon attenuation.

Precision refers to the variation among the individual measurements. If all of the values agree with each other, the overall measurement is *precise* or *reproducible*, even if it isn't accurate. Precision is influenced by the inherent statistical fluctuations due to the Poisson nature of radioactive decay and any further computer processing. For example, conventional 9-point weighted averaging (or "smoothing") improves the precision of each pixel's value.

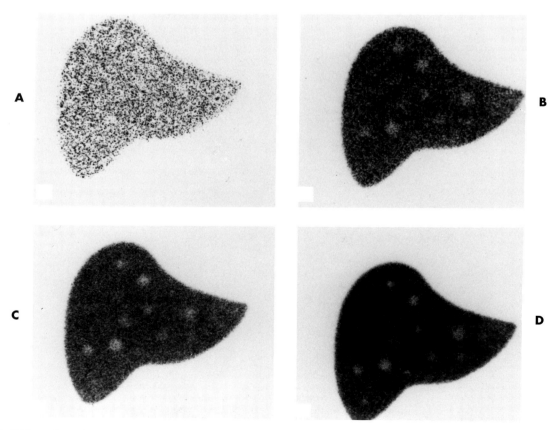

Figure 3-47   Effect of total counts on image quality. All other factors, including spatial resolution, are the same. **A,** 50,000 counts; **B,** 500,000 counts; **C,** 1,000,000 counts; **D,** 2,000,000 counts.

Instrumentation Factors Influencing SNR

To achieve a high signal-to-noise ratio, high resolution and high sensitivity are required. Nuclear medicine imaging forces a compromise between resolution and sensitivity. In 1985 Dr. Gerd Muehllehner published an important study relating these two factors to perceived image quality. Observers viewed computer simulations of the Derenzo phantom and were asked to match images of similar image quality. ("Image quality" in this context was based on the viewers' *perceived* ability to discriminate the hot spots from the background; such a task would be influenced by the complicated interplay between image contrast and noise.) Dr. Muehllehner found that an improvement in resolution of 2 mm (e.g., from 10 mm to 8 mm) resulted in comparable image quality with only about one fourth as many counts. In 1992 Dr. Fred Fahey and co-workers confirmed and extended Dr. Muehllehner's findings in a phantom study with a multicamera SPECT system. These findings are consistent with the view that the image's signal-to-noise ratio dominates perceived image quality and that the ratio may be increased by either increasing contrast (through improved spatial resolution) or decreasing noise (through increased sensitivity).

In practice, the technologist will find the concept of SNR very helpful in optimizing acquisition and processing protocols. By keeping in mind that the goal is to maximize an image's SNR, an optimum choice of collimator, for example, can be found that preserves contrast (through good enough spatial resolution) while providing sufficient sensitivity to keep image noise to an acceptably low level. Similarly, an optimum reconstruction filter can be chosen. Usually the choice that maximizes SNR is in between the highest resolution choice and the highest sensitivity choice.

Conclusion

Nuclear medicine has always been a technology-intensive discipline in medicine. At present, with the emphasis on high-performance imaging devices and state-of-the-art computing, the technologist may be intimidated or overwhelmed with the knowledge and skills he or she is expected to possess. The basic principles of radiation physics, detection, digital computing, and image processing apply across the board to all clinical imaging. Thus the technologist is strongly encouraged to take the time and effort to fully learn these important principles and to become a fully participating member of the imaging team. A good technologist provides a unique and indispensable role and is valued accordingly.

SUGGESTED READINGS

Cho ZH, Jones JP, Singh M: *Foundations of medical imaging,* New York, 1993, John Wiley.

Goris ML, Briandet PA: A clinical and mathematical introduction to computer processing of scintigraphic images, New York, 1983, Raven Press.

Hendee WR: Radioactive isotopes in biological research, New York, 1973, John Wiley.

Rao DV, Chandra R, Graham MC: *Physics of nuclear medicine,* New York, 1984, American Institute of Physics.

Rollo FD: *Nuclear medicine physics, instrumentation, and agents,* St. Louis, 1977, Mosby.

Sandler MP, Coleman RE, Wackers FJTh, et al: *Diagnostic nuclear medicine,* ed 3, Baltimore, 1996, Williams & Wilkins.

Sorenson JA, Phelps ME: *Physics in nuclear medicine,* ed 2, Orlando, 1987, Grune & Stratton.

Swenberg CE, Conklin JJ: *Imaging techniques in biology and medicine,* San Diego, 1988, Academic Press.

Wagner HN, Szabo Z, Buchanan JW: *Principles of nuclear medicine,* ed 2, Philadelphia, 1995, WB Saunders.

Wang CH, Willis DL, Loveland WD: *Radiotracer methodology in the biological, environmental, and physical sciences,* Englewood Cliffs, NJ, 1975, Prentice-Hall.

Paul E. Christian

Computer Science

Objectives

Describe the representation of data in decimal, binary, octal, and hexadecimal format.

Explain the function of the CPU.

Describe the operation and use of input/output devices.

Explain the principles and use of data storage media.

Describe the operation of disk drives.

Discuss the use, advantages, and limitations of data storage media.

Explain the operation of ADCs and the camera/computer interface.

List environmental factors for computers.

Define and discuss operating system.

Differentiate between high-level and machine code programs.

Discuss computer programming and programming languages.

Diagram and explain digital storage of images.

Discuss the advantages and disadvantages of different image size matrices.

Explain the acquisition of gated cardiac data.

Describe image processing operations.

Calculate a nine-point smooth for a 3×3 matrix.

Perform image region of interest placement and curve generation.

Explain the principles of normalization, and calculate normalized background-corrected counts.

Describe frequency space representation of images.

Discuss the principles of SPECT reconstruction.

Explain the use of frequency space filters to remove noise from SPECT images.

Diagram computer network configurations.

Discuss uses for nonimaging computers.

Define the Internet, and discuss nuclear medicine applications.

Computer: An electronic machine that stores instructions and information to perform rapid and complex calculations or to store, manipulate, and retrieve information.

By this definition the computer is distinguished from the calculator, a device used to make a simple computation. In addition, the computer is capable not only of storing information (numbers, data, images, or text) but also of following a set of instructions to make complex calculations and manipulate the information in some specific order. This can be as simple as adding two numbers or as complicated as performing reconstruction of single photon emission computed tomography (SPECT) images. Not only are calculations performed, but also information can be evaluated, such as performing logical evaluations and sorting information in a database.

Computers have become an integral part of the nuclear medicine department, not only with applications to imaging, but also to less demanding but repetitive tasks such as billing, scheduling, patient reports, nuclear pharmacy records, and administrative and general office applications. However, this chapter concentrates primarily on the application of computers to acquire, store, and process images. Image processing is discussed in general, and specific applications are presented in later, clinical chapters.

HISTORY

Long ago, humankind realized the value of a device to help manipulate numbers. Around 1500 BC the Chinese invented the abacus, a device whose beads could be moved to add, subtract, multiply, and divide. For hundreds of years, few ways were found to improve number processing. By the mid-1600s Blaise Pascal and Baron von Leibniz had devised adding machines that, through a series of gears and dials, performed lengthy calculations. In 1804 Joseph Jacquard devised a technique of automating patterns to be woven into material. Jacquard's loom used a series of rods that "read" the perforations in a series of cards, which dictated the pattern to be woven. This device was therefore the first encoding of instructions to a machine.

From 1822 to 1834 Charles Babbage constructed a device he called the *difference engine*. This mechanical instrument used a complex grouping of gears, rods, and wheels to perform a series of calculations according to a predefined instruction set. A more advanced design, the *analytical engine,* which was never completed, established the expression of all-purpose programming with the ability to follow a list of instructions with numbers as long as 50 digits. His assistant, Ada Lovelace, carefully documented the rules for encoding the instructions and wrote the first example of programs that could be used to control a computing machine.

In 1889 Herman Hollerith invented a machine that could sort, collate, and count information on punched cards. This machine was used to compile statistical information from the 1890 census. The company that Hollerith founded later became International Business Machines (IBM). Many types of mechanical calculating machines were developed in that era.

John Atanasoff and Clifford Berry in 1939 devised a prototype computer that used a binary numbering sys-

tem. He had recognized that electronic circuits were well suited to handle binary (1 or 0 or on/off) representations of numbers.

Although several electromechanical computing devices were built in the mid-1940s, a fully electronic digital computer was not operational until 1946. ENIAC (Electronic Numerical Integrator and Calculator) was the first electronic digital computer and was used to calculate artillery-aiming tables for the U.S. Army and to solve problems for production of the hydrogen bomb. This room-sized computer used thousands of vacuum tubes and required programming by manual connection of hundreds of wires. In 1951 Remington-Rand became the world's first large-scale manufacturer of computers when it introduced the UNIVAC-I.

Although the transistor was invented in 1947, it was not fully developed nor was it generally available until the mid-1950s. Additional development of these semiconductor devices was the placement of many components on a single circuit, or *chip*. These devices, called integrated circuits, created a revolution in computers over the next decade, with current technology being able to put millions of transistors on a single chip. Since the introduction of the integrated circuit, the transistor density on a chip has nearly doubled every 18 months.

In 1965 Digital Equipment Corporation introduced the PDP-8, the first successful minicomputer. Before this, computers had been room-sized machines requiring operation by many programmers and electronics technicians. The introduction of these minicomputers allowed thousands of small manufacturing plants, businesses, and scientific laboratories to purchase relatively low-cost systems with high reliability.

The first microprocessor, or computer on a single circuit board, was introduced in 1971. Around that time the performance of the computers was increasing dramatically, while costs for these systems were dropping sharply. In 1973 IBM introduced the first low-cost high-speed magnetic storage device, the Winchester disk. This device allowed rapid storage and recall of large amounts of data, replacing the much slower tape drive. The Motorola 6800 microprocessor was released in 1975, representing the first low-cost computer on a chip. The foundation for the market of personal computers was established in 1977 when Steve Jobs and Steve Wozniak presented the first Apple Computer; that year the TRS-80 and Commodore personal computers also were released. IBM followed in 1981, manufacturing its first personal computer.

In the last 20 years significant improvement has been seen in microprocessor technology. Very large-scale integration (VLSI) circuits have made possible the application of microprocessors into a variety of devices used in nuclear medicine. Devices internal to camera operation, such as energy, linearity, and uniformity correction circuits, are a product of microprocessor technology. The introduction of chips that have megabits of memory and operate at very high speeds with millions of switching operations per second has added significantly to imaging instrumentation performance.

The first introduction of computers into nuclear medicine imaging occurred in the late 1960s and early 1970s. Minicomputers were used to store the output from scintillation cameras and rectilinear scanners. At that time imaging was limited to static and dynamic studies, therefore the relatively unsophisticated and low-speed computers were able to manage all imaging requirements. These early computer systems were limited to single-function applications (i.e., only one acquisition or processing function could be performed at one time). In the mid-1970s, direct memory access and multitasking operations were implemented into minicomputers, which allowed image data to be processed while another study was being acquired. In 1977 capability to perform multigated cardiac studies had been defined; this brought a tremendous new application for nuclear medicine imaging computers and started the proliferation of computers into the community hospital. During that time the performance and memory requirements of nuclear medicine computers were beginning to increase; however, outside of handling the pixel arrays of the images, the computing requirements of these systems were relatively modest.

The commercial availability of SPECT cameras in the early 1980s brought the first computationally intense applications to nuclear medicine in performing filtered back-projection reconstruction. It became immediately apparent that the time demands for reconstructing SPECT images were not feasible with minicomputers, and array processors were attached to perform SPECT reconstructions in a reasonable time. Within the last few years, memory and computing power have further increased, allowing use of windows environments on image processing workstations. These powerful new systems allow the operator to interact with the computer using a mouse in each of several windows on the screen, each window running different programs and all programs being executed simultaneously.

DATA REPRESENTATION

The most fundamental building block of all computers is the transistor; essentially the transistor is a switch that can be placed only in the "on" or "off" positions. Information stored by this switch is therefore *binary* and can be used to represent a 0 or 1. Also, the binary state can be used to signify a logical condition of true or false. All numbers and all logical conditions within the computer are represented in the binary form. The binary configuration, 0 or 1, is called a *binary digit* or *bit*.

Our customary decimal counting system of values 0 through 9 is not sufficient to represent all the numbers;

therefore we use additional columns to represent powers of 10 (10, 100, 1000, etc.). In binary counting, each column is represented by powers of 2 (2^0, 2^1, 2^2, etc. or 1, 2, 4, 8, etc.).

The binary counting method is used for number representation in the computer, although other systems can also be employed by the computer within the system. Counting systems containing 8 bits (octal) or 16 bits (hexadecimal) can also be employed. The equivalent values to usual decimal counting follow.

Decimal	1024	512	256	128	64	32	16	8	4	2	0 or 1
Binary power	2^{10}	2^9	2^8	2^7	2^6	2^5	2^4	2^3	2^2	2^1	2^0
0	0	0	0	0	0	0	0	0	0	0	0
1	0	0	0	0	0	0	0	0	0	0	1
2	0	0	0	0	0	0	0	0	0	1	0
3	0	0	0	0	0	0	0	0	0	1	1
4	0	0	0	0	0	0	0	0	1	0	0
5	0	0	0	0	0	0	0	0	1	0	1
10	0	0	0	0	0	0	0	1	0	1	0
15	0	0	0	0	0	0	0	1	1	1	1
16	0	0	0	0	0	0	1	0	0	0	0
60	0	0	0	0	0	1	1	1	1	0	0
128	0	0	0	1	0	0	0	0	0	0	0
200	0	0	0	1	1	0	0	1	0	0	0
350	0	0	1	0	1	0	1	1	1	1	0

The decimal number 21 is represented as the sum of decimal numbers—16 + 4 + 1:

$$
\begin{aligned}
1 \times 2^4 &= 16 \\
0 \times 2^3 &= 0 \\
1 \times 2^2 &= 4 \\
0 \times 2^1 &= 0 \\
1 \times 2^0 &= \underline{1} \\
&\quad 21
\end{aligned}
$$

or all powers of 2 or in binary—resulting in 0 000 000 000 010 101. Note that 16 numbers are present in these examples, all zeros or ones. Most computers process numbers in groups of 16, 32, or 64 bits.

In hexadecimal counting (base 16) the usual decimal numbers 0 thru 9 are supplemented with letters to obtain the full representation of numbers until the next column is needed. Sometimes computer users see numbers or need to enter certain codes that are in either octal or hexadecimal characterization.

Decimal	Octal	Hexadecimal
0	0	0
1	1	1
2	2	2
3	3	3
4	4	4
5	5	5
6	6	6
7	7	7

Decimal	Octal	Hexadecimal
8	10	8
9	11	9
10	12	A
11	13	B
12	14	C
13	15	D
14	16	E
15	17	F
16	20	10
17	21	11
18	22	12
19	23	13
20	24	14

As mentioned, a bit represents a limited amount of information, and a series of bits is needed to encode larger numbers. Groups of eight bits form a *byte*. The maximum number that can be stored in a byte is 2^8, or 256 entries. Since the first number is 0, numbers from 0 to 255 can be stored in a single byte. Two bytes can be put together to form a word; a word is therefore 16 bits in length and is capable of storing a number as large as 2^{16}, or 65,536. Words are frequently used to represent the number of counts in a single image picture element, called a *pixel*. The range of counts that could be stored in a single word is 0 to 65,535. The most basic storage element of information on a magnetic tape or disk is to store the data in groups of bytes, called a *block*. For example, a disk sector might store a block of 256, 512, or 1024 bytes. Information, whether numbers, text, or executable programs, is called a *file*. The size of a file can be listed as the number of bytes needed to store the information.

Memory requirements are usually indicated as thousands of bytes, or kilobytes. When discussing the size of memory or the size of a file on disk, the prefix kilo- does not refer to the usual definition of 1000, it refers to 1024. Therefore 4 kilobytes of memory is 4 × 1024, or 4096.

To effectively communicate with the computer, humans need to exchange information not as zeros and ones or other numeric representation but as standard written alphanumeric symbols. A set of numbers to represent alphanumeric characters has been established as the American Standard Code for Information Interchange (ASCII). Using this standard code, a byte can represent a letter of the alphabet, a number, punctuation character, or keyboard control character. Text files for word processing can be stored with one byte of information for each character of the document. In addition, ASCII code allows concise communication between the computer operator via the keyboard, computer, and display monitor, allowing the direct translation from alphanumeric characters into binary information. Text files, programs, and data all appear as binary information inside the computer. The confu-

sion of data or text files for programs creates havoc within the computer and can halt operation of the system.

HARDWARE

Central Processing Unit

The nucleus of the computer is called the central processing unit, or CPU (Figure 4-1). Its three primary functions are to regulate the system operation and perform computations, to interact with memory to execute programs and store data, and to coordinate the control of input and output devices. The CPU as the central management area for program execution has two primary components: the control unit (CU) and the arithmetic logic unit (ALU).

The execution of instructions and other operations is performed by transistors. Their switching from one state to another is controlled by a high-speed clock that "ticks" at rates up to about 200 million times per second (200 MHz). With each clock cycle the control unit coordinates the steps necessary to complete each instruction. Each instruction activates other areas within the CPU to perform operations, activates the ALU, and directs communication with memory and other devices. The ALU performs all arithmetic and executes all logic operations.

Memory

Since the CPU acts as the brain of the computer, it retains information by storing it in memory. Memory can be thought of as a group of mailboxes; each memory element has a specific address to store a single byte or word until it is needed. Memory consists of two types: read-only memory (ROM) and random access memory (RAM). The contents of ROM are permanent and re-

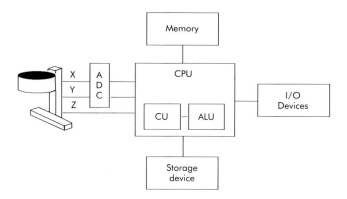

Figure 4-1 Nuclear medicine computer with the camera interfaced via an ADC to digitize x and y signals. The CPU controls the communication of information to the memory, input/output devices, and storage devices, disks, and tape.

main in memory even when the machine is turned off. RAM is sometimes referred to as "read-and-write memory" and can be changed. When a program is loaded into the computer from an external storage device or when data are input into the computer, it resides in RAM. When the computer is turned off, information stored in RAM is lost.

ROM chips reside with the CPU and are used to store the instructions that "boot" the computer and read the first set of instructions from disk. It can also contain information that tests various internal components of the system, identifies and checks the amount of available memory, and identifies external devices.

When a computer is turned on, the electrical signal follows a permanently programmed path to the CPU and ROM chips that start the boot program. Additional ROM chips contain the basic input/output system (BIOS). The BIOS chips check the disk drive to locate the operating system, such as DOS or UNIX. The BIOS instructions then load and start the operating system program found on disk. The BIOS also communicates with other areas, such as the memory, keyboard, monitor, and disks.

RAM chips provide the computer with its tremendous flexibility in performing a wide variety of functions. Outside of being developed to perform computations, the computer is the only tool ever made that was not devised to perform a specific function. RAM therefore provides the capability to contain programs, data, documents, graphics, and spreadsheets, all stored as zeroes and ones. Certain types of RAM chips also contain programs that store flood uniformity and energy correction matrices inside the scintillation camera.

The speed at which information can be stored and retrieved from memory greatly affects the speed of the CPU. Faster RAM chips are more expensive, and the fastest memory might not always be used in the CPU. Slow memory might require the processor to sit idle for several clock cycles while it waits for requested data to be passed to it. A solution to this problem is the addition of fast external RAM *cache memory*. Cache memory is typically built in as part of the main circuitry of the CPU. The cache memory fetches data from RAM and delivers it to the CPU. The first time data are retrieved might take several clock cycles, during which the CPU is idle. The cache also stores a copy of the data retrieved in its high-speed memory chips. As soon as the cache detects that the CPU is idle, it fetches data, or instructions, from memory addresses adjacent to the address for the data the software requested originally. The next time the software asks for data to be sent to the CPU, the cache checks to see if the data have already been stored in its high-speed memory and then delivers the requested data immediately.

For slightly more than the last decade, nuclear medicine computers have employed the capability to bypass the CPU during image acquisition. This is accomplished using direct memory access, or DMA, which employs both hardware and software to allow data to be directly passed into memory. DMA therefore does not require the interruption of another program running in the CPU to store counts or images as they are acquired. In early nuclear medicine computers the scintillation events from the camera were acquired faster than the information could be processed and stored in the computer. DMA takes the CPU out of the loop for data acquisition, allowing counts to be stored in image arrays at very high count rates. DMA also allowed computers to acquire one image while processing another simultaneously.

The computing power required to perform processing on early nuclear medicine computers was fairly minimal. Since the implementation of SPECT, slice reconstructions from two-dimensional images have brought about tremendous computational demands on the CPU. On some nuclear medicine computers the reconstruction of a single 64×64 transverse slice can take several seconds to reconstruct. A special device called an array processor speeds reconstruction times to less than 1 sec per slice. The array processor is a specially designed computer with very fast memory, adders, multipliers, etc. organized to perform computations on image array elements in a parallel manner. Present nuclear medicine computers can reconstruct all slices of a SPECT acquisition in a matter of seconds without the use of array processors.

The internal architecture of ordinary computers relies on several clock cycles to execute each instruction. In an automobile manufacturing plant this would be like completely building each car before starting the next. An innovative variation in computer design is the reduced-instruction set computer (RISC). RISC architecture computers essentially implement an assembly line approach to completing tasks within the CPU. A combination of hardware and software efficiently reorganizes the list of tasks into more efficient instructions. The instructions are then carried out in an assembly line fashion, or *pipeline processing*. Pipeline processing permits loading of the next instruction while preceding orders are being carried out. The efficiency of the assembly line and faster execution of simple instructions produces a tremendous gain in speed. There has been a tremendous growth of RISC computers in the last 5 years because of their overwhelming speed in performing image processing and handling graphics. A long list of operations on each data element and a large number of data elements, such as an image or series of images, are efficiently handled by RISC systems. Repeated computations such as those involved in SPECT slice reconstruction can be performed quickly on RISC machines. At this time some RISC machines can perform many millions of operations per second. It is likely they will dominate nuclear medicine computing in the future, and as prices drop on RISC architecture machines, they will have a significant impact on personal computers within the next few years.

Input/Output Devices

Input/output, or I/O, technology is the practical application of computer science. I/O devices allow us to enter or execute instructions, provide access to data, then finally obtain the results of the program with a meaningful output of results. Since computers understand or communicate only in zeros and ones, I/O devices also provide the means by which humans communicate with the computer.

Bus. The communication of the CPU with the outside world is first done internally in the machine by communication with the right circuit board to the device. Information to and from this circuit board flows through several parallel signal lines, called a *bus*. There are usually 16, 32, or 64 lines on a bus, over which all bits of a word travel in parallel. The number of bits and the speed with which information can be transmitted over the bus significantly affect the speed with which the CPU can communicate not only with memory but also with the I/O devices.

Video display terminal. The most common type of communication device is the keyboard and video display terminal (VDT) (Figure 4-2). The typewriter-like keyboard allows alphabetic and numeric characters to be entered into the computer. In addition, the keyboard of a computer has additional keys not found on a typewriter, such as control (CTRL), alternate (ALT), escape (ESC), and arrow keys to move the cursor. In addition, most keyboards have a series of 10-12 function keys that can be defined by different programs to perform special functions. Replacing the electronic typewriter carriage return is an enter or return key on the right-hand side, which indicates that a typed command or line of instructions has been completed for execution.

Besides the keyboard, the display monitor composes the other half of the VDT. Nuclear medicine systems use a high-quality monitor or cathode ray tube (CRT) similar to a television. A simple monochrome CRT streaks an electron beam across the flat front of the glass tube coated with a layer of phosphors, which glow for a short time after being struck by electrons. A video monitor sweeps the electron beam across this screen and repeats this sweep on the next row. Electromagnetic fields bend the path of the electron stream to draw each scan line on the screen. The screen is painted or refreshed about 60 times per second. The intensity of the electron beam is varied to create different intensities in each picture element, or pixel. High-resolution monitors create an array of about 1000 pixels across and 1000 pixels down.

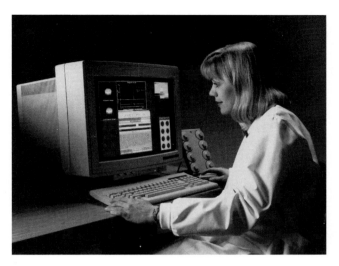

Figure 4-2 Computer operator console, or workstation, allows the operator to communicate with the CPU by keyboard and mouse. (Courtesy Ohio Imaging Division, Picker International, Inc., Bedford Heights, Ohio.)

Color images are generated from a CRT with three electron guns, one for each of the colors—red, green, and blue. Three different phosphor materials that are red, green, and blue are used on the CRT face; the stronger the electron beam, the more light is produced. Different colors are produced by varying the intensity of each beam. Many thousands of colors can be created. Hard copy films are created by taking a short time-exposed picture of a high-resolution CRT display.

Mouse. In 1968 Douglas Engelbart created a pointing device for computer users to interact with information on the screen. Because of its small size and tail-like cable, the device was nicknamed a *mouse*. Although the mouse never can replace a keyboard, it allows rapid interaction with screen information for pointing to and selecting information from a menu or direct interaction with graphics, such as drawing a region of interest. The mouse has become very popular in recent years because it enables the user to point to various graphic displays or windows and to quickly point to and select items from a displayed list.

A mechanical mouse contains a ball that protrudes from a hole in the bottom of the housing. As the housing is moved, the ball rotates and turns two rollers mounted at a 90-degree angle from one another. These rollers turn potentiometers that measure the amount of vertical and horizontal movement.

A trackball is another pointing device that works very much like a mechanical mouse; in fact, it could be thought of as a mouse turned upside down. Instead of the ball rolling along a surface, the user rolls the ball within the housing to turn the rollers that measure the indicated movement in two directions.

An optical mouse has no moving parts. It is used with a special pad covered with a grid of horizontal and vertical lines. A light from a tiny built-in lamp illuminates the grid surface, and a lens focuses the image of the lines onto a photodetector. As the mouse is moved, the photocathode converts the grid information into cursor movements that are translated to the screen. A mouse, whether mechanical or optical, usually has two or three buttons to activate the functions of the screen cursor. The mouse is used to position the cursor, and the buttons are used to activate functions.

Some computers have a joystick, a shaft that can move in either the x or y direction. As the shaft is moved in its cradle, a potentiometer measures the indicated x and y deflection, which is translated to the screen cursor. Similar to the mouse, a button activates functions at the present cursor location.

A light pen can also be used to identify locations on the CRT. A photodetector on its front detects the sweeping electron beam of the CRT. The location is indicated by the photosensor by measuring the time required for the beam to sweep to the position detected by the light pen. A bright spot can be illuminated on the screen at this point. Light pens are valuable for drawing regions of interest on images; however, they have few other practical applications.

Printers. In the past, printers have been used in nuclear medicine computer systems primarily for presenting text information. Daisy wheel printers and dot matrix printers were inexpensive and were used extensively a few years ago. Dot matrix printers use a print head containing a small linear array of 9 to 24 pins. These printing pins are aligned vertically, and each is attached to an individual electromagnet, or solenoid. Each alphanumeric character is generated by activating the solenoids to print the character as a small array, activating only those pins necessary to create one small vertical column. The pins strike a ribbon coated with ink, forcing by impact the translation of ink to paper. Dot matrix printers can print 200 to 600 characters per second. The quality of output from these devices limits their application to text or graphic information only.

In the last few years amazing new technology has almost completely replaced dot matrix printers. Laser printers and ink-jet printers are common in the office environment. The laser printer rapidly turns a beam of laser light on and off; this beam is then reflected onto a print drum coated with an organic photoconducting material. As the drum turns, the image of the page is transferred to the drum, which then picks up a fine black powder, or toner. As the drum continues turning, it is pressed against a sheet of paper, and a small electrostatic charge transfers the toner image to paper. Heat and pressure from rollers bind the image to the paper.

Ink-jet printers use a small print head with a small vertical array of holes or nozzles, finer than human hair. An electric pulse flows through thin resistors at the bottom of each nozzle chamber. The heat from the resistor heats the ink to several hundred degrees for a tiny fraction of a second, boiling off a tiny bubble of vapor that strikes the paper. One line on the paper is created by sweeping the ink-jet nozzle across the page.

Printers can produce black and white or color images on paper. Printer technology has changed vastly over the last few years, allowing high-quality images with many shades of gray or many different colors to be produced at reasonable cost. The best application for paper output of images at present is for short-term use, such as sending an image from a study to the referring physician or placing an image in the patient's chart. The quality of these printed images can deteriorate with time, and the paper can crinkle inadvertently.

Modem. A modem can be used to connect computers over a standard telephone line. The word modem comes from two terms: *mo*dulate and *dem*odulate. The modem produces a continuous frequency, or carrier wave, to transmit information. Once two modems are connected and the carrier signal is established between the two units, the wave of the carrier is either amplitude, frequency, or phase modulated to carry binary information. Data packets, a group of bits, are transmitted and the two modems communicate check signals to ensure that data are received accurately. The speed of data transmission is measured in the number of bits transmitted per second, called a *baud*. Modems most commonly communicate at 300, 1200, 2400, 4800, 9600, 14,400, 19,200 or 28,800 baud. These transmission rates will allow instructions, simple programs, and small image files to be transferred from one system to another within a few minutes; however, modems are not amenable to transferring large files.

Data Storage

Disks. The most common form of data storage is the magnetic disk. Magnetic disks, either floppy or hard, have storage capacities ranging from a few hundred kilobytes (10^3 bytes) to several gigabytes (10^9 bytes). The primary disk on most computers is a hard disk made of an aluminum platter coated on both sides with a thin layer of ferromagnetic material. Microscopically small areas can be magnetized to store a zero or one to encode binary data. The disk is organized into concentric circles called tracks and pie-shaped areas called sectors (Figure 4-3).

These divisions organize the disk so data can be recorded in a logical manner and accessed quickly. Before disks can be used, they are formatted to create the magnetic tracks and sectors. A hard disk (Figure 4-4, *top*) spins at a speed as high as 3600 revolutions per

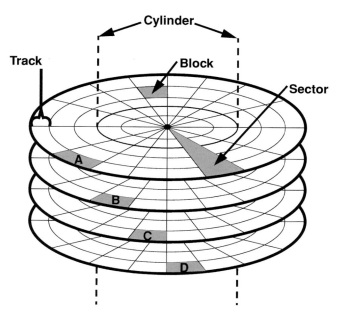

Figure 4-3 Disks are laid out into concentric rings called tracks and pie-shaped sectors that identify locations for storing data. A specific sector on a specific track identifies one block of data, which can be 256, 512, or 1024 bytes. Multiplatter disks may also have vertical cylinders of data on a track. Disks can quickly write data by not having to move the read/write heads from a track by writing to multiple platters in sequence denoted as *A, B, C, D.*

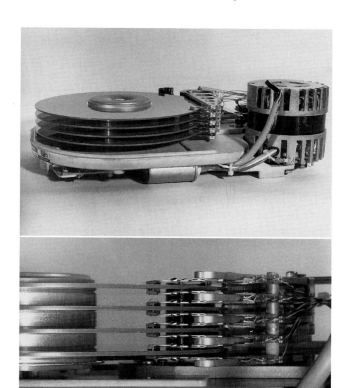

Figure 4-4 *Top,* Winchester disk drive shown here has four platters with read/write heads on both sides of each platter. An actuator arm positions the heads in and out while the disk rotates at high speed, allowing data to be written and retrieved very quickly. *Bottom,* Each platter has a set of read/write heads on each side in extremely close proximity to the disk.

min. A pair of small electromagnets called read/write heads (Figure 4-4, *bottom*) located on an access arm are positioned close to the disk. The read/write heads can be quickly positioned by a stepper motor over the various tracks. As the disk rotates, the read/write heads bring each sector on a particular track past the heads. Binary data can therefore be written to or read from the disk at very high speed. Access time or seek time to a particular track or sector can be a small fraction of a second on hard disks, sometimes a few thousandths.

The distance between the disk surface and the read/write heads is about 10 microinches; therefore hard disk systems usually are sealed to protect them from dust particles, fingerprints, and other foreign material. The heads literally fly over the surface of the disk on a thin cushion of air. Contact between the disk and the read/write heads is called a "head crash"; at this high speed it can damage either the heads or the disk surface.

The most common hard disk system is a Winchester disk. Large storage capacity Winchester disks usually have multiple platters (Figure 4-4), and each platter can be formatted into several hundred tracks. The capacity of a Winchester disk is several megabytes to several gigabytes. Most nuclear medicine computers performing SPECT imaging need a hard disk that can hold at least several hundred megabytes to allow room for the operating system and sufficient space for storing

many patient data sets. Data are laid onto the disk in blocks of information. A block usually consists of 256 bytes; however, some disk systems have larger size blocks—512 or 1024 bytes.

The location of files (information) on the disk is identified by a directory or file allocation table usually found at the beginning of the disk. The file allocation table stores information about the disk's structure, the track and sector location, and length of each file. Each time a file is to be read or written, the operating system orders the hard disk controller to move the read/write heads to the disk file allocation table. The operating system reads the table to determine the location of an existing file or to find available space in which to write a new file. Some nuclear medicine computers require that a single file of images be written onto a continuous sequence of blocks on the disk. The fastest way to write data onto a multiplatter disk is to write on several platters, one after another onto the same track so that time is not lost in mechanically moving the actuator arm to change tracks. Figure 4-3 shows the use of several blocks and platters creating a vertical cylinder of disk space for rapid access. Dynamic and SPECT studies therefore require a significant amount of disk space. Most new systems break up a file into clusters of data strewn onto various regions on the disk. When the operator deletes a file, the computer simply erases the file location from the directory, although the information remains on disk until it is overwritten. Some systems allow recovery of deleted files by reestablishing the information in the directory.

Floppy disks. Floppy disks allow files to be stored on a convenient medium that can be transferred to another computer or archived for later use. Floppy, or flexible, disks are made of mylar coated with ferromagnetic material and come in a variety of sizes—8, 5¼, and 3½ inches. The larger disks are of older technology and typically could store only about 1 megabyte of information. Present technology allows storage of about 2 megabytes of information on a 3½-inch diskette. Floppy disks spin at a rate of about 360 revolutions per min, and the seek time of the read heads to obtain data is a large fraction of a second. The read/write heads on a floppy drive with its single flexible platter are actually contacted by the read/write heads; therefore the disk eventually wears out after many hours of use. Information stored on floppy disks can be archived for several years.

Optical disks. Optical disk drives provide the latest technology to write large amounts of data on a very small area of disk. The first types of optical disks were nonerasable and were called "Write Once Read Many" (WORM) drives. WORM drives use an intense laser beam focused onto the polished surface disk to essentially burn the surface to encode a bit. WORM drives are best suited for storing large quantities of data that will be kept for a long time. The platters in these optical drives can be changed once the disk is filled.

Magneto-optical drives provide an erasable medium for optical encoding of data. The disk is coated with an aluminum substrate protected by a sheet of plastic. An intense laser beam rapidly heats a tiny spot on the disk so the crystals in the alloy can be aligned by the magnetic field of a write head. Bits are stored by magnetically aligning the crystals so that a reflected laser beam encodes binary data. A low-intensity laser beam is used to read the data. Magneto-optical disks are about 5 inches in diameter and contain tens of thousands of tracks for writing data. Although the interchangeable disks cost less than $100, they can store 500 megabytes to 1 gigabyte and are valuable for archiving images.

Magnetic tape. Magnetic tape represented the most common medium for archiving data on early computers. Nine-track tapes provided a common medium for transferring data between different manufacturers' computers. Nine magnetic tracks are laid down side by side on the tape, which is about ½ inch wide. Eight bits, in addition to an error checking track, allow data to be written at 800, 1600, or 6250 bits per inch. A large number of imaging studies can be stored on one tape; however, the time required to move to the correct area of the tape where a file is written can be excessive, waiting many minutes to write or retrieve data. Large quantities of data can be stored very inexpensively.

High-speed cartridge tapes are available on many systems, writing data to a narrow tape at high speed. These tapes can store about 150 megabytes of information at a cost of $25 per tape. Although smaller and more convenient than a 9-track tape, they are still slow in writing and retrieving archived data. Video-8 data cartridges are used on some systems to allow very large amounts of data (hundreds of megabytes) to be archived.

Camera Interface

The output from the scintillation camera detector provides three signals for each gamma ray scintillation event. The x and y signals represent the location of the gamma ray interaction in the detector, and the z signal measures the gamma ray energy. These three signals are analog signals, simply electronic pulses that must be converted into numbers to be transferred into the computer. The camera interface uses two analog-to-digital converters (ADCs) to digitize the x and y signals. Voltage pulses are converted using a successive approximation technique. The incoming pulse is compared to the largest bit in the digital word to represent the data. If the pulse is larger than this most significant bit, the bit is set to 1. Each bit in the digital representation, from the largest to the smallest, is tested against the incoming voltage until the last bit has been set. The resulting digital value is the closest digital approximation to the input analog signal.

Successive approximation ADCs are very fast, and camera position signals are digitized to an accuracy much finer than that of the image matrix into which the image data is stored. In the modern digital scintillation camera the computer is interfaced directly with the camera, and there is no separate noncomputerized operating console for the camera. In these cameras, not only the x and y signals but also the energy z signal is digitized, in addition to other inputs such as an electrocardiogram (ECG) physiologic trigger used in performing gated cardiac studies. ADCs are fast enough that there is no loss in storing counts waiting for them to transform electronic pulses into the digital format. Once the digitized information comes through the camera interface, the DMA transmits the data directly to its assigned memory location without interrupting the activities of the CPU.

Care and Quality Assurance

Imaging computers require certain environmental considerations to ensure reliable performance. The integration of the scintillation camera and computer has, in many cases, mandated the computer to be in close proximity to the camera and, in some situations, it must be in the same room. The considerations in computer operation are temperature, humidity, electromagnetic fields, power, and cleanliness. Imaging computers generate significant heat, in most cases 6000-12,000 BTU per hour. Appropriate air-conditioning must be installed to maintain a temperature near 70° F to prevent overheating. This thermal output must be added to that of other equipment, such as a scintillation camera, in the same room. Neither computers nor scintillation cameras should be in rooms where there is a potential for significant temperature change within a short time. The humidity in the room should also be moderate; approximately 50% relative humidity is desirable. Either very high or very low humidity can adversely affect operation of the computer and its peripheral components.

Computers and magnetic storage media should be remote from any significant sources of electromagnetic fields. Magnets should be kept away from magnetic tapes or disks that could be erased inadvertently.

The voltage applied to circuit boards and components on the boards is very small and can be significantly affected by voltage spikes that occur on the alternating current line. It is best to have computers on their own circuit where they are not influenced by other pieces of equipment that might be plugged into the same circuit and create current fluctuations or electrical noise. Some institutions experience unacceptable voltage spikes or brownouts; a power conditioner might need to be added to prevent transient interruptions in the power source. Computers, and in particular their internal circuit boards, can be very sensitive to static electricity.

Cleanliness of the environment for imaging computers is important. Dust and dirt create problems with power supplies, circuit boards, and in particular disk drives. Figure 4-5 shows the relative size of dirt, dust particles, and fingerprints on the surface of hard disks. Floppy diskettes and magnetic tapes are somewhat less susceptible than hard disks; however, the quality of storage media can be affected by improper care. Most sensitive areas of imaging computers are protected by air filters over the cooling fans. Air filters should be cleaned monthly.

Imaging computers require some quality assurance testing to guarantee performance. A test image, flood, or resolution performed daily should be used to evaluate image size, linearity, and uniformity. Misadjustments of the image size or shape are identified as distortions in the test image. The high count rate of some imaging situations requires validation of the count rate performance of the camera interface and ADCs. The dead-time losses in flow studies or first-pass cardiac angiograms can cause significant clinical errors in results. High-resolution phantom images can also help identify proper computer image acquisition.

The input of a physiologic signal from an ECG requires correct triggering to ensure proper gated car-

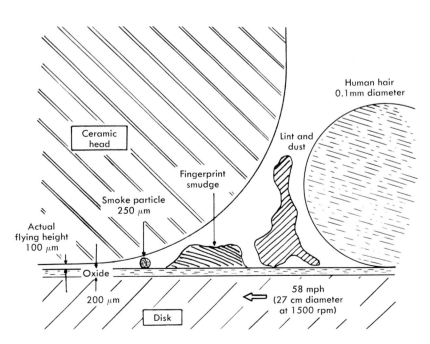

Figure 4-5 Smoke, fingerprints, dust particles, and human hair can all cause disk "crashes"; it is important to store and operate disks in a clean atmosphere.

diac studies. The function of the ECG input is to identify the QRS complex from the patient's cardiac cycle. Expensive nuclear cardiology phantoms and testing equipment are commercially available to check the ECG input and verify ejection fraction values. If this test equipment is not available, other simple tests can ensure proper performance of the computer. The biomedical engineering department in most hospitals has an ECG simulator that can be connected to the ECG input of the nuclear medicine computer to evaluate proper gating. A common technique to validate camera performance is to use a radioactive source to flood the camera detector while acquiring a test gated acquisition. Set a region of interest over the source on the acquired images and generate a time-activity curve. The resultant curve should show constant counts throughout the time-activity curve.

Verification of gating can be done as follows. Set a specific RR interval for acquisition slightly longer than the rate generated by the ECG simulator and acquire the flood images. Generating the time-activity curve should show a decrease in counts in the last one or two frames of the gated study. This occurs because the R wave from the following beat is detected before all image frames of the gated study have time to complete acquisition.

Computer quality control and care procedures should be established and followed regularly. Daily acquisition of a test image, either flood or resolution, should be recorded according to a standard protocol. In addition, daily care should include maintaining an orderly and neat environment in the area of the computer. Air filters should be cleaned monthly and floppy disk drive read/write heads should be cleaned using a commercially available and manufacturer-approved technique.

Most tests to ensure proper function of the computer system itself are beyond the training of personnel in nuclear medicine. Service personnel should troubleshoot problems and run diagnostic software to evaluate and potentially pinpoint system malfunctions. Service personnel should clean the inside of the computer regularly, run diagnostics to evaluate internal systems performance, and check the input and output to peripheral devices. With proper maintenance the hardware and software components of the imaging computer should allow uptime of the system greater than 99%.

SOFTWARE

Software refers to the set of instructions or programs that provide control over the calculations and subsystems of the computer. Control instructions and calculations have no physical hardware and therefore are appropriately named software. For instructions to be followed, they must first be placed into the memory of the computer. Software enables the computer to perform calculations, word processing, game playing, or image processing. Software also provides the interface between the human user and the hardware and peripheral devices to accomplish the desired tasks.

There are three principal types of software: systems software, programming software, and user programs. Systems software comprises the programs and files necessary for the internal operation of the computer and its peripheral devices, as well as the operating system and utility programs necessary to manipulate files. Programming software contains an editor (similar to a word processing program for placing instructions into a file), support libraries, and a compiler to convert the instruction file into an executable program. User programs are the instructions to execute the applications needed by the user, such as word processing, accounting, image acquisition, and image processing.

Operating System

Systems software usually is referred to as the operating system—a set of programs used to control, assist, and run other programs on the computer system. The operating system provides the link between the human user and the internal workings of the computer and its peripheral devices. The instructions in a computer, called a *program*, can be executed only when they reside in memory. On early computer systems it was extremely laborious and time consuming to load the program or instructions into the computer before the program could be executed. After many years the idea of an operating system or master control program to load and run other programs was developed. The operating system is like a toolbox; it contains subprograms that interact with disks, the graphics display, modem, and camera interface and allows us to list programs and files on disks in addition to loading and executing programs. Other programs in the operating system allow us to create, copy, and delete files; to create, modify, and store data; and to run the editor to write programs, convert the instructions into an understandable format by the computer, and execute the new instructions.

When the computer is turned on, a set of instructions that reside in ROM chips is executed to pull up the system by its bootstraps, in other words, to boot the system. Operating systems are large programs and are stored on disk. A disk-operating system (DOS) has a monitor or executive program loaded from disk with the portions of the operating system not needed by memory retained on disk until they are needed. Most personal computers and many nuclear medicine computers have DOS-type operating systems. Examples of operating systems are RT-11 for Digital Equipment Corporation computers; RDOS for Data General Systems; MS-DOS for IBM personal computers and clones; Systems-7 for the Apple Macintosh; and UNIX for a variety of higher level machines.

The operating system is responsible principally for controlling the internal functions of the computer in running programs. Most personal computers and early nuclear medicine computers could run only one program at a time. Early nuclear medicine computers were limited either to image acquisition, image processing, or another applications program at one time. More advanced operating systems can provide foreground and background operations apparently simultaneously. A foreground operation is a process that has priority for execution, such as an image acquisition program. When utilizing DMA, an acquisition program should have minimal requirements of the CPU; therefore, a background program can be running to perform some other type of operation such as image display. When the foreground program is not tying up the computer, the CPU works on the background program until it is interrupted again by foreground requirements.

The operating system manages the computer's activities, interfacing with the various devices and coordinating the systems. In addition, the operating system furnishes the user with a variety of programs needed for maintaining files on the computer. Disk and tape directories can be created and programs and files can be listed, created, deleted, copied, moved, and typed. The operating system also loads programs into memory for execution.

A further enhancement of operating systems is a multitasking environment. Each of several tasks is allowed a portion of memory for the program and to store data required for each program operation. Tasks are assigned priorities, as with the foreground/background operating system. In some senses it is similar to a time-sharing system whereby jobs are swapped back and forth. Each user is given the impression of working alone on the system; however, the increased number and complexity of tasks create a slower response of the computer system.

Programming Languages

Machine-oriented language. The only instructions understood by the computer are represented by a series of zeros and ones, information that is virtually incomprehensible to humans. This form of instructions is machine language. Instructions at this level are extremely basic and perform only the most rudimentary tasks. Assembly language programs are written in short, very specific tasks. Simple instructions are followed one at a time to fetch instructions, decide on the operation to be performed, get values from memory, move these values to locations where operations can be performed,

and so on. In assembly language even simple instructions such as adding two numbers and printing the result would require many simple steps.

High-level programming languages. High-level languages are those in which instructions can be written in terms that more closely resemble English language communication. High-level languages allow programmers the ability to concentrate on writing the program without having to deal with the specifics of machine hardware and devices.

An editor is a program that allows keyboard entry of written material to create, modify, and save a written file that will become the program. The editor therefore is similar to a word processing program, allowing only entry of information, without any guarantee that the program will execute properly, or even execute at all.

There are two general classifications of high-level languages—interpreted and compiled. Normally an interpreted program does not exist as a file of zeroes and ones that represent instructions the CPU can directly execute. An interpreted language is one in which the program is interpreted into machine code, and one line of instructions is executed at a time. Any results are saved, and the next line of the program is then interpreted and executed, and so on. As one would expect, this language runs very slowly, since the instructions must be interpreted before they can be executed. Interpreted languages therefore do not lend themselves to large problems such as image processing. They do have an advantage; in working with small amounts of data the programs are effective and can be quickly changed without the need to recompile and link.

BASIC. A common example of an interpreted language is Beginners All-purpose Symbolic Instruction Code (BASIC). BASIC was readily available on some early personal computers, with the program available from programmable ROMS (PROMs). To write a program in BASIC, the lines of instructions within the program are numbered and executed according to the line number. BASIC and similar programs used for image processing usually have some assembly language subroutines available to perform elementary image processing functions quickly (such as image addition, smoothing, region of interest, curve generation, SPECT reconstruction). This allows fairly rapid image manipulation with the flexibility of rapid programming changes.

A simple example program written in BASIC is shown below to use the decay equation to calculate the activity and volume of radioactivity needed for a clinical procedure at several time intervals. In the example, assume we are using ^{99m}Tc and that we enter the specific activity in mCi/ml at time zero into the computer. Then we have the computer print the specific activity and volume needed for a patient dose of 10 mCi at time intervals of 1 hr for a period of 4 hr. In BASIC this program could be written as:

```
10        REM Tc-99m DECAY EQUATION
          PROGRAM
20        T2 = 6
30        D = 10
40        INPUT "Enter the specific activity
          (mCi/ml) = ", A0
50        PRINT "Time(hr) Sp. Act.(mCi/ml)
          Vol.(ml)"
60        FOR T = 1 TO 4
70        A = A0 * EXP (-0.693 * T / T2)
80        V = D / A
90        PRINT, T, A, V
100       NEXT T
110       STOP
```

The program sets the half-life $(T2)$ to 6, the dose (D) to 10, and prompts the user to enter the specific activity stored in a variable called $A0$. A control command, *FOR* and *NEXT*, sets up a loop to perform the calculation and printing of the results $(T, A$ and $V)$ for delay periods of 1, 2, 3, and 4 hr. When executed, the program output appears as:

Enter the specific activity (mCi/ml) = 13.7

Time(hr)	Sp.Act.(mCi/ml)	Vol.(ml)
1	12.205611	0.819295
2	10.874230	0.919605
3	9.688076	1.032197
4	8.631306	1.158573

In contrast to the interpreted language, compiled languages are used to create programs that execute directly and are therefore much faster. A compiler is a program that translates the written English file of instructions into an intermediate object code file. The compiler therefore translates the English version of the program into a form that is ready to accept subroutines to allow the program's instructions to interact with the CPU and peripheral devices. The linker is a program used to incorporate these library functions into the program, which then outputs an executable version of the program. This executable version now consists of zeros and ones, machine language instructions the computer can understand and perform.

FORTRAN. *Fo*rmula *trans*lation (FORTRAN) is a scientific high-level language that is well established and available on a wide variety of systems from personal computers to mainframes. It has been widely used in nuclear medicine systems for commercial, research, and clinical applications. FORTRAN is a powerful language for performing computations dealing with large amounts of numeric data and for performing complex calculations. However, it is poor at dealing with data contained as text, with formal rules for the syntax that

handles text. The example decay program shown in BASIC appears as follows when it is written in FORTRAN.

```
C    Tc-99m DECAY EQUATION PROGRAM
     REAL A, A0, T2, D, V
     INTEGER T
     T2 = 6
     D = 10
     PRINT*, 'Enter the specific activity (mCi/ml) = '
     READ*, A0
     PRINT*, 'Time(hr) Sp. Act.(mCi/ml) Vol.(ml)'
     DO 20 T = 1, 4
     A = A0 * EXP (-0.693 * T / T2)
     V = D / A
     PRINT*, T, A, V
20   CONTINUE
     END
```

The program is in many respects similar to the BASIC program. The lines that define and perform calculations are nearly identical. However, the lines that define variables and input and print data must deal with the strict syntax rules of FORTRAN to define, read, and write information.

COBOL. Many other high-level programming languages have been written for specific applications. Common Business Oriented Languages (COBOL) has been used for many years to permit easy handling of textual data with relatively modest requirements for complex numeric calculations.

Pascal. This is a language that provides a different approach to the logic of programming. Pascal uses a top-down approach in which the program's main objectives are defined as modules, and the details of the calculations are defined within each module.

C. This high-level language uses a wide variety of functions to perform many tasks that with other languages can be performed only with assembly code routines. The capability of C to interact more directly with the CPU and peripheral devices provides great power in performing complex applications such as graphics. Many windows and workstation environments are written in C because of this power. An example of a decay program written in C follows.

```
#include <stdio.h>
#include <math.h>
main ( )
{
/* Tc-99m DECAY EQUATION PROGRAM */
float A, A0, T2, D, V;
int T;
T2 = 6;
D = 10;
printf("Enter the specific activity (mCi/ml) = ");
```

```
scanf("%f", &A0);
printf("Time(hr) Sp.Act.(mCi/ml) Vol.(ml) =\n");
for (T = 1; T < =4; T++)
{
A = A0 * exp(-0.693 * T / T2);
V = D / A;
printf("%d \t%f \t%f \n", T, A, V );
}
}
```

Note that the lines of the instructions for performing calculations are similar in C, BASIC, and FORTRAN. However, the commands and syntax formality for each language are unique. The control loop also uses a *for* statement that runs for the values of 1 through 4. The commands to enter *(scanf)* and print are unique. Programs written in C are also more transportable between different computer manufacturer systems than some of the other languages. For these reasons C has become a popular language in which much of the commercial software on 32-bit computers has been written.

IMAGE ACQUISITION

Capturing images from the scintillation camera first requires the conversion of analog x, y, and z pulses into digital information. As previously mentioned, digitization is accomplished by the ADCs to provide a quantitative location of the scintillation event. The digital location information locates the appropriate pixel into which the gamma event can be recorded. If the output is from an analog scintillation camera, separate from the computer, the energy pulse has already been processed by a pulse height analyzer and determined to be within the selected energy range. If the particular system is a digital camera/computer, then the digitized z pulse is compared to the selected window settings for pulse height analysis. If the z pulse has been determined to be within the appropriate window, the scintillation event is recorded in the pixel identified by the x and y locations, adding one to the current pixel value (Figure 4-6). Scintillation events are stored in the proper pixel locations until the acquisition time has elapsed or the selected number of counts or count density has been reached.

At present, image matrices are represented as a square matrix with the camera field of view inscribed within the square. The camera field of view shape therefore inscribes a circle, hexagon, square, or rectangle within the matrix (see Figure 4-6), depending on camera shape. The image density for each pixel is determined by the number of gamma ray counts stored within a pixel. For image display the highest pixel count is assigned the brightest intensity on the CRT display, with other pixel counts assigned to appropriate intermediate intensities. Prior to acquisition the image pixel

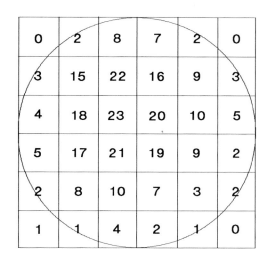

Figure 4-6 Scintillation detector *(circle)* gamma events are input to an array of pixels in the computer. Counts are accumulated by each pixel to store a representation of the image. Arrays of 64 × 64, 128 × 128, and 256 × 256 are most commonly used to store digital images.

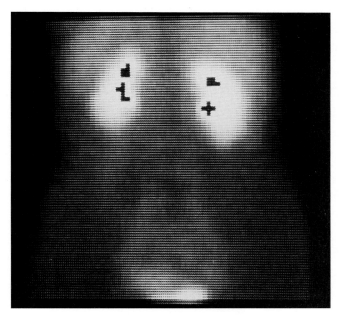

Figure 4-7 Each pixel can store only a limited number of counts; pixel overflow results when the number of counts exceeds the maximum value a pixel can hold. This kidney scan shows pixel overflow in the area of the renal pelvis.

data depth can be selected as an acquisition parameter. A pixel able to contain only 1 byte (8 bits) of information allows the storage of 256 different numbers, 0 to 255. If the counts per pixel reach the maximum of 255, pixel rollover may occur when the 256th count is reached and the pixel value goes back to 0 (Figure 4-7). Pixel rollover is prevented on some systems with the maximum of 255 being retained; however, counts above 255 are not recorded and quantitative information is lost. Acquiring data with a pixel depth in word mode (16 bits) lessens the likelihood of reaching the maximum count of 65,535. A consequence of storing higher density images is that they take twice as much memory and disk space for storage.

Most computer systems allow the selection of 64 × 64, 128 × 128, 256 × 256, or 512 × 512 matrices. Static image acquisition usually contains sufficient counts to produce a high spatial resolution image. If a large field of view camera (400 mm) has a full width at half maximum (FWHM) resolution of 4 mm, then high-resolution images should be stored in a matrix size of at least 100 pixels (400 mm/4 mm). A camera can visualize about 2 bars per the FWHM value. The selected image matrix should be multiplied by this value (2) to get a 200-pixel matrix. Static images acquired in a 256 × 256 matrix therefore are visually indistinguishable from analog images; that is, no evidence of the image matrix is seen. Figure 4-8, A to C, shows a bone scan image displayed as 256 × 256, 128 × 128, 64 × 64 images, respectively. The image resolution deteriorates as the selected acquisition matrix size gets smaller. In Figure 4-8, D, the 64 × 64 data have been used to interpolate intermediate pixels to create a 256 × 256 display image. Note that the interpolated image appears as a smoothed version of the 64 × 64 data without recovering the resolution available with 256 × 256 acquired data.

Dynamic images do not usually contain enough counts to warrant the use of high-resolution matrices; dynamic studies are performed to record physiologic information. The time per image is therefore critical to ensure that meaningful physiologic information is not missed by acquiring images too slowly. Blood flow studies of organs such as the kidneys and brain should be acquired at one frame/sec. The series of images should be continued for a long enough period to obtain valuable information and to not miss the injection bolus. Image resolution for these studies typically uses a 64 × 64 or 128 × 128 matrix. More rapid physiologic phenomena, such as first pass cardiac studies, need acquisition framing rates of 25 frames/sec in a 64 × 64 matrix.

Slower functional processes that take place over a period of many minutes, such as kidney function, need frame rates of 20-30 sec with an image resolution of 64 × 64 or 128 × 128 pixels. Hepatobiliary images require acquisition at 1-3 min/frame, and the high count

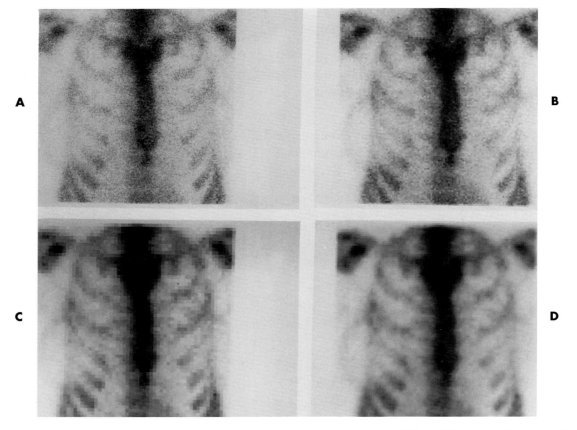

Figure 4-8 Digitized bone scan is shown in high-resolution 256 × 256 matrix **(A),** a 128 × 128 matrix **(B),** and a 64 × 64 matrix **(C).** Both the 256 × 256 and 128 × 128 matrices are adequate for high-resolution imaging; the 64 × 64 matrix begins to lose detail because the pixel size is much larger than the resolution of the camera. Interpolation of the 64 × 64 image data into a 256 × 256 **(D)** matrix fails to recover image resolution, although the image might be more esthetically pleasing.

density allows image matrices of 128×128 or 256×256 to be recorded. Again, the data storage requirements must be considered. A word mode study of 60 1-minute images in a 256×256 matrix requires 7,864,320 bytes (60 frames $\times$ 256 $\times$ 256 $\times$ 2 bytes per word).

Gated blood pool studies and SPECT image files are similar in size and storage format to dynamic studies. SPECT image files from a single detector camera can be acquired as 60 images of 64×64 pixels, or 245,760 words. Significant file space might be required when using multidetector SPECT cameras and acquiring 120 images in a high-resolution matrix of 128×128 pixels using 3,932,160 bytes.

On some computer systems dynamic, gated, or SPECT image files must be stored on sequential data blocks on the disk. When many image files have been acquired and deleted, there might not be enough sequential blocks of available storage, and data acquisition will not be allowed until appropriate space is available. In this case the disk must be "squeezed" to move data so there are no free data blocks between files. Most newer systems do not require contiguous blocks, and information from one file can be distributed into several groups of blocks spread over the disk. The file allocation table on the disk keeps track of the location of the various parts of the file and is totally transparent to the user. Disks that can distribute information in this way cannot be squeezed.

The acquisition of whole-body images into a digital form requires a very high-resolution matrix. The minimum matrix length should be at least a 512-pixel array; however, high-resolution cameras should use a 1024-2048 image matrix. Information acquired into an image matrix size smaller than these arrays has image resolution far below those acquired by spot film imaging.

Many types of imaging are applied to small organs, such as thyroid and heart, compared to the size of the detector. In acquiring computer images of these organs it is sometimes helpful to use hardware magnification, or zoom, to improve the resolution of the acquired image matrix in addition to presenting a larger image for viewing. When the hardware zoom mode is turned on, the x and y signals from the gamma camera are amplified by the zoom factor to fill the image matrix from the center point of the camera, and the outside perimeter of the image is lost. Although zooming increases resolution, there is a decrease in the number of counts per pixel, resulting in a noisier image.

Magnification of areas on digitized images can also be performed. Most commonly it is used to improve the visual display, although there is no increase in resolution. Software zoom is commonly applied to increasing the size of the heart on SPECT myocardial perfusion imaging, since the patient's whole chest fills the field of view; however, the only area of interest is the myocardium. In addition, software zoom of areas on a digitized bone scan also might be useful in better appreciation of small detail such as the vertebrae or hip joints.

Data acquisition of the gated radionuclide ventriculogram (RVG) requires synchronization of dynamic data acquisition with the cardiac cycle. More commonly known as multiple gated acquisition (MUGA), the RR interval of the ECG is divided equally into a series of images. Sixteen to 32 images are used to acquire the data through the length of time for one cardiac cycle. An additional input to the computer to receive the R wave signal from an ECG is required. Data are acquired each time an R wave occurs. The time for each image frame is selected by dividing 60 seconds by the heart rate times the number of images in the sequence. For a 24-frame study, with a heart rate of 60, each frame represents only 42 milliseconds of data acquisition. With the detection of an R wave, acquisition begins with image data rapidly filling each frame in the sequence. If a new R wave is detected before the last frame is reached, acquisition into the first frame of the sequence begins again. Data from several hundred cardiac cycles are required to obtain a statistically accurate image. Images acquired in a 64×64 matrix with a hardware magnification are typically acquired for approximately 5 million counts. Usually this is accomplished in under 10 minutes per view.

The technique just described acquires all data as R waves are detected. In patients with arrhythmias the quality of the data is compromised by premature ventricular contractions (PVCs) and the compensatory beats that follow PVCs. One technique to filter out bad beats is *dual buffering*, which allows information from a single cardiac cycle to be held in temporary image memory buffers. Before this information is added to the final set of data, the length of the cardiac cycle is determined to see if the RR interval is within a selected percentage of the patient's normal cardiac cycle. Heart rates outside the window indicate the buffer should be cleared, and no data from this cardiac cycle is saved. While the first beat was being evaluated, images from the following beat were placed into the second buffer for RR interval evaluation. Data acquisition therefore alternates back and forth between the two buffers, evaluating RR intervals and placing only good cardiac intervals into the save file of images.

Another mechanism for capturing gated cardiac data is list mode acquisition. In list mode the arrival of a z pulse indicates a gamma ray of proper energy has been detected. A timing mark is then stored along with the x and y locations of the scintillation event. In addition, when R waves are detected from the physiologic trigger, a physiologic marker is also placed in the list of data. List mode acquisition requires a significant amount of disk space (several megabytes) to store a single study. The advantage of this technique is that, after data have been acquired as a list of gamma ray events, the data can be evaluated, the desired RR interval can be selected from the acquired data, and images can be constructed only from those of desired heart rate. If the reformatted data are found unacceptable, a new RR interval can be selected and a new series of images can be formatted.

Data obtained from a gated cardiac study are most commonly evaluated by generating a time-activity curve of counts in the left ventricle. If the RR interval has been selected inappropriately, with too many R waves arriving early, image data do not fill the last images of the dynamic sequence equally; therefore counts in the last few frames can be artificially low and the volume curve can tail off at the end. Also, if too many beats have been obtained from inadequately acquired data, the cardiac ejection fraction value may be wrong.

In recent years, gated SPECT myocardial perfusion studies have proven to be helpful in evaluating not only myocardial perfusion, but this technique also displays the slice image as an ECG-gated cinematic study. Thus, not only is perfusion evaluated by the radiopharmaceutical concentration, but diminished perfusion also is correlated with corresponding decreased myocardial wall motion and thinning associated with myocardial infarction.

IMAGE DISPLAY AND PROCESSING

Gamma ray scintillation events that occur at specific detector locations are stored as digital images by accumulating gamma ray counts. As we have discussed, each pixel is stored as a byte or word, and an image is represented as an array or matrix of pixels. Once the information is stored, the image is displayed on a high-resolution CRT. Each pixel on the image is assigned a gray scale value based on the number of counts. Images are typically displayed with the brightest pixel assigned to the maximum display intensity. Display screens and software usually allow images to be displayed as either black on white or white on black. Although the human eye can differentiate fewer than 100 shades of gray, most computer systems generate an 8-bit image, assigning display intensities from 0 to 255. The maximum pixel count is therefore assigned a display intensity of 255 and all other pixels are assigned scaled values from 255 down to 0. Some display systems may be assigned only 64 shades of gray, which is sufficient for viewing. Display artifacts can arise when too few shades of gray are assigned to the display. For example, an image displaying only 16 shades of gray shows the discrete count thresholds that will generate isocount lines where changes in count rate across the image jump from one count threshold to another.

The relationship between the number of counts and display intensity is usually linear (Figure 4-9), which

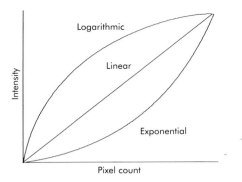

Figure 4-9 Gray-scale intensity can be assigned as a linear relationship relative to the pixel count. An exponential relationship suppresses low counts, providing background subtraction. A logarithmic relationship enhances low-count intensities.

provides a uniform shading between all count levels. Most computers also allow a logarithmic and an exponential relationship between pixel count and intensity. An exponential relationship suppresses the number of gray scales assigned to low-count values while expanding the number of shades of gray assigned to higher pixel counts (see Figure 4-9). This, in effect, reduces the low-count pixels, removing background. Conversely, the logarithmic relationship assigns more gray levels to low-count pixels and compresses the number of shades of gray assigned to high pixel values, enhancing differences in low-count densities.

Background subtraction is another enhancement technique to allow better appreciation of slight differences in count differences. Background enhancement selects a count threshold that is set to the lowest intensity and reassigns intensities between the threshold and the maximum pixel count.

The use of color is another technique to provide image enhancement. Typically a selected color table is used to enhance the differences between pixel count densities and to provide some visual background erase. The red, green, and blue guns of the CRT can be assigned intensity values from 0 to 255 and can be mixed to generate over 16 million colors. A color table that has only ten different colors with discrete steps has the same effect of creating isocontour colors in the image as black and white images with limited shades of gray. The most effective color tables are those that have gradual and continuous shades of color. For example, the colors of the rainbow—from violet through red, representing low- to high-count values, respectively—provide some esthetically pleasing images. Another commonly used color table, the "hot iron" table, assigns gray scales from black to dark red through orange and white for the hottest pixel values. The result is an enhancement similar to an exponential scale to suppress low-count densities.

Image Algebra

The simplest image processing operations are those representing mathematical operations of add, subtract, multiply, and divide. Nuclear medicine computers allow images to be manipulated with these simple functions. For example, a dynamic flow study originally acquired at 1 frame per second can be reformatted through the addition of three images into one to create a dynamic set with each image representing 3 seconds. Image addition is usually performed to improve the count density of images or to compress a sequence of dynamic images into a smaller number of frames, which can be used more easily to identify time-activity changes within the images. Subtraction is commonly applied to an image matrix in one of two ways: subtraction of a numeric value from all pixels, and subtraction of one image from another. Subtraction of a number from the pixel count from each pixel of an image is used to perform background subtraction as an alternative to gray scale enhancement. This technique might be applied to an image where body background is to be eliminated from the image. Subtraction of one frame from another has many clinical uses, such as creation of a cardiac stroke volume image by subtracting the end-systolic image from the end-diastolic image, which leaves only the counts representing areas of myocardial contraction. Another example of frame subtraction is parathyroid imaging, where a technetium image of the thyroid is subtracted from a thallium image of the thyroid and parathyroids. The resultant image is a picture of only parathyroid tissue.

Other simple image manipulations are performed to shift an image a given number of pixels in the x or y direction or to rotate an image about its center point to correct alignment. Image manipulation is also necessary to move images from one position to another with any file of several images.

Image Smoothing

Image smoothing is performed to reduce noise from the random effects of radionuclide counting. The simplest technique is to average the counts of a given pixel with that of its eight surrounding neighbors and replace the center pixel count with the new value.

A most common type of simple image smoothing is a 9-point smooth, a filtering technique to modify a specific pixel value according to the values of its neighbors. The 9-point smooth uses a 3×3 matrix centered over each pixel in the image. The filter weighting values 4, 2, and 1 multiply the center and adjacent pixel values to allow the original value and closest pixels to have more influence on the result of filtering (Figure 4-10). The new computed value after filtering is placed into the pixel location of a new filtered image. Nine-point smoothing blends pixel values with its neighbors, creating a smoother, more esthetic image (Figure 4-10).

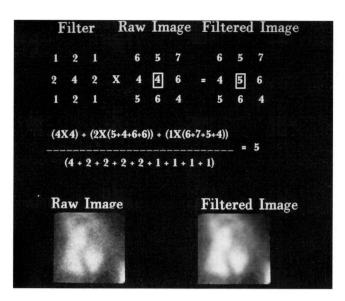

Figure 4-10   A 9-point smooth filter with values of 4, 2, and 1 is applied to the center pixel value *(4)* of a 3×3 pixel area of the raw image. Multiplying the raw image center point by 4, the side values by 2, and the corner pixel values by 1, and then dividing by the filter sum produces a new value *(5)*, which is placed into the filtered image. Raw and 9-point smoothed gated cardiac images are shown at bottom.

However, this smoothing results in a slight loss of resolution, and detail is slightly blurred. Filters can be based not only on a 3×3 matrix but also on a 5×5, 7×7, or larger filter matrix. In addition, filters with negative values around the edges can enhance or sharpen the edges of organs. These filters are sometimes used in applications for automatic edge detection programs.

Filtering of dynamic image sets can use a temporal filter, which performs weighted averaging of an image with those that occur just prior to and just following in a dynamic image sequence. For example, Figure 4-11 shows an example of filtering frame *B* by multiplying the original frame *B* by a weighting value of 2 and adding one times the preceding frame *A* and one times the following image, frame *C*. Temporal filtering is applied most frequently to gated cardiac images with the filter applied in a closed loop. Temporal filtering removes noise without a loss of spatial resolution, as occurs with the 9-point smooth.

Cinematic Display

A dynamic sequence of images may be displayed as a continuous loop movie known as a cinematic display. The images to be displayed are formatted into an area of memory known as a buffer so that information can be retrieved quickly. On some systems there might be insufficient memory, and a display buffer is created on disk. Dynamic studies, gated blood pool images, and SPECT images can all be displayed in a cinematic

Raw images

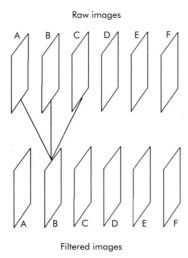

Filtered images

Figure 4-11 Dynamic series of images can be temporally smoothed by adding the previous and following images. Image *B* in the filtered image set is composed of an average of *A, B,* and *C* from the raw images.

mode. The rate at which images are displayed can be changed; for example, the beating heart from a gated blood pool study can be displayed live time in a closed loop to provide an image of the beating heart. Longer dynamic studies, such as 30-minute kidney studies, can be displayed to compress the set of images into a few seconds. The observer therefore has a better appreciation of physiologic changes that occur over a long time.

Image Quantitation

Digital nuclear medicine images are many times acquired to derive quantitative information. Counts in a particular area can be extracted from the image by defining a region of interest (ROI). An ROI is defined on the displayed image using a mouse, joystick, track ball, or light pen. ROIs can be defined as a rectangle or ellipse or manually drawn as an irregular shape. The ROI program usually allows an option to display or print the counts within the region, the number of pixels in the region, and the average count per pixel. Most computer systems allow 16-32 regions to be drawn on a single image. When defining ROIs, the area defined should be physiologically meaningful; for example, when drawing an ROI over the kidney, should the area include the whole kidney and renal pelvis, cortex, and collecting system or simply the cortex? Different information can be extracted from the images, depending on how the ROI has been defined. Some clinical programs perform automated ROI definition. These programs can use a specific count threshold, maximum slope, isocount level, second derivative, or other criteria to identify the edge of an organ. A combination of techniques such as isocount level mixed with the profile maximum slope (second derivative) can be used in

automatically defining the region of the left ventricle on a gated blood pool study.

Some nuclear medicine computer systems allow ROIs to be manipulated just as images can be manipulated. It might be desirable to add or subtract regions. For example, a region defining the renal pelvis could be subtracted from a region defining the whole kidney, leaving the area of the renal cortex. ROIs can be saved with the patient's study to allow reprocessing the information at a later time with the originally defined regions.

Curves

Quantitative information from a single image is derived by setting an ROI and obtaining the ROI counts. The ROI counts in sequential images from a dynamic study can be used to plot the radioactivity versus time change or time-activity curve. Physiologic information from dynamic studies might be appreciated more easily by generating time-activity curves. Curve displays are widely applied to a variety of clinical applications. Curves provide useful information in evaluating the accumulation and washout of radiopharmaceutical from the kidney, changes in left ventricular volume on gated studies (Figure 4-12), and changes in radionuclide distribution on gastrointestinal studies. Curves should be displayed to best demonstrate diagnostic information. When multiple curves are displayed on the same graph, such as the individual kidneys in a renal study, it is important that the curves be properly distinguished one from another and correctly labeled as to their region—left kidney, right kidney, etc. Curve display software many times allows the user to select the options for the format of the display: a continuous line versus dots at each data point, the intensity or color of the curves, and display of axis labels. Curve information should also be scaled properly; that is, the extent of the data range along both the x and y axes changes the appreciation of changes in radioactivity. The appropriate scale of each axis should allow the observer to most accurately view changes of clinical significance in the study. For example, a renal scan with a y axis that is very short would display only a small change in radioactivity in a normal renal study.

The manipulation of curves is also valuable in data interpretation. Simple algebraic functions are useful for applications such as adding curves from two separate regions, performing subtraction of a background curve from an organ curve, or multiplying one curve to match the scaling of another curve.

Due to statistical limitations in counts, it is sometimes helpful to smooth curve data. Commonly a 1-2-1 weighted smooth is done for each curve point with its preceding and following neighbors. Another technique to reduce noise in curve data is to fit the curve points to a mathematical formula that allows additional quan-

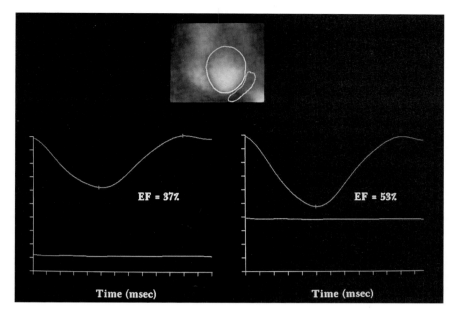

Figure 4-12 Regions of interest of the left ventricle and background can be drawn and time activity curves generated. Curves on the left demonstrate the left ventricle curve *(upper)* and background curve *(lower)*. The background curve contains less activity and is smaller. Curves on the right show a higher background curve *(lower)* after area normalization. With normalization of the background counts, the ejection fraction is correctly computed at 53%.

titative information to be derived. Most commonly, a straight line linear fit or an exponential function is fitted to the data. The fitted curve can then allow quantitative numbers to be measured, such as the slope of a linear function or the half-time of an exponential curve.

Normalization

Normalization is a concept in nuclear medicine that implies that a measurement has been brought to a standard. For instance, two images with different maximum counts may have their intensities normalized if the image with the lowest maximum count is multiplied so that the maximum count matches the second image. The two images, therefore, would be displayed with the same maximum intensity. Normalization is most commonly applied to two ROIs or curves. For example, the counts in ROI-1 are normalized to a second, larger ROI-2 by multiplying ROI-1 counts by a ratio of the number of pixels in ROI-2 divided by the number of ROI-1 pixels. Region normalization is performed most commonly to subtract background counts of one region from the counts from a different size region.

As an example, consider the subtraction of background in calculating left ventricular ejection fraction (EF) from a gated blood pool study (see Figure 4-12). Assume that the counts in an end-diastolic (ED) ROI are 89,485 and in the end-systolic (ES) ROI there are 56,375 counts. We can calculate the left ventricle ejection fraction using the equation: EF = (ED − ES)/

ED × 100. In our example and ignoring background, the ejection fraction would be

$$(89,485 - 56,375)/89,485 \times 100 = 37\%$$

This value is erroneously low, since body background has not been subtracted. Let us assume the end-diastolic ROI contains 89,485 counts with an area of 586 pixels, that the end-systolic counts are 56,375 in 416 pixels, and that a background region contains 9134 counts in 89 pixels. To subtract the proper amount of background activity from the end-diastolic ROI, the area covered by the ROIs must be of the same size, thus the process of region count normalization. Since the background region is smaller than the left ventricle region, the background region counts are multiplied by a ratio of the region sizes (number of left ventricle pixels per number of background pixels).

Normalized background counts =

$$\frac{\text{Background} \times \text{Number of heart pixels}}{\text{Number of background pixels}}$$

The background region contains 9134 counts in 89 pixels, and the end-diastolic heart region contains 586 pixels; the normalized end-diastolic background becomes 9134 × (586/89), or 60,140 counts. This can be subtracted from the end-diastolic count of 89,485, giving a background subtracted end-diastolic count of 29,345. The same normalization calculation can be made for the end-systolic region, which contains 56,375 counts in 416 pixels; the normalized background is 9134 × (416/89), or 42,693 counts. Subtracting this

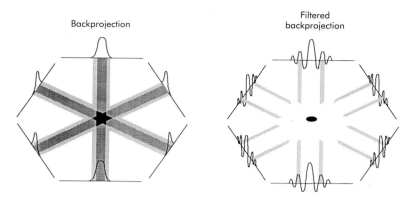

Figure 4-13   Back-projection *(left)* in SPECT reconstruction creates a streak or star artifact. Filtered back-projection *(right)* creates negative values on the sides of high count areas that cancel positive values and remove the star artifact.

normalized background from the end-systolic left ventricle counts gives a net of 13,682 counts. With these normalized background-subtracted values, a background-corrected ejection fraction is calculated as

$$(29,345 - 13,682)/29,345 \times 100 = 53\%$$

With proper subtraction of background, the ejection fraction value has now been significantly changed.

These same principles of normalization can be applied to curve mathematics. Multiplying the background curve by the ratio of the organ region size divided by a smaller background region size properly increases the background curve for subtraction, significantly changing the ejection fraction value. Note that the background curve on the lower right of Figure 4-12 is increased after correct scaling by normalization and that the EF values have changed.

SPECT IMAGING

SPECT imaging is performed by obtaining planar images with the scintillation camera from many angles around the patient. Images are acquired from 360 degrees around the patient, except in myocardial perfusion studies, where 180-degree right anterior oblique to left posterior oblique images over the anterior chest are acquired. Images are acquired in 64 × 64 resolution for most studies for single detector cameras or low count images from multiple detector systems. Images of 128 × 128 resolution can be acquired on high count studies. The planar projection SPECT images are first viewed cinematically to ensure no significant patient motion has occurred. Image data are then backprojected (Figure 4-13, *left*) to overlay areas of increased activity and create a transverse slice image. Back-projection produces a streak or star artifact that results from data being laid onto the slice image from various projections. A technique called filtered backprojection reduces the streak artifact. In the recon-

struction process a frequency space filter is used to modify the projection data, in essence creating negative values on each side of areas of increased counts. These negative numbers, when combined with positive values, cancel each other out, eliminating streak artifacts (Figure 4-13, *right*). Streaks are also reduced by obtaining images from many angles, about 120 images in 360 degrees, essentially viewing objects from more angles.

Frequency Space and Filtering

SPECT reconstruction and filtering will be best understood after discussing the representation of images as a group of frequencies. The representation of objects as a frequency or a spectrum of frequencies is an unusual concept. A simple example is shown in Figure 4-14. This figure represents the count profile of an image with 0.5 centimeter bars and with spaces 0.5 centimeters wide. The counts in the profile of the bar appear as square blocks of activity, which can be approximated by the pattern of a wave with a specific wavelength and amplitude. The wavelength replicates the spacing of the bar pattern, and the amplitude replicates the height or in this case the number of counts. Therefore a simplistic representation of the bar pattern image would be frequency 1 cycle per centimeter with an amplitude of 200.

Image filtering to reduce noise depends on the information content of the image (e.g., counts, collimator, scatter, object distance, background activity). In frequency space filtering there will always be a trade-off or balance between reducing noise and degrading resolution, and vice versa.

Image information can be represented in frequency space by graphically plotting the frequency on the horizontal axis and the wave amplitude on the vertical axis. In Figure 4-15 a square count profile *(top)* of an object can be roughly estimated by using a single wave with a specific wavelength and specific height or amplitude. To the right of the single wave in Figure 4-15 is the fre-

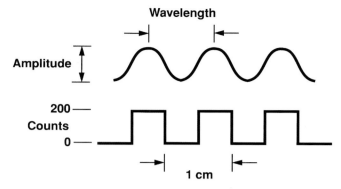

Figure 4-14   A simple application of frequencies would be in estimating the count profile of a parallel line bar phantom as represented at the bottom of the diagram, where 0.5 cm bars and spaces are shown in this count profile. A frequency space estimate of this pattern would be a sinusoidal pattern with wavelength of 1 cm and an amplitude that would correspond to 200 units. The total bar pattern image can now be roughly estimated by specifying a frequency of 1 cycle/cm with amplitude of 200.

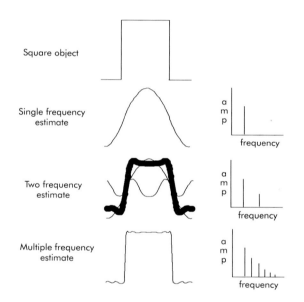

Figure 4-15   Count profile of a square object can be roughly estimated as a single frequency, or wave. The diagram on the right and top represents a single frequency with a specific amplitude to estimate the square object. Two frequencies can be added together *(dark curve)* to better estimate the profile of the original square object. Many frequencies *(bottom)* can be added to more accurately represent the original square profile. The group of frequencies in the lower right curve generate a frequency spectrum of the original object.

quency space graph, showing a single frequency with a specific amplitude, thus representing a very rough estimate of the original square object. An improved representation is made by adding a second wave of higher frequency, also with a specific amplitude. The dark line in Figure 4-15 shows two frequencies added, which bet-

ter represent the original square object. When multiple waves are combined, they provide an accurate representation of the original object *(bottom)*. The group of frequencies *(bottom right)* that now represent this object form a continuous curve—the frequency spectrum of the object. A mathematical process called the *Fourier transform* accomplishes the conversion of the image into its wave components. An inverse process called the inverse Fourier transform transfers the frequency group back into the x,y coordinate system, reconstructing the image. Images in the usual spatial domain are represented as counts in a pixel; in the frequency domain images are represented as amplitudes of various frequencies. The Fourier transform is computationally intense and is usually performed in an array processor to save time.

Frequency space can be thought of as analogous to a piano keyboard. The low keys create long frequency tones, and the upper keys create high frequencies. The combination of several frequencies, such as playing a chord, generates a certain sound. Changing a single frequency, such as changing one note in the chord, creates a sound with a different impression. Images are similarly characterized by properly mixing frequencies. Any object can be represented by a group of sine or cosine waves.

When images are converted to frequency space, objects or organs in the image are represented as a group of low and middle frequencies (Figure 4-16, *top*). The pixel-to-pixel count differences due to variations in counting statistics is represented as a group of high frequencies that we call noise. Figure 4-16 *(top)* shows body background activity as low frequencies, that is, constant activity (long wavelengths) in the body. The significant advantage of converting images to frequency space should now become clear; noise is represented by high frequencies, somewhat separate from the frequencies that represent the object organ of interest.

Filtering, or the reduction of noise, occurs in frequency space by reducing high-frequency information. Noise is reduced by multiplying the frequency space curve by a filter curve (Figure 4-16, *bottom*). The filter values at the low and middle frequencies multiply the object frequencies to retain the organs of interest in the image. The filter values at higher frequencies drop to zero, multiplying high frequencies by zero or very small values, thus eliminating noise.

Filters are mathematical formulas that generate the curve shape, and cutoff values determine the dropoff point of the filter. Cutoff frequency is a common parameter used to generate and characterize filter shapes. Commonly used are the ramp, von Hann (or Hanning), Butterworth, Parzen, Hamming, Wiener, and Metz filters. All these filters have the same basic purpose—to increase the amplitudes of the object frequencies and reduce the amplitude of the high frequencies. The ramp filter (Figure 4-17) is the highest

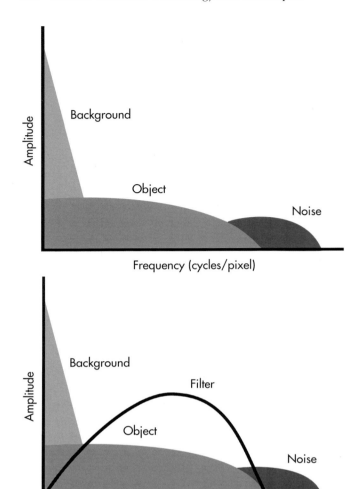

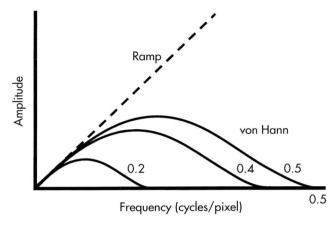

Figure 4-17 A ramp filter is the highest resolution frequency space filter but also creates the largest amount of noise due to its high values due to its great amplitude at high frequencies. Von Hann filters with a cut-off frequency of 0.2, 0.4, and 0.5 cycles per pixel represent commonly used low-pass filters.

Figure 4-16 *Top,* Frequencies representing an image include high frequencies that are the noise in the image and middle and low frequencies that represent the object and uniform body background. *Bottom,* The frequency space filter, when selected with the right cutoff frequency or point where it drops back down to zero amplitude, enhances the object while multiplying the noise frequency by zero to eliminate the noise.

resolution filter but also significantly multiplies high frequencies, producing a noisy image. There is a group of filters classified as low pass, which includes von Hann, Hamming, Butterworth, Parzen and others. Low-pass filters let low frequencies through. Each of these filters is actually a family of filters, defined by various cutoff frequencies. For example, a low-pass filter with a higher cutoff frequency will produce a higher resolution but a noisier image. Using a von Hann filter with a cutoff frequency of 0.2 cycles per pixel produces a smooth image because image frequencies higher than 0.2 are multiplied by small filter values (or zero), therefore reducing noise. A von Hann filter with a cutoff frequency of 0.4 cycle per pixel (Figure 4-17) includes more high frequencies and produces a high-resolution image with little reduction in noise. Frequency space

filtering must balance high resolution against noise reduction. Low-count images must remove many high frequencies and therefore must be smooth, low-resolution images. High-resolution filtered images can be obtained with high-count images.

Butterworth filters are in several aspects the best of the group of low-pass filters. This is because the mathematical formula contains not only a cutoff frequency parameter but also another parameter called the order that adjusts the downslope or roll off of the upper part of the filter. Figure 4-18 *(top)* shows two Butterworth filters, both with an order 4 but with cutoff frequencies of 0.2 and 0.4 cycles/pixel. Butterworth filters with a cut-off frequency of 0.2 and orders of 3, 4, and 5 (Figure 4-18, *bottom*) show steeper downslopes as the order increases. A steeper downslope will produce a higher resolution image.

Another group of filters is adaptive filters, sometimes called restorative filters. Adaptive filters (Metz and Wiener) are powerful filtering techniques in that they use some criteria about the resolution capabilities of the camera and collimator within the mathematical filter function. These filters differ from low-pass filters by not only suppressing noise, but they also prevent blurring and the smoothing of edges of objects. Both Metz and Wiener filters are a family of curves with a multiplier value to create different curve shapes and control the point at which the downslope occurs (Figure 4-19).

Filtering and Tomographic Reconstruction

Many of the filters used for frequency space filtering can also be used in the filtered back-projection reconstruction algorithm. Finding proper filtering for each type of patient study to reduce noise and obtain high

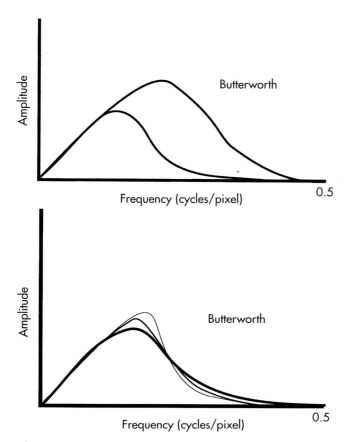

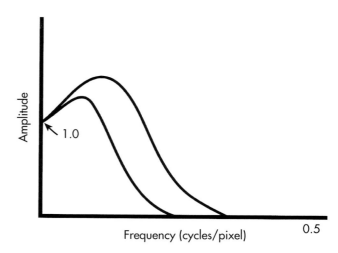

Figure 4-19 Adaptive filters, such as the Wiener, start with amplitude values of 1 and can be controlled by a parameter to enhance middle frequency to provide good smoothing and constant count areas. The roll off portion of the curve provides excellent edge retention of objects with good contrast.

Figure 4-18 The Butterworth filter has two parameters to define the shape of this low-pass filter. The order controls the down slope and cut-off frequency defines the width or spread of the filter. The top curves represent Butterworth filters with order 4 and cut-off frequencies of 0.2 and 0.4. The bottom curves all have the same cut-off frequency (0.2) and orders of 3, 4, and 5.

resolution remains a matter of personal preference in the final image appearance. There is a continual choice between obtaining a high-resolution image and obtaining a smooth image; increasing smoothing through filtering reduces resolution.

Image filtering is usually employed twice in SPECT reconstruction. On most computer systems filtering is performed first as a prefiltering function to remove noise from the planar projection images; then filtering is also incorporated into the reconstruction algorithm. The resultant image quality is influenced directly by image acquisition parameters (matrix size, number of stops, counts per image) and filtering. Although a ramp filter provides the highest resolution SPECT reconstruction, the slices contain a significant amount of noise; therefore optimum prefiltering or postfiltering of slices is an important factor in obtaining high-resolution SPECT. As an example of SPECT reconstruction, processing a ^{201}Tl myocardial study usually begins with a prefiltering of the images prior to reconstruction. Prefiltering is performed most commonly using a

low-pass filter for noise reduction. During reconstruction, a second filter is used in the filtered back-projection reconstruction. Studies such as thallium scans have very poor statistics in the planar images, and filtering is needed to provide an esthetic and interpretable set of slice images. SPECT imaging of the liver requires smooth slices, since abnormalities usually are seen as cold defects in a uniform area of radiopharmaceutical distribution. SPECT imaging of the lumbar spine on a bone scan has many counts and excellent resolution, whereas filters that retain the higher frequencies yield high-resolution slice images.

Prefiltering with low-pass filters using a small cutoff frequency (0.1 cycle per pixel) results in images slightly oversmoothed with some loss in resolution. When the image filter includes too many high frequencies, filtering and filtered back-projection algorithms create a mottled pattern in areas that should have uniform radionuclide distribution. Studies in which high counts are obtained with high-resolution collimators, such as bone imaging of the spine or brain imaging with ^{99m}Tc HMPAO, require the use of a low-pass filter with a fairly high cutoff frequency (0.35-0.5 cycles per pixel). With proper filter selection, these high-count studies yield images with high resolution and little noise. Multiple-detector scintillation cameras obviously have higher sensitivity than single-detector SPECT cameras and yield images with higher count statistics and higher resolution. In addition, the recent implementation of convergent collimators such as fan beam, astigmatic, and cone beam geometries also has improved sensitivity. Many more counts are obtained by these systems.

The speed of some new nuclear medicine computers will, in the near future, allow the use of reconstruction algorithms other than filtered back-projection techniques. These new computers have many megabytes of memory, and their ultrafast processors can execute computationally intense algorithms, such as maximum likelihood (ML), expectation maximization (EM), and conjugate gradient. These new algorithms give improved image quality with a reduction in streak artifacts.

Iterative Reconstruction Algorithms

More complex reconstruction algorithms, called *iterative reconstruction algorithms* have been introduced on some commercial systems in recent years. Iterative reconstruction techniques incorporate much more information about the physics of the imaging situation into the algorithm. Therefore these algorithms are computationally much more intense and may require several minutes to reconstruct. All iterative algorithms, as this name implies, consist of computing a series of improving images of the three-dimensional distribution of activity. Most algorithms will provide clinically useful images after about 20 iterations. There are specific categories of iterative algorithms, such as maximum likelihood, expectation maximization, conjugate gradient, and maximum a priori (MAP). Each filter has its own distinct advantages.

Reconstructions using iterative techniques have no streak artifacts that are produced by back-projection algorithms. Iterative reconstructed images have improved resolution compared to filtered back-projection, and the edges of organs look sharp with good image contrast. Therefore little postreconstruction filtering is required to produce clinical quality images.

Three-Dimensional Display

Although commercial SPECT systems have been available for over 10 years, techniques to view the vast amount of data contained in a series of slice images have remained limited. Surface display and volume rendering are two techniques for three-dimensional viewing. Surface displays are created by selecting a count threshold for generating a three-dimensional isocount surface. The problem, therefore, becomes to correctly set this threshold to include only clinically useful information; the proper threshold setting, therefore, is critical for proper clinical interpretation of the three-dimensional object. Since this display shows only a solid outer surface of the organ, information inside the organ is not seen; therefore the most suitable organs for surface displays are thin organs with cold abnormalities, such as the heart (Figure 4-20) and brain cortex. A very smooth set of slice images creates a smoother surface than the reconstructed slices for directed viewing. Volume rendering is a display technique that pro-

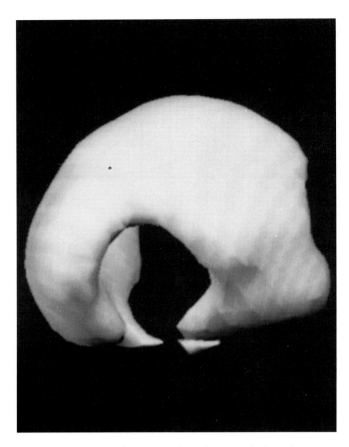

Figure 4-20 Three-dimensional surface renderings from SPECT data create an anatomic and pleasing display. This ^{201}Tl scan shows an inferoapical defect as seen from the 45 LAO projection.

vides a translucent appearance to a three-dimensional volume. A stack of reconstructed transverse slices (an image volume) are reprojected into planar images from multiple directions around the object volume like the original planar images (Figure 4-21, *A*). In this reprojection process the maximum pixel count along each projection line is selected as the maximum activity that would be seen for an individual pixel. This projection of the highest concentration of radioactivity provides the image a translucent appearance and also produces an image with very little noise. This technique is excellent for identifying hot abnormalities in SPECT image data and can be applied to a variety of studies, such as finding hot lesions on bone SPECT and identifying hepatic hemangiomas on labeled red cell studies (Figure 4-21, *B*). The volume rendered projections are viewed cinematically to produce a dramatic and esthetically pleasing display.

CLINICAL APPLICATIONS

Most hospitals use clinical applications programs provided by a computer manufacturer. Before commercial sale of this software, the company must provide evi-

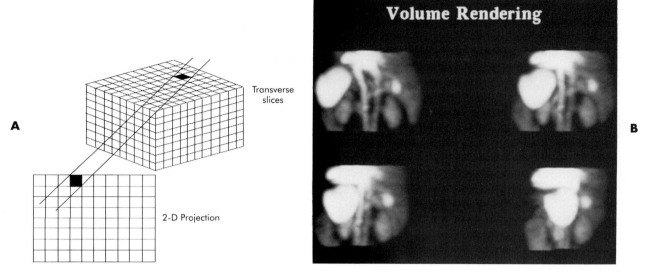

Figure 4-21 **A,** Volume rendering displays are generated from a stack of transverse slices by reprojecting the data into two-dimensional projections for cinematic viewing. The highest count pixel along the path for reprojection is placed into the 2-D image. **B,** Volume rendered translucent display of a hepatic hemangioma study shows the exact anatomic location of a hot lesion in the liver as seen from four different angles.

dence to the Food and Drug Administration of clinical utility along with a description of the program. The accuracy of derived values can vary slightly from one computer system to the next. For example, if we took one patient-gated blood pool study and processed it on several different brands of computers, we would find some variation in the left ventricular ejection fraction value. These variations come from how automated or manual edge detection techniques are implemented, background placement is selected, and so on. We trust that there is not enough variation to change the diagnosis of the patient. Validation of program results is important along with establishing normal values of quantitative results.

Clinical applications programs designed specifically for use in your own hospital can be written in a programming language such as C or Fortran, or you can create a *macro protocol.* A macro is a chain of simple computer operations that are combined to form a practical and meaningful method of evaluating image data. For example, a simple macro can be written to perform image normalization and subtraction of ^{201}Tl-^{99m}Tc thyroid images for parathyroid localization. More involved macros, such as for a renal study, perform a long sequence of operations, such as adding frames of a flow study, displaying the summed image, setting ROIs, generating curves, subtracting normalized background, displaying curves, and performing calculations. Clinical programs or macro protocols should be carefully planned and written to ensure accuracy of the results. Errors or bugs should be identified and removed to ensure that accurate and clinically useful information is being obtained. Any calculated values should be tested on several sets of data to validate the results.

Workstations

Image viewing is most conveniently handled on a multitasking workstation with a graphic user interface. Graphic workstations (see Figure 4-2) usually have a large screen, at least 19 inches, for displaying both images and text. The ease of use and speed of handling image files are very important and are implemented using a windows environment (Figure 4-22), which allows a separate task to be performed in each of several windows. The computer operator manipulates each window by moving the mouse to point a cursor to boxes in the window. Interaction is done with the mouse buttons and keyboard to select various options for processing and display. With several windows open on the screen, the operator can display a study in one window, perform SPECT reconstruction in a different window, and in another window perform data archiving, all simultaneously. Windows environments have also become popular on powerful personal computers and permit several programs to be accessed at the same time.

Nonimaging Computer Applications

Personal computers have found many applications in the nuclear medicine department to perform common business activities. A variety of commercial software programs for word processing, accounting, spreadsheets, and database management have a variety of administrative and patient applications. Unique programs for patient scheduling and generating reports of patient studies are also available. Nuclear pharmacy calculations and records can be automated and accurate records kept using commercially available database programs. Some database software provides access of data

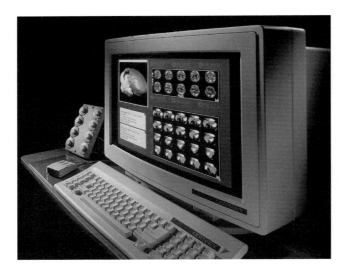

Figure 4-22 Workstation with windows environment provides the ability to perform several processes simultaneously. The mouse is used to move the cursor between windows for interaction with the different processes. (Courtesy Ohio Imaging Division, Picker International, Inc., Bedford Heights, Ohio.)

fields from other records to grant cross-referencing capabilities. For instance, quality control records containing the lot number of a radiopharmaceutical can be referenced to a record of patient doses administered from that lot number.

Networks

Networking of computers in nuclear medicine not only has become common but is also an important enhancement to the nuclear medicine clinic. The connection of two or more computers from the same manufacturer is often simple, and the transfer of images and programs can be performed with ease. However, initial complications may occur when networking systems come from different manufacturers; hardware differences, communications problems, and different image file formats are common challenges. Standard networking protocols such as Ethernet allow reliable communication between systems. Files are usually pushed from one system to another by communications software, which takes only a few seconds to transfer an image file. Additional programs might be required to convert image files properly from one manufacturer's format to that of another.

Several different configurations can be used for networking imaging computers. Figure 4-23 shows four possible arrangements of networks: central host computer, bus network, star network, and ring network. Host networking connects several computers to a larger central host computer for storing and processing all data. The host computer usually has more than one processing terminal for image manipulation and display. Large-capacity disks, optical disks, and tape are available for image storage and archiving. A bus network connects several computers along a single communications line. Each computer has a unique name, and the destination computer is specified when transferring files. A star network connects several computers through a central point. A ring configuration provides a network whereby files are passed around the ring to the destination computer.

PACS

In many departments all nuclear medicine images are acquired digitally and are transferred from one system to another. Physicians can also view and interpret images directly from the computer screen, thus eliminating the need for film. Such a system is called a picture archiving and communications system (PACS). The filmless nuclear medicine department should have hardware and procedures in place to allow archiving of image data, a backup copy of these data, and enough storage capacity to keep many patient studies available for immediate retrieval. Image data should be kept several years, consistent with the practice for maintaining a film library for a specified period.

The Internet

The Internet, or the "information super highway" can be most simply described as a network of networks. At present, there are approximately 80,000 computer networks that are connected together to form the Internet. The Internet was born over 20 years ago from a U.S. Defense Department project to connect various military research sites. The computers send information in an envelope called an Internet Protocol (IP) packet of data to a specific "address." During the 1970s and 1980s this network expanded to include military, government, educational, and commercial computer centers. Although no one owns the Internet, there are organizations that promote the global exchange of information and provide technical direction and management.

The organization of computers on the Internet is controlled by an addressing system. Your own postal mailing address for your residence or business has information from the largest geographic area to a specific city, street, and number. Internet addresses have a set of names and numbers associated for both the computer and computer network. A location such as med.utah.edu indicates direction of the information to the education network domain, the University of Utah, and specifically to the Medical Center computer. Likewise, the information could have been directed to 155.100.78. Data files to be transferred on the Internet are broken up into small, manageably sized data packets that may actually be routed in different directions

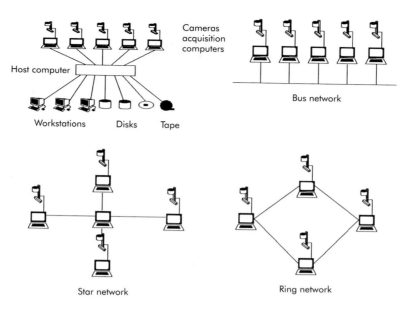

Figure 4-23 Nuclear medicine networks can have a variety of configurations. *Upper left*, Acquisition computers send images to a central host computer, which acts as a server for workstations and peripheral devices. *Upper right*, Bus network, such as Ethernet, allows a line for communication between imaging computers. *Lower left*, Star network allows connection through a central machine. *Lower right*, Ring network allows data to be passed around a closed loop.

on the Internet but arrive and are reorganized into their original format at their destination. The transmission and reorganization of a file is transparent to the computer user and is part of the beauty of the software that uses the Internet Protocol.

Computers within large institutions may be directly connected to the Internet or their network may be connected to the Internet. Access to the Internet may also be provided using either standard telephone lines or special high-speed data lines that connect to another computer that resides on the Internet. Home service is most commonly provided through a commercial network provider for which you pay a nominal monthly fee and pay for your connection time. Often, nuclear medicine computers may not be connected to the Internet due to the concern over security issues. Any computer directly connected to the Internet should have appropriate security of user accounts and protection of data. Computer network system administrators may prevent unauthorized access to sensitive patient data and protect programs.

The Internet provides computer users with the ability to exchange and obtain information. Electronic mail (e-mail) uses a standard format of data called Simple Mail Transfer Protocol (SMTP) to allow various types of computers and software to send and receive mail. As previously mentioned, electronic mail must be addressed not only to a specific computer on a certain Internet domain but also to a specific individual account.

The transfer of information files can be done using ftp (File Transfer Protocol). This protocol uses a stan-

dard transfer method of data between Internet sites. Users may use ftp to enter computers where they have permission to look at a listing of files in different directories and *get* or *put* files. To use ftp, the user must have a fairly specific idea of the computer to be accessed and file directory to be reviewed to obtain the desired information. In the early 1990s a more friendly way of locating information was developed. One of these methods is using software called *Gopher*. Gopher was developed at the University of Minnesota to allow individuals to find specific documents without knowing the exact location of the information. Gopher uses a client-server mode, which connects to an institution's own Gopher server that provides menus of publicly available information. Gopher servers are linked together to provide a wide range of information to be searched and obtained. Other types of networking search programs such as Archie and Veronica allow users to access information that is indexed by key word and title on a regular basis.

The most rapidly expanding part of the Internet is the World Wide Web (WWW or W3). The WWW is based on *hypertext* documents. Hypertext documents have "links" to other documents on the same computer or information at another location, which could be in another city or even country. Hypertext documents differ from other types of connectivity on the Internet in that they provide not only text but also image files, video files, and sound files, which are transferred at the click of a mouse button. A hypertext document is written in a special format language called hypertext markup language (html). Special formatting codes within these documents instruct the local computer to display a certain size font and text, where to position an image file on the page, etc. Links to other documents appear as colored text or small icons, which are activated by clicking on them with the mouse button. This may access a video file, an image or sound file, or may simply connect to another document.

Access to the World Wide Web is obtained using "browser" software that interprets hypertext documents. Browsers like Mosaic, Netscape, and Internet Explorer are common favorites and for personal computers are very reasonably priced. Browser software also contains access to search engines where the user may type in words that describe any topic of interest, and a list of sites using hypertext links is presented on the screen. The user may then move around or "surf" through documents at various sites to locate information.

The World Wide Web provides tremendous opportunities for locating or exchanging information between web sites. For example, a Nuclear Medicine Department could create a web server with documents relevant to its research, continuing education programs, or teaching files, all of which can be available on line to anyone with access to the Internet. At this time many large teaching hospitals have web sites with a variety of information.

SUGGESTED READINGS

English RJ, Brown SE: *SPECT: single photon emission computed tomography: a primer,* ed 2, New York, 1988, Society of Nuclear Medicine.

Erickson JJ: Nuclear medicine computer systems—hardware, *J Nucl Med Technol* 13:97-102, 1985.

Erickson JJ: Nuclear medicine computer systems—software, *J Nucl Med Technol* 13:140-149, 1985.

Erickson JJ, Rollo FD, ed: *Digital nuclear medicine,* Philadelphia, 1983, Lippincott.

Glowniak JV: An introduction to the Internet, part 1: history, organization, and function, *J Nucl Med Technol* 23:56-64, 1995.

Glowniak JV: An introduction to the Internet, part 2: obtaining access. *J Nucl Med Technol* 23:150-157, 1995.

Glowniak JV: An introduction to the Internet, part 3: Internet services, *J Nucl Med Technol* 23:231-248, 1995.

Glowniak JV: An introduction to the Internet, part 4: medical resources, *J Nucl Med Technol* 24:1996.

Harkness B, Christian P, Rowell K: *Clinical computers in nuclear medicine,* New York, 1992, Society of Nuclear Medicine.

Lee K: *Computers in nuclear medicine: a practical approach,* New York, 1991, Society of Nuclear Medicine.

Robert L. Dressler, Jay A. Spicer

chapter 5

Laboratory Science

Objectives

Use laboratory glassware appropriately including beakers, flasks, graduated cylinders, pipets, and burets.

Use an analytical balance to perform mass measurements accurately.

Use and calibrate a centrifuge to separate solids from liquids.

Use a pH meter.

Describe the electronic structure of atoms.

Explain the structure of the periodic chart of elements, and discuss characteristics of various groups.

Explain ionic and covalent bonds.

Use the laws of constant composition and multiple proportions.

Describe the gram atomic weights, gram molecular weights, and the mole.

Describe molarity, molality, and normality.

Explain the characteristics and production of colloids.

Demonstrate and use chemical reaction equations.

Describe oxidation-reduction reactions and electrolytic reactions.

Define acids, bases, and neutralizing reactions.

Define and measure pH.

Explain the mechanisms of buffering solutions.

Describe the simple nomenclature of organic compounds.

*I*n the beginning humans were created as a fusion of two components, one spiritual and the other chemical. As has been and is now, the well-being of each component is vital to life. Although our spiritual involvement with patients is of utmost importance, one must possess a knowledge of the chemical component of life for the successful practice of nuclear medicine.

The following discussion of the chemical principles, fundamental to an understanding of life and the diagnostic processes used in the hope of maintaining a healthy life, is not to be considered as the complete or necessary knowledge required. Because of limitations of space, the following discussion of chemistry is brief and often inadequate. Our hope and intention are that the individual instructors using this text will recognize the points that require further elucidation and will use their knowledge and talents to do so.

GLASSWARE AND INSTRUMENTATION

Glassware

The fundamental part of any scientific laboratory is the equipment, the most basic of which is the glassware. Figure 5-1 shows those items most commonly used in routine laboratory manipulations.

Beakers, flasks, and graduated cylinders. The most frequently used type of glassware is the beaker. Beakers range in capacity from a few milliliters to several liters and are utilized in the preparation of solutions and as weighing vessels when a high degree of accuracy is not required.

Erlenmeyer flasks are also used in these procedures and, because of their conic shape and small mouth, offer the advantage that solutions can be prepared by swirling the contents of the flask with little risk of spilling. This feature also makes the Erlenmeyer flask an ideal vessel for the substance in titrations. Neither the beaker nor the flask provides the accuracy ($\pm 5\%$ to 10%) required for precise volume measurement.

Volume measurements requiring an accuracy of $\pm 1\%$ to 2% can be achieved by the use of the appropriate graduated cylinder (Figure 5-1). However, many laboratory procedures require the preparation of solutions accurate in concentration to $\pm 0.001\%$. This precision can be attained by use of a volumetric flask. Flasks marked TC are calibrated "to contain" a specific volume, depending on the size of the flask, and allow volume measurement within the accuracy limits noted above.

Pipets and burets. In the normal course of laboratory work many occasions arise where a precise volume of a solution or solvents is required and an appropriate-sized volumetric flask is not available. In such cases a small (< 5 ml) or nonintegral volume is usually required, and one must resort to the use of a pipet or buret.

Pipets (Figure 5-1) are transfer vessels used to measure and deliver a precise volume of solution or pure liquid. They are generally of two types: those that must be filled and drained manually, and automatic pipets, which measure and deliver a fixed volume when activated.

The ordinary pipets, which require manipulation, are of two styles: one is calibrated to deliver a fixed volume, whereas the other type is graduated and may be used to deliver any increment of volume up to the full capacity of the pipet. Both styles are available in sizes ranging from microvolumes (a fraction of a milliliter) to those having a capacity of several hundred milliliters.

Care must be exercised in the use of pipets, since some are calibrated to deliver the stated volume by nor-

mal drainage (some solution remains in the tip of the pipet), and others are calibrated to deliver the entire volume drawn into the pipet and thus require "blowing out" of the last traces of the solution. The blow-out pipets are identified by one or two bands placed near the top.

Automatic pipets are especially important to the radioimmunoassay laboratory where accurately known volumes of radioactive solutions are required.

Procedures, such as titrations (p. 149), in which an accurately measured but unknown volume of solution must be determined, are conveniently performed by use of a buret. The buret, being graduated, allows a direct reading of the volume used in reaching the end point, the point at which the added titrant has reacted with the entire quantity of substance present in the sample.

Instrumentation

Just as certain types of glassware are important to the laboratory, so also are several instruments. All nuclear pharmacy or radioassay laboratories must be equipped with a minimum of three instruments: an analytic balance, a centrifuge, and a pH meter.

The analytic balance. The analytic balance (Figure 5-2) is vital to any laboratory where mass measurements of solids are routinely required, usually in small quantities (< 1 g). The balance shown in Figure 5-2 allows mass measurements accurate to ± 0.1 mg.

The balance is designed so that as the units on the weight dials are changed the instrument automatically adds or removes weights from a knife-edge counterbalance inside the instrument. Newer, currently available analytic balances are automatic taring and provide a direct digital readout of weight. If handled with care, the balance will give dependable results with a minimum of service.

The centrifuge. Quite often it is necessary to separate solids from liquids, such as red blood cells from the plasma. When such separations are necessary, a centrifuge is used (Figure 5-3).

The centrifuge is composed of a balanced motor and shaft on which cups or holders are mounted. A container holding the mixture to be separated is placed in one cup and a counterbalance container (having the same weight as the sample container) is placed in the cup opposite the sample.

The centrifuge exerts a strong centrifugal force on the sample by spinning the material at relatively high speeds (500 to 1500 rpm) and, as in the case of blood, the heavier red blood cells settle to the bottom of the container, leaving the lighter plasma on top. One can then draw off the plasma, thus effecting a separation of the two components.

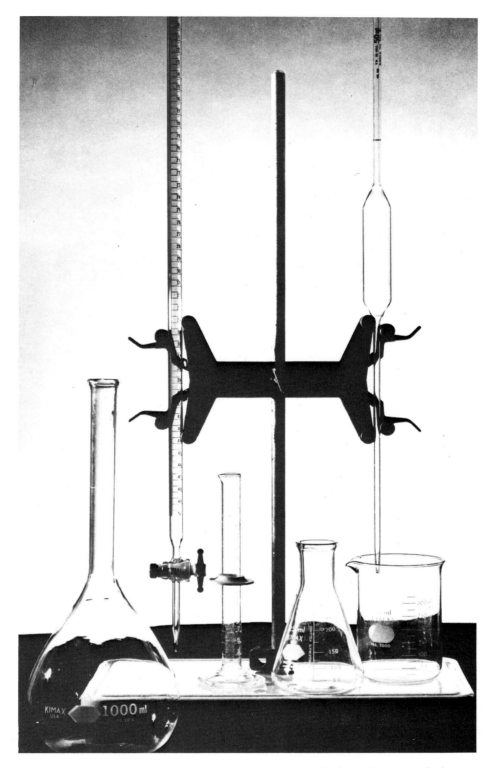

Figure 5-1   Glassware. *Left to right,* Volumetric flask, buret, graduated cylinder, Erlenmeyer flask, pipet, and beaker.

The pH meter. The measurement of pH is generally accomplished by two methods, one of which provides reasonably accurate values and the other, more precise values. The less sensitive method makes use of a paper containing a universal indicator. The universal indica- tor is a mixture of organic dyes, which themselves are acids and bases, and it undergoes changes in color upon being converted from one form to the other, that is, acid to base or base to acid. These color changes occur at specific pH values.

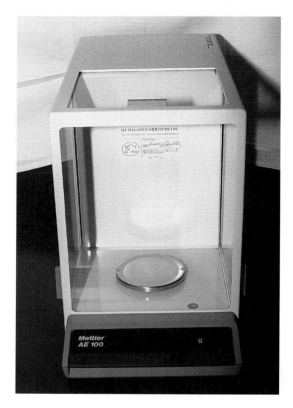

Figure 5-2 Analytic balance.

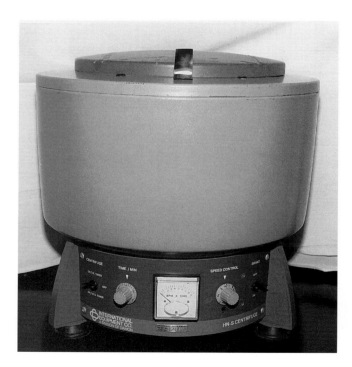

Figure 5-3 Centrifuge.

Accurate pH values, which are usually necessary in radioimmunoassay analysis or the preparation of radiopharmaceuticals, are determined by use of a pH meter (Figure 5-4).

A pH meter has two electrodes. Note that the one in Figure 5-4 contains both electrodes in a single probe. One electrode of known potential (a calomel electrode) serves as a reference and involves the following electrode reaction:

$$2Hg + 2Cl^- \rightleftharpoons Hg_2Cl_2 + 2e^-$$

This reaction has a constant potential of -0.27 V. The second electrode (a glass electrode) consists of a meter wire dipped into a solution of known pH, and this solution is separated by a thin glass membrane from the solution whose pH is to be determined. The potential across the glass membrane, and thus the half-cell voltage of this electrode, is a function of the pH of the solution outside the membrane. A third component of a pH meter is a voltmeter or potentiometer capable of measuring voltages accurate to at least ± 0.01 V. The voltmeter or potentiometer is designed, based upon the potential difference of the two electrodes, to give a reading in pH units.

ELEMENTS AND COMPOUNDS

In introducing the study of chemistry, as it applies to nuclear medicine and nuclear pharmacy as well as any other discipline, it is desirable to define the word *chemistry*. Chemistry can best be defined as the study of matter and the changes that matter undergoes.

All matter exists in one of three physical states—solid, liquid, or gas. Each substance differs in physical and chemical properties from all other substances.

Physical properties are the attributes characteristic of a substance, such as odor, color, hardness, luster, density, and structure. These properties depend on the conditions imposed upon the substance and may be affected by a change in temperature, pressure, or radiation. However, a substance, be it an element or a compound, that has undergone a change in physical properties because of a change in conditions, will exhibit the initial properties when the substance is returned to the original condition. For example, sulfur, which is a yellow solid at room temperature, becomes a liquid when heated to 113° C and returns to the yellow solid when allowed to cool. Physical changes are readily reversible.

In contrast to a change in physical properties, chemical change results in a complex and deep-seated change. Chemical change always results in the formation of one or more "new" substances, each of which has chemical and physical properties unique to itself.

Most chemical changes are reversible only with great difficulty, and many, for example, the burning of wood or paper, are irreversible.

Electronic Structure

Since each element has unique chemical and physical properties, it is logical to ask why this is so. To answer

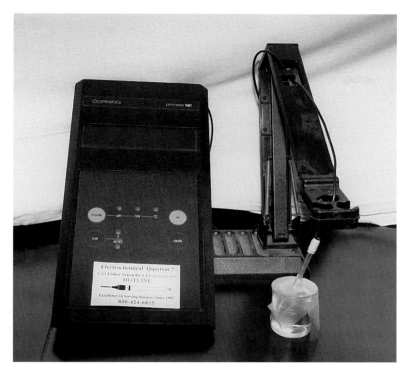

Figure 5-4 pH meter.

this question, one must probe the very nature of the elements: their constitution and behavior.

Experimental evidence has shown that all elements are made up of minute particles called atoms and that an atom is the smallest unit of an element that can exist and still maintain the properties of the element. All atoms of a given element are identical in chemical properties, and the atoms of each element differ in properties from the atoms of all other elements. To understand why this is so requires a knowledge of the structure of atoms and the components necessary to their formation.

Structurally, all atoms can be described as a sphere composed of two parts. One part is a small compact nucleus located at the center of the sphere; the second part, a region of space surrounding the nucleus, is populated by small particles called electrons.

The nucleus is composed, mainly, of two types of particles, protons (p^+) and neutrons (n^0). Protons are small particles, each of which has a charge of $+1$, whereas neutrons, also small particles, have no charge and are therefore neutral. Since it is known that like charges repel, one must wonder what forces hold the protons together in the nucleus. This question cannot be adequately explained in this discussion; suffice it to say that there are other particles within the nucleus that overcome these repulsive forces and act as a "nuclear glue."

The mass of an atom is, for all practical purposes, contained in the nucleus and is equal to the sum of the masses of the protons and neutrons. Each proton

and neutron has arbitrarily been given a value of one atomic mass unit (1 amu), which has been found by experiment to be equal to 1.67×10^{-24} g. By definition, the number of protons in the nucleus of an atom is the same as the atomic number of the element. Since the mass of the neutron is known to be essentially the same as that of the proton, all the mass of the atom is attributed to the protons and neutrons, and the sum of the two is equal to the atomic mass of the atom, expressed in atomic mass units. Thus the atomic mass minus the atomic number equals the number of neutrons present in the nucleus.

The net charge of an atom of an element is zero; that is, it is neutral. Therefore, since we know that protons have a positive charge ($+1$), there must be one negative charge present for each proton in the nucleus. These negatively charged particles are called electrons (e^-), each of which has a net charge of -1. For most purposes, the mass of the electron is considered to be zero, since, when compared to the mass of the proton and neutron, its mass is negligible (5.5×10^{-4} amu). The number of electrons present in an atom, being equal to the number of protons, also signifies that the number of electrons is equal to the atomic number.

As noted earlier, electrons are found in the space surrounding the nucleus. However, they are not found at fixed points but are circulating about the nucleus and occupy specific regions with respect to the nucleus and with respect to other electrons (Figure 5-5). The relative distance of an electron from the nucleus, and the shape and the orientation of the region it occupies, with respect to other regions, has been determined by a combination of spectroscopic evidence and a mathematic treatment known as *quantum mechanics*. However, the results of these treatments are useful in that they allow a description of each electron of an atom in terms of its general position, its relative energy, and the shape of the region that it will occupy. Each electron can be described by a set of four quantum numbers (note that lowercase letters refer to single particles, whereas capital letters refer to systems):

1. The principal quantum number is designated by the letter *n*, which can have a positive integral value, with the exception of zero, that is, 1, 2, 3, and so on. This quantum number indicates the relative distance from the nucleus at which the electron is found and also its relative energy. These are major energy levels and are often called shells.

2. The secondary quantum number is designated by ℓ. The values of ℓ have a range of positive,

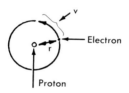

Figure 5-5 Bohr's model of hydrogen atom. *v*, Velocity of electron; *r*, average radius of orbit of electron about nucleus.

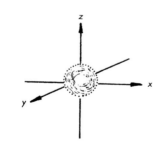

Figure 5-6 Atomic s orbitals.

integral numbers from zero to $n - 1$; that is, if $n = 3$, then $ℓ = 0$, 1, and 2. This quantum number describes the geometric shape of the subenergy level in which the electron is found. These subenergy levels are found within a major energy level and are usually referred to as orbitals.

3. The magnetic quantum number is designated by *m*. The numerical value of *m* can vary from negative ℓ to positive ℓ, that is, if $ℓ = 1$, then $m = -1$, 0, +1. This quantum number defines the orientation of the orbital in space; that is, an s orbital being spherically symmetric (Figure 5-6) has no discernible orientation. However, orientations of the three p orbitals are mutually perpendicular along the x, y, and z axes (Figure 5-7).

4. The spin quantum number is designated *s*. This quantum number can have only one of two numeric values, +½ or −½. This is so because only two electrons may occupy the same orbital (the Pauli exclusion principle) and must have opposite spins. Electrons, being negatively charged, are mutually repulsive. However, evidence has shown that electrons are not simply charged particles moving in space but are also spinning about an axis while undergoing translational motion. The spin of the electron gives rise to a magnetic field, and the fields arising (as north and south poles of a magnet are attracting) consequently reduce the degree of repulsion from like charges. This permits two electrons having common *n*, ℓ, and *m* quantum numbers to occupy the same orbital.

The quantum numbers used to identify an electron do not describe the energy of the electron quantitatively. However, the larger the *n* and ℓ values for the electron, the further the electron will be from the nucleus, and consequently these electrons will have a greater energy than those electrons of lower *n* and ℓ values. Also, the number of orbitals of equivalent energy contained within a major energy level is given by $m = -ℓ$ to $+ℓ$. For example, the second major energy level, $n = 2$, contains two types of subenergy levels. When $ℓ = 0$, $m = 0$, indicating that only one orbital of

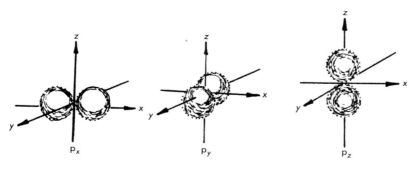

Figure 5-7 Atomic p orbitals.

this type is present, which is termed an *s orbital*. However, when $\ell = 1$ and $m = -1$, 0, and $+1$, indicating that there are three orbitals of this type, each of equivalent energy, they are called *p orbitals*. Thus the second energy level is composed of a total of four subenergy levels or orbitals. For higher values of *n*, in addition to s and p orbitals, there are also d and f orbitals.

From the foregoing discussion it follows that no two electrons can have the same set of quantum numbers; this is known as the *Pauli exclusion principle* (Table 5-1).

An examination of Table 5-1 indicates that the total number of electrons that a given shell *(n)* can accommodate is equal to $2n^2$.

At this point it is necessary to describe the order in which the major and subenergy levels will be filled by electrons. An electron will always enter the lowest energy level available, and obviously the greater the attraction between an electron and the nucleus, the lower the energy of the electron will be. Thus the first electron will enter the 1s orbital of the first energy level, and the second electron, differing in quantum number from the first electron only in the sign of the spin quantum number, will also enter the 1s orbital; these electrons will be paired. Recalling that a given shell can accommodate $2n^2$ electrons, in this case $n = 1$ and $2n^2 = 2$, we find that the first energy level is filled.

The next electron must now enter the second energy level, $n = 2$, and will occupy the 2s orbital; the same will be true for the next electron. The 2s orbital now containing two electrons, whose spins are paired, is filled, and the next electron must enter one of the three 2p orbitals. One might expect the next electron to enter the same p orbital to give paired electrons; however, spectroscopic evidence indicates that this electron enters one of the two remaining empty p orbitals and has the same spin number as the first p electron. This behavior is summarized by Hund's rule, which states that for an atom where orbitals of equal energies are being filled, the electrons will remain unpaired until each orbital is half filled, that is, one electron in each of the orbitals.

To facilitate the assignment of electrons to the lowest energy orbital available, the following sequence is helpful:

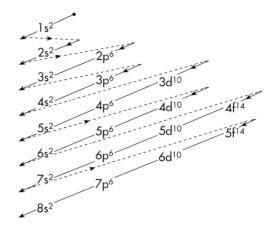

The arrows and broken lines indicate the proper order of filling. The symbols and their significance are as follows:

EXAMPLE: Given the term $4p^3$ indicate the *n, ℓ, m,* and *s* values.

1. $n = 4$, the fourth energy level.
2. Since p electrons are involved, $\ell = 1$.
3. With ℓ being 1, $m = -1$, 0, $+1$ (the three p orbitals), each of which can accommodate 2 electrons for a total of 6.
4. The superscript 3 denotes the presence of 3 electrons in the p orbitals. Following Hund's rule, each orbital (p_x, p_y, p_z) will contain 1 electron, all of which will have parallel spins ($s = +\frac{1}{2}$).

Had the electrons cited in the example been the electrons of highest energy in a neutral atom, the element to which they belong would be known. These being the highest energy electrons would indicate that all orbitals of lower energy had been filled. Thus, by counting the number of electrons (using the diagram above) and recalling that the number of electrons is equal to the atomic number of the element, we find that the element corresponding to the atom has an atomic mass of 33. The periodic chart (Figure 5-8) shows element number 33 to be arsenic (As).

Table 5-1	Relationship of quantum numbers													
Shell *(n)*	1		2							3				
Subshell *(l)*	0	0		1		0		1				2		
m value	0	0	−1	0	+1	0	−1	0	+1	−2	−1	0	+1	+2
s value	±½	±½	±½	±½	±½	±½	±½	±½	±½	±½	±½	±½	±½	±½
Number of electrons*	⇅	⇅	⇅	⇅	⇅	⇅	⇅	⇅	⇅	⇅	⇅	⇅	⇅	⇅

*↑ denotes e⁻ with +½ spin; ↓ denotes e⁻ with −½ spin.

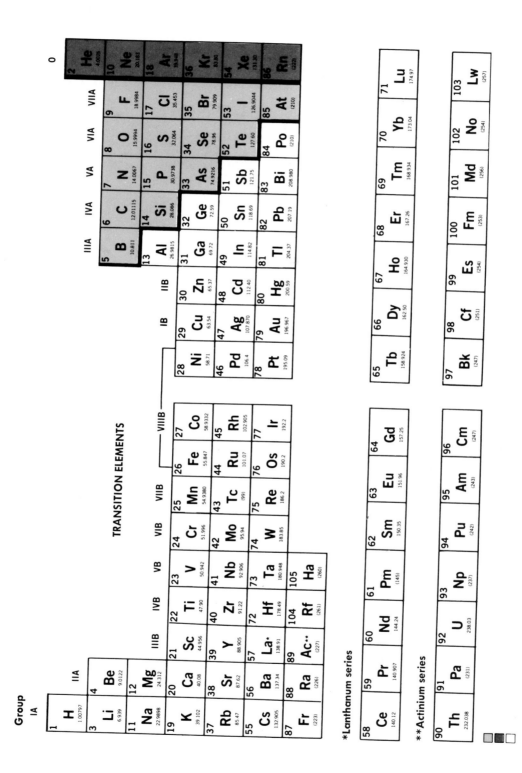

Figure 5-8 Periodic table of elements. (Courtesy Sheehan DC, Hrapchak BB: *Theory and practice of histotechnology,* St. Louis, 1980, Mosby.)

Periodic Chart of the Elements

Early in the nineteenth century chemists noted a relationship between atomic weight and properties of the elements. Even though many of the elements had not yet been discovered, chemists were able to recognize those elements having similar properties and group them into families. Later in the century, about 1870, several chemists segregated the known elements into groups (families) and showed that properties were a function of atomic number rather than atomic weight and that the properties of a given element, both physical and chemical, were similar to those elements having an atomic number differing by 8, 18, 32, and so on. For example, lithium (atomic number 3), sodium (atomic number 11), potassium (atomic number 19), and rubidium (atomic number 37) exhibited similar physical properties in being shiny, ductile, malleable, and good conductors of electrical current. Chemically, these elements are similar in that they form compounds with other elements in the same proportions. Thus *one* atom of Li or Na reacts with *one* atom of fluorine, forming lithium fluoride (LiF) or sodium fluoride (NaF), but *two* atoms of Li or Na react with *one* atom of oxygen to form lithium oxide (Li_2O) or sodium oxide (Na_2O). Other families such as fluorine, chlorine, bromine, iodine, and astatine, or oxygen, sulfur, selenium, tellurium, and polonium are groups of elements exhibiting similar chemical and physical properties.

The periodic chart contains the elements known at this time (Figure 5-8). Elements of similar properties, as discussed above, are grouped together in columns (placed vertically) to form a family having the same electron configuration in the outermost shell; for example, Li, Na, and so on, each contain *one* electron in the outer shell, whereas F, Cl, and so on, each contain *seven* electrons in the outer shell. However, the elements in a row (placed horizontally) differ from each other in chemical and most physical properties. From a consideration of the electron configuration of the elements as discussed earlier it is apparent that the elements in a given row differ in electron configuration from all other elements contained in that row. Thus sodium (Na), having one electron in the 3s atomic orbital, differs from the element of next higher atomic number, magnesium (Mg), which has two electrons in the 3s atomic orbital, and so on.

The information contained in the periodic chart is not restricted to electron configuration of the outer shell but also indicates the complete electronic structure and the relative atomic mass of each element. Each element is identified by its chemical symbol, as shown in Figure 5-9. The number above the chemical symbol is the atomic number (Z number) of the element and the number below the symbol is the average atomic mass (A number) of the element. For example, the element fluorine (Figure 5-9) has an atomic number, or Z number, of 9, which indicates the number of protons

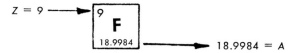

Figure 5-9 Periodic chart representation of fluorine.

and electrons present in the atom. The number 18.9984 shown below the symbol indicates the average atomic mass, or A number, of the element. Recalling that the atomic mass number minus the atomic number gives the number of neutrons present in the nucleus and that the masses of the neutron and proton are essentially identical, one would expect the atomic mass of an element to be an integer. Obviously, the value for fluorine or any other element is not integral and indicates that all atoms of an element are not identical. The nonintegral atomic mass arises from the fact that all atoms of a given element do not contain the same number of neutrons. If some atoms contain a greater or lesser number of neutrons in the nucleus than do other atoms, the average atomic mass of a collection of such atoms will not be integral. Atoms that differ only in the number of neutrons present in the nucleus are called *isotopes*.

Stable Electron Configurations—the Noble Gases

Chemists of the nineteenth century also noted that certain elements were unreactive and would not combine with other elements to give compounds. It is now known that these elements are all members of the eighth group shown in the periodic chart and constitute a family of elements. These elements all exist in the gaseous state under normal conditions and, being inert, are commonly referred to as the *noble gases*. Referring to the periodic chart (Figure 5-8), note that each of the noble gases contains eight electrons in the outer shell, indicating that for these elements the s and p orbitals within the outer shell are completely filled.

Elements other than the noble gases combine with other elements and do so in such a way that the resulting electron configuration of the elements undergoing reaction is changed to an electron configuration of the noble gases. *This gives a stable electron configuration to each element, one that all elements strive to attain.* For this to be true, the reacting elements must either donate to, accept from, or share electrons with another element. For example, sodium, having an electron configuration of $1s^2 2s^2 2p^6 3s^1$, differs in electron configuration from the noble gas neon (Ne) (in which the second energy level is completely filled, $1s^2 2s^2 2p^6$) by one electron; that is, sodium contains one more electron, $3s^1$. Therefore, for sodium to attain an electron configuration identical with neon it must donate (transfer) the 3s electron to another element.

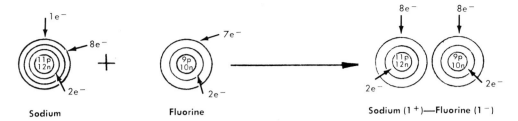

Figure 5-10 Reaction of sodium atom and fluorine atom to produce ionic compound.

Assuming that sodium is undergoing a reaction with fluorine (F), $1s^2 2s^2 2p^5$, we note that the electron configuration of fluorine differs from that of the noble gas neon by one electron. However, fluorine needs to acquire one electron to attain noble gas configuration, *whereas sodium had only to donate one electron to achieve the same electron structure.* We may now write an equation for the reaction of one atom of sodium with one atom of fluorine (Figure 5-10).

Upon comparing the electron structures of sodium (1+), fluorine, (1−) and neon (neutral) we see that they are identical; that is, *each* has an electron structure of $1s^2 2s^2 2p^6$. Note, at this point, that only electrons were involved in this reaction and that the sodium atom in transferring an electron to the fluorine atom acquires a net charge of 1+ and the fluorine atom in accepting the electron from sodium acquires a net charge of 1− (compare the number of protons in the nucleus to the total number of electrons present for sodium and fluorine in the products).

Although the foregoing was a rather simple example, an understanding of the chemistry of most elements can be explained in the same manner. *Most elements undergo reaction by donating, accepting, or sharing electrons so as to attain the electron configuration of a noble gas.* The transition metals are an exception to the rule.

Ionic Compounds

The reaction of sodium with fluorine, discussed in the preceding section, involved a complete transfer of electrons and resulted in the formation of charged particles called *ions.* In those reactions involving a complete transfer of electrons, the ion resulting from the element donating electrons is called a *cation,* in this case a sodium ion (Na^{1+}), and the element accepting electrons is called an *anion* (fluoride ion, F^{1-}). The elements occupying the left-hand part of the periodic chart are known as metals and tend to undergo chemical reaction by donating electrons. Conversely, the non-metals, occupying the right-hand part of the periodic chart, tend to undergo chemical reaction by accepting electrons. Each metallic element differs from the other metals in its ability to donate electrons, and the non-metallic elements differ from each other in their ability to accept electrons. The ability of an element to ac-

Table 5-2	Electronegativity values of selected elements					
H						
2.1						
Li	Be	B	C	N	O	F
1.0	1.5	2	2.5	3.0	3.5	4.0
Na	Mg	Al	Si	P	S	Cl
0.9	1.2	1.5	1.8	2.1	2.5	3.0
K	Ca	Sc	Ge	As	Se	Br
0.8	1.0	1.3	1.8	2.0	2.4	2.8
Rb	Sr	Y	Sn	Sb	Te	I
0.8	1.0	1.2	1.8	1.9	2.1	2.5

cept electrons is known as its *electronegativity,* with the element having the greatest ability to accept electrons (fluorine) arbitrarily being assigned a value of 4. This is the Pauling scale; others exist and are in common use. The ability of all other elements to accept electrons is compared numerically to fluorine. These values are shown in Table 5-2.

Thus in the foregoing reaction between sodium and fluorine, the fluorine atom (electronegativity 4.0) readily acquires an electron from sodium (electronegativity 0.9), resulting in ions, both of which are isoelectronic with neon. Elements that tend to react by transfer of electrons must differ in electronegativity by approximately 2.5 electronegativity units.

At this point we must note that the sodium and fluorine ion produced in this reaction, although having an electron configuration identical with that of neon, differs from the noble gas in that sodium still contains 11 protons in its nucleus and fluorine retains its nine protons. The sodium ion produced now possesses one more proton in its nucleus than it has electrons in the energy levels surrounding it; therefore sodium in this state must have a net charge of 1+. Similarly fluorine, now containing one additional electron, must have a net charge of 1−. Since opposite charges attract each other, it should not be surprising that the resulting ions approach each other and are held together by these electrostatic attractions to form an ionic compound. *All elements that undergo reactions to form ions result in the formation of ionic compounds.*

Covalent Compounds

Elements whose electronegativities differ by less than 2.5 also undergo reaction to attain electron configurations identical with one of the noble gases. However, in this case neither element is sufficiently electronegative to completely acquire the electrons of the second element, the result being that they react in a manner so as to share the electrons in their valence shell (valence electrons are those in the outermost shell). For example, in the reaction of carbon (electronegativity 2.5) with chlorine (electronegativity 3.0), the compound formed *has no charge.* Letting circles (o) and crosses (x) indicate the electrons involved in the reaction and understanding that the electrons of lower energy (in shells closer to the nucleus) are still present, we can represent the reaction as follows:

$$
\overset{\text{o}}{\underset{\text{o}}{\text{o}}}\text{C}\text{o} + 4\,^{x}\!\overset{xx}{\underset{xx}{\text{Cl}}}{}^{x}_{x} \rightarrow
{}^{x}_{x}\overset{\overset{xx}{\text{Cl}}{}^{x}_{x}}{\underset{{}^{x}_{x}\underset{xx}{\text{Cl}}{}^{x}_{x}}{\overset{xx}{\text{Cl}}{}^{x}_{x}\,\overset{ox}{\underset{xo}{\text{C}}}\,\overset{xx}{\text{Cl}}{}^{x}_{x}}}
$$

Even though the chlorine and the carbon atoms have not reacted by electron transfer, each of the atoms has attained the electron configuration of a noble gas by sharing its valence electrons. Unlike sodium fluoride (NaF), the compound carbon tetrachloride (CCl_4), formed in this reaction, is a molecule in which the four chlorine atoms and the carbon atom are bound to each other and function as one unit. The product CCl_4 is called a *molecule.* The bond, in this case, rather than being ionic as that of NaF, is *covalent. All compounds that are formed by the sharing of electrons rather than the transfer of electrons are said to have covalent bonds.*

Even though these bonds are described as being covalent, it is apparent that the electronegativities of the two elements (see Table 5-2) are not the same; therefore the electrons used in forming the bonds between the carbon atom and the four chlorine atoms cannot be shared equally. This leads to the conclusion that the electron pair in each of these bonds is more strongly attracted to chlorine than to carbon. Covalent bonds formed from two different elements of unequal electronegativity must be *polar covalent,* meaning that the electrons forming the bond are more strongly attracted to one atom than to the other.

Those elements of essentially the same electronegativity react to form bonds that are completely covalent; that is, the electrons of the bond are shared equally between the two atoms. For example oxygen, which composes 20% of the earth's atmosphere, exists as the molecule O_2. It is apparent that the electronegativity of each oxygen atom in the molecule is the same; therefore the electrons that bond these atoms cannot be attracted more strongly by one atom than by the other. This results in an equal sharing of electrons, *and the bond is completely covalent.* Other examples of nonpolar

covalent bonds are nitrogen (N_2, which is 80% of the earth's atmosphere), hydrogen (H_2), and the halogens (F_2, Cl_2, Br_2, I_2). As we shall find in a subsequent discussion, the carbon-hydrogen bond in organic molecules is essentially nonpolar covalent because both carbon and hydrogen have electronegativity values of approximately 2.5.

Coordinate Covalent Bonds

Those compounds containing coordinate covalent bonds are similar to those compounds containing covalent bonds in that the bonding electrons are shared by two atoms. However, the electrons used in forming these bonds are donated by *one atom only.* As an example, let us consider the reaction in which a molecule of sulfuric acid is formed from the following elements:

$$
2\text{H}_{\square} + \overset{oo}{\underset{oo}{\text{o}\,\text{S}\,\text{o}}} + 4\,^{x}\!\overset{xx}{\underset{xx}{\text{O}}}{}^{x} \rightarrow
\text{H}_{\square}^{x}\overset{xx}{\text{O}}{}^{o}_{x}\overset{\overset{xx}{\overset{x}{\text{O}}{}^{x}_{x}}{\underset{oo}{\text{o}}}}{\underset{\underset{xx}{\overset{x}{\text{O}}{}^{x}_{x}}{\underset{oo}{\text{o}}}}{\text{S}}}\,^{o}_{x}\overset{xx}{\text{O}}{}^{x}_{\square}\text{H}
$$

or

$$
\begin{array}{c}
\text{O} \\
\uparrow \\
\text{H}\!-\!\text{O}\!-\!\text{S}\!-\!\text{O}\!-\!\text{H} \\
\downarrow \\
\text{O}
\end{array}
$$

The symbol — represents a covalent bond, and ↑ represents a coordinate covalent bond in which the arrow points toward the atom that did not contribute any electrons to bond formation.

Considering each bond in the sulfuric acid molecule, and the electrons used in forming each bond, it is apparent that the hydrogen-oxygen bonds and two of the sulfur-oxygen bonds are polar covalent, whereas the remaining two sulfur-oxygen bonds are coordinate covalent bonds, in that the electrons used in forming these bonds are contributed by the sulfur atom only.

Complex Ions and Chelates

The formation of coordinate covalent bonds need not occur by reaction of neutral elements as shown in the preceding section. There are many reactions in which a coordinate covalent bond is formed by the interaction of a neutral molecule with an ion. In reactions of this type the driving force, or reason for reaction, is that an atom contained within the neutral molecule has not attained the electron configuration of a noble gas. In previous discussions the metals were assumed to react by transfer of their electrons to form ionic compounds. However, elements such as aluminum (Al) have been found to form compounds in which the bonds are largely polar covalent. This being true, it is apparent that the aluminum atom needs three electrons to at-

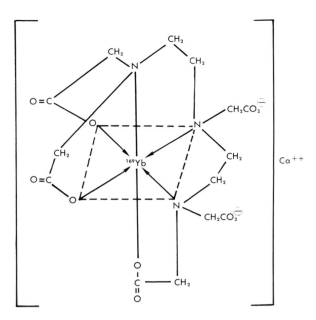

Figure 5-11 Ytterbium-pentetic acid (Yb-DTPA) complex. *Arrows,* Coordinate covalent bonds; *dotted line,* plane through these atoms.

tain the noble gas configuration of argon (Ar). Consequently aluminum chloride ($AlCl_3$), in a nonpolar solvent, reacts with anhydrous chloride gas (Cl_2) according to the following equation:

The electrons used in forming the fourth chlorine-aluminum bond are donated by the chloride ion, resulting in the formation of a coordinate covalent bond. The ions that provide the bonding electrons are called *ligands*.

A second example of coordinate covalent bond formation is that in which a positive ion undergoes reaction with a neutral molecule, as illustrated in the following reaction:

The products resulting from reactions of neutral molecules with either a cation or an anion are called *complex ions*.

Although elements such as aluminum and nitrogen can share one pair of electrons with simple ions to form complex ions, other elements, especially the transition elements, must accept two or more pairs of electrons to attain a noble gas electron configuration. These complexes are especially important in nuclear medicine and in many cases involve the formation of chelates in which the electron pairs (two or more pairs)

are donated by functional groups present in the ligand molecule. The term *chelate,* from the Greek word *chēlē* (claw), is reserved for these ligands. The complex ytterbium-pentetic acid (Yb-DTPA) (Figure 5-11), used as a cisternographic imaging agent, is an excellent example of a chelate. In this case the electrons used in forming the coordinate covalent bonds are donated by the functional groups present in the penetetic acid molecule.

Although the structure of many complex ions of technetium are still under investigation, it is reasonable to assume that their structures are similar to those formed by ytterbium.

LAWS OF CONSTANT COMPOSITION AND MULTIPLE PROPORTION

The fact that elements generally react with other elements to attain a noble gas electron configuration leads to the conclusion that any two elements that undergo reaction must do so in a definite ratio of atoms, that is, one Na to one F and one C to four Cl. It then follows that the elements must also react to definite ratios by weight. This is stated by the *law of constant composition:* A compound, regardless of its origin or method of preparation, always contains the same elements in the same proportions by weight.

In some cases, depending on reaction conditions, an element will combine with another to give products that differ in the ratio of atoms of the two elements. For example, sodium usually reacts with oxygen to form sodium oxide (Na_2O), but under other conditions they react to form sodium peroxide (Na_2O_2). However, in each case the ratio of sodium to oxygen is definite. This is stated by the *law of multiple proportions:* When two elements combine to form two or more different compounds, the ratio of the mass of one element that combines with a fixed mass of a second element is a simple ratio of whole numbers, for example, 2:1 or 3:2.

Sample Problems

EXAMPLE 1: When subjected to quantitative elemental analysis, two samples of a compound containing only carbon and oxygen give the following data:

	Weight of sample	Weight of C found	Weight of O found
Sample 1:	0.7335 g	0.2002 g	0.5333 g
Sample 2:	0.6162 g	0.1682 g	0.4480 g

Do these data uphold the law of constant composition? If the law is upheld, the percentage of carbon and oxygen must be the same in each sample. To determine this, the ratio of the weight of each element to the total weight of the sample must be equal to the ratio of the percent of the element to 100%.

Sample 1:

$$\text{Percent carbon} = \frac{0.2002}{0.7335} = \frac{\% \text{ C}}{100\%} \quad \% \text{ C} = 27.29$$

$$\text{Percent oxygen} = \frac{0.5333}{0.7335} = \frac{\% \text{ O}}{100\%} \quad \% \text{ O} = 72.71$$

Sample 2:

$$\text{Percent carbon} = \frac{0.1682}{0.6162} = \frac{x\% \text{ C}}{100\%} \quad \% \text{ C} = 27.29$$

$$\text{Percent oxygen} = \frac{0.4480}{0.6162} = \frac{x\% \text{ O}}{100\%} \quad \% \text{ O} = 72.71$$

The percentage of carbon and oxygen being the same for both samples indicates that they are of identical composition and thus support the law of constant composition.

EXAMPLE 2: A third sample, obtained from a different source, was also found to contain only carbon and oxygen and gave the following data upon analysis:

	Weight of sample	Weight of C found	Weight of O found
Sample 3:	0.3599 g	0.1543 g	0.2056 g

Show that these data illustrate the law of multiple proportions. Follow the procedure used in example 1.

Sample 3:

$$\text{Percent carbon} = \frac{0.1543}{0.3599} = \frac{\% \text{ C}}{100\%} \quad \% \text{ C} = 42.87$$

$$\text{Percent oxygen} = \frac{0.2056}{0.3599} = \frac{\% \text{ O}}{100\%} \quad \% \text{ O} = 57.13$$

Obviously this composition indicates that sample 3 was obtained from a compound different from that of samples 1 and 2. Although the samples differ in composition, the law of multiple proportions states that the ratios of the masses of the elements in each compound should be related as simple whole numbers. Thus:

$$\textit{For sample 1:} \quad \frac{\% \text{ O}}{\% \text{ C}} = \frac{72.71}{27.49} = 2.66$$

$$\textit{For sample 3:} \quad \frac{\% \text{ O}}{\% \text{ C}} = \frac{57.13}{42.87} = 1.33$$

Therefore the ratios of oxygen to carbon in sample 1 and sample 3 are related by the ratio of 2.66:1.33 or 2:1.

GRAM ATOMIC WEIGHTS, GRAM MOLECULAR WEIGHTS, AND THE MOLE CONCEPT

The chemistry discussed thus far has been based on the interactions of individual atoms. Although this description is a valid one, the isolation and use of single atoms in the laboratory is neither practical nor possible. The smallest sample that can be accurately measured in the laboratory will contain 10^{15} to 10^{17} atoms or molecules.

For a reaction to be accurately described by a chemical equation, it is necessary only that the number of atoms or molecules of the reactants be present in the *ratio* given by the coefficients for these substances. In the following reaction, the ratio of hydrogen (H_2) molecules to oxygen (O_2) molecules must be 2:1.

$$2H_2 + 1O_2 \rightarrow 2H_2O$$

The chemist, being unable to count the number of atoms or molecules necessary for a given reaction, must resort to an indirect method to achieve this ratio. The fact that each element possesses a unique atomic mass (see Figure 5-8) indicates that even though equal weights of hydrogen and oxygen could be measured, the number of molecules of hydrogen present in the sample would be 16 times that of the oxygen molecules; that is, one hydrogen molecule has a weight of 2 relative to a weight of 32 for one oxygen molecule. A convenient method that allows the measurement of the required quantities of the reactants by accurate weighing of each substance is based directly upon their gram atomic weight (gaw) or gram molecular weight (gmw). By definition, these are the weights in grams that are numerically equal to the atomic weights (amu) or molecular weights (the sum of the atomic weights of all atoms present in the molecule) of the elements or compounds involved. From this definition it is apparent that 1 gmw of any two substances will contain the same number of atoms or molecules. The number of atoms or molecules in 1 gaw or gmw has been shown by experiment to be 6.02×10^{23}. This number is called *Avogadro's number,* and 1 gaw or gmw of any substance is commonly referred to as 1 *mole.*

These concepts are illustrated in the following examples:

EXAMPLE 1: How many moles (gram atomic weights) of chromium (Cr) are contained in 28 g? From the periodic chart the atomic weight of chromium is found to be 52 amu; therefore the weight of Cr contained in 1 mole (gaw) is 52 g.

$$\frac{1\ mole}{52\ g} = \frac{x\ mole}{28\ g}$$

$$x = \frac{(28\ g)(1\ mole)}{52\ g}$$

$$x = \frac{28}{52}\ mole$$

$$x = 0.538\ mole$$

EXAMPLE 2: How many grams are contained in 0.59 moles (gram molecular weights) of sulfuric acid? Sulfuric acid, H_2SO_4, being a molecule, requires that we first determine its molecular weight.

$$2\ H \times\ 1\ amu = 2\ amu$$
$$1\ S \times 32\ amu = 32\ amu$$
$$\underline{4\ O \times 16\ amu = 64\ amu}$$
$$Molecular\ weight = 98\ amu$$

Therefore 1 mole (gmw) would contain 98 g of sulfuric acid, and

$$\frac{98\ g}{1\ mole} = \frac{x\ g}{0.59\ mole}$$

$$x = \frac{(98\ g)(0.59\ mole)}{1\ mole}$$

$$x = (98\ g)(0.59)$$
$$x = 57.82\ g$$

EXAMPLE 3: How many molecules are contained in 0.50 mole of nitrogen (N_2)? One mole (gmw) of N_2 (28 g) would contain Avogadro's number of molecules (6.02×10^{23}), therefore

$$\frac{6.02 \times 10^{23}\ molecules}{1\ mole} = \frac{x\ molecules}{0.50\ mole}$$

$$x = \frac{(0.50\ mole)(6.02 \times 10^{23}\ molecules)}{1\ mole}$$

$$x = (0.50)(6.02 \times 10^{23})\ molecules$$
$$x = 3.01 \times 10^{23}\ molecules$$

EXAMPLE 4: How many moles of water (H_2O) are present in a sample containing 5×10^{12} molecules? One mole of H_2O contains 6.02×10^{23} molecules, therefore

$$\frac{1\ mole}{6.02 \times 10^{23}\ molecules} = \frac{x\ mole}{5.0 \times 10^{12}\ molecules}$$

$$x = \frac{(1\ mole)(5.0 \times 10^{12}\ molecules)}{6.02 \times 10^{23}\ molecules}$$

$$x = \frac{(5.0 \times 10^{12})\ mole}{6.02 \times 10^{23}}$$

$$x = 0.83 \times 10^{-11}\ mole$$
$$x = 8.3 \times 10^{-12}\ mole$$

EMPIRICAL AND MOLECULAR FORMULAS

All substances now known were initially obtained from natural resources or chemical reactions, and in many cases their elemental composition and structures were unknown. The elements present in such compounds must be determined by *qualitative chemical analysis,* and the relative amount of each element by *quantitative chemical analysis.* The information obtained in these analyses is useful in determining the empirical formula of a substance.

The ratio of the elements contained in a substance (the relative number of each kind of atom present) is indicated by the empirical formula. However, the empirical formula may not truly reflect the molecular formula of the substance, which may be a whole number multiple of the empirical formula. For instance, the organic substance oxalic acid, which is a constituent of some plants, has an empirical formula of CHO_2 but a molecular formula of $C_2H_2O_4$.

EXAMPLE: A compound, upon analysis, was found to have the following composition by weight:

$$Carbon\ (C) = 50.7\%$$
$$Hydrogen\ (H) = 4.25\%$$
$$Oxygen\ (O) = 45.1\%$$

What is the empirical example of the compound?

Since percentage is based upon 100, it may be assumed that a 100 g sample of the compound would contain

$$50.7\ g\ C$$
$$4.25\ g\ H$$
$$45.1\ g\ O$$

Also knowing that a definite atomic weight (and gram atomic weight) is a unique property of each element, the relative abundance of each element is obtained by the following:

$$Carbon:\ \frac{50.7\ g}{12\ g} = \frac{x\ gaw}{1\ gaw}$$

$$x = \frac{50.7\ g}{12\ g}\ (1\ gaw)$$

$$x = 4.23\ gaw$$

$$Hydrogen:\ \frac{4.25\ g}{1\ g} = \frac{x\ gaw}{1\ gaw}$$

$$x = \frac{(4.25\ g)(1\ gaw)}{1\ g}$$

$$x = 4.25\ gaw$$

Oxygen: $\dfrac{45.1\ g}{16\ g} = \dfrac{x\ gaw}{1\ gaw}$

$$x = \dfrac{(45.1)(1\ gaw)}{16\ g}$$

$$x = \dfrac{45.1}{16}\ gaw$$

$$x = 2.82\ gaw$$

However, each element must be present in an integral value of its atomic weight, or gram atomic weight. To obtain integral values for each element, we must divide the above values of the gram atomic weight by the smallest value obtained. Thus:

Oxygen: $\dfrac{2.82\ gaw}{2.82\ gaw} = 1$

Carbon: $\dfrac{4.23\ gaw}{2.82\ gaw} = 1.5$

Hydrogen: $\dfrac{4.25\ gaw}{2.82\ gaw} = 1.5$

These values indicate that the empirical formula of the compound is $C_{1.5}H_{1.5}O_1$. Obviously, these values are not integral and the actual number of atoms present in the molecule must be a multiple of these. Multiplying the value for each element by 2 results in an empirical formula of $C_3H_3O_2$, indicating an integral or whole number value for each element.

Further analysis of the above substance indicates its molecular weight to be 142. What is the molecular formula of the compound?

The molecular weight of the compound is derived from the following empirical formula:

Carbon	(3) (12) =	36
Hydrogen	(3) (1) =	3
Oxygen	(2) (16) =	32
Empirical weight	=	71

Inasmuch as the molecular formula must be a multiple of the empirical formula, that is, $^{142}\!/_{71} = 2$, the molecular formula is $C_6H_6O_4$.

Empirical or molecular formulas may be characteristic of several different compounds and provide no information pertinent to the structure of the molecule.

SOLUTIONS AND COLLOIDS

Much of the chemistry encountered in nuclear medicine involves solutions. A solution is a homogeneous mixture of two substances: the *solute* can be a gas, liquid, or solid, and the *solvent*, generally a liquid. One must choose a solvent that will dissolve the solute and yet not undergo chemical reaction with the solute.

In working with solutions one must know the concentration of solute in a given volume of solution and therefore must be familiar with the methods and units used in defining concentrations.

Molarity

Molarity expresses the number of moles of solute contained in 1 L of solution.

$$\text{Molarity (M)} = \dfrac{\text{Number of moles of solute}}{\text{Number of liters of solution}}$$

Sample Problems

EXAMPLE 1: What is the molarity of a solution prepared by dissolving 16 g of barium chloride ($BaCl_2$) in sufficient water to give a total volume of 450 ml?

Step 1: How many moles of $BaCl_2$ are in the 16 g sample?

$$1\ \text{mole}\ (BaCl_2) = 137.5\ g + 2(35.5\ g)$$
$$1\ \text{mole}\ (BaCl_2) = 208.5\ g$$

$$\dfrac{1\ \text{mole}}{208.5\ g} = \dfrac{x\ \text{mole}}{16.0\ g}$$

$$x = \dfrac{(16.0\ g)(1\ \text{mole})}{208.5\ g}$$

$$x = \dfrac{16.0\ \text{mole}}{208.5}$$

$$x = 0.077\ \text{mole}$$

Step 2: Molarity (M) $= \dfrac{\text{mole}}{\text{liter}}$

$$M = \dfrac{0.077\ \text{mole}}{0.450\ L}$$

$$M = \dfrac{0.171\ \text{mole}}{L\ (\text{molar})}$$

EXAMPLE 2: How would 20 L of 6.0 M sodium hydroxide (NaOH) solution be prepared from solid NaOH?

Step 1: How many grams of NaOH are in 6.0 moles?

$$1\ \text{mole}\ (NaOH) = 23\ g + 16\ g + 1\ g$$
$$1\ \text{mole}\ (NaOH) = 40\ g$$

$$\dfrac{x\ g}{6.0\ \text{moles}} = \dfrac{40\ g}{1\ \text{mole}}$$

$$x = \dfrac{(40\ g)(6.0\ \text{moles})}{1\ \text{mole}}$$

$$x = (40)(6.0)\ g$$
$$x = 240\ g\ \text{in}\ 6.0\ \text{moles of NaOH}$$

Step 2: One liter of 6.0 molar (M) solution requires 240 g of NaOH. Therefore for 20 L of 6.0 M solution, (20) (240 g) = 4800 g of NaOH dissolved in sufficient water to give a total volume of 20 L.

EXAMPLE 3: How could the solution prepared in example 2 be used to obtain 1.0 L of 0.50 M NaOH solution?

Step 1: The 6.0 M NaOH must be diluted with additional water. What volume of the 6.0 M solution contains 0.50 moles of NaOH?

$$\frac{1.0 \text{ L}}{6.0 \text{ mole}} = \frac{x \text{ L}}{0.50 \text{ mole}}$$
$$\text{(NaOH)} \qquad \text{(NaOH)}$$

$$x = \frac{(1.0 \text{ L})(0.50 \text{ M})}{(6.0 \text{ M})}$$

$$x = \frac{0.50 \text{ L}}{6.0}$$

$$x = 0.083 \text{ L}$$

Step 2: If 0.083 L of 6.0 M NaOH contains 0.50 moles of NaOH, then to obtain a 0.50 M solution, one must add enough water to bring the volume to exactly 1.0 L.

Molality

A *molal* solution is defined as the number of moles of solute contained in 1 kilogram (kg) of solvent.

$$\text{Molality (m)} = \frac{\text{Number of moles of solute}}{\text{Number of kilograms of solvent}}$$

Whereas 1 L of a *molar* solution is prepared by the addition of sufficient solvent to the solute to give a total volume of 1 L, a *molal* solution is prepared when the solute is dissolved in 1 kg (in the case of water, 1 L) of solvent. The total volume of a 1 molal solution will generally be greater than that of a 1 molar solution.

EXAMPLE: Calculate the molality of a solute prepared by dissolving 20.4 g of sodium chloride (NaCl) in 192 g of H_2O.

Step 1: How many grams are contained in 1 mole of NaCl?

$$1 \text{ mole (NaCl)} = 23 \text{ g} + 35.5 \text{ g}$$
$$1 \text{ mole (NaCl)} = 58.5 \text{ g}$$

Step 2: How many moles are contained in 20.4 g of NaCl?

$$\frac{1 \text{ mole}}{58.5 \text{ g}} = \frac{x \text{ mole}}{20.4 \text{ g}}$$

$$x = \frac{(20.4 \text{ g})(1 \text{ mole})}{58.5 \text{ g}}$$

$$x = \frac{(20.4)}{58.5} \text{ mole}$$

$$x = 0.349 \text{ mole}$$

Step 3: From the definition of molality:

$$m = \frac{0.349 \text{ mole}}{0.192 \text{ kg}}$$

$$m = 1.82 \text{ molal solution}$$

It should be noted that most solutions are usually expressed in terms of molarity rather than molality.

Normality

A third method of expressing concentration, and one that is in general more useful than that of molarity or molality, is in terms of normality (N). Normality is defined as the number of equivalents (Eq) of solute per liter of solution. The number of equivalents present in a solution, rather than being defined as the number of moles of solute per liter, is defined as the number of moles of reactant species contained in 1 mole of the solute. For example, as we have discussed earlier, in the reaction $H^+ + {}^-OH \rightarrow H_2O$ the reactants must arise from two different substances, one of which provides H^+ and another that provides ^-OH (conventionally OH^-, also ionically OH^-). Those compounds that give H^+ ions are called acids, as we shall discuss later. Two of the most common acids are hydrochloric acid (HCl) and sulfuric acid (H_2SO_4). Both of these acids may be considered to be completely ionized in aqueous solution to give the H^+ ion and the corresponding anions. It should be apparent that ionization of 1 mole of HCl will give rise to 1 mole of H^+ ion, whereas the ionization of 1 mole of H_2SO_4 will give rise to 2 moles of H^+ ion. Thus in comparing HCl with H_2SO_4, we note that 0.5 mole of H_2SO_4 will provide the same number of H^+ ions that would be provided by 1 mole of HCl. Therefore the weight of H_2SO_4 that will provide 1 Eq of H^+ ion (1 mole) is half of its molecular weight: $98 \text{ g}/2 = 49$ g, whereas the weight of HCl required to produce 1 Eq (1 mole) of H^+ is equal to its molecular weight (36.5 g). Similarly, the substances that provide OH^- ion (called bases) will have equivalent weights dictated by the number of moles of OH^- that will be provided by 1 mole of the base. Thus:

$$\text{Normality (N)} = \frac{\text{Number of equivalents}}{\text{Number of liters of solvent}}$$

and

$$\text{Normality (N)} =$$
$$\frac{\text{(Moles of solute)("Moles" of reactant provided)}}{1 \text{ L of solution}} =$$
$$\frac{\text{Equivalents}}{\text{Liter}} = \frac{\text{Eq}}{\text{L}}$$

A second type of reaction to utilize *normal* solutions is that in which an oxidation-reduction is involved. This type is yet to be discussed, and suffice it to say at this point that the equivalent weight of a reagent in an oxidation-reduction reaction is determined by the number of electrons that it accepts or donates.

How are equivalent weights calculated? The equivalent weight, in grams, of an acid is calculated when the gram molecular weight of the acid is divided by the number of potential hydrogen ions contained in the molecule. For a base the gram molecular weight is divided by the number of hydroxide ions.

Problems

EXAMPLE 1: What is the equivalent weight of HCl?

$$\text{Equivalent weight} = \frac{\text{gmw}}{\text{Number of H}^+ \text{ ions}}$$

$$\text{Equivalent weight} = \frac{36.5 \text{ g}}{1} = 36.5 \text{ g}$$

EXAMPLE 2: What is the equivalent weight of H_2SO_4?

$$\text{Equivalent weight} = \frac{\text{gmw}}{\text{Number of H}^+ \text{ ions}}$$

$$\text{Equivalent weight} = \frac{98 \text{ g}}{2}$$

$$\text{Equivalent weight} = 49 \text{ g}$$

EXAMPLE 3: What is the equivalent weight of 1 mole of calcium hydroxide, $Ca(OH)_2$?

$$\text{Equivalent weight} = \frac{\text{gmw}}{\text{Number of OH}^- \text{ ions}}$$

$$\text{Equivalent weight} = \frac{74 \text{ g}}{2}$$

$$\text{Equivalent weight} = 37 \text{ g}$$

From the foregoing discussion it is evident that the normality of a solution must be a whole number multiple of a corresponding molar solution.

EXAMPLE 4: What is the normality of a 90 ml sample of a solution that contains 10 g of NaOH?

Step 1:

$$1 \text{ equivalent weight of NaOH} = \frac{1 \text{ gmw of NaOH}}{1 \text{ OH}^- \text{ ion}}$$

$$1 \text{ equivalent weight} = \frac{40 \text{ g}}{1} = 40 \text{ g of NaOH}$$

Step 2: The number of equivalents of NaOH in solution:

$$\frac{1 \text{ Eq}}{40 \text{ g}} = \frac{x \text{ Eq}}{10 \text{ g}}$$

$$x = \frac{(1 \text{ Eq})(10 \text{ g})}{40 \text{ g}}$$

$$x = \frac{10}{40} \text{ Eq} = 0.25 \text{ Eq of NaOH}$$

Step 3: Normality equals equivalents/liter, therefore

$$N = \frac{\text{Eq}}{\text{L}} = \frac{0.25}{0.09}$$

$$N = 2.78 \text{ normal}$$

Note: Since normality equals molarity for NaOH, this solution is both 2.78 N and 2.78 M.

EXAMPLE 5: What are the normality and molarity of 100 ml of an aqueous solution containing 50.0 g of phosphoric acid (H_3PO_4)?

Step 1: How many grams of H_3PO_4 are contained in 1 gew (gram equivalent weight)?

$$1 \text{ gew} = \frac{1 \text{ gmw}}{\text{Number of H}^+ \text{ ions}}$$

$$1 \text{ gew} = \frac{98.0 \text{ g}}{3} = 32.7 \text{ g of } H_3PO_4$$

Step 2: What is the number of equivalents in 50 g of H_3PO_4?

$$\frac{1 \text{ Eq}}{32.7 \text{ g}} = \frac{x \text{ Eq}}{50.0 \text{ g}}$$

$$x = \frac{(1 \text{ Eq})(50.0 \text{ g})}{32.7 \text{ g}}$$

$$x = \frac{50.0 \text{ g}}{32.7 \text{ g}} = 1.53 \text{ Eq of } H_3PO_4$$

Step 3: Normality, by definition:

$$N = \frac{1.53 \text{ Eq}}{0.100 \text{ L}}$$

$$N = 15.3 \text{ normal}$$

Step 4: Since H_3PO_4 is triprotic (3 H^+ ions), the molarity of this solution will be

$$m = \frac{N}{3} = \frac{15.3}{3}$$

$$m = 5.10 \text{ molar } H_3PO_4$$

Colloids

A second type of mixture, one that is important in nuclear medicine, is the *colloid*. Unlike true solutions, colloids consist of minute particles that are suspended in a dispersing medium. Colloid particles vary in shape and range in size from 10^{-9} to 10^{-7} m in diameter. Although several important types of colloids exist, we restrict our discussion to the colloid in which a solid is dispersed in a liquid—a *sol*.

Although one might expect the particles to settle out on standing, the dispersed colloid particles remain suspended in the dispersing medium indefinitely. This behavior is attributed to a constant bombardment of the dispersed particles by the molecules of the dispersing medium; thus the colloid particles are in constant motion. This phenomenon is called *Brownian movement* and may be observed with the proper type of microscope.

Unlike true solutions, colloids exhibit an optical effect characterized by the scattering of light when a narrow beam is passed through them. The scattering of light is attributable to the deflection of light by the colloid particles and is called the *Tyndall effect.*

A third property characteristic of colloids is an electrical charge effect in which charged particles such as ions are bound or adsorbed on the surface of the colloid particle. An important example, probably involving this effect, is the ^{99m}Tc-labeled sulfur colloid used for liver imaging.

CHEMICAL REACTIONS AND EQUATIONS

The ability to predict chemical reactions and to correctly write and understand the chemical equations describing the reactions is of utmost theoretical and practical importance. The basis for one type of chemical reaction, the combination reaction, in which two elements react to produce one substance, and the chemical equations describing this reaction are discussed previously in this chapter. In addition to combination reactions, several other types of chemical reactions must be considered, which are as follows:

1. Metathesis or double decomposition
2. Oxidation-reduction
   a. Replacement
   b. Electrochemical

Since all reactions are described by a chemical equation, it is necessary that the terms and symbols used in writing equations be learned. The symbols indicating the physical state of substances involved in a reaction are as follows:

1. A gas is indicated by (g) and may alternatively be indicated by the symbol (↑), for example, O_2(g) or O_2(↑).
2. A liquid is designated by (l), for example, H_2O(l).
3. A solid is indicated by (s) or, if there is a product precipitating from solution, by the symbol (↓), for example, $BaSO_4$(↓).
4. The symbol → separates the reactants from the products of the reaction.

A correct chemical equation also requires that the equation be balanced; that is, the number of atoms of each element appearing as reactants must be found in equal number in the products. The steps as one proceeds in completing and balancing an equation are as follows:

1. Determine the correct formulas for those compounds obtained as products from a knowledge of the valence or oxidation numbers of the elements of the charge on ions involved in the reaction. The valence or oxidation number of monatomic ions is equal to the net charge of the cation or anion. The charge of many complex ions is not readily discernible and should be committed to memory. Once determined, the formula of a compound cannot be changed in subsequent balancing operations (Table 5-3).
2. Balance those ions of elements other than hydrogen, oxygen, and polyatomic ions.
3. *Then* balance the hydrogen and oxygen atoms.
4. The correct coefficients for reactants and products must be the smallest whole number possible, for example:

$$2H_2 + O_2 \rightarrow 2H_2O$$

not

$$4H_2 + 2O_2 \rightarrow 4H_2O$$

5. Finally, the sum of the charges of the reactants must equal the sum of the charges of products.

Table 5-3   Common ions, their symbols and charge

Ion	Chemical symbol	Charge
Hydroxide	OH^-	$1-$
Nitrate	NO_3^-	$1-$
Nitrite	NO_2^-	$1-$
Phosphate	PO_4^{3-}	$3-$
Carbonate	CO_3^{2-}	$2-$
Bicarbonate	HCO_3^-	$1-$
Sulfite	SO_3^{2-}	$2-$
Sulfate	SO_4^{2-}	$2-$
Bisulfate	HSO_4^-	$1-$
Ammonium	NH_4^+	$1+$
Stannous or tin (II)	SN^{2+}	$2+$
Stannic or tin (IV)	SN^{4+}	$4+$
Ferrous or iron (II)	Fe^{2+} (FeO)	$2+$
Ferric or iron (III)	Fe^{3+} (Fe_2O_3)	$3+$
Cuprous or copper (I)	Cu^+ (Cu_2O)	$1+$
Cupric or copper (II)	Cu^{2+} (CuO)	$2+$
Permanganate	MnO_4^-	$1-$
Manganese (IV)	MN^{4+} (MnO_2)	$4+$
Manganese (II)	Mn^{2+} (MnO)	$2+$
Pertechnetate	TcO_4^-	$1-$
Technetium (IV)	Tc^{4+} (TcO_2)	$4+$
Chromate	CoO_4^{2-}	$2-$
Chromium (III)	Cr^{3+}	$3+$
Mercurous	Hg^+	$1+$
Mercuric	Hg^{2+}	$2+$
Cyanide	CN^-	$1-$
Thiocyanate	SCN^-	$1-$

The balanced equation specifies the ratio or quantity of reactants required and the ratio or quantity of products produced. This is called the *stoichiometry* (element-equality) of the reaction. The following example illustrates the foregoing steps and the stoichiometry of a reaction:

EXAMPLE: Complete and balance the following equation:

$$Fe(OH)_3 + H_2SO_4 \rightarrow$$

Step 1: From Table 5-3, the hydroxide ion has a charge of $1-$. Therefore the iron present in $Fe(OH)_3$ must have a charge of $3+$. Similarly, for H_2SO_4 each hydrogen has a charge of $1+$ and so the sulfate anion must have a charge of $2-$. Products formed in this reaction must involve an interchange of cations and anions by the two reactants. Therefore ferric ion combines with sulfate ion, and hydrogen ion combines with hydroxide ion. *All products formed must be neutral, that is, have no charge.* Iron having a $3+$ charge and sulfate having a $2-$ charge dictates that the correct formula for this product must be $Fe_2(SO_4)_3$. The remaining product is H_2O, and the equation showing both reactants and products is as follows:

$$Fe(OH)_3 + H_2SO_4 \rightarrow Fe_2(SO_4)_3 + H_2O \text{ (unbalanced)}$$

Step 2: Since each reactant and product contains hydrogen or oxygen or both, those compounds containing iron may be used in stating the balancing procedure.
Reactant: 1 Fe^{3+}
Product: 2 Fe^{3+}
Therefore:

$$2\,Fe(OH)_3 + H_2SO_4 \rightarrow Fe_2(SO_4)_3 + H_2O \text{ (unbalanced)}$$

It is now convenient to balance the polyatomic sulfate ion.
Reactant: 1 SO_4^{2-}
Product: 3 SO_4^{2-}
Therefore:

$$2\,Fe(OH)_3 + 3\,H_2SO_4 \rightarrow Fe_2(SO_4)_3 + H_2O \text{ (unbalanced)}$$

Step 3: Complete the balancing of elements, considering hydrogen and oxygen.
Reactants: 12 H^+
Product: 2 H^+
Thus:

$$2\,Fe(OH)_3 + 3\,H_2SO_4 \rightarrow Fe_2(SO_4)_3 + 6\,H_2O \text{ (balanced)}$$

Check the oxygen, other than those contained in sulfate ions.
Reactant: 6 O^{2-}
Product: 6 O^{2-}

Step 4: The coefficients of reactants and products cannot be reduced to smaller whole numbers; therefore they are correct as written in step 3.
Step 5: Since all compounds, reactants, and products are electrically neutral, the sum of the charges of the reactants equals that of the products and the equation, complete and balanced, is that shown in step 3.

The stoichiometry of the balanced equation states that two molecules or moles of $Fe(OH)_3$ react with three molecules or moles of H_2SO_4 to yield one molecule or mole of $Fe_2(SO_4)_3$ and six molecules or moles of H_2O.

All balanced equations give the information shown in the foregoing example. The value of the chemical equation lies in the fact that it is the basis for calculating the amount of product produced from a given quantity of reactants and, conversely, allows calculation of the quantities of reactants required to produce a desired quantity of products.

Metathesis Reactions

The term *metathesis* means mutual exchange and is often referred to as double decomposition. When two compounds undergo metathesis, both compounds are decomposed and two new compounds are formed. The positive ions of each compound react with the negative ions of the other compound, as shown in the following equation:

$$A^+B^- + C^+D^- \rightarrow A^+D^- + C^+B^-$$

These reactions generally involve ionic compounds as reactants and nearly always give ionic products, one of which is usually a solid.

EXAMPLES: Predict the products obtained in the following reactions and balance the equations:

1. $CdSO_4 + KOH \rightarrow$
2. $Pb(NO_3)_2 + H_2S \rightarrow$

(See Table 5-3 for ionic charges.)
Double decomposition would give

1. $CdSO_4 + KOH \rightarrow Cd(OH)_2 \downarrow + K_2SO_4$ (unbalanced)
2. $Pb(NO_3)_2 + H_2S \rightarrow PbS \downarrow + HNO_3$ (unbalanced)

Balance equation 1.
Reactant: 1 Cd^{2+}
Product: 1 CD^{2+}; therefore the reactant KOH must be multiplied by 2 to balance K^+ ions.

$$CdSO_4 + 2KOH \rightarrow Cd(OH)_2 \downarrow + K_2SO_4$$

Inspection of this equation shows that both SO_4^{2-} and OH^- ions occur in equal numbers in both the reactants and the products, and the equation as shown is balanced.
Balance equation 2.
Reactant: 1 Pb^{2+}
Product: 1 Pb^{2+}; therefore Pb^{2+} ions are balanced.
  Thus:
Reactant: 1 S^{2-}
Product: 1 S^{2-}; therefore S^{2-} ions are balanced.

Thus:

Reactant: $2 \ NO_3^{1-}$

Product: $1 \ NO_3^{1-}$; therefore the product HNO_3 must be multiplied by 2 to balance NO_3^{1-} ions.

$$Pb(NO_3)_2 + H_2S \rightarrow PbS \downarrow + 2HNO_3$$

Inspection shows that the H^+ ions occur in equal numbers in both the reactants and products, and the equation as shown is balanced.

Oxidation-Reduction Reactions

Oxidation-reduction reactions, commonly called *redox* reactions, are those reactions in which certain atoms gain or lose electrons and thus undergo a change of oxidation number. The oxidation number of a monatomic ion is its charge. For example, the oxidation number of F^- ion is -1 (or it can be expressed $1-$). If the oxidation number changed during a reaction ($2F^- \rightarrow F_2 + 2e^-$), an oxidation or reduction has occurred (F^-, oxidation number -1, has undergone oxidation to give neutral F_2). The process of oxidation always involves the loss of electrons, and consequently the oxidation number of the element involved changes in a positive direction. For example, the ion Fe^{2+} readily undergoes oxidation by loss of an electron to give Fe^{3+}. For each reactant undergoing oxidation there must be a second reactant that undergoes reduction. The reactant undergoing reduction must gain one or more electrons, and thus its oxidation number changes in a negative direction. For example, if the foregoing reaction, in which Fe^{2+} was oxidized to Fe^{3+}, is reversed so that $Fe^{3+} + 1e^- \rightarrow Fe^{2+}$, than a reduction has occurred. Changes in oxidation number generally occur within the limits of ± 5 as indicated below.

Oxidation

$\longrightarrow$

$-5 \ -4 \ -3 \ -2 \ -1 \ 0 \ +1 \ +2 \ +3 \ +4 \ +5$

$\longleftarrow$

Reduction

Confusing as it may seem, an oxidizing agent is a reactant that, by acquiring electrons from a second reactant, causes an increase in oxidation number of the second reactant. Conversely, a reducing agent is the reactant that donates electrons and brings about a reduction of the oxidation number of the other reactant (the oxidizing agent). This change is illustrated in the equation below.

In all redox reactions the total number of electrons lost by the reducing agent must equal the total number of electrons gained by the oxidizing agent.

The oxidation states of substances involved in redox reactions are undergoing change, and many equations cannot be balanced by simple inspection. However, the total ionic charge of the reactants must be equal to that of the products, and the number of atoms of each element in the reactants must equal the number of atoms of the same elements in the products. In balancing redox equations, one must observe several rules.

1. The oxidation state of all elements is zero; that is, the number of electrons and protons are equal and the charge is zero.
2. The oxidation state of a monatomic ion is equal to the charge of that ion. Some elements maintain the same oxidation number in the majority of compounds in which they are found, as shown in Table 5-4.
3. The sum of all oxidation numbers of the atoms of a compound must equal zero.

Those elements generally exhibiting only one oxidation state are shown in Table 5-4.

For example, chlorine in the compound $HClO_3$ (chloric acid) has an oxidation number of $+5$. In determining the oxidation number of chlorine from the formula one must make use of Table 5-4, which states that oxygen always has an oxidation number of -2 and that hydrogen, in most compounds, has an oxidation number of $+1$. Since there are three oxygens in the $HClO_3$ molecule, the sum of the oxidation numbers for oxygen is required to be $3(-2)$, or -6, and hydrogen has an oxidation number of $+1$. Since rule 3 states that the sum of all oxidation numbers for each compound must equal zero, and the sum of the oxidation numbers of hydrogen and oxygen ($+1 + [-6]$) equals -5, the oxidation number of chlorine must be $+5$. Note that the oxidation number of the atoms involved in a compound is determined by their electronegativity and the electronegativity of the elements to which they are bonded.

Having established the rules for balancing redox equations, let us consider the use of these rules in the following examples. The most convenient method of balancing charge is by use of half-reactions. Half-reactions involve only the ions undergoing a change in oxidation number during reaction.

EXAMPLE 1: Balance the following equation:

$$HNO_3 + H_2S \rightarrow NO + S + H_2O \text{ (unbalanced)}$$

Determine the oxidation state of each atom on both sides of the equation to find which atoms have undergone a change of oxidation number.

Oxidation number = 0	Oxidation number = 0	Oxidation number = +2 (or $^{++}$)	Oxidation number = −2 (or $^=$)
Ca	+ S	$\rightarrow$ Ca^{++}	+ S$^=$
Reducing agent	**Oxidizing agent**	**Oxidized**	**Reduced**

Table 5-4	Elements generally exhibiting one oxidation state	
Element	**Common oxidation number**	**Rare oxidation number**
Hydrogen	$+1$ (H^+)	-1 (H^-)
Alkali metals (Na, K, and so on)	$+1$ (Na^+)	
Alkaline earth metals (Mg, Ca, and so on)	$+2$ (Mg^{++})	
Oxygen	-2 ($O^=$)	-1 (O^-), $+2$ (O^{++})
Fluorine	-1 (F^-)	
Chlorine, bromine, and iodine	-1 (Cl^-)	Cl: $+1, +3, +5, +7$ Br: $+1, +3, +5$ I: $+1, +5, +7$

Consider each compound separately.

$$\begin{array}{ccc} +1 \; +5 \; 3(-2) & 2(+1) \; -2 & \\ H \; N \quad O_3 \; + & H_2 \quad S \rightarrow & \\ +2 \; -2 & 0 & 2(+1) \; -2 \\ N \quad O \; + & S \; + & H_2 \quad O \; (unbalanced) \end{array}$$

In arriving at these oxidation numbers the use of the foregoing rules and Table 5-4 tells us that hydrogen always has the oxidation numbers of $+1$ and oxygen -2. The sum of the oxidation numbers of hydrogen atoms in HNO_3 is $+1$ and, since there are three oxygen atoms in this substance, the sum for oxygen atoms is $3(-2) = -6$. Rule 3 states that the sum of the oxidation numbers for the HNO_3 molecule must be zero; therefore nitrogen must have an oxidation number of $+5$; that is, the equation (hydrogen $+1$, plus oxygen $-6 = -5$) requires that the oxidation number of nitrogen be $+5$.

$$H(+1) \; N(+5) \; O_3(-6) \text{ or } (+1) + (+5) + (-6) = 0$$

The equation states that the product containing nitrogen is NO and, using the procedure just described, we find that nitrogen in the product has an oxidation number of $+2$.

$$\begin{array}{cc} +2 \; -2 & \\ N \quad O \text{ or } (+2) + (-2) = 0 \end{array}$$

Therefore the half-reaction in which nitrogen is involved is as follows:

$$N^{5+} + 3e^- \rightarrow N^{2+}$$

Similarly, it is found that sulfur occurs as a reactant in H_2S, having an oxidation number of -2.

$$\begin{array}{cc} 2(+1) \; -2 & \\ H_2 \quad S \text{ or } (+2) + (-2) = 0 \end{array}$$

Sulfur occurs in the product in the elemental form, and by rule 1 is must have an oxidation number of zero. The half-reaction involving sulfur is

$$S^{2-} - 2e^- \rightarrow S^0$$

Inspection of the equation shows that the oxidation numbers of hydrogen and oxygen remain the same in both the reactants and products; that is, they do not change.

Considering the half-reactions and recalling that the number of electrons acquired by the oxidizing agent must equal the number of electrons donated by the reducing agent, we may readily note that the half-reaction involving nitrogen must be multiplied by 2 and the half-reaction involving sulfur be multiplied by 3. The six electrons donated by sulfur must equal the six electrons accepted by nitrogen.

$$2(N^{5+} + 3e^- \rightarrow N^{2+})$$
$$3(S^2 - 2e^- \rightarrow S^0)$$

Applying the coefficients of the half-reactions, the full equation in which nitrogen and sulfur are balanced must be written as

$$2HNO_3 + 3H_2S \rightarrow 2NO + 3S + H_2O \; (unbalanced)$$

The atoms of the remaining elements must now be balanced, and balancing must be done by inspection.

Nitrogens are balanced.
Sulfurs are balanced.
Reactant: 8 H's
Product: 2 H's

Multiplying H_2O (the product) by 4 balances H's and gives the equation

$$2HNO_3 + 3H_2S \rightarrow 2NO + 3S + 4H_2O$$

Inspection shows that the oxygens are also balanced and the equation has been balanced by a simple inspection process. Let us consider a second example of a redox reaction.

EXAMPLE 2:

$$K_2Cr_2O_7 + HCl$$
$$\rightarrow KCl + CrCl_3 + H_2O + Cl_2 \; (unbalanced)$$

Following the process outlined in the preceding example, we find that the elements undergoing oxidation and reduction are as follows:

$$2(Cr^{6+} + 3e^- \rightarrow Cr^{2+}) \text{ reduction (oxidizing agent)}$$
$$3(Cl^- - 2e^- \rightarrow Cl_2^0) \text{ oxidation (reducing agent)}$$

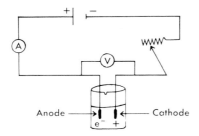

Figure 5-12 Oxidation-reduction involving use of electric current. *A,* Amperage; *V,* voltage.

Note that all the Cl^- ion in the reaction does not undergo oxidation, as some is used in forming the products KCl and $CrCl_3$ in which the oxidation number of -1 is retained.

Multiplying, to balance changes in oxidation number, gives

$$K_2Cr_2O_7 + 6HCl \rightarrow$$
$$KCl + 2CrCl_3 + H_2O + 3Cl_2 \text{ (unbalanced)}$$

Balancing the remaining elements gives

$$K_2Cr_2O_7 + 14\ HCl \rightarrow$$
$$2KCl + 2CrCl_3 + 7H_2O + 3Cl_2 \text{ (balanced)}$$

Electrolytic Reactions

A special type of oxidation-reduction is that involving an electric current supplied by an external source and using an electrolytic cell (Figure 5-12).

The anode is highly electron deficient and may be thought of as being positive in charge, whereas the cathode is rich in electrons and therefore has a large negative charge. This being the case, positive ions (cations) in solution or in the liquid state migrate to the cathode and are reduced by a transfer of electrons from the cathode to the cation. Conversely, the anions, being negatively charged, migrate to the anode and in transferring electrons to the anode undergo oxidation. These processes are summarized as follows:

Cathode: $A^+ + le^- \rightarrow A^0$ (reduction)
Anode: $B^- - le^- \rightarrow B^0$ (oxidation)

Electrolysis is utilized primarily in the industrial production of certain elements such as elemental sodium and chlorine. A second important process involving electrolysis is that of electroplating, in which elemental chromium, nickel, or silver is deposited or plated on the surface of other metals as a protective or decorative coating.

ACIDS AND BASES

An understanding of the chemistry and theory of acids and bases is vital to the practice of nuclear medicine,

since the acidity of the body fluids must remain essentially constant. All compounds and, more important, solutions of the compounds are acidic, basic, or neutral. The properties of acids and bases are given below.

Acids	Bases
1. Taste sour	1. Taste bitter
2. Cause certain organic dyes, called indicators, to change color; for example, blue litmus paper in the presence of an acid changes to red.	2. Cause certain organic dyes, called indicators, to change color; for example, red litmus paper in the presence of a base changes to blue.
3. Release CO_2 from carbonate salts.	3. Feel slick (slimy).
4. Common acidic materials: vinegar, citrus juices, soda (seltzer and all carbonated beverages).	4. Common bases: aqueous ammonia solution, soap, and lye (NaOH).

Concepts of Acids and Bases

Acids and bases have been defined in the historic evolution of chemistry by the Arrhenius (1884), Brönsted-Lowry (1923), and Lewis (1923) concepts. Each of these concepts remains useful in the current understanding of acid-base chemistry.

Arrhenius defined an acid as a substance that yields hydrogen ion (H^+) or hydronium ion (H_3^+O) when dissolved in water, and bases as those substances that yield hydroxide ions (OH^-) when dissolved in water.

The Brönsted-Lowry concept provides a more general definition of acids and bases. It defines an acid as a substance that can provide (or donate) a proton (H^+) to a second substance, which, by definition is a base. For example, acetic acid can donate a proton directly to a base such as ammonia.

$$CH_3COOH + NH_3 \rightarrow CH_3COO^- + NH_4^+$$
Acid **Base** **Acetate** **Ammonium**
ion **ion**

Brönsted-Lowry acids and bases are not restricted to aqueous solutions, as are Arrhenius acids and bases; therefore this concept is valid for any solvent system. Thus the following reaction can occur:

$$H_2SO_4 + NaCl \rightarrow HCl + HSO_4^-$$
Acid **Base** **Acid** **Base**

Sulfuric acid is used as both a reactant and a solvent.

Lewis, in 1923, proposed a still more general definition of acids and bases. The Lewis concept defines an acid as any compound that can *accept* an *electron pair* and a base as any compound that can *donate* an *electron pair.* Acid-base reactions of this type often involve the formation of a coordinate covalent bond and are illustrated by the reaction of boron trifluoride with ammonia as follows:

Acid Base

Boron trifluoride, having an empty orbital, can accept the two nonbonding electrons of the nitrogen in ammonia (recall that the second energy level can accommodate eight electrons).

Neutralization Reactions

The majority of reactions that have been discussed previously cannot be classified as neutralization reactions. The process of neutralization involves the reaction of acids with bases as defined by the Arrhenius concept, H^+ or H_3^+O and OH^-. The products of neutralization are invariably a salt and water. If equal quantities, as defined by normality of an acid and base, are mixed, the resulting solution is neither acidic nor basic. The discipline of medicine makes use of acids and bases, not only in clinical diagnostic procedures, but also as agents in treating certain injuries and disorders. Antacids, containing aluminum and magnesium hydroxides, are commonly used to neutralize excess stomach acid (HCl). Sodium bicarbonate (a base) finds use as a neutralizing agent in the treatment of acid burns, and picric acid is often used to accelerate the rate of mitosis.

A general equation describing the neutralization process may be written as follows:

$$HA + BOH \rightarrow AB + H_2O$$
$$\text{Acid} + \text{Base} \rightarrow \text{A salt} + \text{Water}$$

The driving force for all neutralization reactions is the formation of the stable water molecule, and equations for these reactions can be balanced by simple inspection.

$$H_2SO_4 + NaOH \rightarrow Na_2SO_4 + H_2O \text{ (unbalanced)}$$

Inspection gives the following:
1. SO_4^{2-} ions are balanced
2. *Reactant:* 1 Na^+
   Product: 2 Na^+
3. Multiplying the reactant NaOH by 2 gives

$$H_2SO_4 + 2NaOH \rightarrow Na_2SO_4 + H_2O \text{ (unbalanced)}$$

4. Multiplying the product H_2O by 2 to balance hydrogen gives

$$H_2SO_4 + 2NaOH \rightarrow Na_2SO_4 + 2H_2O$$

Inspection shows that the oxygen atoms are balanced; therefore the equation is balanced.

Calculations

Laboratory procedures using neutralization reactions are quite common and are generally used in determining unknown quantities of acids or bases present in biologic or chemical samples. A useful relationship for calculation of the quantity of an acid or base in a given sample is

$$V_1N_1 = V_2N_2$$

V_1 = Volume of the standard solution (prepared in the laboratory)
N_1 = Normality of the standard solution
V_2 = Volume of the unknown solution
N_2 = Normality of the unknown solution

The usefulness of this equation becomes readily apparent when one applies it to the evaluation of results of neutralization reactions obtained by titrimetric procedures. Since the normality of the standardized solution of acid or base (equivalents per liter or equivalents per milliliter) is known, one can titrate a known volume or weight of a sample containing an unknown quantity of acid or base and, by the use of the volume-normality relationship given above, ascertain the quantity of acid or base present in the sample.

Titrations are performed by taking an aliquot (V_2, a precisely measured volume) of the solution containing an unknown quantity (N_2 in the foregoing equation) of acid or base and placing it in a titration vessel, usually an Erlenmeyer flask. A standard solution of acid or base whose concentration is precisely known is then carefully delivered into the titration flask by use of a buret. The point at which neutralization occurs, the end point, is detected by use of an organic indicator that changes color when neutralization occurs. The volume, V_1, of standard acid or base required to exactly neutralize the substance in the "unknown" is read from the buret. At this point the values of V_1, N_1, and V_2 are known, and by use of the relationship $V_1N_1 = V_2N_2$, the number of equivalents (N_2) of the substance contained in the unknown can be calculated. The following examples illustrate the usefulness of titrimetric procedures as analytic tools.

EXAMPLE 1: What is the normality of a hydrochloric acid solution, 25 ml of which requires 37 ml of 0.30 N NaOH solution for neutralization?

$$V_1 \text{ (NaOH)} = 37 \text{ ml}$$
$$N_1 \text{ (NaOH)} = 0.30 \text{ N}$$
$$V_2 \text{ (HCl)} = 25 \text{ ml}$$
$$N_2 \text{ (HCl)} = ?$$

Using $V_1N_1 = V_2N_2$, solve for N_2.

$$(37 \text{ ml})(0.30 \text{ N}) = (25 \text{ ml})(N_2)$$

$$N_2 = \frac{(37 \text{ ml})(0.30 \text{ N})}{25 \text{ ml}}$$

$$N_2 = \frac{11.1}{25} \text{ N}$$

$$N_2 = 0.44 \text{ N}$$

EXAMPLE 2: Given 30.0 ml of 0.25 M H_3PO_4 (phosphoric acid) solution, what volume of 0.25 M $Ca(OH)_2$ (calcium hydroxide) solution would be required for neutralization?

Step 1: Since the equation is valid only when concentrations are expressed as normalities, we must first find the normality of both the H_3PO_4 and $Ca(OH)_2$ solutions. H_3PO_4 is a triprotic acid (3 H^+ ions), therefore

$$\text{Normality} = 3 \text{ (Molarity)}$$

or

$$N = 3 \text{ (0.25 M)}$$
$$N = 0.75 \text{ for } H_3PO_4$$

$Ca(OH)_2$ is a dibasic (2 OH^- ions) base, therefore

$$\text{Normality} = 2 \text{ (Molarity)}$$

or

$$N = 2 \text{ (0.25 M)}$$
$$N = 0.50 \text{ for } Ca(OH)_2$$

Step 2: Using $V_1N_1 = V_2N_2$

$$V_1 \text{ (}H_3PO_4\text{)} = 30.0 \text{ ml}$$
$$N_1 \text{ (}H_3PO_4\text{)} = 0.75 \text{ N}$$
$$V_2 \text{ (Ca[OH]}_2\text{)} = ?$$
$$N_2 \text{ (Ca[OH]}_2\text{)} = 0.50 \text{ N}$$
$$(30.0 \text{ ml})(0.75 \text{ N}) = (V_2)(0.50 \text{ N})$$

$$V_2 = \frac{(30.0 \text{ ml})(0.75 \text{ N})}{0.50 \text{ N}}$$

$$V_2 = \frac{22.5}{0.50} \text{ ml}$$

$$V_2 = 45.0 \text{ ml of } Ca(OH)_2$$

Strong Versus Weak Acids and Bases

The foregoing discussion of acids and bases implied that all acids and bases dissociate completely in aqueous medium giving either a H_3O^+ ion or a OH^- ion. In reality, only *strong acids* such as HCl, HBr, HI, H_2SO_4, and HNO_3 may be considered to be completely ionized in aqueous solutions; thus:

$$H_2SO_4 + 2H_2O \rightarrow 2H_3O^+ + SO_4^{2-}$$

The common bases NaOH and KOH are *strong bases* and dissociate completely when dissolved in water; thus:

$$NaOH + H_2O \rightarrow Na^+ + OH^- + H_2O$$

Many acids are defined as being *weak*, in that they do not completely dissociate in water because the conjugate base of the acid is of nearly the same base strength as water. Some of the common weak acids are acetic acid, carbonic acid, phenol, water, and boric acid. For example, less than 0.5% of the acetic acid molecules in a 1 M solution undergo reaction with water to produce H_3O^+ ion, the remaining 99.5% of the molecules remain undissociated. Equations for such reactions are written as follows:

$$CH_3COOH + H_2O \rightleftharpoons CH_3COO^- + H_3O^+$$

The double arrow separating reactants and products indicates that a dynamic equilibrium is established in which the rate of the reverse reaction, thus:

$$H_3O^+ + CH_3COO^- \rightarrow CH_3COOH + H_2O$$

is equal to the rate of the forward reaction

$$CH_3COOH + H_2O \rightarrow CH_3COO^- + H_3O^+$$

Thus at equilibrium the concentration of each species in the solution remains constant. The disproportionate length of the arrows in the equation simply indicates that the acetic acid remains largely undissociated.

A similar situation exists for aqueous solutions of *weak bases*, for example, NH_3, Na_2CO_3, and H_2O. Thus a 0.1 M solution of NH_3 in water undergoes reaction to the extent of 0.5%.

$$NH_3 + H_2O \rightleftharpoons NH_4^+ + OH^-$$

EQUILIBRIUMS AND EQUILIBRIUM CONSTANT

The extent of dissociation of weak acids and bases and the resulting equilibriums have been studied exhaustively. These studies have resulted in a mathematic statement that allows calculation of the degree of dissociation. The mathematic expression describing the general equilibrium reaction

$$HY + H_2O \rightleftharpoons Y^- + H_3O^+$$

is expressed as follows:

$$K_{HY} = \frac{[Y^-][H_3O^+]}{[HY][H_2O]}$$

Note: The brackets [ ] indicate concentration of the species in moles per liter.

The equation states that the mathematic product of the concentrations of the reaction products divided by the mathematic product of the concentrations of the reactants is a constant (this is valid only at a given temperature). For example, the equilibrium expression for

$$NH_3 + H_2O \rightleftharpoons NH_4^+ + OH^-$$

is expressed as follows:

$$K_{NH_3} = \frac{[NH_4^+][OH^-]}{[NH_3][H_2O]}$$

Inasmuch as water is present in large excess in most solutions, its concentration remains essentially constant; therefore the term for the concentration of water is incorporated with the equilibrium constant and the mathematic expression is normally

$$K_{NH_3} = \frac{[NH_4^+][OH^-]}{[NH_3]}$$

Experiments have shown that K_{NH_3} is equal to 1.8×10^{-5}m at 25° C. In general, the larger the numeric value of K, the stronger the acid or base, depending on whether H_3O^+ or OH^- ion is one of the products.

A most important equilibrium reaction is that involving pure water because reactions involving acids and bases are normally conducted in aqueous medium. Even though water is neutral, it was classified as both a weak acid and a weak base in the preceding section.

Experiments have shown that water undergoes autoionization, in which one molecule of water functions as an acid and a second molecule functions as a base, giving the following equation:

$$H_2O + H_2O \rightleftharpoons H_3O^+ + OH^-$$

It is apparent that, even though autoionization is occurring, water is neutral because the concentration of H_3O^+ ion is exactly equal to the concentration of OH^- ion. The equilibrium expression for water is

$$K = \frac{[OH^-][H_3O^+]}{[H_2O]}$$

or

$$K_W = [H_2O]K = [OH^-][H_3O^+]$$

The concentration of water being constant gives

$$K_W = [OH^-][H_3O^+]$$

K_W has been determined experimentally to be 1×10^{-14}M². For pure water

$$[H_3O^+] = [OH^-] = \sqrt{1 \times 10^{-14}} = 1 \times 10^{-7}M$$

THE pH CONCEPT

Following the logic of the preceding discussion, an aqueous solution, no matter whether acidic, basic, or neutral, must have a concentration of H_3O^+ and OH^- ions, the product of which must equal 1×10^{-14}.

$$K_W = [H_3O^+][OH^-] = 1 \times 10^{-14} \text{ M}^2$$

Any solution in which $[H_3O^+]$ is equal to $[OH^-]$ must be neutral, and any solution in which $[OH^-]$ and $[H_3O^+]$ are unequal must be either basic or acidic. However, at all times $[H_3O^+] \times [OH^-]$ equals 1×10^{-14}M². As with the solutions discussed previously, the concentration of H_3O^+ is expressed as moles/liter. This has been further simplified and is commonly expressed in terms of pH (from the French *puissance d'hydrogène*, meaning power of hydrogen) as a number between 0 and 14.

The pH of a solution is defined as being equal to the negative log of the $[H_3O^+]$; thus:

$$pH = -\log [H_3O^+]$$

and a neutral solution having a concentration of H_3O^+ equal to 10^{-7} has a pH of 7.

$$pH = -\log [H_3O^+] = -\log 10^{-7} = 7$$

For those solutions in which $[H_3O^+]$ is larger than 10^{-7}, the solution will contain a concentration of H_3O^+ ions greater than that of OH^- ions and will therefore be acidic. Whenever the $[H_3O^+]$ is greater than $[OH^-]$, the pH will be less than 7, and for those solutions in which the $[H_3O^+]$ is less than $[OH^-]$, the pH will be greater than 7 and the solution will be basic.

Values of pH
1, 2, 3, 4, 5, 6   **7**   8, 9, 10, 11, 12, 13, 14
Acidic   Neutral   Basic

In an analogous manner, the pOH of a solution is the negative log of $[OH^-]$; therefore, knowing that pH is equal to $-\log [H_3O^+]$ and that K_W is equal to 1×10^{-14}, we find that pOH must equal $14 - $ pH. For example, if a solution is found to have a $[H_3O^+]$ of 1×10^{-3}M, the pH of the solution will be $-\log (1 \times 10^{-3})$, or 3, and the pOH therefore must be $14 - 3$, or 11.

EXAMPLE 1: What is the pH of a solution that has a $[H_3O^+]$ of 2.3×10^{-5} M? Using the relationship $pH = -\log [H_3O^+]$, we proceed as follows:

$$pH = -\log (2.3 \times 10^{-5})$$
$$pH = -(\log 2.3 + \log 10^{-5})$$
$$pH = -(0.36 + [-5] \log 10)$$
$$pH = -(0.36 - 5)$$
$$pH = -(-4.64)$$
$$pH = 4.64 \text{ (The solution is acidic.)}$$

EXAMPLE 2: A solution is found to have a concentration of OH^- equaling 3.0×10^{-8} M. What is its pH?

a. Using $pOH = -\log [OH^-]$, find pOH.

$$pOH = -\log (3.0 \times 10^{-8})$$
$$pOH = -(\log 3.0 + [-8] \log 10)$$
$$pOH = -(0.477 + [-8])$$
$$pOH = -(-7.523)$$
$$pOH = 7.52$$

b. Using pH + pOH = 14, find pH.

$$pH + 7.52 = 14$$
$$pH = 14 - 7.52$$
$$pH = 6.48 \text{ (The solution is acidic.)}$$

EXAMPLE 3: Find the $[H_3O^+]$ of a solution that has a pH of 9.8 using pH = $-\log [H_3O^+]$.

$$9.8 = -\log [H_3O^+]$$
$$\log [H_3O^+] = -10 + 0.2$$

Using antilogs, find the $[H_3O^+]$.

$$[H_3O^+] = (\text{antilog } 0.2)(\text{antilog} - 10)$$
$$[H_3O^+] = 1.58 \times 10^{-10} \text{ M}$$

EXAMPLE 4: Given the following information for a solution of acetic acid:

$$K_a = 1.8 \times 10^{-5}$$
$$[HOAc] = 0.5 \text{ M (HOAc is acetic acid.)}$$

Find the pH of the solution.

a. The equilibrium reaction is

$$HOAc \rightleftharpoons H^+ + OAc^-$$
$$0.5 \text{ M} \quad x \text{ M} + \quad x \text{ M}$$

We know that

$$K_a = \frac{[H^+][OAc^-]}{[HOAc]}$$

Assuming that x M of HOAC dissociates, the concentrations at equilibrium are

$$[HOAC] = 0.5 - x$$
$$[H^+] = x$$
$$[OAc] = x$$

Thus:

$$1.8 \times 10^{-5} = \frac{x^2}{5 \times 10^{-1} - x} = \frac{x^2}{5 \times 10^{-1}}$$

HOAc, being a weak acid, is largely undissociated, and x, compared to 5.0×10^{-1}, is very small and may be eliminated from the denominator without seriously affecting the value calculated for x.

$$x^2 = (1.8 \times 10^{-5})(5 \times 10^{-1})$$
$$x^2 = 9 \times 10^{-6}$$
$$x = 3 \times 10^{-3} \text{ M} = [H^+] = [OAc^-]$$

b. Using pH = $-\log [H_3O^+]$, proceed as follows:

$$pH = -\log (3 \times 10^{-3})$$
$$pH = -(\log 3 + [-3] \log 10)$$
$$pH = -(-2.52)$$
$$pH = 2.52 \text{ (The solution is acidic.)}$$

BUFFER SOLUTIONS

All biologic systems are dependent on fluids that are maintained within very narrow limits of pH. For example, human blood must be maintained within a pH range of 7.3 to 7.5 and therefore requires a means by which these pH limits can be maintained. The mechanism by which this is achieved is referred to as *buffering* and involves a solution that contains a mixture of substances, some that are acidic and others that are basic. Again, with blood being used as an example, the substances involved in the buffering effect are carbonates, bicarbonates, carbonic acid, the phosphates (PO_4^{3-}, HPO_4^{2-}, and $H_2PO_4^-$), and certain proteins that function by maintaining the pH of blood in the range of 7.3 to 7.5.

A relatively simple buffer system is one consisting of a mixture of acetic acid and its conjugate base acetate ion. To understand how this system can function to maintain a pH within a small range, we must recall that acetic acid, being a weak acid, is described by an equilibrium expression. Let us examine what occurs when a "foreign" acid or base is introduced into the acetic acid–acetate ion buffer system.

$$HOAc \rightleftharpoons H^+ + OAc^- \quad K_a =$$
$$1.8 \times 10^{-5} = \frac{[H^+][OAc^-]}{[HOAc]}$$

This equation shows that undissociated acetic acid is present and is available to react with any base entering the system. For example, if a small quantity of sodium hydroxide is added to the system (HOAc + NaOH → NaOAc + H_2O), the concentration of acetic acid will decrease while the concentration of acetate ion will increase. Conversely, when an acid such as HCl is added to the system (NaOAc + HCl → HOAc + NaCl), the concentration of acetic acid increases while the concentration of acetate ion is decreased. The concentration of the buffer system components will undergo change, but the expression governing the equilibrium will still be valid.

Although buffer solutions will not maintain a fairly constant pH if large quantities of acids or bases are added to them, it is remarkable how much they can accommodate without an appreciable change in pH. This is illustrated in the following example:

EXAMPLE: Consider 1 L of the acetate buffer that is 0.1 M in acetic acid and 0.1 M in sodium acetate.

$$HOAc \rightleftharpoons H^+ + OAc^- \quad K_a = 1.8 \times 10^{-5}$$
$$0.1 \text{ M} \quad x \text{ M} + x \text{ M}$$
$$NaOAc \rightarrow Na^+ + OAc^- \text{ (100\% ionized)}$$
$$0.1 \text{ M} \quad 0.1 \text{ M} \quad 0.1 \text{ M}$$

a. Calculate the pH of the following buffer solution:

$$K_a = \frac{[H_+][OAc^-]}{[HOAc]} = \frac{[H^+](1 \times 10^{-1} + x)}{(1 \times 10^{-1} - x)} = 1.8 \times 10^{-5}$$

Since the acetic acid contributes a negligible amount of the total quantity of OAc^-, the $[OAc^- + x]$ may be assumed to be 0.1 M. Similarly the $[HOAc - x]$ may be assumed to be 0.1 M; therefore

$$1.8 \times 10^{-5} = \frac{[H^+](1 \times 10^{-1})}{(1 \times 10^{-1})}$$

and

$$[H^+] = 1.8 \times 10^{-5} \text{ M}$$

The pH of the solution will be, to a first approximation, as follows:

$$
\begin{aligned}
pH = -\log [H^+] &= -\log (1.8 \times 10^{-5}) \\
pH &= -(\log 1.8 + [-5] \log 10) \\
pH &= -(0.26 - 5) \\
pH &= 4.74
\end{aligned}
$$

b. Calculate the pH of the solution after addition of 0.1 mole of HCl, assuming that the increase in total volume of the buffer solution will be negligible.

$$
\begin{array}{ccccc}
HCl & + & NaOAc & \rightarrow & NaCl & + & HOAc \\
0.01 \text{ M} & & 0.01 \text{ M} & & 0.01 \text{ M} & & 0.01 \text{ M}
\end{array}
$$

The reaction states that for each equivalent of HCl added, 1 equivalent of OAc^- will be consumed, thus forming an equivalent of HOAc. The concentrations now become

$$
\begin{array}{ccccc}
HOAc & \rightleftharpoons & H^+ & + & OAc^- \\
(0.1 \text{ M} + 0.01 \text{ M}) & & x \text{ M} & + & (0.1 - 0.01 \text{ M})
\end{array}
$$

Following the same rationale as used in part (a), calculate the $[H^+]$.

$$K_a = \frac{[H^+][OAc^-]}{[HOAc]}$$

$$\frac{[H^+](0.09)}{(0.11)} = 1.8 \times 10^{-5}$$

$$[H^+] = \frac{(1.1 \times 10^{-1})(1.8 \times 10^{-5})}{(9 \times 10^{-2})}$$

$$[H^+] = 0.22 \times 10^{-4} = 2.2 \times 10^{-5} \text{ M}$$

Thus:

$$
\begin{aligned}
pH = -\log[H^+] &= -\log(2.2 \times 10^{-5}) \\
pH &= -(\log 2.2 + [-5] \log 10) \\
pH &= -(0.34 - 5) \\
pH &= 4.66
\end{aligned}
$$

Comparing the pH of the original buffer solution, 4.74, with the pH of the solution after addition of 0.01 mole of HCl, 4.66, we see that the pH has changed by only 0.08. As a problem to solve, what change in pH would be expected if 0.01 mole of NaOH had been added to the original solution?

Similarly the buffer systems involved in maintaining a narrow pH range for blood involve simple acid-base reactions such as those just described.

ORGANIC COMPOUNDS

The chemistry that has been discussed in the preceding sections has involved, with the exception of acetic acid, substances that are referred to as being inorganic. Inorganic substances comprise all those elements and compounds derived from elements other than carbon, the number of which can be counted in the thousands. Organic chemistry is best defined as the chemistry of carbon, and organic compounds recorded in the literature are numbered in the millions. Carbon differs from all other elements in its unique ability to form strong covalent bonds to other carbon atoms, thus resulting in myriads of compounds ranging from those of low molecular weight to highly complex molecules containing thousands of carbon atoms. Obviously, a thorough discussion of organic chemistry is beyond the scope of this chapter; however, the importance of organic chemistry, as applied to nuclear medicine specifically and all living systems generally, requires some foundation in this subject.

Historically, organic chemistry as a discipline is relatively young, since philosophic and theologic thought held that organic substances, being found primarily in living systems, required a vital force for their creation and that humans would never accomplish the creation or synthesis of these substances. In 1828 the German chemist Friedrich Wöhler, while working with the inorganic substance ammonium cyanate (NH_4^+ CNO^-), found that when it was heated it was converted to the nonionic organic substance urea

$$(H_2N-\overset{\overset{\displaystyle O}{\|}}{C}-NH_2)$$

which is a metabolic product excreted in the urine. This discovery gave rise to great controversy in the scientific community, and serious investigation in organic chemistry did not occur until the mid-1800s.

Types of Organic Compounds and Nomenclature

Organic compounds are divided into families or homologous series in which all members of a given family exhibit essentially the same type of chemical reactivity. Each family of simple organic compounds is characterized by a *functional group*, the most reactive site of the molecule, which determines the chemical reactions that all members of the family will undergo. The main families of organic compounds and their characteristic functional groups are given in Table 5-5.

As we have previously noted, each compound possesses a name unique to itself; this is also the case with organic compounds. Although many organic compounds, especially those isolated as naturally occurring products in the early years of organic chemistry, are still

Table 5-5 Families of organic compounds and their functional groups

Family	Structure	IUPAC name	Suffix	Functional group
Alkanes		Methane	*–ane*	(None)
Alkenes		Ethene	*–ene*	
Alkynes	H—C≡C—H	Ethyne	*–yne*	—C≡C—
Arenes (aromatic compounds)		Benzene	*–ene*	—C—H
Alcohols		Ethanol	*–ol*	—O—H
Phenols		Phenol	*–ol*	—O—H
Ethers		Diethylether	*–ether*	—O—
Halides		Bromomethane	The substituents *chloro-, fluoro-,* etc. are prefixed to parent alkane.	—X(F, Cl, Br, I)
Aldehydes		Ethanal	*–al*	O=C—H
Ketones		2-Propanone	*–one*	O=C—

Table 5-5 Families of organic compounds and their functional groups—cont'd

Family	Structure	IUPAC name	Suffix	Functional group
Carboxylic acids	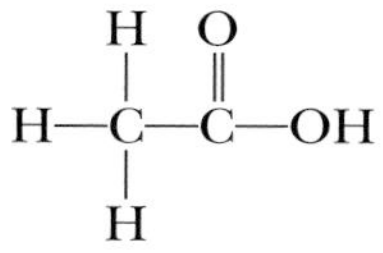 H—C—C—OH (with H, O as shown)	Ethanoic acid	*–oic*	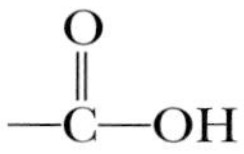 —C—OH (with O)
Esters	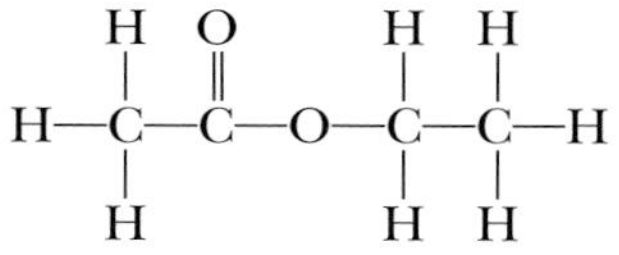 H—C—C—O—C—C—H	Ethyl ethanoate	*–oate*	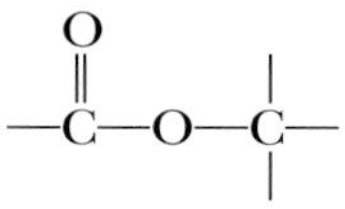 —C—O—C—
Amides	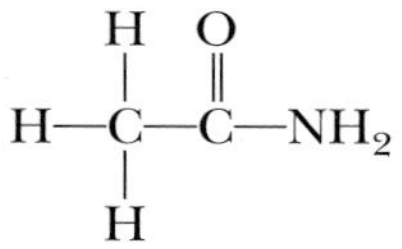 H—C—C—NH_2	Ethanamide	*–amide*	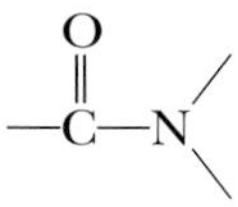 —C—N
Amines	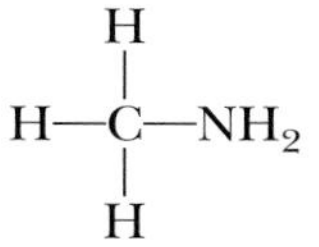 H—C—NH_2	Methamine	*–amine*	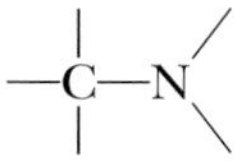 —C—N
Thiols	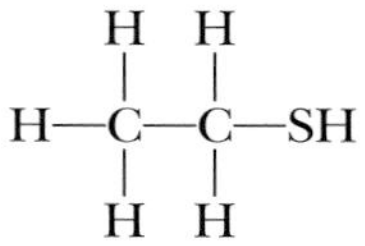 H—C—C—SH	Ethanethiol	*–thiol*	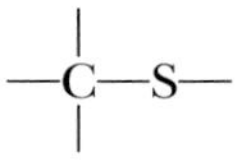 —C—S—

referred to by the names (common or trivial names) given them by their discoverers, the multitude of organic compounds now known requires a systematic method of naming them. Currently, the generally accepted rules for naming organic compounds are those set down by the International Union of Pure and Applied Chemistry (IUPAC). Using alkanes as an example, the IUPAC rules are as follows.

Those molecules in which all the carbon atoms are bonded so as to form a continuous chain are called "normal" alkanes (Table 5-6). All other alkanes are named as though they had been derived from the hydrocarbon with the longest continuous chain, this being the parent compound (rule 1).

EXAMPLE:

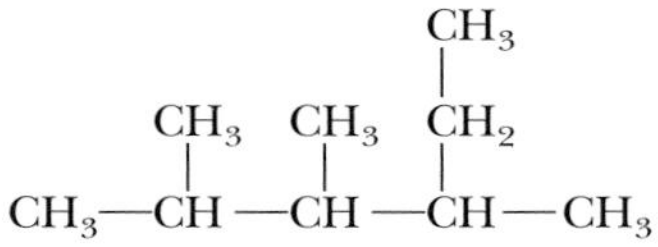

$$CH_3—CH—CH—CH—CH_3$$
(with CH_3, CH_3, CH_2, CH_3 branches)

Rule 1: The longest chain consists of six carbon atoms; therefore the parent hydrocarbon is *hexane.* However, unlike hexane there are three branches in the above molecule in which CH_3 groups have been substi-

tuted for hydrogens of the parent compound. The CH_3 groups belong to a family of alkyl groups, which are derived from the alkanes by removal of one hydrogen. These are named by replacement of the -ane ending of the alkane by -yl (Table 5-7).

Rule 2: The carbon atoms of the parent structure are numbered from the end that will give the *lowest numbers* to those carbons to which the alkyl groups are attached.

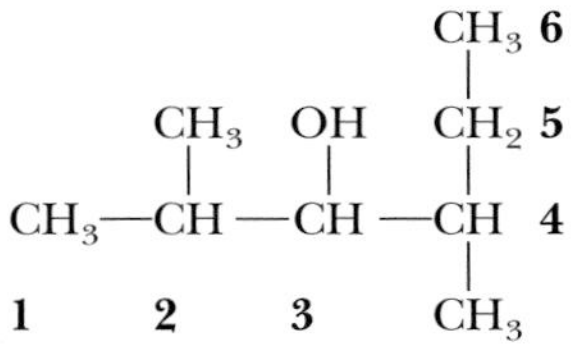

$$CH_3—CH—CH—CH$$
(numbered 1 2 3 4, with CH_3, OH, CH_2 5, CH_3 6, CH_3 branches)

Number as above and *not* as follows.

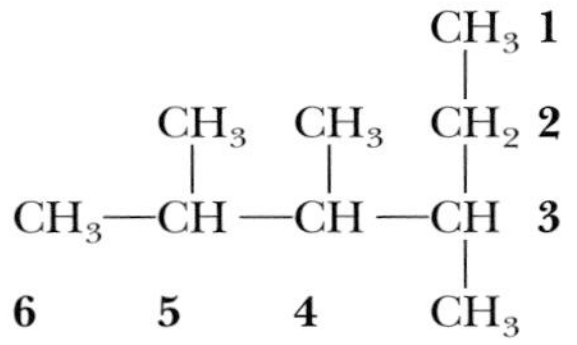

$$CH_3—CH—CH—CH$$
(numbered 6 5 4 3, with CH_3, CH_3, CH_2 2, CH_3 1, CH_3 branches)

Rule 3: The groups attached to the parent structure are given both a name and a number to indicate their

Table 5-6 Normal alkanes (C_nH_{2n+2})

Number of carbons	Name	Expanded formula	Condensed formula
1	Methane	(see structure)	CH_4
2	Ethane	(see structure)	$CH_3—CH_3$
3	Propane	(see structure)	$CH_3—CH_2—CH_3$
4	Butane	(see structure)	$CH_3—(CH_2)_2—CH_3$
5	Pentane	(see structure)	$CH_3—(CH_2)_3—CH_3$
6	Hexane	(see structure)	$CH_3—(CH_2)_4—CH_3$

Starting with pentane, the alkanes are named systematically with a numeric prefix indicating the number of carbon atoms, that is, pent-, hex-, hept-, oct-, non-, dec-, undec-, dodec-, tridec-, tetradec-, pentadec-, hexadec-, heptadec-, octadec-, nonadec-, eicos- (20), heneicos- (21), docos-, tricos-, tetracos-, and so on.

point of attachment. If the same group occurs as a substituent in the molecule more than once, then the prefixes di-, tri, tetra-, and so on, are used to specify the number of times this group appears. If more than one type of group is attached to the parent compound, these groups are named in alphabetic order. Therefore the correct name for the above compound is "2,3,4-trimethylhexane."

Note that a comma (with no space) is used between numbers and a hyphen between the number and the name of the substituent.

Note in Table 5-7 that the isobutyl and *tert*-butyl groups were not shown to be derived from one of the normal alkanes. The names given these groups arise from an older nomenclature in which both of the alkanes containing four carbon atoms were called butanes. This pair of structural isomers consists of the normal butane and a second compound having the structure that is called isobutane. Inspection of the structure

of isobutane shows that two alkyl groups can be derived, depending on the hydrogen that is removed. The prefixes secondary and tertiary are used to indicate the carbon through which the alkyl substituent is attached. If the carbon of the alkyl group, at the point of attachment, is bonded to only one other carbon, the alkyl group is designated as primary; if bonded to two other carbons, the alkyl group is secondary; and it is tertiary if bonded to three other carbons, for example, the *sec*-butyl and *tert*-butyl groups.

The IUPAC rules for naming all organic compounds follow, in general, the above rules with the following modifications: (1) the ending (suffix) of the name is

Table 5-7 Alkyl groups derived from the alkanes by removal of one hydrogen

	Common alkyl groups	Derived from
Methyl	$CH_3—$	Methane
Ethyl	$CH_3—CH_2—$	Ethane
Propyl	$CH_3—CH_2—CH_2—$	Propane
Isopropyl	$CH_3—\overset{\mid}{C}H—CH_3$	Propane
Butyl	$CH_3—CH_2—CH_2—CH_2—$	Butane
sec-Butyl	$CH_3—\overset{\mid}{C}H—CH_2—CH_3—$	Butane
Isobutyl	$\overset{CH_3}{\underset{CH_3}{\diagdown}}HC—CH_2—$	Butane
tert-Butyl	$CH_3—\overset{CH_3}{\underset{CH_3}{\overset{\mid}{\underset{\mid}{C}}}}—$	Butane

dictated by the main functional group present in the compounds, (2) the longest continuous chain (parent compound) must contain the main functional group, and (3) the chain is numbered so that the main functional group receives the lowest possible number.

EXAMPLE:

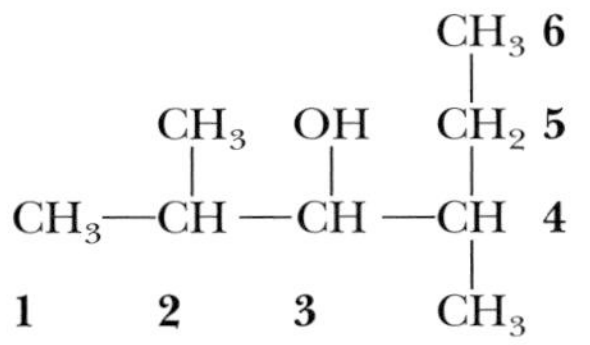

$$\underset{1 \quad\quad 2 \quad\quad 3 \quad\;\; CH_3}{CH_3—\underset{\mid}{\underset{CH_3}{C}H}—\underset{\mid}{\underset{OH}{C}H}—\underset{\mid}{\underset{CH_2\;5}{\overset{CH_3\;6}{C}H\;4}}}$$

2,4-Dimethyl-3-hexanol

Alkanes. Also called saturated hydrocarbons, these compounds are a major source of energy but are of little importance in nuclear medicine. Perhaps the greatest utility in nuclear medicine would be their use as solvents; however, as a point of interest the saturated hydrocarbon cyclopropane

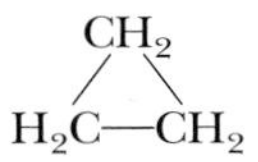

$$\overset{CH_2}{\underset{H_2C—CH_2}{\diagup\!\diagdown}}$$

(with the prefix "cyclo-" indicating a ring or cyclic system) has found use as a general anesthetic.

Alkenes. This family of hydrocarbons, which contains a carbon-carbon double bond (C=C) is a potentially

useful group of substances in labeling procedures. Although several substances are currently under investigation, their usefulness as imaging agents has yet to be proved. Potential agents may arise through addition of radioactive reagents to the carbon-carbon double bond.

$$R—HC{=}CH—R' + HI \rightarrow R—\overset{H}{\underset{H}{\overset{\mid}{\underset{\mid}{C}}}}—\overset{H}{\underset{I}{\overset{\mid}{\underset{\mid}{C}}}}—R'$$

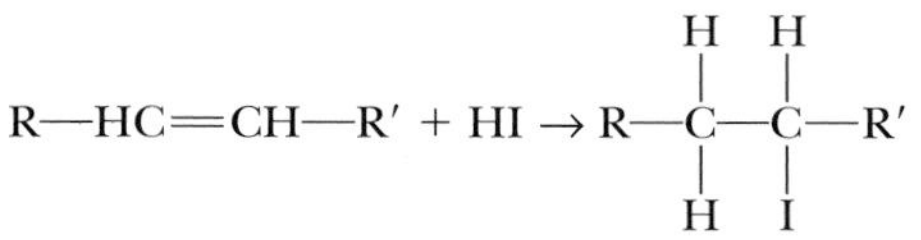

The alkynes, having chemical properties similar to the alkenes, are also of interest as potential sources of radiopharmaceuticals.

Arenes and aromatic compounds. This family of compounds contains at least one aromatic ring, which is characterized by benzene, the simplest of the aromatic compounds.

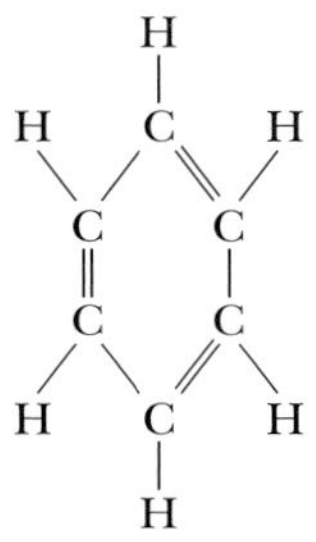

The chemistry of these compounds differs greatly from that of the alkenes and alkynes in that, rather than addition reactions, they undergo substitution reactions in which one or more hydrogens are replaced by another atom or group, for example, the iodination of benzene is

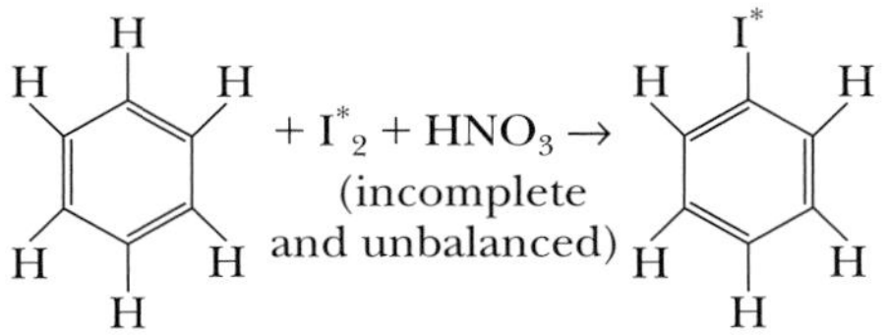

$+ I^*_2 + HNO_3 \rightarrow$ (incomplete and unbalanced)

This reaction is found to be especially useful in the preparation of *ortho*-iodohippuric acid, which has found use as a renal function agent.

Among other aromatic substances containing a radioactive halogen are the estrogens, which have been approved for experimental imaging procedures in humans.

An especially important radiolabeled aromatic compound used for determination of thyroid function is T_3.

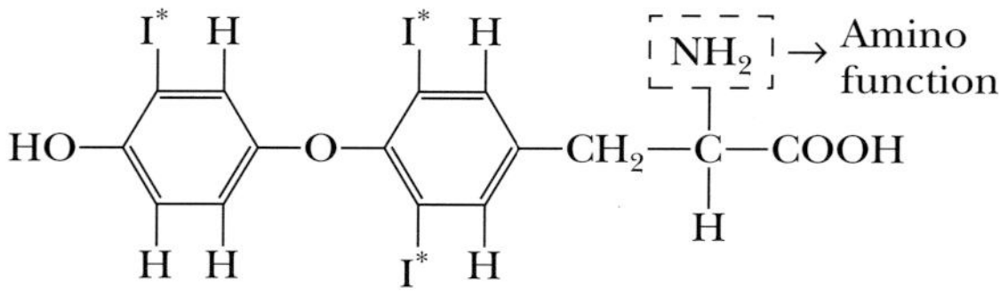

3,5,3'–Triiodothyronine (T₃)

Alcohols and phenols. Alcohols and phenols contain the functional group —OH. Inspection of the structures of rose bengal and T_3 shows that each contains a phenolic hydroxyl (—OH) function as a part of the molecule. Likewise, brominated estrone, mentioned in the preceding section, also contains this functional group.

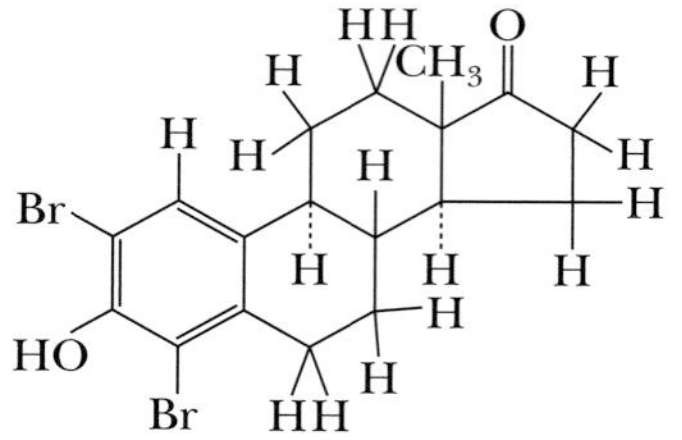

2,4–Dibromoestrone

Molecules containing this structural feature are highly important in preparation of radiopharmaceuticals.

Ethers. The ether linkage, R—O—R, also occurs in rose bengal and T_3, and its importance as a structural feature, as with the phenolic —OH function, lies in its ability to facilitate substitution reactions in which radioactive halogens are introduced into the aromatic ring.

Halides. Radiopharmaceuticals that contain halogens, especially those containing radioactive bromine or iodine, again for example, rose bengal, T_3, and brominated estrogen, are of utmost importance and have great effectiveness in the practice of nuclear medicine solely because of the presence of the radioactive halogen in these molecules. However, the functional molecules are of equal importance in that they determine the organ or site in which the total radioactive substance is localized.

Aldehydes and ketones. The carbonyl function

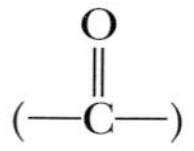

$$(-\overset{\overset{\displaystyle O}{\|}}{C}-)$$

is common to both aldehydes and ketones. The presence of this functional group is not especially important to the labeling of organic molecules, but, as noted in the preceding section, its presence is vital in determining the biodistribution of the radioactive substance.

Carboxylic acids. Several compounds containing the carboxyl function have been noted in previous sections. In addition, pentetic acid (DTPA) forms a complex with ^{169}ytterbium to give ^{169}Yb-pentetic acid (^{169}Yb-DTPA), a cisternographic imaging agent.

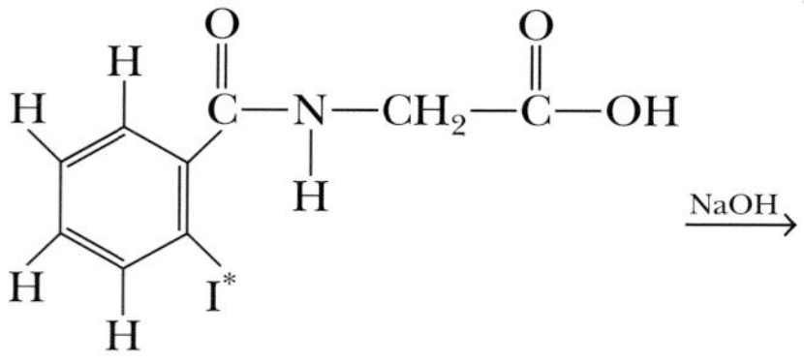

o-**Iodohippuric acid**

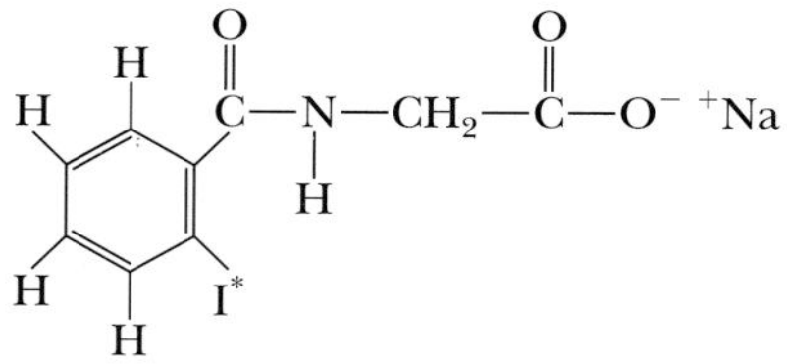

Hippuran

The sodium salt of *o*-iodohippuric acid, hippuran, in filtering through the glomeruli of the kidneys, provides an effective means of evaluating kidney function, especially important in patients who have received a kidney transplant.

Esters, functioning as derivatives of carboxylic acids, are formed by means of an acid-catalyzed condensation reaction between a carboxylic acid and an alcohol. These substances have not as yet been found to be useful as precursors to radiopharmaceuticals.

$$R-\overset{\overset{\displaystyle O}{\|}}{C}-OH + R'-OH \overset{H^+}{\rightarrow} R-\overset{\overset{\displaystyle O}{\|}}{C}-O-R' + H_2O$$

Amides. Hippuran (previous section), in addition to the carboxylate group, also contains an amide function.

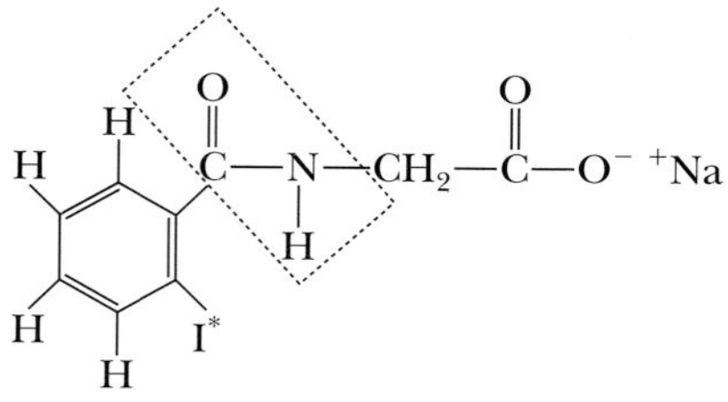

Hippuran, showing the amide function

Components of all biologic tissues have amide functions, which usually are referred to as peptide linkages. The protein human serum albumin (HSA), whose structure is not completely known, when labeled with ^{99m}Tc, is used as a blood pool imaging agent.

Amines and thiols. Amines and thiols are the nitrogen and sulfur analogs of the alcohols. Substances in which the amino groups ($-NH_2$) are an important structural component are the proteins and amino acids from which they are derived.

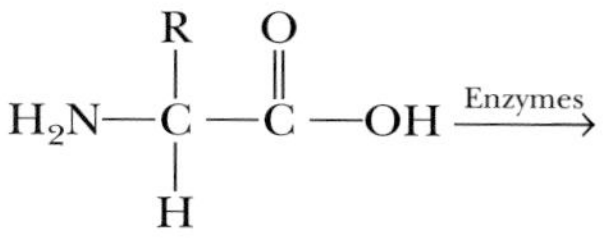

$$H_2N-\underset{\underset{H}{|}}{\overset{\overset{R}{|}}{C}}-\overset{\overset{O}{\|}}{C}-OH \xrightarrow{\text{Enzymes}}$$

Amino acid

$$H_2N\left[\underset{\underset{H}{|}}{\overset{\overset{R}{|}}{C}}-\overset{\overset{O}{\|}}{C}-\underset{\underset{H}{|}}{N}-\underset{\underset{H}{|}}{\overset{\overset{R}{|}}{C}}\right]_x\overset{\overset{O}{\|}}{C}-OH + xH_2O$$

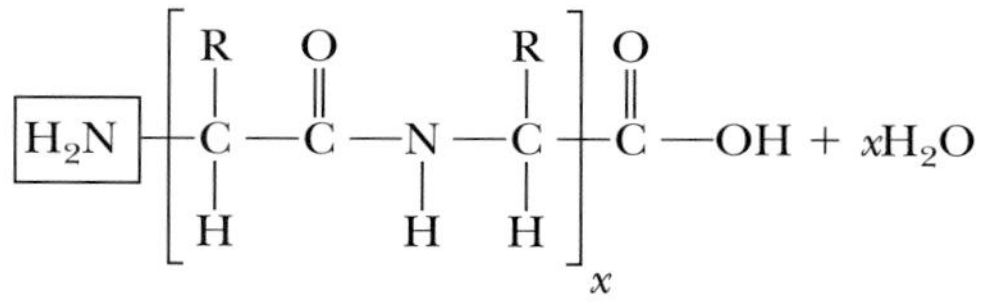

Protein

Of the compounds useful in nuclear medicine, one of the most important is pentetic acid (DTPA; see the previous carboxylic acids).

CONCLUSION

The foregoing comments, in which the significance of the various organic functional groups to nuclear medicine have been noted, should not be considered by the student to be a complete description of the chemistry of these compounds. A thorough understanding of each of the radiopharmaceutical compounds requires not only a knowledge of their structure and biologic fate, but also ultimately a knowledge of the chemical processes by which they are prepared. A discussion of the procedures used in preparing these substances is contained in Chapter 6. Of course, a thorough understanding of the theoretical and preparative techniques of organic chemistry as related to nuclear medicine and to an insight into the chemical basis of life is an unending quest.

SUGGESTED READINGS

Chang, R: *Chemistry,* ed 3, New York, 1988, McGraw-Hill.

Harris, DC: *Quantitative chemical analysis,* ed 3, New York, 1991, WH Freeman.

Wade LG Jr: *Organic chemistry,* ed 2, New York, 1990, Prentice Hall.

chapter *6*

Sally W. Schwarz, Carolyn J. Anderson, Joanna B. Downer

Radiochemistry and Radiopharmacology

Objectives

Discuss nuclear stability and its relationship to radioactive decay.

Describe the basic mechanisms for radionuclide production in a reactor.

Describe the fundamentals of particle accelerator operation and the production of radionuclides using particle accelerators.

Describe generator kinetics in the production of radionuclides, and detail the difference between transient and secular equilibrium.

Diagram a wet column and dry column molybdenum-technetium generator, and explain the elution process.

Describe the chemical properties of the pertechnetate ion.

Explain the technetium labeling processes used by reduction methods.

Discuss the chemical and labeling processes of gallium and indium radiopharmaceuticals.

Describe the pharmacokinetics of thallium as a myocardial perfusion imaging agent.

Explain iodination techniques.

List and describe the properties of PET radiopharmaceuticals and advantages of using these compounds.

Describe the differences between quality control relative to radionuclide purity, radiochemical purity, and chemical impurities.

Describe how particle sizes are measured.

Discuss the difference between sterile compounds and compounds containing pyrogens and tests for ensuring these properties.

PRODUCTION OF RADIONUCLIDES

Nuclear Stability

There are approximately 275 different nuclei that have shown no evidence of radioactive decay and hence are considered stable with respect to this type of transformation. Figure 6-1 shows the relationship of the number of neutrons to the number of protons in the known stable nuclei. In the light elements, stability is achieved when the numbers of neutrons and protons are approximately equal. As the elements become heavier, the ratio of neutrons to protons (N/P ratio) for nuclear stability increases from 1 to about 1.5. If a nucleus has an N/P ratio too high for stability (neutron rich), it will undergo radioactive decay in a manner such that the N/P ratio decreases to approach the line of stability. The consequence is the production of a negative beta particle (β^-) as shown by the following example:

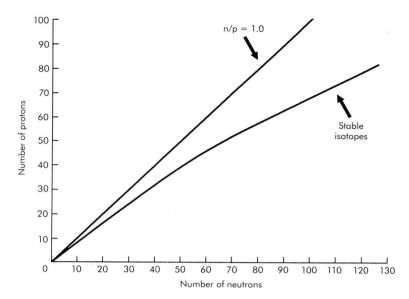

Figure 6-1 Neutron-proton ratio in stable isotopes becomes greater than 1 as the mass increases.

$$n \rightarrow p + e^- + \bar{\nu} \; (\beta^- \text{ decay})$$

If the N/P ratio is too low for stability, then radioactive decay occurs in a manner that will reduce the number of protons and increase the number of neutrons by the net conversion of a proton to a neutron. This is accomplished through either positron emission (β^+) or absorption by the nucleus of an orbital electron (electron capture, or EC). Examples are shown in the following reactions:

$$p \rightarrow n + e^+ + \nu \; (\beta^+ \text{ decay})$$
$$p + e^- \rightarrow n + \nu \; (\text{electron capture})$$

Beta decay often leaves the daughter nucleus in an excited state. This excitation energy is removed either by gamma-ray emission or by a process called internal conversion. Generally, emission of a gamma ray occurs immediately after the beta decay (within 10^{-12} sec), but in some cases the nucleus may remain in the higher energy state for a measurable length of time. When this occurs, the excited nucleus is said to be in a metastable state, indicated by the letter "m." An example is ^{99m}Tc, which decays with a half-life of 6 hr to ^{99}Tc. The transition of a radionuclide from an upper energy state to a lower energy state by the emission of gamma rays is referred to as an *isomeric transition.*

If a nucleus is capable of emitting a gamma ray, there is also a probability that the photon may eject an electron from an extranuclear shell. This process is an alternative to isomeric transition and is known as *internal conversion.* As an upper level electron undergoes a transition to occupy the lower energy electron site, an x ray is emitted, characteristic of the electron shell that is being filled. In a process similar to internal conversion, these x rays may cause the ejection of an additional outer shell electron known as an *Auger electron.*

The process continues until all inner shell vacancies have been filled by "cascading" electrons from outer shells, with corresponding emissions of x rays or Auger electrons.

Positron decay leaves the daughter nuclide two electron mass units lower than the parent, requiring at least 1.022 MeV (2×0.511 MeV/electron) of transition energy. Once released from the nucleus, the β^+ reacts with an electron, resulting in the release of two 0.511 MeV photons, which are called annihilation radiation, emitted in opposite directions. Some positron-emitting radionuclides decay to excited states of the daughter nuclide. These excited daughter nuclides can further decay by isomeric transitions as discussed earlier.

Alpha decay occurs primarily for nuclei heavier than lead. In alpha decay the proton number is reduced by 2 and the mass by 4 units. It is represented by the following equation:

$$^A_Z X \rightarrow ^{(A-4)}_{(Z-2)} Y + {}^4He$$

The probability of alpha decay is greater for nuclei with an even number of neutrons or protons than for nuclei with an odd number. Radionuclides that decay by alpha emission are not useful in nuclear medicine imaging but may have future therapeutic applications.

Radionuclides used to label radiopharmaceuticals for nuclear medicine imaging should decay by either gamma or positron (β^+) emission. Gamma radiation emitted from radiopharmaceuticals readily penetrates tissues and escapes from the body, allowing external detection by gamma cameras. Positron-emitting radionuclides produce two 0.511 MeV gamma photons emitted in opposite directions from the positron-electron annihilation. The angle of nearly 180 degrees of the emitted 0.511 MeV photons is exploited in positron emission tomography (PET) to allow electronic collimation of the radiation and determination of the three-dimensional location of the decay event.

Reactor-Produced Radionuclides

The two major principles of a nuclear reactor are that neutrons induce fission in uranium and that the number of neutrons released by this fission is greater than one. Thus:

$$^{235}U + n \rightarrow \text{fission products} + \nu n$$

For each neutron consumed, an average of 2.5 new neutrons (νn) are released with an energy of 1.5 eV. These new neutrons can be used to fission other ^{235}U nuclei, leading to the release of more neutrons, self-propagating the reaction. These nuclear chain reactions are controlled by the use of moderators and neutron absorbers (materials used to reduce neutron energy [thermalize] to 0.025 eV) in a reactor so that an equilibrium state is reached. Radionuclides can be produced in a nuclear reactor by two methods: (1) irradiation of material within the neutron flux (neutrons $\times$ cm^{-2} $\times$ sec^{-1}) or (2) separation and collection of the fission products.

Thermal neutron reactions. The neutrons around the core of a nuclear reactor are low-energy (thermal) neutrons that typically induce the following types of nuclear reactions:

$$^{A}_{Z}X + n \rightarrow ^{A+1}_{Z}X + \gamma \qquad \text{(1)}$$

$$^{A}_{Z}X + n \rightarrow ^{A}_{Z-1}Y + p \qquad \text{(2)}$$

In a reaction of the first type of reaction the target atom $^{A}_{Z}X$ with atomic number Z and atomic mass A absorbs a neutron, and energy is emitted in the form of gamma rays. This is written as an (n,γ) reaction. The following are examples:

$$^{98}Mo(n,\gamma)^{99}Mo$$
$$^{112}Sn(n,\gamma)^{113}Sn$$

In the second type of reaction a proton is emitted after absorption of a neutron by the target atom. Since this changes the atomic number of the nucleus, an isotope of a different element (Y) is formed. Examples of this type of nuclear reaction (n,p) are as follows:

$$^{14}N(n,p)^{14}C$$
$$^{3}He(n,p)^{3}H$$

The (n,γ) reaction forms a radioisotope from a stable isotope of the same element, precluding production of high specific activity material. The specific activity is defined as the decay rate (dpm) of a radioactive isotope per gram of that same element. In an n,p reaction the product nuclide is an isotope of a different element, enabling the production of high specific activity,

carrier-free (no stable isotope of the same element) radioisotopes.

The previously described reactions will produce neutron-rich products, decaying primarily by β^- emission. Radionuclides that decay by β^- emission are not generally used in imaging. However, products of (n,γ) reactions include parent isotopes used in nuclear generators. In a radionuclide generator the daughter radionuclide is the isotope of interest and is usually separated from the parent isotope by column chromatography. Examples of the parent-daughter system of radionuclide generators are as follows:

$$^{98}Mo(n,\gamma)^{99}Mo \xrightarrow{t_{1/2} = 67 \text{ hours}} {}^{99m}Tc$$
$$^{112}Sn(n,\gamma)^{113}Sn \xrightarrow{t_{1/2} = 115 \text{ days}} {}^{113m}In$$
$$^{124}Xe(n,\gamma)^{125}Xe \xrightarrow{t_{1/2} = 17 \text{ hours}} {}^{125}I$$

Fission product separation. The fission process itself results in the formation of lighter radionuclides of unequal mass, some of which are used in nuclear medicine (^{99}Mo, ^{131}I, ^{133}Xe) (Figure 6-2). The neutron interacts with the ^{235}U nucleus to form unstable ^{236}U, which then undergoes fission. An example of a fission reaction occurring in a nuclear reactor is as follows:

$$n + ^{235}_{92}U \rightarrow ^{236}_{92}U \rightarrow ^{89}_{36}Kr + ^{144}_{56}Ba + 3n$$

Similar to products of (n,γ) reactions, fission products tend to decay by β^- emission, and only a limited number have found use in nuclear medicine. However, un-

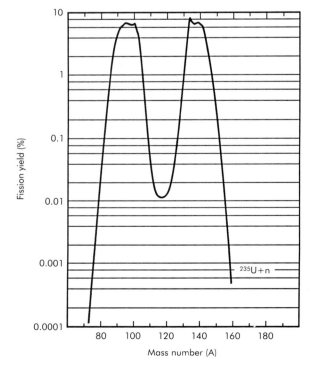

Figure 6-2 Relative yields of fission products of various mass formed after uranium fission.

like radionuclides formed from (n,γ) reactions, fission products can be produced carrier free. For example, fission-produced ^{99}Mo is formed from uranium, whereas thermal neutron-produced ^{99}Mo is made from bombarding a ^{98}Mo target. Unfortunately, a major problem associated with fission-produced radionuclides is the difficulty in chemically separating the product of interest from the others formed to obtain a radiochemically pure preparation.

Accelerator-Produced Radionuclides

Accelerators are devices that increase the energy of charged particles to enable a nuclear reaction upon impact with a target. Either a cyclotron or a linear accelerator can be used to produce radionuclides, depending on the type of nuclear reaction and the yield desired. In linear accelerators, ions are repeatedly accelerated through small potential differences. The accelerator tube consists of a series of cylindrical electrodes called *drift tubes*. A high-frequency alternating voltage is applied between the two electrodes, resulting in acceleration of the ions at each gap between electrodes. Acceleration to high energies requires relatively long acceleration tubes, creating obvious size-related problems for general use of these machines.

The invention of the cyclotron in 1930 was a successful attempt to overcome the difficulties associated with the length of high-energy linear accelerators. The basic principles of the cyclotron are shown in Figure 6-3. The particles are accelerated in spiral paths inside two semicircular flat evacuated metallic cylinders called dees. The dees are placed between the two poles of a magnet so that the magnetic field operates on the ion beam, constraining it to a circular path. At the gap between the dees the ions experience acceleration due to the imposition of an electrical potential difference, re-

sulting in a deflection from the original path. The beam particles originate from the ion source at the center of the cyclotron, acquiring energy for each passage across the gap. Eventually the high-energy particle beam reaches the periphery of the dees where it is deflected onto an external target. Fixed-frequency cyclotrons can accelerate positively charged ions up to about 50 MeV for protons. Techniques have now been developed to use cyclotrons at much higher energies. Linear accelerators can accelerate particles up to energies of several hundred MeV.

The majority of cyclotrons built before 1980 accelerated positively charged ion species, H^+. Medical cyclotrons currently marketed by CTI PET Systems (Knoxville, Tennessee), IBA (Louvain, Belgium), and Scanditronix (Uppsala, Sweden) accelerate negative ions (H^-). This design allows for a simple deflection system, in which the beam is extracted by interaction with a very thin carbon foil. The carbon foil strips electrons from H^-, resulting in the formation of positively charged H^+, which changes direction without a final magnetic deflection. The H^+ beam then bombards the target in a manner similar to that in a positively charged ion cyclotron. It is also possible to extract the beam at two points, allowing production of two radioisotopes simultaneously.

For the production of short-lived positron-emitting radionuclides, more compact and less expensive linear accelerators with energy capabilities in the 3-4 MeV range are being developed by a number of companies. At present, these accelerators can generate only ^{15}O, although the goal is eventually to produce other radionuclides such as ^{11}C, ^{13}N, and ^{18}F. Science Research Laboratories (Summerville, Massachusetts) has developed an electrostatic linear accelerator, the Tandem Cascade Accelerator, which uses high-current bombardment with a relatively low-energy beam. The Tan-

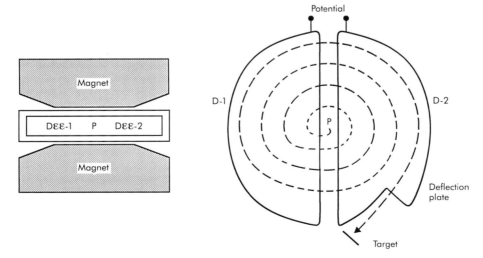

Figure 6-3 Schematic diagram of the operation of a positive ion cyclotron. (From Kowalsky RJ, Perry JR: *Radiopharmaceuticals in nuclear medicine practice,* Norwalk, Conn, 1987, Appleton & Lange.)

dem Cascade Accelerator is less than half the cost and also less than one fifth the weight of a cyclotron. IBA has designed a compact accelerator distributed by CTI PET Systems. It is a 3.2 MeV deuteron (^{2}H) machine that produces only ^{15}O. An alternate approach is to use a radiofrequency quadrupole (RFQ) accelerator to accelerate ^{3}He for radiopharmaceutical production. Due to the mass to charge ratio of ^{3}He, a much smaller accelerator is needed for ^{3}He than deuterons or protons. Science Applications International Corporation (San Diego, California) has designed such an accelerator.

The cost of radionuclide production depends upon the method employed. In a reactor there are many positions for thermal neutron irradiation of samples, allowing several isotopes to be produced simultaneously. This allows the cost of operation to be divided among several reactor-produced radionuclides. The overall price of fission products produced in a nuclear reactor is largely associated with the extensive separation process. Alternatively, the cost of accelerator-produced isotopes is quite high. Since the machine is utilized to produce a single radionuclide, the entire cost of operating the accelerator must be charged for each production.

Generator Systems

Certain parent-daughter systems involve a long-lived parent radionuclide that decays to a short-lived daughter. Since the parent and daughter nuclides are not isotopes of the same element, chemical separation is possible. The long-lived parent produces a continuous supply of the relatively short-lived daughter radionuclide and is therefore called a generator. The generator systems used in nuclear medicine are listed in Table 6-1.

There are two types of parent-daughter relationships, known as transient and secular equilibrium. In a transient equilibrium system the half-life of the parent is a factor 10-100 times greater than that of the daughter, whereas in secular equilibrium the half-life of the parent is 100-1000 times greater than that of the daughter. The ^{99}Mo-^{99m}Tc generator, where ^{99}Mo has a 67-hr half-life and ^{99m}Tc has a 6-hr half-life, is an example of transient equilibrium (Figure 6-4). The generator system ^{113}Sn($t_{1/2} = 115$ days) $- ^{113m}$In($t_{1/2} = 1.7$ hr),

shown in Figure 6-5, is an example of secular equilibrium. The time required to reach equilibrium dictates how frequently each generator can be eluted and depends on the half-lives of the parent and daughter.

Equations governing generator systems. Assuming there is initially no daughter activity present in a generator, the daughter activity at any given time can be calculated from the following general equation:

$$A_2 = \frac{\lambda_2}{\lambda_2 - \lambda_1} \times A_1^0(e^{-\lambda_1 t} - e^{-\lambda_2 t}) \qquad (3)$$

where A_1^0 is the parent activity at time zero, A_2 is the daughter activity at time t, and λ_1 and λ_2 are the decay constants for the parent and daughter, respectively. This general equation can be simplified for the special cases of transient and secular equilibrium. In both cases a state of radioactive equilibrium is reached after a certain time in which the decay rates of the parent and daughter are equal.

In the case of transient equilibrium, as the time t becomes sufficiently large, $e^{-\lambda_2 t}$ is negligible compared with $e^{-\lambda_1 t}$, and the equation can be simplified as follows:

$$A_2 = \frac{\lambda_2}{\lambda_2 - \lambda_1} \times A_1^0 e^{-\lambda_1 t} \qquad (4)$$

Since $A_1 = A_1^0 e^{-\lambda_1 t}$, where A_1 is the parent activity at time t, this equation can be rewritten as

$$A_2 = \frac{\lambda_2}{\lambda_2 - \lambda_1} A_1 \qquad (5)$$

Assuming the parent only decays to the daughter, at equilibrium the daughter activity will be greater than the parent activity by the factor $\lambda_2/(\lambda_2 - \lambda_1)$. At equilibrium, both activities then appear to decay with the half-life of the parent. In the specific case of the ^{99}Mo-^{99m}Tc generator there is only 86% decay of the ^{99}Mo to ^{99m}Tc. This makes the factor (0.86) $\lambda_2/(\lambda_2 - \lambda_1)$, which simplifies to (0.86 × 1.1). Therefore the actual ^{99m}Tc activity present at transient equilibrium is 0.946 times the ^{99}Mo activity.

Table 6-1 Decay properties for parent and daughter radionuclides of several generators			
Generator	**Parent $t_{1/2}$**	**Daughter $t_{1/2}$**	**Daughter E_γ (%)**
^{99}Mo-^{99m}Tc	2.78 d	6 hr	140 keV (90)
^{81}Rb-^{81m}Kr	4.7 hr	13 sec	190 keV (65)
^{113}Sn-^{113m}In	115 d	1.7 hr	393 keV (64)
^{68}Ge-^{68}Ga	280 d	68 min	511 keV (176)
^{62}Zn-^{62}Cu	9.3 hr	9.8 min	511 keV (196)
^{82}Sr-^{82}Rb	25 d	1.3 min	511 keV (192)

In the case of secular equilibrium, the parent activity does not decrease significantly during many daughter half-lives. The decay constant of the parent (λ_1) is much smaller than that of the daughter (λ_2), and the following approximation can be made:

$$\lambda_2 - \lambda_1 \simeq \lambda_2 \qquad (6)$$

This approximation can be used to further simplify equation 5 to yield the following expression:

$$A_2 = A_1 \qquad (7)$$

Thus, at equilibrium the daughter activity is equal to the parent activity, as shown in Figure 6-5.

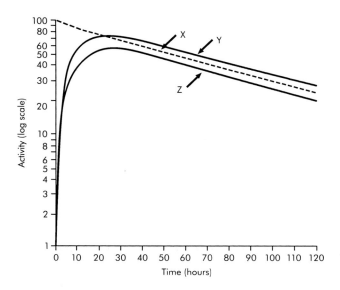

Figure 6-4 Growth and decay of daughter radionuclide in a transient equilibrium situation. At equilibrium, daughter activity *(Y)* actually exceeds parent activity *(X)*. Point *Z* is the daughter activity present in a ^{99}Mo-^{99m}Tc generator. Daughter (^{99m}Tc) activity is less than parent (^{99}Mo), since only 86% of the ^{99}Mo present decays to ^{99m}Tc.

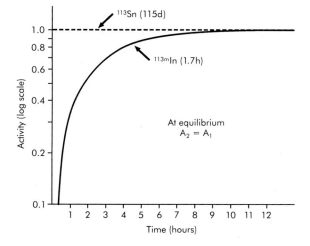

Figure 6-5 Growth and decay in ^{113}Sn-^{113m}In generator as an example of secular equilibrium.

^{99}Mo-^{99m}Tc generator. The ^{99}Mo-^{99m}Tc generator is commonly used in nuclear medicine because of the ideal half-life (6 hr) and optimum energy (140 keV, 90% abundance) of ^{99m}Tc. A large number of radiopharmaceuticals are made with ^{99m}Tc, and they are discussed later in the chapter. Molybenum-99 ($t_{1/2} = 67$ hr) forms the anionic species molybdate (MoO^{2-}) and paramolybdate ($Mo_7O_{24}^{6-}$) in an acidic medium. These anions are loaded on the generator column containing positively charged alumina (Al_2O_3) that has previously been washed with saline (pH 5). The generator is eluted with normal saline (0.9% NaCl), and ^{99m}Tc is produced as pertechnetate (^{99m}TcO$_4^-$).

The two types of ^{99}Mo-^{99m}Tc generators used in nuclear medicine are the wet column and dry column generators (Figure 6-6). The wet column generator contains a reservoir of normal saline that is connected to the alumina column. After elution of this generator, saline remains on the column, leading to the formation of water radiolysis products, which are reducing agents. This causes reduction of the ^{99m}Tc and decreased ^{99m}TcO$_4^-$ yields, since the reduced ^{99m}Tc species do not elute from the column. This problem has been addressed by purging the saline reservoir with O_2. Previous attempts to add oxidizing agents to the column to decrease reduction of ^{99m}Tc species resulted in ^{99m}Tc radiopharmaceutical formulation problems.

The dry column generator system was developed to alleviate poor elution yields of ^{99m}TcO$_4^-$ by removing saline from the column after elution. This decreases the amount of radiolysis products formed. The dry column generator employs a 5-20 ml saline charge, which is applied to an exterior port of the generator. An evacuated vial draws saline through the generator to remove ^{99m}TcO$_4^-$, followed by air to dry the column. Leaving the air on the column promotes oxidation of any reduced ^{99m}Tc species back to the +7 valence state of ^{99m}TcO$_4^-$, which can then be eluted.

^{113}Sn-^{113m}In generator. Indium-113m can be used to prepare a number of radiopharmaceuticals for imaging lungs, liver, brain, and kidneys. Tin-113 is produced in a reactor by neutron irradiation of ^{112}In. The ^{113}Sn is then loaded onto a generator column containing hydrous zirconium oxide. Elution of ^{113m}In ($t_{1/2} = 1.7$ hr) is achieved with 0.05 M HCl. Due to the long half-life of ^{113}Sn (115 days), the ^{113}Sn-^{113m}In generator can be used for 6-12 months, making it one of the most economical generators. The biggest drawback of this generator is that the photon energy of ^{113m}In (393 keV) is not ideal for use with the gamma camera. In the United States the ^{113}Sn-^{113m}In generator has largely been replaced by the ^{99}Mo-^{99m}Tc generator; however, the ^{113}Sn-^{113m}In generator is still useful in developing countries and more isolated regions of the world.

^{82}Sr-^{82}Rb generator. Rubidium-82, a positron-emitting radionuclide, is used primarily as a myocardial perfu-

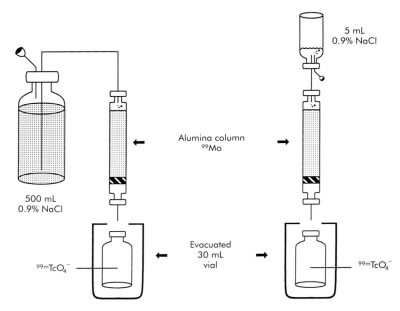

Figure 6-6   Schematic diagram of a wet column ^{99}Mo-^{99m}Tc generator *(left)* that has a 0.9% NaCl reservoir. A dry column ^{99}Mo-^{99m}Tc generator *(right)*.

sion agent for PET imaging. The rubidium cation (Rb$^+$) is an analogue of potassium (K$^+$) and therefore gives a similar biodistribution. Strontium-82 (t$_{1/2}$ = 25 days) is accelerator produced by bombardment on a molybdenum target. Strontium-85 is also produced as a radionuclidic impurity. The allowable limit of ^{85}Sr present in the ^{82}Rb elution is 0.2 μCi/mCi ^{82}Rb. The allowable limit of ^{82}Sr breakthrough is 0.02 μCi/mCi. The generators regularly meet this requirement after a first elution of the generator to waste. The ^{82}Sr is loaded onto a stannic oxide column, and ^{82}Rb (t$_{1/2}$ = 76 sec) is eluted with normal saline (0.9% NaCl). The 76 sec half-life of ^{82}Rb allows rapid repeat imaging studies but poses difficulties in dose preparation for patient administration, and the limited chemistry of this alkali metal ion severely restricts potential applications for this radionuclide in nuclear medicine. In an effort to overcome the short half-life, a calibrated continuous infusion system has been developed, allowing elution of the generator directly into an intravenous catheter. The ^{82}Rb generator is an FDA-approved radiopharmaceutical produced by Medi Physics, an Amersham Company.

^{81}Rb-^{81m}Kr generator.   Krypton-81m, a gamma ray–emitting nuclide with a photon energy of 190 keV (65% abundance), is commonly used as a lung-imaging agent. Rubidium-81 (t$_{1/2}$ = 4.7 hr), cyclotron produced by the reaction ^{79}Br(α,2n)^{81}Rb or ^{82}Kr(p,n)^{81}Rb, is loaded onto a generator column containing a strong cation-exchange resin (Bio Rad AGMP-50). The noble gas ^{81m}Kr (t$_{1/2}$ = 13 sec) is eluted by passing humidified oxygen over the generator column. The ^{81m}Kr and

O$_2$ are delivered to the patient via a nonrebreathing face mask. The major disadvantages of the ^{81}Rb-^{81m}Kr generator are the high cost and the 12-hr expiration time of the generator due to the 4.5 hr half-life of the parent isotope. This limits the use of the generator to the day of delivery only. The generator is an FDA-approved radiopharmaceutical produced by Medi Physics, an Amersham Company.

^{68}Ge-^{68}Ga generator.   Gallium-68 (t$_{1/2}$ = 68 min) emits a 2.92 MeV positron in 89% abundance, making it very useful in PET imaging. The ^{68}Ge-^{68}Ga generator is not FDA approved, and only a few ^{68}Ga radiopharmaceuticals have been investigated clinically. These include ^{68}Ga macroaggregated albumin (MAA), ^{68}Ga citrate, and ^{68}Ga ethylenediaminetetraacetic acid (EDTA). Several generator systems have been developed to separate ^{68}Ga from ^{68}Ge. The early generators consisted of ^{68}Ge adsorbed onto an alumina column. The ^{68}Ga was eluted with a 0.005 M solution of EDTA at pH 7.[8] However, since ^{68}Ga forms such a strong complex with EDTA at neutral pH, it was difficult to dissociate ^{68}Ga from ^{68}Ga-EDTA to allow formation of other complexes. A solvent extraction ^{68}Ge-^{68}Ga generator was later developed that produces a ^{68}Ga-oxine chelate.[5] Although ^{68}Ga-oxine was a weaker chelate than ^{68}Ga-EDTA, problems with the operation of the generator system prevented it from becoming clinically useful. Most recently, a generator yielding ^{68}Ga in an ionic form has been developed.[12] In this generator ^{68}Ge is loaded onto a tin dioxide column and ^{68}Ga is eluted using 1 M HCl. The only problem incurred in this generator is the presence of trace metals, which sometimes

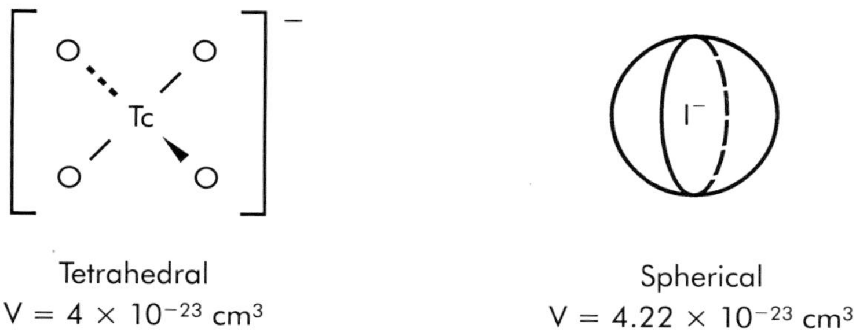

Tetrahedral
$V = 4 \times 10^{-23} \text{ cm}^3$

Spherical
$V = 4.22 \times 10^{-23} \text{ cm}^3$

Figure 6-7   Spatial comparison of TcO_4^- and I^- ions.

reduces the amount of complexation with ^{68}Ga. This is the only ^{68}Ge-^{68}Ga generator produced commercially.

^{62}Zn-^{62}Cu generator. Copper-62, a positron-emitting radionuclide (98% abundance) with a 9.7 min half-life, is an attractive radionuclide for PET imaging. ^{62}Cu-labeled pyruvaldehyde bis(N^4-methylthiosemicarbazone) (^{62}Cu-PTSM) has been used in clinical investigations for heart and brain blood flow measurement.[7] The parent isotope, ^{62}Zn, is cyclotron produced via the ^{63}Cu(p,2n)^{62}Zn reaction. Facilities for the production of ^{62}Zn exist at a number of commercial facilities as well as at several clinical PET centers. The major disadvantage is the short half-life of ^{62}Zn (9.3 hr), which requires generator replacement at 1- or 2-day intervals. Two different ^{62}Zn-^{62}Cu generator systems have been developed. In one design, ^{62}Zn is loaded onto a column containing Dowex 1×8 anion exchange resin, which retains Zn^{2+} and allows Cu^{2+} to be eluted using 0.2N HCl/1.8N NaCl or 2N HCl.[14] The other system employs a column containing a strong cation exchange resin adsorbent (CG-120, Amberlite), and ^{62}Cu is eluted in 0.2 M glycine.[6] The eluant in the latter generator is suitable for direct intravenous injection.

TECHNETIUM RADIOPHARMACEUTICALS

Technetium-99m was discovered in 1937 by Perrier and Segre in a sample of naturally occurring ^{98}Mo that had been irradiated by neutrons and deuterons. It was introduced into nuclear medicine in 1957 with the development of the ^{99}Mo-^{99m}Tc generator at the Brookhaven National Laboratory. The first clinical use of technetium, in 1961 at the University of Chicago, heralded a new era for nuclear medicine. The widespread use of ^{99m}Tc as the radionuclide of choice for a variety of nuclear medicine imaging procedures has been based mainly on its physical properties. These properties include a $t_{1/2}$ of 6 hr, a 140 keV photon (88% abundance), which provides good tissue penetration and imaging capabilities for use with gamma cameras, and no beta decay—providing a low radiation ab-

sorbed dose. Another advantage is its ready availability from the ^{99}Mo-^{99m}Tc generator.

Oxidized Technetium Complexes

Technetium is obtained from a generator in normal saline (0.9% NaCl) as the pertechnetate ion, ^{99m}TcO$_4^-$. In this form Tc is in the +7 valence state as pertechnetate and has all seven of the outer electrons involved in covalent bonding. This is the most stable of all valence states of technetium in aqueous solution. The single negative charge of pertechnetate and the geometry of the compound—oxygens in the four corners of a tetrahedron—give it a charge and size similar to the iodide ion (Figure 6-7). As a result the biodistribution of ^{99m}TcO$_4^-$ is similar to I^-. It concentrates primarily in the thyroid, salivary glands, gastric mucosa, and choroid plexus. Pertechnetate crosses the placental barrier, so the fetal radiation dose must be considered when determining the suitability of a study employing pertechnetate for a pregnant woman. Pertechnetate is excreted primarily via the gastrointestinal tract and the kidneys. It is used for thyroid imaging and first-pass radionuclide angiocardiography. It has also been used in the past for brain imaging.

Pretreatment of a patient with potassium perchlorate, Lugol's solution (a solution of 5% iodine and 10% potassium iodide), or a saturated solution of potassium iodide (SSKI) influences the distribution of technetium. Perchlorate is approximately the same size as pertechnetate and competitively inhibits the uptake of ^{99m}Tc pertechnetate into the thyroid and salivary glands, choroid plexus, and gastric mucosa. Stable iodine-127 is also taken up by these tissues and blocks the uptake of pertechnetate. Activity in the choroid plexus presents a problem in interpreting brain images, so it is advantageous to block the uptake into this tissue using one of these pharmaceuticals.

Other than pertechnetate, the only radiopharmaceutical containing technetium possibly in a +7 valence state is technetium-sulfur colloid. ^{99m}Tc-sulfur colloid (^{99m}Tc-SC) is prepared from commercially available kits that contain sodium thiosulfate, phosphoric or hydrochloric acid, gelatin, and a buffer. Sodium thiosulfate and gelatin are added to an acidified solution of ^{99m}Tc-pertechnetate. The mixture is heated in a boiling water bath for 5-10 min. Following heating, the vial is vented and a buffer is added. ^{99m}Tc-SC exists as ^{99m}Tc-heptasulfide coprecipitated with colloidal sulfur particles, which are generated from acid decomposition of the sodium thiosulfate. The final suspension is maintained at a pH of 5.5-6.0 to avoid conversion of the heptasulfide back to pertechnetate. The particle size range is 10 nm to 2.0 μ. Gelatin is used as a stabilizer to prevent aggregation of the colloidal particles, which would result in lung uptake when injected.

After intravenous injection ^{99m}Tc-SC is rapidly cleared from the blood. Cells of the reticuloendothelial system (RES) phagocytize the colloidal particles. In normal subjects approximately 90% of the ^{99m}Tc-SC is localized in the liver. The remainder of the radiopharmaceutical is sequestered by the RES cells in the spleen and bone marrow.

Filtering of the ^{99m}Tc-SC suspension with a 0.22 μ filter removes the larger colloidal particles. The remaining mini ^{99m}Tc-SC, less than 100 nm in size, can be used for bone marrow imaging and lymphoscintigraphy because the smaller particles are more efficiently phagocytized by the lymph nodes and marrow. Lymphoscintigraphy can also be performed using ^{99m}Tc-antimony sulfur colloid, prepared using a commercially available kit formulation that is not FDA approved. It is available under a physician sponsored investigational new drug application (IND). The average particle size range of ^{99m}Tc-antimony sulfur colloid is 3-30 nm.

A reduced ^{99m}Tc radiopharmaceutical, ^{99m}Tc-albumin colloid (Microlite), is manufactured by DuPont Pharmaceuticals. It is prepared by adding ^{99m}Tc-pertechnetate to the kit and mixing. The particle range is 0.4 to 2.0 μ. This compound has the same indications as ^{99m}Tc-SC. The advantage of this kit formulation over ^{99m}Tc-SC is that it does not require heating.

Reduced Technetium Complexes

To alter the biodistribution of technetium it is necessary to attach it to carriers. First the technetium must be chemically reduced from the +7 valence state to a lower oxidation state, where it is a more reactive species capable of combining with a large number of compounds. This can be accomplished using a number of reducing agents such as stannous chloride, iron ascorbate, or electrolytic methods. Stannous chloride is the reducing agent used most frequently in kit formulations for ^{99m}Tc radiopharmaceuticals.

Blood pool imaging agents. Labeling of red blood cells (RBCs) with ^{99m}Tc provides an intravascular tracer useful for a variety of imaging procedures, including radionuclide ventriculography (RVG) and hemangioma and gastrointestinal bleeding studies. RBCs can be la-

beled with ^{99m}Tc using either in vivo or in vitro methods.

A common method for in vivo labeling of RBCs involves injection of stannous chloride (usually in the form of a pyrophosphate kit reconstituted with 0.9% NaCl) into the patient to "tin" the cells. After 10-15 min ^{99m}Tc-pertechnetate is injected. Despite the speed and ease of in vivo RBC labeling, the low labeling efficiency of 80% results in sufficient free ^{99m}TcO$_4^-$ to complicate interpretation of images in studies such as gastrointestinal bleeding. A modified in vivo RBC labeling method has been developed that improves labeling efficiency. The patient's blood is tinned as in the first method, then a sample of the patient's blood is withdrawn into an anticoagulated syringe containing ^{99m}TcO$_4^-$. After incubation of the syringe at room temperature for 10-15 min, the contents are then reinjected into the patient. This allows ^{99m}Tc labeling of a smaller volume of blood, which results in higher labeling efficiency.

An in vitro method for labeling RBCs with ^{99m}Tc is the use of a commercially available kit, Ultratag (Mallinckrodt). An aliquot of the patient's blood, anticoagulated with heparin or acid-citrate-dextrose (ACD), is removed and added to the reaction vial containing stannous chloride. The stannous chloride diffuses across the RBC membrane. Sodium hypochlorite is then added to the vial to reduce any extracellular stannous chloride. Next, ^{99m}Tc-pertechnetate is added to the kit formulation. It diffuses across the RBC membrane and is reduced and bound intracellularly. The final radiochemical purity of this preparation is over 90%.

Human serum albumin (HSA) labeled with ^{99m}Tc is another intravascular tracer that has been used. Commercially available kits contain the albumin and the stannous chloride reducing agent. Addition of ^{99m}TcO$_4^-$ results in the formation of ^{99m}Tc-HSA, which can be used as a blood pool imaging agent.

Skeletal imaging agents. In 1972 phosphate derivatives were labeled with technetium for skeletal imaging. Before this, skeletal imaging was performed using radioisotopes of strontium (^{85}Sr and ^{87m}Sr) or fluorine-18. These isotopes had either unfavorable decay characteristics, which resulted in high radiation absorbed doses, or undesirably short half-lives. The first technetium phosphate evaluated was an inorganic phosphate, ^{99m}Tc polyphosphate.

There are two basic types of phosphate derivatives: inorganic phosphates that have phosphorus-oxygen bonds (P—O—P), and organic phosphates that have phosphorus-carbon bonds (P—C—P) (Figure 6-8). The inorganic phosphates are composed of differing lengths of the basic POP unit ($[$—P—O—P—$]_n$). When there is only one POP, the phosphate is pyrophosphate; when there is more than one POP unit, it is a polyphosphate. The polyphosphates undergo hy-

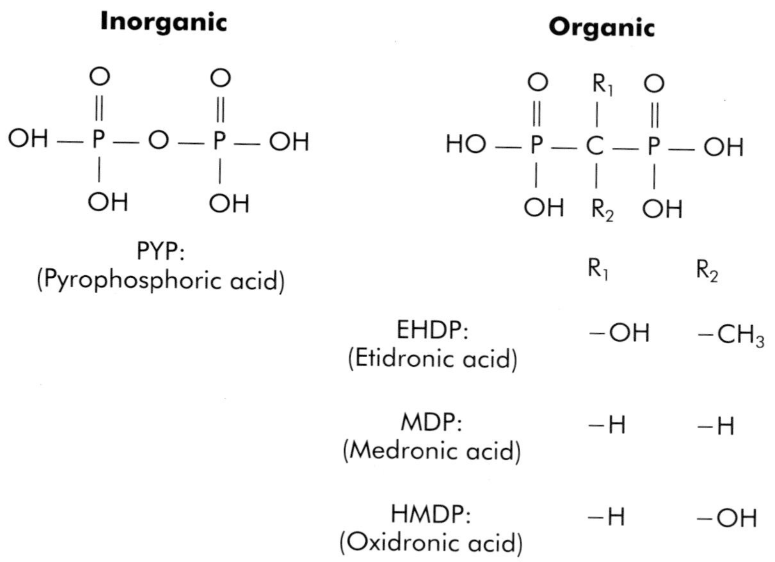

Inorganic

Organic

$$\text{OH} - \overset{\overset{\displaystyle O}{\|}}{\underset{\underset{\displaystyle OH}{|}}{P}} - O - \overset{\overset{\displaystyle O}{\|}}{\underset{\underset{\displaystyle OH}{|}}{P}} - \text{OH}$$

PYP:
(Pyrophosphoric acid)

$$\text{HO} - \overset{\overset{\displaystyle O}{\|}}{\underset{\underset{\displaystyle OH}{|}}{P}} - \overset{\overset{\displaystyle R_1}{|}}{\underset{\underset{\displaystyle R_2}{|}}{C}} - \overset{\overset{\displaystyle O}{\|}}{\underset{\underset{\displaystyle OH}{|}}{P}} - \text{OH}$$

	R_1	R_2
EHDP: (Etidronic acid)	$-OH$	$-CH_3$
MDP: (Medronic acid)	$-H$	$-H$
HMDP: (Oxidronic acid)	$-H$	$-OH$

Figure 6-8 Inorganic and organic phosphate agents used for skeletal imaging.

drolysis in vivo by alkaline phosphatases, which degrade them to the basic P—O—P unit, pyrophosphate. Since the P—C—P bonds of the organic phosphates are more resistant to the phosphatase hydrolysis, these compounds are more stable in vivo. This results in more rapid blood clearance and greater skeletal uptake than with the inorganic phosphates.

Technetium labeling of a phosphate is accomplished by reaction of the phosphate with stannous chloride to form a stannous phosphate chelate, followed by addition of ^{99m}Tc pertechnetate, which is reduced and complexed with the phosphate.

Lung imaging agents. MAA is formed by heat denaturation of the protein in an aqueous solution. Particles formed have diameters of 10-90 μ, with the majority between 10 and 40 μ. All commercially available MAA products utilize stannous chloride as the reducing agent. Since the smallest vessels in the lung vasculature range from 7-10 μ in diameter, labeled macroaggregates greater than 10 μ are readily trapped, allowing for lung visualization through capillary blockade.

Renal imaging agents. ^{99m}Tc-pentetate (DTPA) and ^{99m}Tc-glucoheptonate (GHP) are two chelates used for renal imaging studies (Figure 6-9). These low molecular weight, water-soluble compounds are rapidly eliminated from the body. ^{99m}Tc-DTPA is excreted exclusively by glomerular filtration. ^{99m}Tc-GHP is cleared through glomerular filtration in addition to tubular secretion, with some retention of activity in the renal cortex. These tracers can also be used for brain imaging. DMSA (2,3-dimercaptosuccinic acid) is another chelating agent that has been labeled with ^{99m}Tc and used for renal imaging. The cortical retention of this agent

appears to be superior to other currently available agents, with 50% of the injected activity retained in the renal cortex 1 hr after administration. The commercial kit preparation supplied by Medi-Physics, an Amersham Company, has recently been reformulated. The DMSA kit is light sensitive and should be stored between 2 and 8° C. After preparation the ^{99m}Tc-DMSA has a shelf life of 4 hr and should be stored in the refrigerator.

The technetium renal agent, ^{99m}Tc-mertiatide (mercaptoacetyltriglycine [MAG-3]) (Figure 6-9), has been synthesized as a replacement for ^{131}I-Hippuran. The ^{99m}Tc-mertiatide has rapid blood clearance and renal excretion via tubular secretion and glomerular filtration, similar to ^{131}I-Hippuran.[16] The preferential nuclear properties of ^{99m}Tc make ^{99m}Tc-mertiatide superior to ^{131}I-Hippuran as a renal agent. The kit method of preparing ^{99m}Tc-mertiatide requires boiling for 10 min. The quality control method for the kit formulation employs Sep-Pak chromatography, which is discussed later under quality control.

Cardiac imaging agents. One of the goals of nuclear medicine has been to develop a ^{99m}Tc complex that has a biodistribution similar to ^{201}Tl. Recently several technetium agents taken up by the myocardium in relation to blood flow have been developed (Figure 6-10).

One of these cardiac agents is ^{99m}Tc-methoxyisobutyl isonitrile (MIBI), also known as ^{99m}Tc-sestamibi (Cardiolite). The kit method of production is a 10-min boiled preparation involving a ligand exchange labeling reaction. This results in the formation of a ^{99m}Tc-hexakis-isonitrile complex with ^{99m}Tc in an oxidation state of +1. The method of myocardial localization is not known, although it has been determined that it does not occur via the Na$^+$/K$^+$ pump,

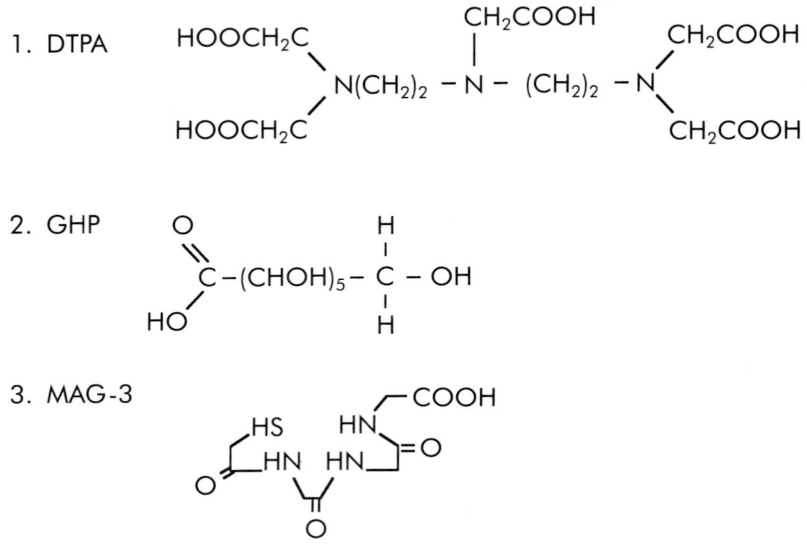

1. DTPA

2. GHP

3. MAG-3

Figure 6-9 Agents used for renal imaging.

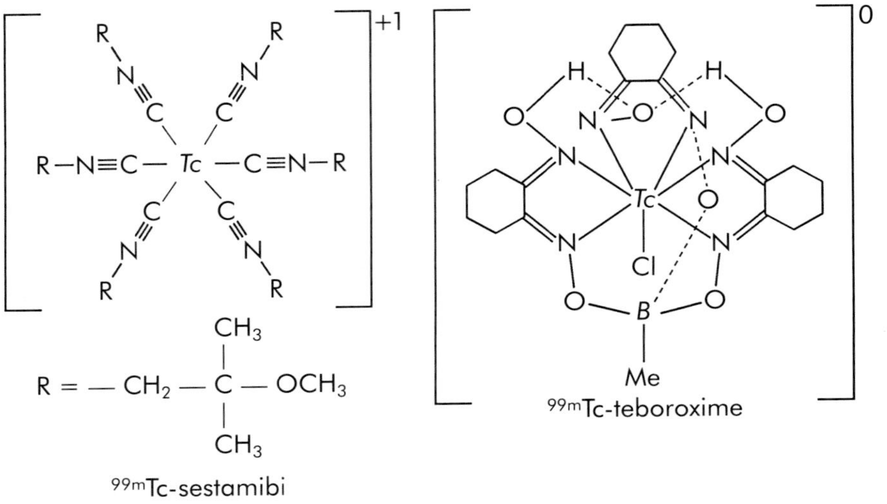

^{99m}Tc-sestamibi

^{99m}Tc-teboroxime

$$R = -CH_2 - \underset{\underset{CH_3}{|}}{\overset{\overset{CH_3}{|}}{C}} - OCH_3$$

Figure 6-10 Two technetium cardiac agents developed as replacements for ^{201}TlCl.

which is the mechanism of uptake for ^{201}Tl.[15] ^{99m}Tc-sestamibi has approximately a 65% cardiac extraction efficiency; minimal or no redistribution occurs. The amount of liver uptake that occurs has presented some problems in reading the resulting cardiac images.[4]

The second commercially available technetium cardiac agent is a neutral boronic acid adduct of a technetium dioxime complex (BATO). This agent, ^{99m}Tc-teboroxime (Cardiotec), is a neutral complex with ^{99m}Tc in a +3 oxidation state. The kit formulation is a 15-min boiled preparation employing a template synthesis, which indicates that the complex is formed around the ^{99m}Tc once it is added to the reaction. The method of uptake into the myocardium has not yet been determined. ^{99m}Tc-teboroxime exhibits 95% ex-

traction efficiency but shows rapid washout from the myocardium.[3] This allows imaging to be initiated as early as 3-4 min after injection but necessitates completion of imaging within 15-20 min due to the rapid clearance.

The most recently available cardiac agent is ^{99m}Tc-tetrofosmin (Myoview), a cationic ^{99m}Tc-complex of an ether-substituted phosphine ligand. The kit formulation of ^{99m}Tc-tetrofosmin involves an exchange reaction during the 15-min, room-temperature incubation. The unreconstituted kit should be stored in the refrigerator, protected from light. The method of quality control is detailed in the section on radiopharmaceutical quality assurance. Uptake into the myocardium reaches a maximum of 1.3% of the injected dose (ID)

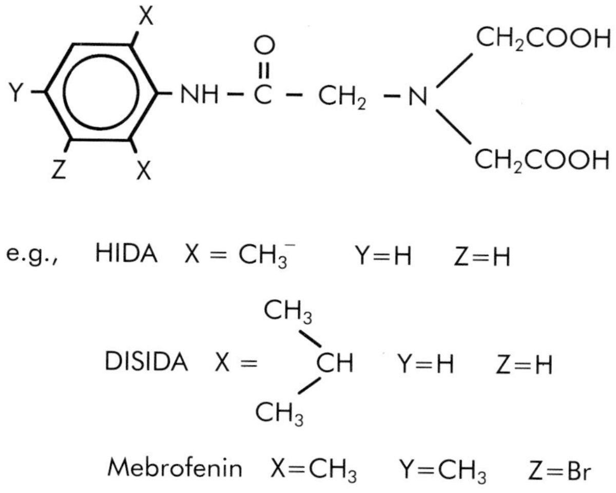

Figure 6-11 ^{99m}Tc-hepatobiliary analogs developed with different groups substituted on the aromatic ring of the iminodiacetic acid structure.

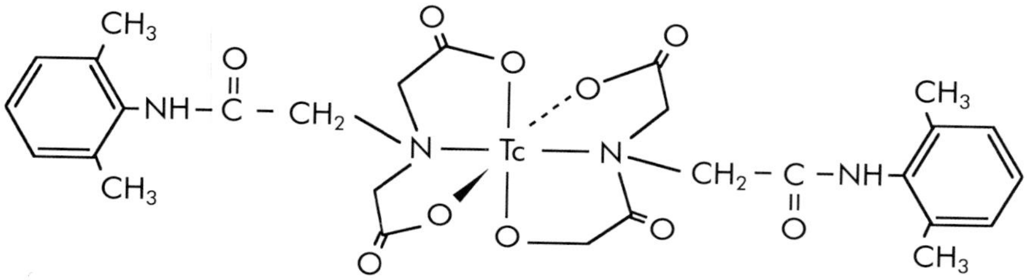

Figure 6-12 Dimeric configuration of Tc-HIDA.

at 5 min postinjection, falling to 1% ID by 2 hr. The mechanism of uptake into the myocardium has not been established. Imaging may be initiated 15 min post injection.

Hepatobiliary imaging agents. A group of *N*-substituted iminodiacetic acid ligands that contain hydrophilic groups for ^{99m}Tc complexation and possess the necessary hepatocellular specificity have been developed. The first of this group of radiopharmaceuticals was ^{99m}Tc-lidofenin (HIDA). A variety of ^{99m}Tc-iminodiacetic acid analogues that have different groups substituted on the aromatic ring have also been developed (Figure 6-11). Generally, the newer agents offer improved hepatocellular specificity, more rapid blood clearance, and reduced renal clearance. These agents provide information regarding hepatocyte function, outline the biliary tract, and provide evidence of bile flow or obstruction. The hepatobiliary imaging agents are removed from the blood by carrier-mediated processes that also transport and excrete bilirubin. The uptake and clearance are therefore affected by increasing levels of bilirubin. The newer agents, ^{99m}Tc-disofenin (Hepatolite) and ^{99m}Tc-mebrofenin (Choletec), show an improvement in competitive uptake of the radio-

pharmaceutical even in cases of significantly elevated bilirubin levels.

Hepatobiliary excretion of a compound has been found to be related to several physicochemical characteristics: (1) a molecular weight of 300-1000; (2) the presence of a strong anionic polar group ionized at plasma pH; (3) the presence of a nonpolar group to decrease renal excretion; (4) lipophilic character; and (5) binding to plasma proteins, which can promote transfer into the hepatocyte. The original work done on ^{99m}Tc-HIDA determined the structural configuration to exist as a dimer (Figure 6-12).[11] The ^{99m}Tc atom serves as a bridge between two ligand molecules. Dimerization is one of the major factors determining the hepatobiliary route of excretion for this radiopharmaceutical.

Brain imaging agents. With the advent of single photon emission computed tomography (SPECT) there was renewed interest in brain imaging. One of the new lipophilic brain agents is ^{99m}Tc-hexamethyl propylamineoxime (HMPAO), also known as exametazime. ^{99m}Tc-exametazime (Cerutec) is rapidly extracted into the brain (about 6% ID at 1 min after injection) then immediately decomposes in vivo to a more polar metabolite that does not diffuse out of the brain. Evidence has been presented to indicate that the conversion to the nondiffusible form can be accomplished by an intracellular reaction with glutathiones.[13] The main problem with the original commercial kit formulation is instability—it must be used within 30 min of preparation, and quality control must be done before injection. A recent modification of the kit formulation of HMPAO is the immediate addition of methylene blue to the kit preparation after the addition of $^{99m}TcO_4^-$ to stabilize the ^{99m}Tc-exametazime. After preparation of ^{99m}Tc-exametazime, the kit can be used for 4 hr. Since the final injectate is a dark blue color and therefore cannot be checked for the presence of particulate matter, it must be injected through a 0.22 μ filter, which is provided by the manufacturer.

Additionally, white blood cells (WBCs) have been labeled with technetium using ^{99m}Tc-exametazime. The original kit formulation, not the stabilized kit formulation, must be used for ^{99m}Tc-WBC labeling. Radiolabeling is accomplished in the presence of plasma, in vitro. Unlike the labeling of WBCs using ^{111}In-oxine, transferrin does not adversely affect the ^{99m}Tc-labeling process. Although diagnostic equivalent images can be obtained with ^{99m}Tc-labeled WBCs, the 6 hr half-life of technetium can make imaging 24 hr after injection difficult, when abscess-background ratios typically are maximized.

A second commercial technetium brain agent is ^{99m}Tc-L,L-ethylcysteinate dimer (ECD). ^{99m}Tc-ECD (Neurolite) has approximately 5% of the injected dose extracted into the brain within 2 min postinjection. This agent shows more rapid brain clearance and a higher brain-soft tissue ratio than ^{99m}Tc-HMPAO.[10] The commercial kit formulation is also stable for 6 hr.

GALLIUM AND INDIUM RADIOPHARMACEUTICALS

The four radionuclides of indium and gallium that have been used in nuclear medicine applications are ^{67}Ga, ^{68}Ga, ^{111}In, and ^{113m}In. As discussed previously, ^{68}Ga and ^{113m}In are generator produced. Cyclotron production of ^{67}Ga ($t_{1/2}$ = 78 hr) and ^{111}In ($t_{1/2}$ = 67 hr) can be accomplished by several different nuclear reactions:

$$^{67}Zn(p,n)\ ^{67}Ga$$
$$^{68}Zn(p,2n)\ ^{67}Ga$$
$$^{111}Cd(p,n)\ ^{111}In$$
$$^{109}Ag(\alpha,2n)\ ^{111}In$$

Analysis of the decay schemes for ^{67}Ga and ^{111}In indicates the following gamma photon energies and abundances: ^{67}Ga, 93 keV (40%), 184 keV (24%), 296 keV (22%), and 388 keV (7%); ^{111}In, 173 keV (89%) and 247 keV (94%). The physical half-lives and decay characteristics of ^{67}Ga and ^{111}In make them well suited for nuclear medicine. The gamma energies of ^{111}In are in the optimum range of detectability for the commercially available gamma cameras, and the abundance of gamma emissions provides 183 photons for every 100 disintegrations. Although the gamma energies of ^{67}Ga are in a range suitable for detection, their abundances are low. Therefore over twice as much ^{67}Ga as ^{111}In would need to be injected to obtain a comparable image.

In aqueous solution gallium and indium exist only as Ga^{3+} and In^{3+}, making radiopharmaceutical production simpler than with ^{99m}Tc, since a reduction does not have to be performed. The solution chemistry of both indium and gallium is similar to that of iron, with In^{3+} and Ga^{3+} forming very strong complexes with the plasma protein transferrin. To see the desired biodistribution using an indium or gallium radiopharmaceutical, a complex must be formed that is stronger than that of the metal with transferrin.

The solubility of indium hydroxides varies with the pH. At values higher than 4.5 indium hydroxide becomes very insoluble. In aqueous solution the free hydrated Ga(III) ion is stable only under acidic conditions. Hydrolysis occurs as the pH is raised, leading to the formation of insoluble gallium hydroxide. Unlike indium hydroxide, gallium hydroxide is amphoteric, dissolving in alkaline as well as acidic solutions. Thus, as pH is raised to ~3, $Ga(OH)_3$ precipitates but then redissolves as $Ga(OH)_4^-$ at pH greater than 7.4.[9]

The most widely used ^{67}Ga radiopharmaceutical is ^{67}Ga-citrate, an agent used for imaging tumors and sites of inflammation. Upon injection of the ^{67}Ga-citrate, greater than 90% of the gallium becomes bound to plasma proteins, particularly transferrin, resulting in slow clearance from the plasma. However, when transferrin is saturated with stable gallium or iron prior to injection of radioactivity, the plasma and urinary clearance are improved. Under these conditions gallium distribution shifts from soft tissue to bone, although uptake by tumors does not seem to be affected. Alternatively, increasing ^{67}Ga protein transferrin binding causes an increase in soft tissue activity and decreased tumor activity. The mechanisms of ^{67}Ga localization in tumors and sites of inflammation are not completely understood, but the uptake of gallium into intracellular components by one or more mechanisms, possibly involving transferrin binding, is strongly indicated.

^{68}Ga is used to prepare radiopharmaceuticals for PET imaging. ^{68}Ga-citrate is used in studies of regional plasma volume. ^{68}Ga-EDTA forms an ionic chelate complex that is excluded from the brain by the blood-brain barrier following intravenous injection in normal subjects and has been used to assess the size and extent of blood-brain barrier disruption in patients with brain tumors. The commercial MAA kits designed for preparation of ^{99m}Tc-MAA have also been used to prepare

^{68}Ga-MAA.[2] The major use for ^{68}Ga-MAA has been as a reference flow marker in PET imaging studies.

Because of the great stability of indium and gallium with transferrin, only very strong chelates can be used in vivo to direct the localization of the radionuclides to other sites. Strong chelators such as EDTA or DTPA can be easily labeled with gallium or indium using citrate or acetate as a transfer ligand. ^{111}In-DTPA has been used for renal and brain imaging and is currently used for cisternography.

Gallium and indium colloids can be prepared easily and conveniently as the insoluble hydroxides. By adding a small amount of ferric chloride to the radionuclide to act as a carrier, increasing the pH, and adding gelatin as a stabilizer, colloids that can be used as liver/spleen-imaging agents are formed. Larger particles prepared in a similar manner can be used for lung imaging.

Platelets and WBCs can be labeled with ^{111}In to provide agents for imaging inflammatory processes and thrombi. A weak complex is formed between the ^{111}In radiometal and 8-hydroxyquinoline (oxine). Since the ^{111}In-oxine complex is weak, the metal rapidly exchanges with transferrin in the plasma. In the absence of plasma, the complex diffuses across the cell membrane and the metal binds to intracellular sites. Isolation of the desired blood component from plasma permits easy labeling of either platelets or WBCs. This is routinely accomplished using centrifugation or sedimentation.

Procedures to label WBCs and platelets with ^{111}In-oxine vary, but the overall process can be summarized as follows:

1. Draw the patient's blood into an anticoagulated syringe and sediment the WBCs or platelets by centrifugation. Remove and save the leukocyte-poor (LPP) or platelet-poor plasma (PPP).
2. Wash the cells with 0.9% NaCl (saline) to remove plasma transferrin. Remove the saline wash, and resuspend the cells in saline.
3. Add ^{111}In-oxine to the cell suspension and incubate 15 min at room temperature.
4. Add a portion of the LPP or PPP to the ^{111}In-labeled WBCs or ^{111}In-labeled platelet preparation. Centrifuge the cells.
5. Resuspend the labeled cells in the remaining LPP or PPP for reinjection.

Overall labeling efficiencies (percentage of ^{111}In bound to cells) for WBCs is 70%-90% and for platelets is 50%-70%. Care must be taken to avoid damaging the cells during the labeling procedure.

^{111}In has also been conjugated to octreotide as an agent for the scintigraphic localization of primary and metastatic somatostatin receptor positive neuroendocrine tumors.[1] Somatostatin is a naturally occurring 14 amino acid peptide responsible for hormonal regulation of a number of organ systems. However, octreotide

(Sandostatin), an eight amino acid analogue of somatostatin, has a much longer biologic half-life and even greater regulatory properties than the native peptide.[10] For these reasons it is a much better target for labeling than somatostatin. A labeled form of octreotide is commercially available as the DTPA chelated compound ^{111}In-DTPA-octreotide (^{111}In-pentetreotide, Octreoscan). The most commonly diagnosed tumors have been carcinoids and gastrinomas, with a lower success rate noted for insulinomas and neuroblastomas. In the kit formulation ^{111}In is complexed using sodium citrate, added to the pentetreotide, and incubated for 30 min at room temperature. Quality control must be performed before patient administration using C_{18} Sep-Pak chromatography.

Monoclonal antibodies (MAb) have been labeled with ^{111}In using bifunctional chelates. The chelating agent is first conjugated to the antibody, and then ^{111}In binds to the conjugated MAb via the chelating agent. The MAb B72.3 (satumomab) is an intact MAb that is directed to a high molecular weight, tumor-associated glycoprotein. The expression of this glycoprotein has been demonstrated in a variety of adenocarcinomas. This MAb has been conjugated using a derivatized DTPA ligand, then radiolabeled with ^{111}In. The kit formulation contains 1 mg of satumomab pendetide (Oncoscint). ^{111}In-acetate is prepared by addition of ^{111}In chloride to a vial of sodium acetate buffer. The ^{111}In-acetate is then transferred to the MAb reaction vial. The vial is incubated for 30 min at room temperature and filtered through a low protein-binding 0.22 μ filter. The preparation should be stored at room temperature and used within 8 hr of preparation. The indication for ^{111}In-satumomab pendetide is determination of the extent and location of extrahepatic malignant disease in cases of colorectal or ovarian carcinoma.

THALLIUM CHLORIDE

^{201}Tl is a monovalent cationic metal used in cardiac imaging. It is ultimately obtained from a ^{201}Pb-^{201}Tl generator. ^{201}Pb is produced by bombarding natural thallium metal with protons, according to the following nuclear reaction:

$$^{203}Tl(p,3n)\,^{201}Pb \xrightarrow[\text{EC}]{t_{1/2}\,9.4\text{ hr}}\,^{201}Tl$$

The ^{201}Pb is then complexed and undesirable target material is removed by ion exchange chromatography. The purified lead radioisotopes are affixed to another column. ^{201}Pb decays by electron capture with a $t_{1/2}$ of 9.4 hr to give ^{201}Tl. A second purification by column chromatography is required to remove the ^{203}Pb radiocontaminant, which is present at the end of purification at a level less than 0.5% per mCi ^{201}Tl at calibration. The ^{201}Tl is isolated carrier-free, has a $t_{1/2}$ of

74 hr, and decays by electron capture with gamma emissions between 140 and 170 keV.

Thallium clears rapidly from the blood, with maximum concentration in the heart at approximately 10-30 min after injection in the resting state and at 5 min after stress induced either by exercise or pharmacologic intervention at the time of administration. Uptake of ^{201}Tl into the myocardium occurs intracellularly in proportion to blood flow. Additionally, adequate tissue oxygenation is required to support ^{201}Tl uptake in myocardial cells, since oxygen supports the Na-K-ATPase concentrating mechanism. Similarities between ^{201}Tl$^+$ and K$^+$ include monovalent charges, comparable ionic radii, and involvement in the membrane Na-K-ATPase pump.

There are a number of pharmacologic stress inducers available for use with ^{201}Tl. Dipyridamole (Persantin) is a coronary vasodilator that has been employed in ^{201}Tl cardiac imaging to simulate exercise stress testing in patients who cannot exercise adequately. The dose employed is 0.142-0.570 mg/kg/min and is infused over 4 min. The most frequent adverse reaction reported was chest pain/angina pectoria. Parenteral aminophylline (50-250 mg over 30-60 sec by slow intravenous injection) should be available during dipyridamole stress testing for relieving adverse reactions such as bronchospasm or chest pain.

Adenosine (Adenocord) is another coronary vasodilator recently made available for use in perfusion imaging. The initial dose of 6 mg is infused as a rapid intravenous bolus. It has a much shorter $t_{1/2}$ in plasma than dipyridamole (<10 sec versus <30 min), which would allow more rapid reversal of the pharmacologic effect. The most common adverse effects are facial flushing and shortness of breath.

IODINATED RADIOPHARMACEUTICALS

Sodium iodide, either ^{123}I- or ^{131}I-labeled, is used for thyroid imaging, uptake measurements, and therapy (in the case of ^{131}I) as a capsule or a solution for oral administration. ^{123}I ($t_{1/2}$ of 13.2 hr) decays by electron capture with emission of a 159 keV gamma (83%), whereas ^{131}I ($t_{1/2}$ of 8 days) decays by β^- emission with subsequent gamma emission of 364 keV (82%). ^{131}I has also been used to label monoclonal antibodies for in vivo tumor imaging and therapy. HSA labeled with ^{125}I ($t_{1/2}$ of 60 days decays by electron capture with a 35 keV gamma) is used to measure plasma volume, and ^{125}I-labeled antibodies are used for radioimmunoassay.

To label proteins, particularly antibodies, with iodine it is important to use mild iodination agents that do not denature the protein. Iodination of proteins involves the formation of positively charged iodine species that react with various groups of the protein. Under general conditions used for iodination, the tyrosine residues in the protein are iodinated to the greatest extent, giving monoiodotyrosine and diiodotyrosine.

The method of iodination chosen depends upon the application. Retention of biologic activity of the protein is probably the most important consideration in the choice of the labeling technique. However, the overall labeling yield is also a key factor in determining the ultimate utility of a method. A variety of methods have been used to oxidize iodide to a positively charged species to effect protein iodination. Some of the most commonly used methods for iodination of proteins are outlined below.

1. I$_2$ iodination (δ indicates partial charge).

2. Iodine monochloride iodination.

3. Chloramine-T iodination. Chloramine-T is a strong oxidizing agent that converts iodide ion to an iodinating species (possibly HOI). The exact mechanism of chloramine-T iodination is unknown.

4. Enzymatic iodination. Various peroxidases have been found to catalyze the iodination of proteins. Lactoperoxidase is most commonly used. In a typical iodination reaction the protein, enzyme, radioiodine, and a small amount of hydrogen peroxide are mixed to effect the labeling.

5. Indirect iodination. Most methods of direct iodination involve the addition of an oxidizing agent to the protein. This can be avoided by first iodinating a molecule with a structure similar to tyrosine, which can then be attached to the protein. N-succinimidyl-3-(4-hydroxyphenyl) propionate (SHPP) is a molecule that has been used for this application. SHPP is initially iodinated, usually by the chloramine-T technique, separated from the iodinating solution, and then added to the protein at pH 5.

6. Iodogen iodination. Iodogen, chloroglycoluril, is a mild iodinating agent that is quite popular.

The iodogen is coated on the reaction vessel or bound to insoluble beads. The protein and radioiodine are added in an aqueous solution. Since the iodogen is not water soluble, it remains bound to the reaction vessel or beads, allowing easy separation of the labeled protein. Other iodinated compounds used in nuclear medicine are ^{131}I-orthoiodohippuran for renal imaging, ^{131}I-metaiodobenzylguanidine (MIBG) for adrenal tumor imaging, ^{123}I-iodoamphetamine for brain imaging, and ^{123}I-labeled fatty acids for myocardial imaging.

Cyclotron production of ^{123}I can be accomplished by several methods. Enriched [124]Te can be bombarded with protons, resulting in the [124]Te(p,2n)[123]I reaction. The most likely contaminant of this reacton is [124]I, which emits a high-energy photon that can affect image resolution. Alternatively, this can be produced by the [127]I(p,5n)[123]I, where the main contaminant is [125]I. This contaminant does not pose a problem in imaging but will deliver a higher radiation dose to the patient due to the $t_{1/2}$ of 65 days. [131]I is obtained predominantly as a chemically separated fission product.

PET RADIOPHARMACEUTICALS

The most frequently used positron-emitting radionuclides for PET imaging are [15]O ($t_{1/2} = 2$ min), [13]N ($t_{1/2} = 10$ min), [11]C ($t_{1/2} = 20$ min), and [18]F ($t_{1/2} = 110$ min). Their decay characteristics are described in Table 6-2. Unlike the radionuclides used in conventional nuclear medicine, these are identical to those found in naturally occurring biomolecules, and therefore the biochemical and physiologic processes in the body can be studied directly. Although fluorine is not usually native, labeling with ^{18}F only minimally changes the structure of a biomolecule, since its size is similar to the hydrogen it replaces. The short half-lives of these isotopes require production and radiopharmaceutical synthesis close to where the PET imaging takes place. This often requires an on-site cyclotron; however, for ^{18}F-labeled radiopharmaceuticals, centralized radiopharmacies that supply regional hospitals and PET centers are becoming more common.

Oxygen-15 Radiopharmaceuticals

Oxygen-15 is cyclotron produced, generally by the [14]N(d,n)[15]O nuclear reaction. With a half-life of 2.04 min, PET radiopharmaceuticals labeled with [15]O are limited to a few simple molecules such as ^{15}O-labeled water (H_2[15]O), ^{15}O-labeled oxygen gas ([15]OO), ^{15}O-labeled carbon dioxide (CO[15]O), and ^{15}O-labeled carbon monoxide (C[15]O). The short half-life and the low radiation absorbed dose allow amounts of activity up to 100 mCi to be administered in imaging procedures, which can be repeated at 8- to 10-min intervals.

[15]O-labeled gas can be used directly to study O_2 metabolism, or the [15]OO can be converted to ^{15}O-labeled CO, CO_2, or H_2O. Labeled carbon oxides are produced by passing the [15]OO through an activated carbon furnace. The furnace temperature determines whether C[15]O or CO[15]O is produced. High specific activity [15]O can be produced that allows ^{15}O-labeled CO to be safely administered to patients by inhalation. Carbon monoxide labeled with [15]O binds to hemoglobin found in the RBC, allowing the study of red blood cell volume.

[15]O-labeled water is usually produced from CO[15]O via the carbonic acid mediated exchange reaction by bubbling CO[15]O through saline. The ^{15}O-labeled water is produced in a form suitable for immediate intravenous injection. This tracer can also be produced by passing labeled oxygen gas and hydrogen gas over a suitable catalyst. The most common use for ^{15}O-labeled water is as a tracer for cerebral and myocardial perfusion.

Nitrogen-13 Radiopharmaceuticals

Nitrogen-13 is cyclotron produced most frequently by the [16]O(p,α)[13]N nuclear reaction. This nuclear reaction is usually performed using a water target to yield ^{13}N in the form of the aqueous nitrate ion [13]NO$_3^-$. The ^{13}N-labeled nitrate ion can be converted to ^{13}N-labeled ammonia by a reaction with a reducing agent such as titanium(III) chloride. ^{13}N-labeled ammonia has been used as a tracer for cerebral and myocardial blood flow, since it undergoes relatively high extraction into these organs and exhibits prolonged retention. A major fraction of the extracted [13]NH$_3$ is metabolically incorporated into amino acids.

[13]N-labeled nitrogen gas, N[13]N, is obtained by proton or deuteron bombardment of carbon dioxide containing a trace of N$_2$ by the [16]O(p,α)[13]N or [12]C(d,n)[13]N nuclear reactions. Labeled N[13]N is used for studying pulmonary ventilation and is superior to the radioactive noble gases [127]Xe or [88m]Kr due to its lower solubility in blood.

Table 6-2 Decay properties of several short-lived positron-emitting radionuclides used in nuclear medicine

Nuclide	$t_{1/2}$ (min)	E_{β^+} max (MeV)	Preferred method of production
[15]O	2	1.72	[14]N(d,n) [15]O
[13]N	10	1.19	[16]O(p,α) [13]N
[11]C	20	0.96	[14]N(p,α) [11]C
[18]F	110	0.64	[18]O(p,n) [18]F

Carbon-11 Radiopharmaceuticals

Carbon-11 is generally produced by the $^{10}B(d,n)^{11}C$ or $^{14}N(p,\alpha)^{11}C$ nuclear reactions. ^{11}C-labeled carbon monoxide (^{11}CO), carbon dioxide ($^{11}CO_2$), and cyanide ($^{11}CN^-$) are the most commonly used synthetic precursors. The number of different ^{11}C-labeled compounds that have been synthesized as radiopharmaceuticals for PET studies is extensive. This chapter briefly discusses a few of the more clinically useful ones.

One compound routinely prepared is ^{11}C-labeled acetate, a tracer used in the study of myocardial metabolism. ^{11}C-glucose is also used to study metabolism. Early methods to prepare ^{11}C-glucose were lengthy compared to the 20 min half-life of ^{11}C; however, modifications have corrected this. The glucose analogue 2-deoxy-D-glucose labeled with ^{11}C in the C-1 position has been synthesized rapidly from the $H^{11}CN$ precursor. This analogue of glucose has similar characteristics except that it fails to undergo intracellular enzymatic glycolysis beyond initial phosphorylation. It is metabolically trapped in brain cells and has been used for measurement of cerebral glucose metabolism.

Fluorine-18 Radiopharmaceuticals

Fluorine-18 is produced by either the $^{18}O(p,n)^{18}F$ or the $^{20}Ne(d,\alpha)^{18}F$ nuclear reaction. The use of a neon gas target containing 1% F_2 provides labeled fluorine gas, $^{18}F^{19}F$. The production of ^{18}F involving F_2 gas is inherently carrier added, and there are practical limits on the specific activity that can be obtained. The proton irradiation of ^{18}O-labeled water is the preferred method of producing ^{18}F. The target is constructed of metals such as silver, copper, titanium, nickel, or stainless steel. The target has small cavities for the target water, which are 0.1-3 ml in volume and covered by thin metal foils. The production of ^{18}F in most ^{18}O-labeled water targets is excellent, with yields of greater than 1 Ci at end of bombardment (EOB). The major problem in producing ^{18}F using ^{18}O-labeled water is the limited

availability and high cost of the enriched isotopic target material. To aid in the conservation of the ^{18}O-labeled water, the recovery of unused target material by ion exchange chromatography is frequently practiced.

The most frequently used and most important ^{18}F-labeled radiopharmaceutical is 2-deoxy-2-[^{18}F]fluoro-D-glucose (FDG). FDG is used predominantly in the study of cerebral and myocardial metabolism. In the brain FDG undergoes carrier-mediated uptake as a glucose analog and serves as a substrate for hexokinase. The ^{18}F radiolabel is metabolically trapped in the cell because phosphorylation cannot proceed past the C-1 carbon (Figure 6-13). In brain imaging studies FDG maps normal brain metabolic activity, whereas in cardiac studies FDG is used to denote ischemic regions where glucose metabolism increases as a consequence of diminished fatty acid metabolism.

^{18}F-labeled spiperone used in the study of brain dopamine receptors is also an attractive molecule for ^{18}F labeling. It can be prepared by a one-step displacement reaction of nitrospiperone, but this reaction gives low yields and is generally unreliable. A multistep synthesis involving a fluorination with $^{18}F^-$ followed by alkylation is the preferred method of preparing ^{18}F-labeled spiperone.

THERAPEUTIC RADIOPHARMACEUTICALS

Sodium ^{32}P-phosphate is an FDA-approved radiopharmaceutical indicated for treatment of polycythemia vera, chronic myelocytic leukemia, chronic lymphocytic leukemia, and for palliation of metastatic bone pain. It is prepared as a solution for intravenous administration. Chromic ^{32}P-phosphate is a suspension of ^{32}P used for intracavity installation for treatment of peritoneal or pleural effusions caused by metastatic disease. Phosphorus-32 decays by β^- emission with a $t_{1/2}$ of 14.3

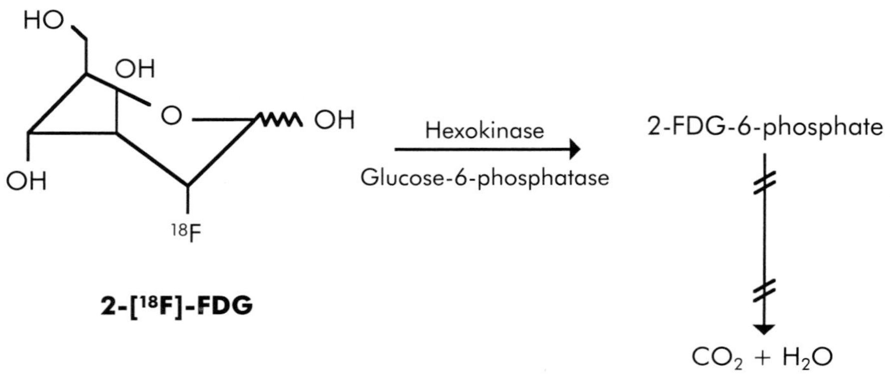

2-[^{18}F]-FDG → (Hexokinase / Glucose-6-phosphatase) → 2-FDG-6-phosphate → $CO_2 + H_2O$

Figure 6-13 FDG undergoes metabolism by hexokinase but is metabolically trapped, since phosphorylization cannot proceed.

days. The major toxicity noted is significant marrow suppression in approximately one third of patients receiving this radiopharmaceutical. The duration of response is 1.5-11 months.

Recently ^{89}Sr-chloride (Metastron) has been approved by the FDA for relief of bone pain in cases of painful skeletal metastases. The compound behaves biologically like calcium and localizes in hydroxyapatite crystal by ion exchange. Strontium uptake occurs preferentially at sites of active osteogenesis. This allows primary bone tumors and areas of metastatic involvement to accumulate significantly higher concentrations of strontium than surrounding normal bone. ^{89}Sr decays by β^- emission with a $t_{1/2}$ of 50.6 days.

Two radiotherapeutic agents are currently under investigation, ^{186}Re-HEDP and ^{153}Sm-EDTMP; ^{186}Re decays by β^- and gamma emission with a $t_{1/2}$ of 90.6 hr and ^{153}Sm decays soley by β^- emission and has a $t_{1/2}$ of 46.3 hr. Both of these beta-emitting radionuclides are complexed with bone-seeking ligands, which localize by chemisorption. The duration of response is 1-12 months. The main toxicity of these radiotherapeutics is mild transient bone marrow supression.

RADIOPHARMACEUTICAL QUALITY ASSURANCE

Radionuclidic Purity

Radionuclidic purity is defined as the proportion of the total radioactivity present as the stated radionuclide. As such, measurement of radionuclidic purity requires determination of the identity and amounts of all radionuclides that are present. Radionuclidic impurities can have significant effects on the overall radiation dose to the patient and the quality of the images obtained. The identities and amounts of radionuclidic impurities found in a radiopharmaceutical depend on the method of radionuclide production used. As an example, ^{99m}Tc obtained from a generator prepared using neutron bombardment-produced ^{99}Mo has different impurities than ^{99m}Tc obtained from a generator containing fission-produced ^{99}Mo. The requirements for radionuclidic purity as listed by the *United States Pharmacopeia XXIII (U.S.P.)* for sodium ^{99m}Tc-pertechnetate solution are listed in Table 6-3.

An assay using a multichannel analyzer for detection and identification of all gamma-emitting radiocontaminants present in a sample is usually performed by the manufacturer. In the case of ^{99m}Tc, one expected radionuclidic impurity is parent ^{99}Mo. It is possible for the user to assay routinely for ^{99}Mo breakthrough using a gamma-ionization dose calibrator and a lead vial holder thick enough to absorb the 140 keV gamma of ^{99m}Tc but allow penetration of the 720 and 740 keV gammas of ^{99}Mo (Figure 6-14). The Nuclear Regulatory Commission (NRC) allowable ^{99}Mo contamination is less than 0.15 μCi/mCi of ^{99m}Tc. NRC regulations require that each elution from a ^{99}Mo-^{99m}Tc generator be tested for ^{99}Mo breakthrough and the records maintained for 3 years.

Radiochemical Purity

Radiochemical purity is defined as the proportion of the stated radionuclide that is present in the stated chemical form. The radiation absorbed dose, the biologic distribution, and thus the quality of the image are directly related to the radiochemical purity. Several chromatographic methods can be used to determine radiochemical purity, including gel-permeation chromatography, gas-liquid chromatography, and paper chromatography. The method applicable to routine in-house quality control of technetium radiopharmaceuticals is paper or instant thin-layer chromatography (ITLC).

Chromatography involves the separation of a chemical mixture into its components along a stationary phase (adsorbent) as a result of different velocities in the mobile phase (migrating solvent). Radiochromatography differs from regular chromatography only

Table 6-3 NRC allowable radionuclidic impurities in ^{99m}Tc-pertechnetate

Neutron bombardment	Fission-separation ^{99}Mo
^{98}Mo(n,γ) ^{99}Mo	
^{99}Mo < 0.15 μCi/mCi ^{99m}Tc	^{99}Mo < 0.15 μCi/mCi ^{99m}Tc
Other gamma-emitting radionuclides:	Other gamma-emitting radionuclides:
0.5 μCi/mCi ^{99m}Tc	^{131}I < 0.05 μCi/mCi ^{99m}Tc
<2.5 μCi/administered dose	^{103}Ru < 0.05 μCi/mCi ^{99m}Tc
	^{89}Sr < 0.0006 μCi/mCi ^{99m}Tc
	^{90}Sr < 0.00006 μCi/mCi ^{99m}Tc
	Remaining $\beta + \gamma$ < 0.1 μCi/mCi ^{99m}Tc
	α < 0.001 μCi/mCi ^{99m}Tc

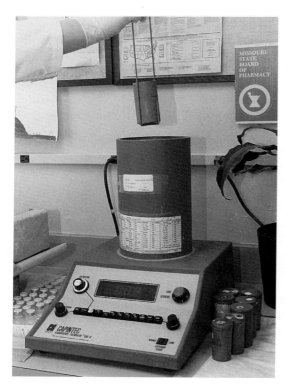

Figure 6-14 Molybdenum-99 assay chamber being placed in a dose calibrator.

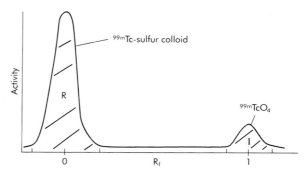

Figure 6-15 Radiochromatogram scan of ^{99m}Tc-sulfur colloid *(R)* indicating the radiochemical purity. The only radiocontaminant present is ^{99m}TcO$_4^-$ *(I)*.

in that the presence of the component is determined by the location of its radioactivity rather than by some other physical or chemical property. The R_f of a compound is defined as the measure of its migration distance.

$$R_f = \frac{\text{Distance of center of spot from origin}}{\text{Distance of solvent front from origin}}$$

Where the $R_f = 1$, the component migrates with the solvent front; where the $R_f = 0$, the component remains at the point of application (origin).

The ideal separation of a component in a solvent system gives an R_f value greater than 0 but less than 1. A component that migrates at the solvent front ($R_f = 1$) or remains at the origin ($R_f = 0$) is not truly separated. However, for routine rapid quality control of technetium radiopharmaceuticals and the separation of known impurities, free pertechnetate (^{99m}TcO$_4^-$) and free reduced technetium (^{99m}TcO$_2$) from the labeled radiopharmaceuticals, R_f values of 1 and 0 are considered acceptable.

A typical thin-layer radiochromatogram of ^{99m}Tc-sulfur colloid with ^{99m}TcO$_4^-$ contaminant is shown in Figure 6-15. The radioactivity associated with the peaks may be measured in several ways. The simplest method, which was used to obtain the data in Figure 6-15, involves the use of a radiochromatogram scanner. In this system the paper chromatography strip is moved across

a detector, a ratemeter indicates the count rate, and the counts are graphically printed out by a strip chart recorder. A manual counting system can also be employed, in which the chromatogram is cut into strips and each strip is counted using a well counter or an ionization dose calibrator.

The radiochemical purity of a radiopharmaceutical preparation can be calculated using the following expression:

Percentage of radiochemical purity

$$= \frac{\text{Area R}}{\text{Area R} + \text{Area I}}$$

$$= \frac{\text{Counts in strip R}}{\text{Counts in strip R} + \text{Counts in strip I (total counts)}}$$

where *R* refers to the radiopharmaceutical and *I* refers to the impurity.

Routine rapid radiochromatography can be performed to evaluate the percentage of radiochemical purity of ^{99m}Tc radiopharmaceuticals. The most commonly employed procedure involves the use of instant thin-layer chromatography silica gel-impregnated (ITLC-SG) glass-fiber sheets as the solid support. These strips are developed in solvents such as saline, acetone, and methyl ethyl ketone (MEK). ^{99m}Tc radiopharmaceuticals can be divided into three groups based on their chromatographic behavior.

1. Oxidized, particulate: This group contains ^{99m}Tc-sulfur colloid. Since the technetium is present in the +7 oxidation state, it is not necessary to analyze for free reduced ^{99m}Tc in these preparations. The chromatographic system used involves a single solvent (saline, acetone, or MEK) to determine the amount of free pertechnetate.

2. Reduced, particulate: This group includes the ^{99m}Tc-labeled lung perfusion imaging agent, MAA. The rapid chromatographic procedures described for sulfur colloid can be used only to

Table 6-4 Chromatographic systems used for quality control of ^{99m}Tc radiopharmaceuticals

Radiopharmaceutical	Solvent	Solid support	R_f		
			Free $^{99m}TcO_4^-$	Free $^{99m}TcO_2$	^{99m}Tc-labeled radiopharmaceutical
Sulfur colloid Albumin colloid	Acetone, saline, or MEK	ITLC-SG	1.0	—	0
MAA	Acetone, saline, or MEK	ITLC-SG	1.0	—	0
PYP	Acetone or MEK	ITLC-SG	1.0	0	0
MDP/HDP DTPA GHP DMSA	Saline	ITLC-SG	1.0	0	1.0
Disofenin	20% NaCl	ITLC-SA	1.0	0	0
Mebrofenin	H_2O	ITLC-SG	1.0	0	1.0
Sestamibi	100% EtOH	Aluminum oxide TLC	0	0	1.0
Teboroxime	Saline	Whatman 31ET	1.0	0	0
	Saline-acetone (1:1)	Whatman 31ET	1.0	0	1.0

ITLC-SA, Silica acid; ITLC-SG, silica gel.

determine free pertechnetate. It is not possible to separate free reduced ^{99m}Tc (which is colloidal at physiologic pH) and the ^{99m}Tc MAA using this rapid system. It is possible, however, to use an indirect method to detect $^{99m}TcO_2$ impurity levels. The radiopharmaceutical is first filtered through a Millipore filter with a 1 μ pore diameter, which retains the ^{99m}Tc MAA but allows the colloidal free reduced ^{99m}Tc to pass through. Once the macroparticles have been removed, rapid chromatography on the filtrate (using either saline, acetone, or MEK) enables the determination of free $^{99m}TcO_4^-$ and $^{99m}TcO_2$.

3. Reduced, soluble: This group contains the soluble, reduced ^{99m}Tc-radiopharmaceuticals, including DTPA, glucoheptonate, methylene diphosphonate, pyrophosphate, DMSA, and albumin. The chromatographic procedure for this group involves two solvents (saline and an organic solvent, such as acetone or MEK) to determine the percentages of free pertechnetate, free reduced technetium, and labeled radiopharmaceutical.

The R_f values of the technetium radiopharmaceutical and the relevant impurities are outlined in Table 6-4 for each of these groups. The steps in a typical chromatographic procedure for a reduced, soluble ^{99m}Tc-radiopharmaceutical are as follows:

1. Place 1 ml of saline in a small glass vial; repeat this procedure with the organic solvent.
2. Mark two 1 cm by 6 cm ITLC chromatography strips at 2 cm and 5 cm with a pencil.
3. Place a small spot of the radiopharmaceutical in the center of each strip (near the mark located 2 cm from the bottom of the strip) using a tuberculin syringe.
4. Place one strip into each solvent before the spot has air dried to prevent air oxidation of the radiopharmaceutical. Allow the solvent front to move up each strip until it has reached the line at 5 cm.
5. Cut the strips in the middle between the pencil markings and count each portion of the strips for activity, or use a radiochromatogram scanner to measure the amount of activity along the intact strips.
6. In the dual solvent system, the percentage of free $^{99m}TcO_4^-$ is calculated from the strip developed in the organic solvent and the percentage of free $^{99m}TcO_2$ is determined using the strip developed in saline. Subtraction of the percentages of these two impurities from 100% yields the overall radiochemical purity of the ^{99m}Tc radiopharmaceutical.

Radiochemical testing using ITLC is easily performed in any nuclear medicine laboratory. Testing each lot of a radiopharmaceutical kit on a weekly basis is a reasonable approach for routine radiochemical testing. Additional testing should be performed if there are questions concerning purity of a given preparation. Several of the newer technetium radiopharma-

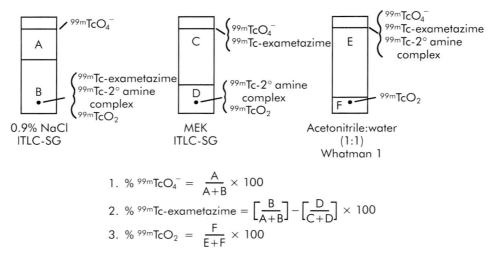

1. $\% \, ^{99m}TcO_4^- = \dfrac{A}{A+B} \times 100$

2. $\% \, ^{99m}Tc\text{-exametazime} = \left[\dfrac{B}{A+B}\right] - \left[\dfrac{D}{C+D}\right] \times 100$

3. $\% \, ^{99m}TcO_2 = \dfrac{F}{E+F} \times 100$

Figure 6-16 Chromatographic system used for radiochemical purity determination for ^{99m}Tc-exametazime and calculation of percentage of radiochemical purity.

ceuticals require more specific types of quality control methods. In the preparation of the lipophilic ^{99m}Tc-exametazime, three radiochemical impurities can be present: a secondary ^{99m}Tc-amine complex, ^{99m}TcO$_4^-$, and reduced hydrolyzed ^{99m}Tc. A combination of three chromatographic systems is necessary for radiochemical purity determination: 0.9% NaCl (ITLC-SG); MEK (ITLC-SG); and acetonitrile-water (1:1). In the 0.9% NaCl (saline) solvent the ^{99m}TcO$_4^-$ migrates at the solvent front, whereas the ^{99m}Tc-exametazime, secondary ^{99m}Tc-amine complex, and free reduced ^{99m}Tc remain at the origin. In the MEK solvent, ^{99m}TcO$_4^-$ and ^{99m}Tc-exametazime migrate at the solvent front, whereas the secondary ^{99m}Tc-amine complex and the free reduced ^{99m}Tc remain at the origin. Use of the acetonitrile-water (1:1) solvent causes ^{99m}TcO$_4^-$, ^{99m}Tc-exametazime, and the secondary ^{99m}Tc-amine complex to migrate with the solvent front, whereas the free reduced ^{99m}Tc remains at the origin. The calculations used for determining the percentage of ^{99m}Tc-exametazime are shown in Figure 6-16.

The radiochemical purity of ^{99m}Tc-mertiatide is determined using Sep-Pak chromatography. Sep-Paks are made of C$_{18}$ hydrocarbon chains that retain nonpolar compounds. Initially the Sep-Pak is prepared by washing with 100% ethanol to remove nonpolar impurities, then with 0.001N HCl to remove polar impurities. A sample of the ^{99m}Tc-mertiatide is then placed on the Sep-Pak and eluted with a 0.001N HCl solution, which elutes any polar impurities present in the preparation. This fraction is retained and labeled fraction 1. Then the Sep-Pak is eluted with an ethanol-saline (1:1) solution, which solubilizes and elutes the ^{99m}Tc-mertiatide. This fraction is labeled 2, and the Sep-Pak is labeled 3. Fractions 1, 2, and 3 are counted in the dose calibrator. Figure 6-17 shows the calculation for ^{99m}Tc-mertiatide purity determination.

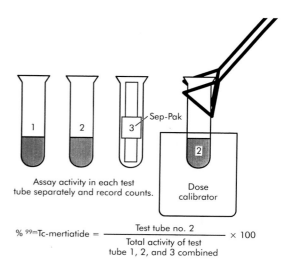

$\% \, ^{99m}Tc\text{-mertiatide} = \dfrac{\text{Test tube no. 2}}{\substack{\text{Total activity of test} \\ \text{tube 1, 2, and 3 combined}}} \times 100$

Figure 6-17 Calculation of percentage of radiochemical purity of ^{99m}Tc-mertiatide.

A single solid support, aluminum oxide, and a single solvent, 100% ethanol, are utilized for quality control of ^{99m}Tc-sestamibi. The ^{99m}Tc-sestamibi migrates at the solvent front. Pertechnetate is thought to form a complex with the aluminum and remains at the origin. The ^{99m}TcO$_2$ also remains at the origin.

Quality control for ^{99m}Tc-teboroxime involves use of a two-solvent system. Solvents and solid supports for this analysis are outlined in Table 6-4.

^{99m}Tc-tetrofosmin quality control requires the ITLC-SG as the solid support, and a 35:65 (v/v) mixture of acetone and dichloromethane. After spotting the ITLC-SG, the solvent is allowed to migrate 15 cm. The strip is removed from the solvent and cut into 3 pieces, each approximately 5 cm in length. The percent ^{99m}Tc-tetrofosmin will be equal to the activity of the center piece of the strip, divided by the total activity of the three pieces, multiplied by 100.

Completion of quality control, involving C_{18} Sep-Pak chromatography, is recommended before patient administration for ^{111}In-pentetreotide. The Sep-Pak is prepared for use by initially flushing with 10 ml of methanol, followed by 10 ml of water. A sample of ^{111}In-pentetreotide is placed on the Sep-Pak and eluted with 5 ml of water. The fraction is labeled fraction 1. The Sep-Pak is then eluted with 5 ml of methanol which solubilizes ^{111}In-pentetreotide. This is labeled fraction 2, and the Sep-Pak is labeled fraction 3. Each fraction is assayed in the dose calibrator, and the percent purity of the ^{111}In-pentetreotide is determined (Fig 6-18).

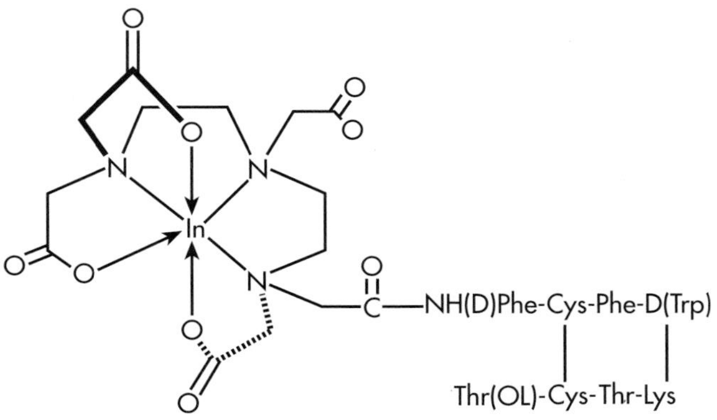

Chemical Impurities

Chemical impurities are all of the nonradioactive substances present in a radiopharmaceutical preparation that either affect labeling or directly cause adverse biologic effects. In microgram concentrations aluminum can affect the formation of ^{99m}Tc-labeled radiopharmaceuticals. The NRC states the concentration of aluminum should not exceed 10 μg/ml. The presence of excess Al^{3+} can cause formation of colloidal ^{99m}Tc-Al particles, resulting in liver uptake, aggregation of sulfur colloid to larger particles with resultant capillary blockade and lung visualization, and ^{99m}Tc-RBC aggregation, which results in uptake of the damaged cells in lungs and spleen.

Aluminum can be detected using a spectrophotometric method. Aluminum solutions of known concentrations are reacted with aluminon reagent (the ammonium salt of aurin tricarboxylic acid), and the absorbance in the visible region of the spectrum is measured. A standard curve is then prepared by plotting the absorbance versus the aluminum concentration; this curve can be used to determine aluminum concentrations of unknown samples. A more convenient method for aluminum determination is the use of a commercially available indicator paper impregnated with aluminon reagent that turns pink when Al^{3+} is present in a spot of the eluate solution. A standard solution of Al^{3+} (10 μg/ml) is used as a color comparison.

Most of the commercially available technetium kits contain stannous ion as the reducing agent. In most cases more stannous ion is contained in each kit than is actually required to reduce and bind the technetium that is added; this excess of stannous ion has been found to cause some problems. For example, liver uptake has been noted on an otherwise normal bone scan, which may be attributable to the formation of ^{99m}Tc-tin colloids. Another problem that can occur with excess stannous ion is inadvertent RBC labeling. As mentioned previously, excess stannous ion injected into a patient receiving a reduced ^{99m}Tc radiopharmaceutical remains in the circulation. This can cause RBC

Figure 6-18 Spatial configuration of ^{111}In-pentetreotide (OctreoScan).

labeling upon subsequent administration of ^{99m}Tc-pertechnetate for brain or thyroid imaging.

Particle Sizing

Particle sizing of MAA is another important quality control test. This microscopic test is conveniently conducted on a hemocytometer grid on which 100-200 particles are sized, and the entire field is scanned for unacceptably large MAA particles or clumping of human albumin microspheres.

Microbiologic Testing

Sterility testing. The objective of sterility testing is to provide assurance that the sterilization process was conducted properly. The sterility test required by the *U.S.P. XXIII* involves inoculation of the product in both fluid thioglycollate and soybean-casein digest media. Fluid thioglycollate provides conditions for growth of aerobic and anaerobic bacteria. Soybean-casein digest medium supports growth of fungi and molds. The official sterility test requires 14 days, but due to the short half-life of ^{99m}Tc, the *U.S.P. XXIII* allows for the release of these radiopharmaceuticals before the completion of the tests. The cold kits used to prepare the ^{99m}Tc radiopharmaceuticals are tested for sterility and pyrogen content.

Pyrogen testing. The *U.S.P. XXIII* also requires pyrogen testing. Pyrogens are any agents that cause a rise in temperature and are generally considered to be heat-stable by-products of the growth of bacteria, yeasts, and molds. The word *pyrogen* is often used to mean bacterial endotoxin. Previously, to test for the presence of pyrogens the *U.S.P. XXIII* required the monitoring of three healthy rabbits for 3 hr after intravenous injection of the test sample. The test was positive if any rabbit showed an increase of 0.6° C or more above the baseline temperature or if the sum of the three temperature increases exceeded 1.4° C.

The *U.S.P. XXIII* now employs the limulus amebocyte lysate (LAL) as the approved method of pyrogen testing. LAL, which is isolated from the horseshoe crab (Limulus), reacts with gram-negative bacterial endotoxins in nanogram or greater concentrations to form an opaque gel. Gram-negative endotoxins are recognized as the most important source of pyrogen contamination, and the LAL test is both a rapid and a very sensitive in vitro method.

Manufacturers are required to perform sterility and apyrogenicity testing on all of their products before release into the marketplace. The short half-life of ^{99m}Tc, however, prohibits testing of ^{99m}Tc-labeled radiopharmaceuticals for sterility and apyrogenicity prior to patient administration. Since this is the case, it is imperative that the user emphasize aseptic technique. The use of laminar airflow enclosures improves the environment for radiopharmaceutical formulation, since these enclosures contain high-efficiency particulate air (HEPA) filters to remove particles of 0.3 μ and larger with an efficiency of 99.97%. Vertical laminar airflow hoods are preferred in a radiopharmacy, since horizontal flow presents a potentially serious contamination hazard to personnel by forcing radioactivity out into the room. If the laminar airflow cabinet is reinforced, it can support a leaded glass shield to provide radiation protection for the technologist during preparation of the radiopharmaceuticals.

REFERENCES

1. Bauer W, Briner U, Doepfner W, et al: SMS 201-995: a very potent and selective octapeptide analogue of somatostatin with prolonged action, *Life Sci* 31:1133, 1982.
2. Brodack JW, Kaiser SL, Welch MJ: Laboratory robotics for the remote synthesis of generator-based positron-emitting radiopharmaceuticals, *LRA* 1:285, 1989.
3. Coleman RE, Maturi M, Nunn AD, et al: Imaging of myocardial perfusion with Tc-99m SQ 3Q217: dog and human studies, *J Nucl Med* 27:893, 1986.
4. Dudczak R, Leitha T, Kletter K, et al: Comparison of Tc-99m-methoxyisobutyl-isonitrile (MIBI) for myocardial imaging in man, *J Nucl Med* 29:794, 1988.
5. Ehrhardt GJ, Welch MJ: A new germanium-68/gallium-68 generator, *J Nucl Med* 19:925, 1978.
6. Fujibayashi Y, Matsumoto K, Yonekura Y, et al: A new zinc-62/copper-62 generator as a copper-62 source for PET radiopharmaceuticals, *J Nucl Med* 30:1938, 1989.
7. Green MA, Mathias CJ, Welch MJ, et al: Copper-62-labeled pyruvaldehyde bis(N^4-methylthiosemicarbazonato) copper (II): synthesis and evaluation as a positron emission tomography tracer for cerebral and myocardial perfusion, *J Nucl Med* 31:1989, 1990.
8. Green MW, Tucker WD: An improved gallium-68 cow, *Int J Appl Radiat Isot* 12:62, 1961.
9. Green MA, Welch MJ: Gallium radiopharmaceutical chemistry, *Nucl Med Biol* 16:435, 1989.
10. Leveille J, Demonceau G, DeRoo M, et al: Characterization of technetium-99m-L,L-ECD for brain perfusion imaging. Part 2. Biodistribution and brain imaging in humans, *J Nucl Med* 30:1902, 1989.
11. Loberg MD, Fields AT: Chemical structure of technetium-99m-labeled N-(216-dimethylphenyl-carbamoylmethyl)-iminodiacetic acid (Tc-HIDA), *Int J Appl Rad Isot* 29:167, 1978.
12. Loc'h C, Maziere B, Comar D: A new generator for ionic gallium-68, *J Nucl Med* 21:171, 1980.
13. Neirinckx RD, Burke JF, Harrison RG, et al: The retention mechanism of technetium-99m-HMPAO: intracellular reaction with glutathione, *J Cereb Blood Flow Metab* 8:54, 1988.
14. Robinson GD, Zielinski FW, Lee AW: Zn-62/Cu-62 generator: a convenient source of copper-62 radiopharmaceuticals, *Int J Appl Rad Isot* 31:111, 1980.
15. Sands H, Delano ML, Gallagher BM: Uptake of hexakis (t-butylisonitrile) technetium (I) and hexakis (isopropylisonitrile) technetium (I) by neonatal rat myocytes and human erythrocytes, *J Nucl Med* 27:404, 1986.
16. Taylor Jr A, Eshima D, Fritzberg AR, et al: Comparison of iodine-131 OIH and technetium-99m MAG$_3$ renal imaging in volunteers, *J Nucl Med* 27:795, 1986.

SUGGESTED READINGS

Choppin G, Rydberg J, Liljenzin JO : *Radiochemistry and nuclear chemistry*, ed 2, Oxford, England, 1995, Butterworth-Heinemann.

Fowler JS, Wolf AP: The synthesis of carbon-11, fluorine-18 and nitrogen-13 labeled radiotracers for biomedical applications. In *Nuclear Science Series, Nuclear Medicine*, Technical Information Center, U.S. Department of Energy, 1982.

Kilbourn MR: Fluorine-18 labeling of radiopharmaceuticals. In *Nuclear Science Series, Nuclear Medicine*, Washington, DC, 1990, National Academy Press.

Kowalsky RJ, Perry JR: *Radiopharmaceuticals in nuclear medicine practice*, Connecticut, 1987, Appleton & Lange.

Krenning EP, Bakker WH, Kooij PPM, et al: Somatostatin receptor scintigraphy with Indium-111-DTPA-D-Phe^1-octreotide in man: metabolism, dosimetry and comparison with Iodine-123-Tyr-Octreotide. *J Nucl Med* 33:652, 1992.

Steigman J, Eckelman WC: Chemistry of technetium in medicine. In *Nuclear Science Series, Nuclear Medicine,* Washington, DC, 1992, National Academy Press.

Swanson DP, Chilton HM, Thrall JH: *Pharmaceuticals in medical imaging,* New York, 1990, Macmillan.

Verbruggen AM: Radiopharmaceuticals: state of the art, *Eur J Nucl Med* 17:346, 1990.

Welch MJ, Kilbourn MR: Positron emitters for imaging. In *Freeman L, ed: Freeman and Johnson's clinical radionuclide imaging,* ed 3, vol 1, Orlando, Fla, 1984, Grune & Stratton.

Marleen M. Moore

Radiation Safety in Nuclear Medicine

chapter 7

Objectives

List and define units of radiation, absorbed dose, and dose equivalent.

Discuss sources of radiation exposure to the general population.

List the regulatory limits for radiation exposure.

Define ALARA and detail a comprehensive ALARA program for nuclear medicine.

Discuss patient radiation exposure, and describe exposure (with examples) to critical organs.

Explain the appropriate use of ionization chambers.

Use Geiger counters and scintillation detectors for laboratory surveys and decontamination procedures.

Describe the appropriate clinical use of the dose calibrator to be in compliance with federal and state regulations.

Discuss the use of personnel monitoring devices.

List the criteria for posting warning signs for exposure to radiation.

Discuss the receipt, disposition, and disposal of radioactive materials and radioactivity.

Discuss the methods of testing for and controlling radioactive contamination.

Define the criteria that constitute a misadministration.

Discuss the necessary precautions when using therapeutic radionuclides.

Describe the effects of ionizing radiation.

INTRODUCTION

The practice of nuclear medicine includes handling radioactive materials and exposure to radiation. To do this safely requires precautions to ensure minimum radiation exposure to personnel and the general population and only appropriate exposure to patients. In addition, procedures must be utilized to prevent contamination from unsealed sources. Federal and state regulations mandate many of these policies and procedures. The medical use of radioactive materials is regulated by the Nuclear Regulatory Commission, either directly or in agreement with states. The practices discussed in this chapter comply with these regulations, which provide for safe use of radioactive materials.

UNITS

A system of measurement is required to determine the amount of radioactivity used and to quantify the resulting radiation. Nuclear medicine now officially uses the system of units known as the Système International d' Unités (SI), which was introduced in Chapter 1. The commonly used traditional system of units and appropriate conversion factors are listed in Table 7-1.

Three important concepts of determining radiation levels are exposure, absorbed dose, and dose equivalent.

Radiation Exposure

X ray and gamma radiations have the property of producing ions, that is, liberating electrical charge when interacting with matter. A common method of determining the intensity of x ray or gamma radiation is to measure the magnitude of the electrical charge (of either sign) liberated in air. The quantity that denotes the amount of electrical charge per unit mass of air is termed the exposure. The definition of exposure (X) is the quotient Q/m, where Q is the sum of the electrical charges of all the ions of one sign produced in a volume of air whose mass is m, that is:

$$X = Q/m$$

There are several important aspects to the concept of exposure.
1. The concept applies only to ionizing electromagnetic radiation, such as x rays and gamma rays, and not to particle radiations, such as beta particles and neutrons.
2. Air is the interacting medium.
3. The measured endpoint is the amount of ionization per unit mass of air.
4. It becomes operationally difficult to fulfill the requirements for measuring exposure for photon energies less than several keV and more than several MeV. Accordingly, the use of this concept is limited to photons with energies of 3 MeV or less.
5. Devices expressly designed to measure exposure are referred to as air ionization chamber instruments.

The concept of exposure is expressed in fundamental units of coulomb/kg of air in SI units. In traditional units, radiation exposure is measured in Roentgens. A roentgen (R) is defined as 2.58×10^{-4} coulomb/kg of air. This is also equivalent to the older definition of 1 electrostatic unit of charge (ESU)/cm^3 of air at standard temperature and pressure.

Absorbed Dose

Radiation damage often depends on the amount of energy absorbed per unit mass of the irradiated material. The quantity that specifies the energy imparted to a material by any type of ionizing radiation per unit mass at the point of interest is termed the absorbed dose. Absorbed dose (D) is defined as the quotient of E/m, where E is the energy absorbed by material of mass m:

$$D = E/m$$

The SI unit for this quantity is the gray (Gy), which is defined as the energy deposition of 1 joule/kg of material. The concept of absorbed dose applies to all categories of ionizing radiation dosimetry, to all materials, and to all forms of ionizing radiation. The traditional unit is the rad, which is defined as energy deposition of 0.01 joule/kg. Thus, 1 Gy = 100 rad.

Dose Equivalent

The dose equivalent concept originated from the observation that different biologic effects can be produced for the same absorbed dose by different types of radiation. The dose equivalent is a computed quantity that expresses a measure of the biologic harm imparted to tissue. The dose equivalent (H) at a point of interest in tissue is defined by the following equation:

$$H = DQN$$

where D is absorbed dose, Q is a modifying quantity called the quality factor, and N is the product of all other appropriate modifying factors that apply to a given situation. The quality factor concept is based on research studies that have shown that the biologic effects of ionizing radiation are not solely determined by the absorbed dose but also by the density of ionization produced along the path of the ionizing particles. A measure of the ion density along the path of an energetic particle is the particle's linear energy transfer (LET), which expresses the energy transfer per unit path length. The LET of an ionizing particle is often

Quantity	Name	Symbol	Relationship to replaced unit
Radiation exposure	X unit	C per kg	3881 Roentgens per X unit
Absorbed dose	Gray	Gy	100 rad per gray
Dose equivalent	Sievert	Sv	100 rem per sievert

Table 7-1 SI derived units adopted for specifying ionizing radiation levels

expressed in the units of keV/mm or keV/μ. The quality factors used for radiation safety purposes have been obtained from measurements of the relative biologic effect (RBE) of specific types of radiation as a function of the LET of the ionizing radiation. The ratio of the absorbed doses of a reference type of radiation and the type of radiation in question that produces the same biologic effect is the RBE. For example, if 20 cGy (20 rad) of x rays (250 kVp lightly filtered x radiation is generally used as the reference radiation for RBE determinations) produce the same biologic endpoint as 1 cGy (1 rad) due to neutron irradiation, the RBE of the neutron radiation is 20. Table 7-2 shows the QF dependence on LET; Table 7-3 lists QF values for several types of ionizing radiation.

Although several modifying factors have been proposed, the only one commonly employed is the quality factor.

The special unit of dose equivalent is the sievert (Sv). The dose equivalent in Sv is numerically equal to the absorbed dose in Gy multiplied by the appropriate modifying factors. The use of this concept is illustrated by the following example:

A radiation worker employed at a cyclotron facility incurs whole body absorbed doses of 2 cGys due to gamma radiation and 0.1 cGy due to fast neutrons. Compute the worker's whole body dose equivalent H.

Table 7-2	Relationship between quality factor and linear energy transfer

LET (keV/μ in water)	QF
3.5 or less	1
3.5-7.0	1-2
7.0-23	2-5
23-53	5-20
53-175	10-20

Table 7-3	Quality factor values for selected types of ionizing radiation

Type of radiation	QF
X rays, gamma rays, beta particles, and electrons	1
Thermal neutrons	5
Neutrons	20
Protons	20
Alpha particles	20

From U.S. Nuclear Regulatory Commission Title 10, Code of Federal Regulations. Part 20. Standards for protection against radiation, *Fed Reg* 56(98):23390, 1991.

$$H \text{ (cSv)} = \Sigma \text{ (absorbed dose in cGy for each type of radiation multiplied by the corresponding QF)}$$
$$= (2 \times 1) \text{ gamma radiation} + (0.1 \times 20) \text{ fast neutrons}$$
$$= 4 \text{ cSv}$$

where the symbol Σ denotes the sum of the terms described in parentheses, and the QF values are taken from Table 7-3. In traditional units the dose equivalent is the rem. This is numerically equal to the absorbed dose in rad multiplied by the quality factor. Thus, 1 Sv = 100 rem.

To provide the example above, it was necessary to go outside of the medical situation. For the radiations used in a medical setting, the quality factor equals one, so the absorbed dose and dose equivalent will be equal. Further, when using traditional units, the exposure in roentgens will be approximately equal to the dose in rad to tissue at that location.

EFFECTIVE DOSE EQUIVALENT

The radiation doses imparted to the various organs of the body due to either external irradiation or the presence of internal radioactivity can vary markedly depending on the type of radiation and, in the case of internal radioactivity, on the biologic characteristics of the material. The International Commission on Radiation Protection (ICRP) has introduced a quantity, the effective dose equivalent, which reflects not only specific organ doses but also the relative radiosensitivity of the organs.[9] The effective dose equivalent (H_E), is defined as

$$H_E = \Sigma w_i H_i$$

where H_i is the dose equivalent of a specified organ and w_i is the corresponding weighting factor. The weighting factor (w_i) represents the ratio of the radiation detriment resulting from a given dose equivalent to a specific organ to the detriment due to a uniform whole body dose equivalent of the same magnitude. The tissue weighting factors are based on the assumption that the health detriment associated with a given dose to a specific organ can be expressed as the product of the probability of harm and the severity of the resultant illness.

The numeric values of the weighting factors recommended by the ICRP are shown in Table 7-4. As an example of the significance of the values, it is assumed that the radiation detriment or risk of a given dose to the red bone marrow is about 12% of the corresponding risk of receiving a uniform dose of the same amount to the whole body. The attraction of the effective whole body dose equivalent is that it provides, in a single computed quantity, a measure or index of the biologic harm of radiation exposure even in those cases in which the body is not uniformly irradiated. Use of the weighting factors shown in Table 7-4 results in indices of both somatic (cancer induction) and genetic risks associated with radiation doses. The weighting factor for the gonads can be omitted, and the resultant recalculated weighting factors can be used to compute cancer-induced risks alone. This approach yields a computed effective dose equivalent that is generally called the *somatic dose index*. For example, the somatic dose index for a diagnostic nuclear medicine procedure requiring the administration of 3 mCi of ^{99m}Tc colloid

has been computed to be 1.7 mSv (170 mrem).[4] This means that the somatic radiation risk of the examination is approximately the same as that associated with a uniform whole body dose equivalent of 1.7 mSv (170 mrem).

SOURCES OF RADIATION EXPOSURE

The primary source of exposure to much of the population is from what is called background radiation. Humans have always been exposed to background levels caused by the following:

1. Terrestrial radiation from the presence of naturally occurring radioactivity in the soil, primarily due to uranium and its by-products. The levels of radiation may vary significantly, depending on the location. For example, the Colorado Plateau in the Rocky Mountains has higher levels of terrestrial radiation due to greater amounts of uranium.
2. Cosmic radiation that results from the interaction of particles from outer space with the atmosphere and high energy photons from outer space. Cosmic radiation levels will be higher at a higher altitude due to less shielding from the atmosphere.
3. Internal radioactivity due to naturally occurring radioactivity deposited in the body. An example is ^{40}K, a naturally occurring isotope of potassium.

The average annual whole body radiation dose

Table 7-4	Organs and weighting factors used for computing effective whole-body dose equivalent*

Organ/tissue	Weighting factor
Gonads	0.25
Breast	0.15
Red bone marrow	0.12
Lungs	0.12
Thyroid	0.03
Bone surfaces	0.03
Whole body	1.0
Remaining tissues†	0.30

*Average for a large population consisting of persons of both sexes and all ages.
†The factor for the remaining tissues is equally (0.06) divided among the remaining five organs or tissues having the highest doses.

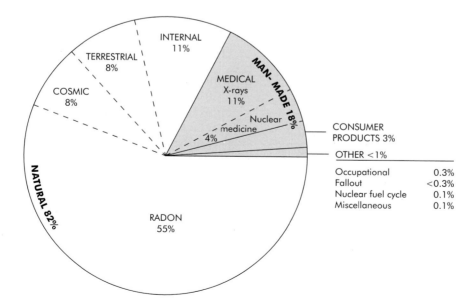

Figure 7-1 Percentage contribution of various radiation sources to the total average effective dose equivalent in the U.S. population. (From Ionizing radiation exposure of the population of the United States, *National Council on Radiation Protection Report No. 93*, Washington, DC, 1987, The Council.)

equivalent in the United States is approximately 0.82 mSv (82 mrem)/yr, varying from about 0.65 mSv (65 mrem)/yr in the Atlantic and Gulf Coast regions to about 1.4 mSv(140 mrem)/yr in the Colorado plateau. Recent estimates of the annual radiation dose to the population have also included the contribution due to radon gas. The estimated whole body dose equivalent due to radon is approximately 2 mSv (200 mrem)/yr, though the tissue of concern is only the lung.[7] Thus, the average total estimated whole body dose equivalent is 3 mSv (300 mrem)/yr, of which 1 mSv(100 mrem)/yr is due to penetrating radiations (Figure 7-1).

The only other significant source of radiation to the general population in the United States is due to medical radiation exposure, presumably for beneficial reasons. As shown in Table 7-5, the average per capita radiation dose equivalent due to medical radiation is approximately 0.53 mSv (53 mrem)/yr.[12] This estimate includes 0.39 mSv (39 mrem)/yr due to diagnostic x rays and 0.14 mSv (14 mrem)/yr due to use of radiopharmaceuticals.

The remaining contributors to the average per capita radiation dose equivalent are consumer products, nuclear industry, weapons testing, and, perhaps of most interest, occupational exposure.[6] Although the average whole body dose equivalent for nuclear medicine personnel is estimated to be 3 mSv (300 mrem)/yr, the numbers of personnel are small (approximately 10,000) compared with the total population. Thus, the dose averaged over the population results in about 0.001 mSv (0.1 mrem) of the occupational exposure contribution. The total annual effective dose equivalent due to both natural and man-made sources in the United States is estimated to be 3.6 mSv (360 mrem)/yr.[12]

Table 7-5	Annual effective dose equivalent in the United States population	
Source	**Dose (mSv)**	**% of total**
Natural sources		
Radon	2.0	55
Other	1.0	27
Medical		
Diagnostic x rays	0.39	11
Radiopharmaceuticals	0.14	4
Occupational	0.009	0.3
Consumer products	0.05-0.13	2.0
Nuclear industry, weapons testing research, etc.	0.0011	1.0
ROUNDED TOTALS	3.6	100

From Ionizing radiation exposure of the population of the United States, *National Council of Radiation Protection Report No. 93*, Washington, DC, 1987, The Council.

RADIATION DOSE RECOMMENDATIONS AND REGULATIONS

The benefits of the use of radiation have been recognized for over a century. The potential for harm was also recognized shortly after radiation was first used for medical and therapeutic uses. Various advisory groups exist to review the use of radiation, evaluate the risk, and make recommendations on safe use, including exposure levels for personnel and the general population. The most prominent international organization is the International Commission on Radiological Protection (ICRP). In the United States, the National Council on Radiation Protection and Measurements (NCRP), a private organization, provides radiation dose recommendations that often serve as the basis for adoption by regulatory agencies.

Regulations for use of radioactive materials and radiation exposure are enforced by a number of federal and state agencies, primarily the Nuclear Regulatory Commission (NRC). This agency is charged by Congress to regulate the use of by-product radioactive materials. This is accomplished either directly or, in many states, indirectly. In "agreement" states the NRC delegates the authority for regulation to the state with the proviso that state regulations may not conflict with federal regulations. In agreement states the regulations extend to use of all radioactive materials, since these states are not restricted to just use of by-product materials.

Other agencies that regulate various portions of the medical use of radioactive materials are the Food and Drug Administration (FDA), Department of Transportation (DOT), Environmental Protection Agency (EPA), and Occupational Safety and Health Administration (OSHA). However, it is the regulations of the NRC with which the worker in nuclear medicine must be familiar.

The NCRP provides recommendations for radiation workers and for areas with sources of radiation that result in exposure to the general population.[16] The current recommendations are shown in Table 7-6. The current federal regulations for radiation workers due to occupational exposure are shown in Table 7-7. These reflect the regulations that were implemented by the NRC in January of 1994.[22] These regulatory and recommended limits are for just external and internal occupational exposure and exclude background level radiation and personal medical exposure.

ALARA Philosophy

The NRC requires that licensees, including those in agreement states, make every reasonable effort to keep radiation exposures and regulated releases of radioactive materials as low as reasonably achievable. This philosophy of "as low as reasonably achievable" is the basis of the acronym ALARA. A statement signed by an institution's administrator who has authority to commit funds must be submitted as part of a license. This commitment assures that resources will be allocated to implement policies and procedures that minimize occupational exposure. It is the belief of the NRC that

medical occupational exposures can be maintained at values of 10% or less of the limits given in the federal regulations.[5,11,19]

PATIENT DOSIMETRY

The amount of activity used for patient studies also results in an absorbed dose. The consideration of what constitutes an acceptable dose for clinical studies is different in that patients receive a benefit from the study via the information provided to the referring physician.

The absorbed dose received depends on the type of radioactivity, the amount of activity administered, the distribution, amount of time in each organ, and the physical relationship to other organs. A straightforward method for calculating the dose has been developed, called the Medical Internal Radiation Dose Committee (MIRD) system. However, in day-to-day operations it is rare that such a dose calculation is needed. In most cases a quick estimate of the dose to one or more organs will suffice. The radiopharmaceutical package insert contains a table that gives doses for the "average" patient as a function of administered activity. A simple calculation using this table and the activity administered provides the approximate dose, which may have been requested by the clinician or patient. In cases where a more accurate dose calculation is required, a medical physicist is often consulted.

| Table 7-6 | Dose-limiting recommendations of the National Council on Radiation Protection |

Category of recommendation	Recommended effective dose equivalent
Occupation exposure	
Whole body (prospective)	50 mSv (5 rem) in any 1 year
Skin	500 mSv (50 rem) in any 1 year
Hands	750 mSv (75 rem) in any 1 year
Forearms	300 mSv (30 rem) in any 1 year
Other organs, tissues, and organ systems	150 mSv (15 rem) in any 1 year
Fetus of radiation worker	5 mSv (0.5 rem) in gestation period
General public or occasionally exposed individuals	Up to 5 mSv (0.5 rem) in any 1 year
Individual (whole body)	
Average to population (genetic and somatic)	1.7 mSv (0.17 rem) in any 1 year
Students (whole body)	1 mSv (0.1 rem) in any 1 year

Modified from Recommendations on limits for exposure to ionizing radiation, *National Council of Radiation Protection Report No. 91*, Washington, DC, 1987, The Council.

RADIATION SAFETY AND LABORATORY INSTRUMENTATION

Instruments used in the Radiation Safety Program are designed to allow detection ranging from extremely small amounts of activity associated with wipe tests to the much higher levels of the exposure rates around generators or patients containing therapeutic amounts of radioactivity. To meet these requirements a variety of instruments are required.

Survey Instruments

Geiger-Mueller (GM) instruments. A portable survey meter utilizing a GM tube is used for area surveys for contamination. The GM tube (see Chapter 3) provides high gas amplification, resulting in an ability to detect individual ionizing events. The GM meter is operated to display the rate at which the individual events are detected, usually using a ratemeter, which is calibrated in counts per minute (cpm). This simplicity of design results in an instrument that is inexpensive and reliable.

The GM probe consists of a gas-filled tube with a metal housing. Usually, one section of the housing is replaced with a thin window, such as mica, which is cov-

| Table 7-7 | Federal dose limits for occupational exposure of radiation workers |

Dose category	Dose equivalent limit per calendar quarter (13 weeks), except for fetus
Whole body, head and trunk, active blood forming organs, lenses of the eyes, and gonads	12.5 mSv (1.25 rem)
Hands, forearms, feet, and ankles	187.5 mSv (18.75 rem)
Skin of whole body	75 mSv (7.50 rem)
Fetus of radiation worker	5 mSv (0.5 rem) during entire gestation period

ered with a removable cap, often plastic. With the cap removed, all except the lowest energy beta particles (e.g., ^{3}H) are able to penetrate the thin window and are readily detected. With the cap in place, only higher energy beta particles and x rays and gamma rays penetrate. A typical commercial meter is shown in Figure 7-2, *A.*

A GM meter is not the best instrument for measuring exposure rates. GM meters are often energy dependent and also have a large dead time, resulting in significant loss at high count rates. However, it is possible to calibrate a GM meter in mR/hr with a calibration source of an energy comparable to the energy of radiations that will be monitored. The unit must be calibrated annually, in accordance with license requirements. At calibration the count rate or exposure reading from a check source, usually attached to the side of the meter, is recorded on a label attached to the meter. Before each use of the meter, a reading of the check source must be obtained to ensure proper operation.

Ionization chamber instruments. Survey instruments operated in the ionization region of the gas amplification curve are designed to measure radiation exposure or exposure rate. These instruments operate in the current mode rather than pulse mode, and so require the detection of a large number of events. Survey meters are unable to detect very small amounts of activity, such as with contamination. Adequate sensitivity for low exposure levels is obtained by using a rather large air-filled chamber (Figure 7-2, *B*). Ionization survey meters may be used accurately to measure high exposure rates and should be used when surveying a large source of radioactivity, such as a generator, or a patient treated with a therapeutic amount of radioactive iodine.

Portable ionization chamber instruments must also be calibrated annually and must have a check source reading obtained at calibration. The check source often is sent separately and mounted in a convenient location in the radiopharmacy when returned. As with GM meters, a reading of the check source is made before each use.

A portable ionization chamber may have a removable cap. This allows detection of the presence of higher energy beta particles, such as those from ^{32}P or ^{89}Sr. The concept of exposure is defined only for x rays and gamma rays, however, so a measurement of beta-particle intensity is not possible.

Scintillation instruments. Scintillation detectors utilizing a sodium iodide crystal are found as portable devices and also as fixed devices such as well counters. As portable devices, a probe consisting of a crystal and photomultiplier tube is connected to electronics similar to that found with a GM tube. The high sensitivity of the scintillation detector makes it particularly useful for detecting very low levels of activity (Figure 7-2, *C*). For quantitative measurements, however, it is necessary to calibrate the detector with the radionuclide of interest and also to use the same geometry. A system such as this may be used, for example, in checking the thyroid of personnel who have cared for ^{131}I-therapy patients.

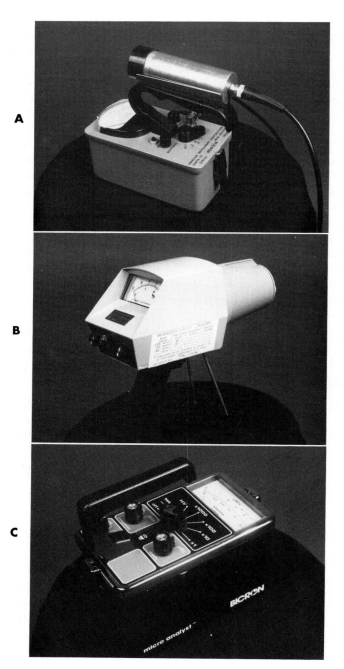

Figure 7-2 Variety of portable radiation survey instruments. **A,** Geiger-Muller (GM) device with an end window probe. **B,** Ionization chamber-based instrument of the "cutie pie" design. **C,** Scintillation detector (NaI) survey instrument.

MEASUREMENT OF RADIOACTIVITY

Well Counter

A sodium iodide well counter is used for determination of radioactivity, usually in dpm, from wipe tests and leak tests. As described in Chapter 3, the well counter may be used to accurately quantitate very small amounts of radioactivity. With a well counter it is necessary to determine the minimum radioactivity that may be detected (MDA) for any radionuclide that will be used. The MDA will depend on the background counting statistics, counting time, and detector efficiency

$$MDA = \frac{4.66 \sim_b + 3}{Kt}$$

where $\sim_b$ is the standard deviation of the background, K is the detector efficiency (with conversion to μCi, and t is the counting time. The conditions of the radioactive materials license require that instruments used for wipe tests be able to detect contamination of less than 0.005 μCi.

Routine quality control of the well counter should also include daily calibration with a standard, usually ^{137}Cs. The gain or high voltage at which proper calibration occurs should be recorded. A 1-minute count at a fixed window width should also be recorded. This allows monitoring for any drift in the system. Monthly, a check of the FWHM of the ^{137}Cs photopeak should be obtained. Spread in the photopeak may be, among other possibilities, indicative of degradation of the crystal. See Chapter 3 for additional discussion of testing.

Radionuclide dose calibrator. The radionuclide dose calibrator is an ionization chamber that allows assay of gamma emitters. The operation and quality control testing for a dose calibrator are described in Chapter 3 and discussed later in this chapter under Operational Radiation Safety.

Airborne Activity Samplers

The concentration of radioactivity in air can be determined with the aid of a variety of equipment in operation, termed air sampling. Such methods as filtration, precipitation, and continuous measurement are used. The devices most commonly used to evaluate airborne activity levels associated with nuclear medicine procedures involving ^{133}Xe gas, labeled aerosols, ^{131}I sodium iodide, and so forth are ion chamber and filtration samplers.

Ion chamber samplers. The method most generally applicable to radioactive gases (e.g., ^{133}Xe) is to continuously draw the air to be sampled through a sensitive ion chamber. The resultant ion current produced due to the radioactivity in the air can be converted directly into the air concentration of the radionuclide. Such monitors continuously draw air through the ion chamber at a known rate, detect the radioactivity, and display the computed concentration, typically in μCi/m^3. Most radioactive gases may be monitored with this type of instrument (Figure 7-3).

Filtration samplers. The presence of either radioiodine or labeled aerosols in air can be monitored by assaying the activity deposited by air in appropriate filtering media when the air is drawn through the filters at a known rate. For example, airborne radioiodine activity is evaluated by drawing a measured quantity of air through activated charcoal filters to efficiently trap the radioiodine. The trapped activity is then assayed by counting the filter contents in a scintillation well counter of known sensitivity for the sampled radionuclide. The quotient of trapped activity to sampled air volume yields the average airborne concentration, provided the trapping efficiency is 100%. The airborne concentration of ^{99m}Tc aerosols can be evaluated by a similar method, except that laminated glass filters are used rather than activated charcoal filters.

Small, compact personal air samplers that allow the wearer to perform work without interference are commercially available. These devices consist of a pump unit in series with a filter—typically, an activated charcoal filter to trap radioiodine or a paper filter to trap radioactive particles.

Air Flow Measuring Devices

A variety of ventilation measurements must be periodically made to demonstrate that certain nuclear medicine procedures involving radioactive gases or volatiles are being performed in a safe environment. For example, the performance of fumehoods is tested by

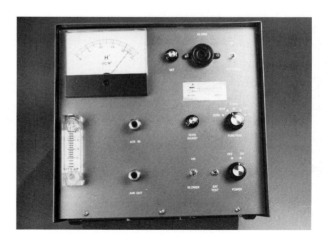

Figure 7-3 Ion chamber air sampler that provides instantaneous readings of airborne activity.

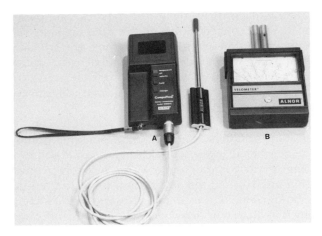

Figure 7-4 Two types of anemometers. **A,** Thermal (hot-wire) anemometer. **B,** Gravitational anemometer.

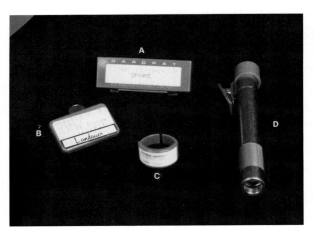

Figure 7-5 Variety of personnel monitoring devices. **A,** Photographic film badge. **B,** Thermoluminescent dosimeter body monitor. **C,** Thermoluminescent dosimeter ring monitor. **D,** Pocket ionization chamber dosimeter.

measuring the average face velocity of the air being drawn through the hood opening. Similarly, the negative pressure required of rooms in which ^{133}Xe gas is used can be established by measuring the rates of ventilation input and output. A variety of instruments are available for making such measurements. These devices, often termed *anemometers,* use either gravitational or thermal methods to measure the linear flow rate (e.g., in feet per minute) of the air movement at the point of measurement. Figure 7-4 shows a variety of anemometers. Air flow measurements are often made by the engineering or safety services staff in the institution.

PERSONNEL DOSIMETERS

Personnel exposed to ionizing radiation are monitored to determine their occupational exposure. Although this primarily consists of monitoring external exposure, it is also necessary to assess the need to monitor internal exposure and, if necessary, incorporate it into a worker's total exposure history. External monitoring can be accomplished by using a photographic film, thermoluminescent, or pocket dosimeter (Figure 7-5).

Photographic Film Dosimeters

Photographic film is sensitive to ionizing radiation, and when it is used as a monitor, the amount of film darkening is a measurement of the radiation exposure. For use as a monitor, a film strip in a light-tight cover is placed in a special holder. The combination of the film strip and the holder constitutes the film monitor and is referred to as a film badge. This film badge has a small, open window that allows the film to be exposed with most x ray and gamma radiations and high energy beta radiations. The film badge also contains a set of plastic and metal filters. Since different types and en-

ergies of radiation will be attenuated differently by these filters, the pattern on the processed film may be used to determine the type, approximate energy, and intensity of the exposure. Since film response is energy dependent, this approximate energy determination allows use of a film energy response calibration curve. Such monitors can be used to measure exposures as low as 0.01 mSv (10 mrem) and as high as several Sv. Although limited by the large size of the film badge, the shape may be adapted so that film badges may be used to monitor the whole body, hands, wrist, etc., depending on where the film badge is worn. Some advantages of film badges include the following:

1. *Permanent record.* The manufacturer of the film badge retains the film. If a suspicious reading is noted, the film may be reread. This is particularly useful when an employee receives an exposure that is of an energy or type of radiation that should not have been encountered, where a review of the film may indicate that the film was worn incorrectly or handled improperly.
2. *Energy and nature of exposure.* The pattern on the film may indicate the angle of exposure, whether the exposure was a series or single event, and the energy, which may be correlated with the employee's working environment.
3. *Cost.* Film badges remain the least expensive way of monitoring personnel. They are inexpensive enough that it is possible to monitor employees who may receive little if any exposure, thus providing both reassurance and an assessment of the working environment.

There are, however, disadvantages to the use of film dosimetry, including:

1. *Energy dependence.* Due to the energy dependence, the film must be properly placed between the filters in the badge holder or errone-

ously high readings will be observed. A reread-ing of the film will identify this if it is noted that no filter pattern is present.

2. *Fading.* Film also fades with time, so it may not be used for extended monitoring. Typically, film cannot be accurately evaluated if returned beyond 3 months.

3. *Size.* The size of film limits the ability to moni-tor fingers or eye level.

Thermoluminescent Dosimeters

A small semiconductor material called a thermolumi-nescent dosimeter (TLD) may also be used to monitor radiation exposure. When radiation interacts with a TLD, the energy is stored in the material. When heated, the energy is released as light, and the amount of light is proportional to the amount of energy stored. The TLD most commonly used for monitoring is lithium fluoride, usually found as chips that are 1/8 inch square. This size is readily incorporated into rings for finger monitoring and plastic-encased clips or elastic bands for attachment to eyeglasses.

The advantages of a TLD are primarily its size and limited energy dependence. In addition, it is relatively insensitive to temperature and humidity and does not fade with time. Where the circumstance warrants, as in low exposure areas, TLD monitors may be utilized for more extensive periods, typically 3 months.

One disadvantage of TLD is that, once it is heated and the reading is recorded, the only permanent record is the reading. It is not possible to reread the TLD should there be a questionable result. The signed, written record maintained by the supplier is, however, a legal document. Another disadvantage is the cost. In situations where dosimeters are exchanged monthly, the TLD is more expensive.

Pocket Dosimeters

When it is necessary to quickly evaluate possible radia-tion exposure, a pocket dosimeter may be used. It may be used as a second monitor in high dose rate opera-tions, to provide immediate information to other per-sonnel such as nurses caring for therapy patients, or to evaluate possible exposure in new operations. There are two general types of pocket dosimeters that may be used. These are small ionization chambers with direct or indirect read and compact GM-based digital dosim-eters.

Pocket ionization chambers are designed to measure the ionization events within an air-filled chamber. Both direct and indirect read chambers are constructed of a cylinder of metal (Figure 7-5, *D*). Direct read chambers operate on the principle of an electroscope. Exposure to radiation results in discharge of the chamber, which may be seen by looking through the chamber and view-

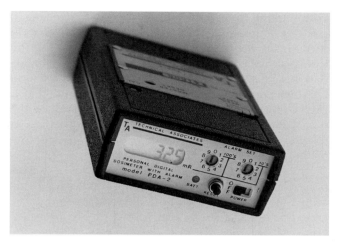

Figure 7-6   Digital pocket dosimeter with numeric readout and adjustments for audio alarm.

ing the position of a hairline on a scale. With indirect read chambers, it is necessary to use a special reader to determine the exposure. This type of dosimeter is subject to erroneous readings due to electrical leakage and being hit or dropped. They are also not accurate for extended exposures.

Digital dosimeters that utilize a GM tube have fea-tures that make them particularly useful (Figure 7-6). The exposure and/or exposure rate may be provided on a digital display, allowing simple evaluation of the radiation field. Many have audible signals, emitting chirps at a frequency proportional to the intensity of the radiation. The units are small, easily fitting into a pocket or clipped onto a belt. They are not subject to erroneous readings due to physical conditions or rough handling by personnel.

PERSONNEL MONITORING

Personnel who are working in areas where there is a reasonable likelihood of receiving a measurable expo-sure to radiation should be issued personnel dosim-eters. The conditions of the radioactive materials license require that dosimeters be issued to personnel who could receive in excess of 10% of the maximum permissible dose (MPD) (i.e., 500 mrem/yr).[22] Many workers are unlikely to receive such a radiation expo-sure but should be monitored to demonstrate compli-ance with institutional ALARA goals, to provide useful information to employees regarding their working en-vironment, and to provide data for the Radiation Safety Officer (RSO) to assess any changes in the working en-vironment.

The primary monitor that is issued should be worn between the neck and waist to monitor the whole body exposure. A film badge is often used for personnel monitoring. The whole body badge monitors the exposure to the trunk. Film badges are usually exchanged monthly, although a more frequent cycle is possible. In addition to the whole body badge, monitors for the hands are issued to workers handling radioactive materials. Ring badges containing a TLD chip are often used for this. The ring badge is worn on the hand that is likely to receive the highest exposure. Furthermore, the ring badge is worn under protective gloves to prevent accidental contamination of the ring that does not reflect exposure to the skin and hand.

The reports that provide the results of personnel monitoring should be reviewed and initialed when received by the RSO. Any unusual exposures should be promptly investigated (Table 7-8). If the exposure exceeds ALARA Level I, it is necessary to evaluate the cause. If the exposure exceeds ALARA Level II, the employee must be notified in writing and an explanation must be generated and corrective action proposed. A summary report of personnel monitoring, giving any Level I or II exposures, should be included in the quarterly Radiation Safety Committee meeting. Depending on the size of the institution, either the original or a duplicate report should be posted for personnel to review and initial. Records of personnel monitoring must be maintained as permanent records.

For the pregnant worker, other conditions may exist. As soon as a worker learns she is pregnant, she should notify her supervisor and the Radiation Safety Officer. The pregnant employee should read the information on the risks of radiation in pregnancy, as contained in USNRC Regulatory Guide 8.36 *Radiation Dose to the Embryo/Fetus*. As a "declared pregnant worker" she will be asked to sign a statement that she is pregnant and has been informed of the risks. The exposure limits are 500 mrem to the fetus during gestation, not to exceed 50 mrem/mo. This is monitored by a separate badge, which should be worn at the abdomen. To provide quicker feedback on exposure, this badge may be exchanged more frequently than the whole body badge. Mutually agreed upon work restrictions may be in effect for a pregnant employee. Unless the worker's exposure will exceed 50 mrem/mo in a particular job, these restrictions should not affect the worker's choice of job assignments, particularly those that may result in financial gain (e.g., on-call). The employer must,

however, provide the pregnant employee with opportunities for work in situations that are likely to result in lower exposures. The worker may also choose not to declare pregnancy, in which case none of these conditions are in effect.

In addition to the monitoring that provides a permanent record, pocket dosimeters are useful in situations where there is the possibility for high exposure in a relatively short period. For example, the pregnant technologist working on-call should be able to obtain immediate exposure information, allowing for a change in working conditions if necessary. These monitors, however, do not provide the permanent record required by regulatory agencies.

Personnel Bioassays

Bioassays of radioactivity are methods used to determine the presence and amount of internal radioactivity resulting in an internal dose. In nuclear medicine the only practice routinely requiring bioassays is the handling of high activity therapeutic amounts of ^{131}I sodium iodide.[20] Personnel who handle therapeutic quantities of unsealed radioactive sodium iodide or who are in the room during patient administration of these amounts must have a thyroid bioassay between 6 and 72 hours following involvement. Personnel handling lesser amounts, such as for hyperthyroid treatments or when handling encapsulated material, need less frequent assays. However, a consistent policy with a 6- to 72-hour time frame helps prevent forgotten bioassays.

The bioassay is performed by taking a count of the level of the thyroid in a manner analogous to a thyroid uptake. Using a sensitivity calculation for ^{131}I, the count is then converted to radioactivity. If an amount of radioiodine greater than a specified trigger limit is detected,[18] follow-up actions are required. The radioiodine procedures are reviewed to determine the cause. The employee is usually restricted from further iodine work until the activity has decreased to an acceptable level.

The contribution of the internal dose equivalent due to internal uptake must also be added to the individual's external dose. This may be done by contacting the

Table 7-8	ALARA investigation levels example reporting levels and timelines		
	Immediately	24 hours	30 days
Eye	75 rem/event	15 rem/event	15 rem/year
Skin or extremity	250 rem/event	50 rem/event	50 rem/year
Single organ	No criteria	No criteria	50 rem/year
Total body	25 rem/event	5 rem/event	5 rem/year

film badge supplier and requesting that the calculated dose be added to the individual's record. Negative findings do not require that any correction to the monitoring record be made.

CONTROL OF PERSONNEL RADIATION EXPOSURE

A major goal of a Radiation Safety Program is to maintain personnel exposures ALARA. Since nuclear medicine involves the handling of unsealed sources, techniques to minimize both external exposure and internal contamination are necessary. With use of the techniques described, the technologist in a busy department should be able to keep whole body exposure to no more than 30 to 40 mrem/mo and prevent internal contamination altogether.

External Exposure Control

External exposure may be minimized by utilizing three principles of radiation protection, as follows:
- Minimize the amount of *time* spent near a source of radiation.
- Maximize the *distance* from a source.
- Place *shielding* between the source and persons to be protected.

There are many situations where an awareness of the time factor may be used to reduce exposure. Tasks should be performed as swiftly as reasonable near radiation sources. New procedures should be evaluated to develop familiarity with the procedure before they are implemented near radioactivity. When positioning patients, technologists should spend only as long as necessary near the imaging table. Studies have shown that the most significant source of whole body exposure is the radiation emanating from the patient during the imaging procedure.[14]

In many situations, distance may be used. The exposure rate around a small source will decrease as the square of the distance, or *inverse square law* (see Chapter 1). Use of the inverse square law has a most dramatic effect when tongs are used to move vials containing large amounts of radioactivity. For example, a small vial containing a 10 mCi ^{131}I capsule will have an exposure rate at the surface (assume 1 cm) of 22 R/hr. If the vial is held for 1 minute, the dose to the fingertips would be

$$22 \text{ R/hr} \times 1/60 \text{ hr}^1 \text{ or } 370 \text{ mR}$$

By holding the vial with 25 cm tongs, as commonly found in hot labs, this skin dose is reduced by $(\frac{1}{25})^2$ or a factor of 625 resulting in a skin dose of approximately 0.6 mR.

When imaging a patient, technologists should re-

main as far from the patient as reasonable, while still providing necessary oversight of the patient's condition and image acquisition.

Shielding may be any material that attenuates the radiation, although lead is most often used. Nuclear medicine makes extensive use of specialized shielding of sources by using syringe shields (Figure 7-7), lead bricks, leaded glass, and lead containers. In this way the amount and weight of the lead is minimized, and the sources may be shielded individually. Other materials may also be used, such as concrete walls, which provide both structural barrier and shielding.

To determine the thickness of a type of shielding material that is needed, the half-value layer (HVL) of that material is useful information. As described in Chapter 1, the HVL is dependent on the material and the energy of radiation. Tables of HVLs are available for commonly used materials and radionuclides (Table 7-9). The HVL needed for shielding may be calculated exactly (see Chapter 1). Often, approximations are useful. For example, 7 HVLs will reduce the incident exposure rate by a factor of roughly 100%.

Examples of effective and necessary shielding are found throughout the hot lab. All materials in storage are locally shielded. When preparing materials, work is performed behind an L-block consisting of a lead base and front and leaded glass for viewing the working area. These are designed based on the highest energy and radioactivity in use. Lead bricks may be used for partial barriers and around areas such as water baths.

Syringe shields are very effective for reduction of exposure to the hands and fingers during patient injection. Most of the exposure to technologists is from ^{99m}Tc. Syringe shields thick enough to protect technologists from the energy and activities of ^{99m}Tc are readily available. Many departments have a standard size shield (e.g., 3 cc) issued to each technologist but

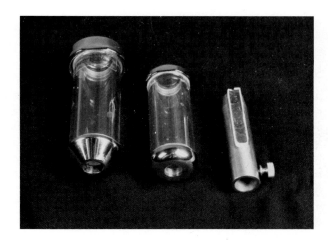

Figure 7-7 Syringe shields used for dose preparation and administration.

Table 7-9	Percentage of radiation transmitted through various half-value layers

Number HVL	Transmitted through an absorber
1	50
2	25
3	12.5
4	6.25
5	3.125
6	1.5625
7	0.78125
8	0.390625
9	0.1953125
10	0.09765625

have other sizes available in lesser quantities (see Figure 7-7). These should be used when preparing kits and must be used during patient injection.

RADIATION SAFETY PROGRAM

A comprehensive Radiation Safety Program consists of policies and procedures to minimize personnel radiation exposure and prevent contamination. Specific procedures and protocols are found in the institutional radioactive materials license. Often these protocols, including necessary forms, are taken directly or with minor modification from either NRC Regulatory Guide 10.8 *Guide for the Preparation of Applications for Medical Use Programs* or similar agreement state documents. These documents provide a very useful resource when developing specific protocols. A more general description of the required procedures and related radiation safety considerations follows.

Radiation Safety Committee and Radiation Safety Officer

A radioactive materials license issued to an institution requires that there be a Radiation Safety Committee and a designated Radiation Safety Officer. The Radiation Safety Committee oversees the use of radioactive materials. The committee must consist of an authorized user from each area using radioactive materials (e.g., nuclear medicine, laboratory, and radiation oncology), a nursing representative, and a representative of the management of the institution. The committee must meet quarterly to review aspects of the Radiation Safety Program. The committee must review the entire Radiation Safety Program annually and suggest changes or improvements.

A Radiation Safety Officer (RSO), who is responsible for implementing the Radiation Safety Program, must be named on the license. The RSO must directly oversee the day-to-day aspects of radiation safety, including maintenance of all required records, reports, and copies of regulations. The RSO reports to the Radiation Safety Committee and must have authority to directly inform the administration of radiation safety concerns so that quick corrective action can occur. The RSO may be a physician who meets specific training or certification criteria, a medical or health physicist, or a radiation safety technologist who has fulfilled rather extensive classroom and training requirements.

General Radiation Safety Practices and Training. All personnel handling radioactive materials must document that they have received acceptable training. In addition, each department must document that all personnel have received training in specific aspects of radiation safety when hired and then annually. A component of a Radiation Safety Program is that every department must have published general rules for safe handling of radioactive materials. These should include the following:
- Wear protective clothing such as laboratory coats.
- Wear disposable gloves while handling radioactive materials.
- Monitor hands for contamination before leaving the area.
- Use syringe shields.
- Do not eat, drink, smoke or apply cosmetics where radioactive material is stored or used.
- Do not store food or drink where radioactive material is stored or used.
- Wear personnel monitoring devices correctly.
- Dispose of radioactive waste in designated receptacles.
- Never pipette by mouth.
- Conduct surveys and wipe tests as required.
- Keep flood sources and other radioactive materials in shielded, labeled containers.
- Assay each patient dose before administration.
- Use a cart or wheelchair to move large sources.

Other aspects of initial and annual training should include a review of the license conditions, rights of radiation workers as given in *Form NRC-3 Notice to Employees* (Figure 7-8), emergency procedures, personnel monitoring reports, and radiation safety procedures specific to the institution. A written record of training, including the date of the training and a legible list of attendees, must be maintained.

Control of Radioactive Materials

Ordering and receiving. All radioactive materials that are ordered must be listed on the radioactive materials license and must not exceed any limits given on the li-

UNITED STATES NUCLEAR REGULATORY COMMISSION
Washington, D.C. 20555

NOTICE TO EMPLOYEES

STANDARDS FOR PROTECTION AGAINST RADIATION (PART 20); NOTICES, INSTRUCTIONS AND REPORTS TO WORKERS; INSPECTIONS (PART 19); EMPLOYEE PROTECTION

WHAT IS THE NUCLEAR REGULATORY COMMISSION?

The Nuclear Regulatory Commission is an independent Federal regulatory agency responsible for licensing and inspecting nuclear power plants and other commercial uses of radioactive materials.

WHAT DOES THE NRC DO?

The NRC's primary responsibility is to ensure that workers and the public are protected from unnecessary or excessive exposure to radiation and that nuclear facilities including power plants are constructed to high quality standards and operated in a safe manner. The NRC does this by establishing requirements in Title 10 of the Code of Federal Regulations (10 CFR) and in licenses issued to nuclear users.

WHAT RESPONSIBILITY DOES MY EMPLOYER HAVE?

Any company that conducts activities licensed by the NRC must comply with the NRC's requirements. If a company violates NRC requirements, it can be fined or have its license modified, suspended or revoked.

Your employer must tell you which NRC radiation requirements apply to your work and must post NRC Notices of Violation involving radiological working conditions.

WHAT IS MY RESPONSIBILITY?

For your own protection and the protection of your co-workers, you should know how NRC requirements relate to your work and should obey them. If you observe violations of the requirements, you should report them.

HOW DO I REPORT VIOLATIONS?

If you believe that violations of NRC rules or of the terms of the license have occurred, you should report them immediately to your supervisor. If you believe that adequate corrective action is not being taken, you may report this to an NRC inspector or the nearest NRC Regional Office.

WHAT IF I WORK IN A RADIATION AREA?

If you work with radioactive materials or in a radiation (controlled) area, the amount of radiation exposure that you may legally receive is limited by NRC Regulations. The limits on your exposure are contained in sections 20.101, 20.103, and 20.104 of Title 10 of the Code of Federal Regulations (10 CFR 20). While those are the maximum allowable limits, your employer should also keep your radiation exposure as far below those limits as is "reasonably achievable."

MAY I GET A RECORD OF MY RADIATION EXPOSURE?

Yes. Your employer is required to tell you, in writing, if you receive any radiation exposure above the limits set in the NRC regulations or your employer's license. In addition, if your job involves radiation, you may request from your employer a record of your annual radiation exposures and a written report of your total exposure when you leave your job.

HOW ARE VIOLATIONS OF NRC REQUIREMENTS IDENTIFIED?

NRC conducts regular inspections at licensed facilities to assure compliance with NRC requirements. In addition, your employer and site contractors conduct their own inspections to assure compliance. All inspectors are protected by Federal law. Interference with them may result in criminal prosecution for a Federal offense.

MAY I TALK WITH AN NRC INSPECTOR?

Yes. Your employer may not prevent you from talking with an NRC inspector and you may talk privately with an inspector and request that your identity remain confidential.

UNITED STATES NUCLEAR REGULATORY COMMISSION REGIONAL OFFICE LOCATIONS

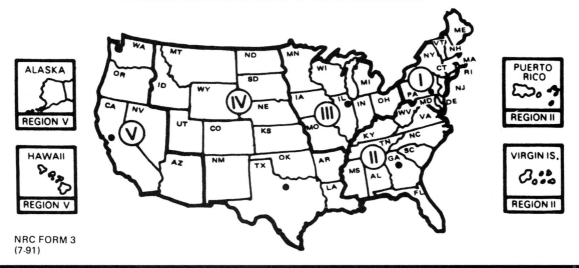

NRC FORM 3
(7-91)

Figure 7-8   U.S. Nuclear Regulatory Commission radiation protection standards Notice to Employees.

Continued

MAY I REQUEST AN INSPECTION?

If you believe that your employer has not corrected violations involving radiological working conditions, you may request an inspection. Your request should be addressed to the nearest NRC Regional Office and must describe the alleged violation in detail. It must be signed by you or your representative.

HOW DO I CONTACT THE NRC?

Notify an NRC inspector on-site or call the nearest NRC Regional office collect. NRC inspectors want to talk to you if you are worried about radiation safety or other aspects of licensed activities, such as the quality of construction or operations at your plant.

CAN I BE FIRED FOR TALKING TO THE NRC?

No. Federal law prohibits an employer from firing or otherwise discriminating against a worker for bringing safety concerns to the attention of the NRC. You may not be fired or discriminated against because you:

- ask the NRC to enforce its rules against your employer;
- testify in an NRC proceeding;

- provide information or are about to provide information to the NRC about violations of requirements;
- are about to ask for or testify, help, or take part in an NRC proceeding.

WHAT FORMS OF DISCRIMINATION ARE PROHIBITED?

No employer may fire you or discriminate against you with respect to pay, benefits, or working conditions because you help the NRC.

HOW AM I PROTECTED FROM DISCRIMINATION?

If you believe that you have been discriminated against for bringing safety concerns to the NRC, you may file a complaint with the U.S. Department of Labor. Your complaint must describe the firing or discrimination and must be filed within 30 days of the occurrence.

Send complaints to:

Office of the Administrator
Wage and Hour Division
Employment Standards Administration
Room S3502
U.S. Department of Labor
200 Constitution Avenue, NW
Washington, DC 20210

or any local office of the Department of Labor, Wage and Hour Division. Check your telephone directory under U.S. Government listings.

WHAT CAN THE LABOR DEPARTMENT DO?

The Department of Labor will notify the employer that a complaint has been filed and will investigate the case.

If the Department of Labor finds that your employer has unlawfully discriminated against you, it may order you to be reinstated, receive back pay, or be compensated for any injury suffered as a result of the discrimination.

WHAT WILL THE NRC DO?

The NRC may assist the Department of Labor in its investigation. NRC may conduct its own investigation where necessary to determine whether unlawful discrimination has prevented the free flow of information to the Commission. Also, if the NRC or Department of Labor finds that unlawful discrimination has occurred, the NRC may issue a Notice of Violation to your employer, impose a fine, or suspend, modify, or revoke your employer's NRC license.

A representative of the Nuclear Regulatory Commission can be contacted at the following addresses and telephone numbers. The Regional Office will accept collect telephone calls from employees who wish to register complaints or concerns about radiological working conditions or other matters regarding compliance with Commission rules and regulations.

Regional Offices

REGION	ADDRESS	TELEPHONE
I	U.S. Nuclear Regulatory Commission Region I 475 Allendale Road King of Prussia, PA 19406-1415	(215) 337-5000
II	U.S. Nuclear Regulatory Commission Region II 101 Marietta St., N.W., Suite 2900 Atlanta, GA 30323	(404) 331-4503
III	U.S. Nuclear Regulatory Commission Region III 799 Roosevelt Road Glen Ellyn, IL 60137	(708) 790-5500
IV	U.S. Nuclear Regulatory Commission Region IV 611 Ryan Plaza Drive, Suite 400 Arlington, TX 76011-8064	(817) 860-8100
V	U.S. Nuclear Regulatory Commission Region V 1450 Maria Lane, Suite 210 Walnut Creek, CA 94596-5368	(510) 975-0200

To report incidents involving fraud, waste or abuse by an NRC employee or NRC contractor,

telephone:

OFFICE OF THE INSPECTOR GENERAL

HOTLINE

1-800-233-3497

Figure 7-8, cont'd. For legend see p. 197.

cense. To meet this requirement the RSO must review radioactive materials orders. Generally, standing orders for general use must be reviewed annually, whereas "special" orders should be reviewed on a case-by-case basis. In addition, manufacturers or commercial radiopharmacies must keep a copy of the license on file and should check that materials ordered are approved on the license.

Procedures for receiving radioactive materials should detail how the delivery will reach the nuclear medicine pharmacy. If packages are received at a loading dock, personnel working in that area must be trained on safe handling techniques, including the need for visual checks of packages and procedures to follow if a package is damaged. Packages received after hours must be delivered to a designated location. Typically, that location either will have a locked, possibly shielded storage space or there will be a protocol in place for security personnel to deliver the package to the radiopharmacy. Again, it is necessary for security personnel to be trained in radiation safety techniques. The most straightforward situation exists where a commercial radiopharmacy delivers radioactive material directly to the nuclear medicine department. Often, this eliminates transport by security or distribution personnel.

Opening packages. Radioactive materials received in the nuclear medicine department must be checked in within 3 hours during normal working hours and, if any are received at other times, as soon as the department reopens. This check should consist of donning disposable gloves to then conduct a visual inspection of the package. If there is any evidence of damage or wetness indicating leakage, the package should be immediately secured and the RSO should be notified. Next, all packages requiring Type I, II, or III Department of Transportation labels must be wipe tested when received. This wipe test must be counted with a system capable of detecting 2000 dpm. The package should then be opened, and a second visual check should be made to ensure that the contents are what was indicated on the packing slip and that there is no damage. Indications of damage would be breakage, less liquid than expected, or discoloration of the packing material. If indications of damage are observed, the package should be secured and the RSO should be contacted. Finally, the contents should be removed and the empty shipping package should be surveyed for contamination with a low-range GM meter. Before disposal, all radioactive symbols must be defaced. During all of these steps, good radiation safety practices should be used, such as wearing disposable gloves and using tongs to move the source. Records of receipt of the material and the findings of the wipe test must be maintained.

Dose calibrator testing. The dose calibrator, used to assay doses of prepared radiopharmaceuticals, must be tested to verify proper function. The required tests and frequency are listed in Table 7-10.

These tests (see Chapter 3) will ensure that an assay is accurate and reproducible. On installation and annually, certified standards should be assayed to test for accuracy of the unit. The recorded radioactivity must be within 10% of the limits of the National Institute of Standards and Technology (NIST) for traceable certified radioactivity. Also on installation, the variation in recorded radioactivity with geometry should be evaluated. Keeping the radioactivity constant, the volume in a vial and also in a syringe will be varied and the reading should be noted. The variation between the standard vial reading and a syringe reading should also be determined. The linearity should be tested quarterly to ensure that readings are accurate for the range of radioactivities that are assayed. Finally, before patient doses are assayed each day, the constancy of response should be checked using a long-lived source, such as ^{137}Cs. For this test the most commonly used setting, usually ^{99m}Tc, should be checked daily, and other commonly used settings should be checked weekly. A schedule of the required times for the other tests should be placed in a conspicuous place on the calibrator. The results of testing should be reviewed and signed by the RSO.

Radionuclide generator testing. Each eluate of a ^{99}Mo/^{99m}Tc generator must be tested to determine the contamination levels of the parent radionuclide, ^{99}Mo. The maximum contamination level that is acceptable for human administration is 0.15 μCi of ^{99}Mo per mCi of ^{99m}Tc. This level must not be exceeded during the shelf

Table 7-10 Dose calibrator tests

Test	Test frequency
Accuracy test using two or more standards of certified radioactivity.	At installation and at least annually thereafter.
Linearity tests through the range of radioactivities assayed.	At installation and at least quarterly thereafter.
Geometric or volume-of-source dependence evaluation for each of the source configurations used.	At installation and before implementation of new source configurations.
Constancy-of-response tests using a long-lived reference source.	Once each day of use before use.

life of a prepared radiopharmaceutical (e.g., 6 hours after preparation). The molybdenum radioactivity is usually determined by placing the eluate vial in a specially designed lead holder that attenuates effectively all the lower energy ^{99m}Tc photons, while allowing transmission of some percentage of the higher energy ^{99}Mo photons. The total radioactivity of molybdenum should then be determined; the method used depends on the calibrator used. The concentration must be calculated, and the acceptability of the eluate must be verified. A record of the radioactivity of ^{99m}Tc and of ^{99}Mo, the ratio, time and date of measurement, and the name of the person conducting the test must be maintained. The procedure manual should contain a description of the method used for molybdenum contamination. A list of authorized personnel trained in the procedure should be maintained.

Measurement and records of radiopharmaceutical use. Before administration, each patient dose must be assayed. For beta emitters, such as ^{89}Sr, this may be done by measurements and calculations or by obtaining the dose in unit form from an approved manufacturer or preparer. Records must be maintained that include identification of the radiopharmaceutical, identification of the patient, the results of the assay, the date and time of the assay, and identification of the individual preparing the dose. In addition, the syringe must be labeled to identify its contents and either its use (i.e., the clinical procedure) or the patient. This labeling is an important way of preventing administration of the wrong radiopharmaceutical, particularly in departments where more than one technologist may handle the dose.

Administration of patient dose. Syringe shields in sizes to fit the syringes used must be available in the department for use in the preparation and administration of radiopharmaceuticals. If possible, each technologist should have a syringe shield in the most commonly used size. Use of syringe shields significantly reduces exposure to the hands and eyes and should be used at all times. Disposable gloves must also be worn. These serve two purposes: protecting the hands from radioactive contamination and serving as a barrier to infectious diseases (Figure 7-9).

Infection control procedures, as required by the OSHA Laboratory Standards Act, also require methods to prevent infectious diseases from needle sticks. Needles used for patient injections must not be recapped by hand. Many departments use needle boxes for immediate, safe disposal.

Daily and weekly surveys for exposure and contamination. Area surveys for external radiation exposure lev-

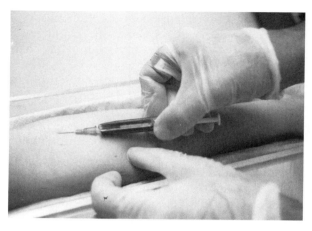

Figure 7-9 Proper technique for administration of radiopharmaceutical.

els and removable contamination must be performed regularly in all areas of the nuclear medicine department.

At the end of each day when radioactive materials are used, a survey of external exposure levels must be performed. This includes weekends or holidays when a procedure is performed on-call. All areas where radioactive materials have been prepared or used, radiopharmacy lab, injection room, and applicable imaging rooms, must be surveyed and the results must be recorded. A portable survey instrument, either an ionization chamber or a wide-range GM meter or both, with a range of 0.1 mR/hr to 1 R/hr, should be used. The readings should be recorded in mR/hr. A background level reading in an area known to be free of radiation should also be recorded. Action levels, which are typically two or three times the average levels for that area, should be established. If a reading exceeds the action level, corrective action, such as checking that all sources are in lead storage or removing a flood source from a room, must be taken and the action taken should be recorded on the survey form. A survey of all wastebaskets may prevent contaminated materials from being disposed of via this route.

Surveys to detect removable contamination must be performed weekly. A wipe should be made with a filter paper disk or cotton swab over an area 10 cm × 10 cm on designated areas. These areas should be where it is more likely that contamination will be found, such as the floor near the camera or treadmill, work surfaces, and telephones. Wipes should be performed in each area of use. The wipes should then be counted in a well counter. Wipe test results in counts per minute should then be converted to disintegrations per minute, using the counting efficiency that has been determined for the counter. Results should be recorded in dpm/100 cm^2. Action levels must also be established for wipe test results. If an area exceeds 200 dpm/100 cm^2, decontamination must be performed[21] and the area must be wipe tested again. Action levels for intervention by the Radiation Safety Officer are often established so that the source of the contamination may be investigated.

Posting of Signs and Notices

Certain signs should be posted near the entrance to each room where radioactive material is used or stored to inform individuals entering the area of the presence of a potential hazard and to denote radiologic safety evaluation and control of the area. Signs commonly employed include the following:

Sign	Intended use
	To signify areas in which radioactive material is used or stored in amounts exceeding quantities specified by state and federal regulatory agencies, typically when the quantities exceed 10 times the quantity specified in Appendix C of Part 20 of the NRC regulations.[17]
	To signify areas accessible to personnel in which a major portion of the body of a person could receive more than 5 mrem in 1 hour and more than 100 mrem in 5 consecutive days.
	To denote areas accessible to personnel in which a major portion of the body of a person could receive a dose in excess of 100 mrem in any 1 hour.
CAUTION ☢ AIRBORNE RADIOACTIVITY AREA	To signify that the airborne activity level in the area may transiently exceed the restricted area limit or may exceed 25% of the restricted area limit when averaged over 1 week.

Each of these signs must bear the three-bladed symbol, which is the international warning symbol for ionizing radiation. Generally, the trefoil is magenta against a yellow background.

Various other signs and notices are often posted near the entrance of or in areas where radioactive material is used or stored. These include notices to radiation workers that provide information as required by federal or state regulatory agencies, for example, the NRC *Form NRC-3 Notice to Employees* (see Figure 7-8); signs that provide instructions for the actions necessary in the case of an accident or emergency; and signs that provide the evacuation time necessary for a room in which an accidental release of gaseous activity has occurred.

CONTAMINATION CONTROL

Sealed Source Leak Tests and Inventory

Sealed sources used for dose calibrator testing and for camera quality control must be inventoried and leak tested for removable contamination. A written inventory and exposure survey of the source storage area must be performed quarterly. The inventory should be taken and the leak test should be performed every 6 months. The inventory and leak test must include all photon-emitting sources of greater than 100 μCi. A general procedure for the test is as follows:

1. Wipe the source with a dampened cotton swab or paper wipe held with forceps. Place wipe material in a marked test tube. Obtain a background level sample with the same wipe material.
2. Using a wide window, count in a well counter that is capable of detecting a minimum of .005 μCi of radioactivity.
3. Record the results. Calculate the removable radioactivity.
4. Any sealed source with more than 0.005 μCi removable radioactivity of the source material must be removed and stored. The appropriate regulatory agency must be notified.

Note that if radioactivity is detected, external contamination rather than leakage must be ruled out. If counting is done in a multichannel analyzer, there must be confirmation that the observed counts are at the photopeak of the sealed source and not a clinical nuclide.

Sources no longer in use, such as ^{57}Co sources too weak for the intended use, may be placed in long-term storage until disposed of. If the source is taped shut with the date recorded and a note indicating that it is not in use, a leak test is not required.

Control and Evaluation of Airborne Activity

Special efforts are required to evaluate and document that radioactive materials, which are either volatile or potentially volatile, are safely controlled. Considerations should include safety precautions that are practiced while the materials are used or stored, evaluations of concentrations of the materials breathed by workers in restricted areas, and evaluations of the airborne concentrations in applicable nonrestricted areas including points of release to the atmosphere. Such efforts are indicated not only for radioactive gases, like ^{133}Xe, but also for dispersible materials, like ^{99m}Tc DTPA aerosols and for materials with a volatile component, the best example of which is ^{131}I sodium iodide. The evaluations or surveys are often calculations based on certain physical measurements, that is, ventilation or discharge rates and knowledge of the quantities of materials periodically used by the nuclear medicine facility.

Storing and Using Radioactive Gases and Other Dispersible or Volatile Materials

Rooms in which gaseous radioactive material is used and the nuclear pharmacy should be maintained at a negative pressure with respect to the surrounding areas. Maintaining such an area at negative pressure means that the direction of airflow at the boundaries of the room is into the room. Thus, airborne activities generated within the room are removed by the exhaust system that maintains the negative pressure and the activity should not, to any appreciable extent, passively diffuse into the surrounding nonrestricted areas like corridors or waiting areas. The exhaust system serving areas in which volatile radioactive materials are used or stored should serve only those areas (a dedicated system), should provide enough ventilation to sufficiently dilute radioactivity released within the room, and should exhaust the radioactivity at release points properly located away from the general population, for example, on the rooftop of the building and away from any air intakes. Measurements should be made to demonstrate that the airflow at the boundaries of such rooms is toward the room, and measurements should be periodically made thereafter, about every 6 months, to show that the situation is unchanged.

It is important to properly store radioactive gases and volatiles. Containers of ^{133}Xe are generally stored in a fumehood so that any inadvertent leakage of activity is routed away from the immediate work area. Optimum storage of ^{131}I sodium iodide solution intended for oral administration involves several considerations. Although the fraction of the vial activity that is gaseous is kept at a low value (about 0.0001 to 0.001) by maintaining it at a basic pH, the volatile fraction can be further reduced by keeping the stored vials refrigerated and in the dark. According to manufacturers of ^{131}I sodium iodide, the basic pH minimizes the labeled I_2 species, whereas reduced temperature assists in controlling the volatile HI component. Also, when preparing the radioactivity for patient administration, it is important to minimize agitation or handling of the vial and to avoid exposure of the contents to bright light.

It is generally recommended that information be posted in imaging rooms in which ^{133}Xe is used that specifies the period of time that the room should be evacuated by personnel following an accidental release of gas within the room. A common criterion used to calculate the evacuation time is to delay reentry until the average concentration of ^{133}Xe in the room has decreased to the occupational limits specified for restricted areas. (This criterion is very conservative, since the airborne activity to which radiation workers are exposed in restricted areas may be averaged over the 520 working hours of a calendar quarter to demonstrate compliance with the specified limit of airborne activity concentration.) Such a calculation employs the volume of room air into which the activity was released and the net ventilation rate of the room. In equation form the time of evacuation can be expressed as

$$T = (V/Q) \ln (A/CV)$$

where T is the time of evacuation in minutes, A is the released activity of ^{133}Xe in mCi, V is the room air volume in ml (1 ft^3 = 28,300 ml), Q is the net ventilation rate of the room in ml/min, and C is the airborne activity concentration limit of ^{133}Xe in the air of a restricted area (3×10^{-5} μCi/ml).

As an example, compute the evacuation time that should be posted in a ^{133}Xe imaging room if the greatest radioactivity used is 30 mCi, the dimensions of the room are 10 ft $\times$ 12 ft $\times$ 8 ft, and the net ventilation rate of the room is 250 ft^3/min.

$$T = V/Q \ln (A/CV)$$

where
$V = 960$ ft^3 = 2.7×10^7 ml
$Q = 250$ ft^3/min = 7.1×10^6 ml/min
$C = 3 \times 10^{-5}$ μCi/ml
$A = 30$ mCi = 3×10^4 μCi

$$T = \frac{2.7 \times 10^7 \text{ ml}}{7.1 \times 10^6 \text{ ml/min}} \frac{3 \times 10^4 \text{ } \mu\text{Ci}}{(3 \times 10^{-5} \text{ } \mu\text{Ci/ml})(2.7 \times 10^7 \text{ ml})}$$

$T = 3.8 \ln 37$ min
$T = 13.7$ min

Evaluation of the average concentrations of airborne activity in nonrestricted areas should also be performed and documented. The practice of maintaining rooms in which gaseous activities are used at a negative pressure with respect to the surrounding nonrestricted areas helps to ensure that the airborne levels in those areas are at acceptably low values. However, it is prudent to periodically document the low levels by conducting airborne activity surveys to measure the levels (refer to the Radiation Safety Instruments and Devices section of this chapter for descriptions of various airborne sampling devices). Such surveys, usually conducted during representative use of the gaseous or volatile radionuclide, permit the evaluation of the peak or worst-case airborne concentration levels. If the measured peak levels are less than the nonrestricted area concentration limit for a specific radionuclide, then there is compliance. If the transient peak levels are significantly higher than the nonrestricted area limit, however, a calculation should be made over an extended time—from a month to a year—to demonstrate that the time-averaged concentration is less than the applicable limit.

A special case is the evaluation of the average concentration at the site where a ventilation system serving a gaseous activity use area, such as a ^{133}Xe imaging room, releases the air to the atmosphere. For the release site to be a nonrestricted area the average airborne activity of the exhaust must be less than the nonrestricted area limit for the radionuclide under consideration. Calculation of the average concentration requires knowledge of the discharge rate of the exhaust and the activity released from the site in a given period. The following example illustrates such a calculation.

A room used for ^{133}Xe examinations has a continuously operating ventilation system whose measured discharge rate is 2000 ft^3/min, and it is assumed that all of the administered activity for an average patient workload of 12 examinations per week is released from the ventilation exhaust. If the average administered activity is 10 mCi per patient, show that the average concentration at the release point, based on a representative week, is less than the USNRC limit for ^{133}Xe in the air of a nonrestricted area, 3×10^{-7} μCi/ml (a useful conversion factor is 28,300 ml/ft^3).

The total estimated release of activity per week is

$$(12 \text{ patients/wk})(10 \text{ mCi/patient}) =$$
$$120 \text{ mCi/wk} = 1.2 \times 10^5 \text{ } \mu\text{Ci/wk}$$

The total volume of air released per week is

$$(2000 \text{ ft}^3/\text{min})(10,080 \text{ min/wk})(28,300 \text{ ml/ft}^3) =$$
$$5.7 \times 10^{11} \text{ ml/wk}$$

The average concentration for the week is then

$$c = \frac{1.2 \times 10^5 \text{ } \mu\text{Ci/wk}}{5.7 \times 10^{11} \text{ ml/wk}} = 2.1 \times 10^{-7} \text{ } \mu\text{Ci/ml}$$

The computed average in this example represents 70% of the NRC limit. Thus, although such a situation satisfies the Commission's regulation, it provides a small margin of safety and does not fulfill the ALARA goal of licensees voluntarily reducing environmental releases to 10% or less of the legal requirements. When results indicate that air concentrations are in excess of the desired level, several corrective actions can be taken. These include increasing the discharge rate, decreasing the released activity by utilizing activated charcoal filters to trap most of the radioactive xenon, and considering the location of the exhaust (e.g., on a rooftop) as a restricted area. However, the last approach is often operationally burdensome—the boundary of the restricted area must be clearly established and posted—and access to the location must be restricted.

When charcoal filters are used to reduce the con-

centration released to the atmosphere, the user must be able to demonstrate that the filters are effective and are performing as assumed. Measurements to determine the trapping efficiency and whether a filter has become saturated should be periodically performed.

Spills and Accidents

With even the most careful attention to radiation safety procedures, it is possible for an accident to occur, usually a spill. Since this may also include personnel contamination, procedures for handling personnel and area control and decontamination must be posted in any area where unsealed radioactive material is routinely handled. If there is a possibility that a spill could occur resulting in an immediate room shutdown, the procedure should be posted in more than one location.

A procedure to handle a radioactive spill should include the following:

1. *Clear the area.* Have anyone else in the immediate area move to a more distant location and remain there until checked for contamination. If there is any chance of shoe contamination of these people, have them remove their shoes at a boundary quickly defined as the clean area. If there are noncontaminated personnel present, ask one of them to assist.
2. *Notify* a supervisor or the Radiation Safety Officer. The posted form must clearly list current notification numbers.
3. *Contain the spill* with absorbent paper. If the radioactive material is high activity, attempt to shield the source if this can be done quickly.
4. *Evaluate the severity* to determine the best way to decontaminate and whether assistance from the Radiation Safety Office should be obtained.
5. *Decontaminate personnel.* Removing and bagging outer clothing, including shoes, will remove most contamination. Skin contamination is removed by gentle washing with tepid water and soap or a commercial decontaminating agent. Do not irritate or abrade the skin, which may cause absorption of the contaminant. Check the effectiveness with a low-range GM survey meter, and continue until the radiation level is acceptable. Residual radioactivity on the hands may be removed by using powder-lined gloves taped at the wrist, causing the radioactivity to be released with sweat.
6. *Decontaminate the spill area,* using personnel and radiation safety precautions appropriate for the radioactivity and type of radionuclide. For low-activity spills, immediately start using absorbent paper. Work from the outside to the center of the spill. If necessary, wash with small amounts

of decontaminant, making sure that the liquid does not spread the contamination. Place all contaminated materials in a plastic bag, label it, and place it in radioactive waste. For high-activity spills with greater possibility for high exposure to personnel, it is reasonable to plan the decontamination procedure before starting, including an assessment of the exposure rate. Depending on the findings, it may be necessary to use more than one person or to allow some time for decay.

7. *Survey* using a low-range GM tube. Record the findings, noting the location and reading. When no additional contamination is removable, take wipe tests to confirm successful decontamination. Record these results and location.

8. *Write up a report,* describing the accident and steps taken to clean up the spill.

An all too common spill may occur when injecting the patient who is being stressed on a treadmill. The radioactive material often lands on the treadmill and may also land on the patient. In this case, stop the treadmill, have the patient step off (if possible onto a towel or absorbent paper), and contain the radioactivity. Have the patient step out of his/her shoes to a clean area, and decontaminate the skin if necessary. Decontaminate the treadmill as much as possible. If any radioactivity remains, as often happens, have patients wear booties until no radioactivity is detectable on the treadmill.

Radioactive Waste Disposal

The objective of radioactive waste management is to prevent human contact with concentrations of material or radiation levels significantly above background level. Most of the waste material generated in nuclear medicine may be disposed of by holding the material in storage for extensive decay, diluting and dispersing the material to the atmosphere or sanitary sewer system, or returning the spent material to the manufacturer or supplier. Rarely, these techniques are not appropriate, and materials are concentrated and shipped for land burial. Recommended techniques for safe disposal follow. As with all aspects of nuclear medicine, records of the disposal must be maintained by the department.

Return to manufacturer or supplier. This method is very useful for long-lived materials found in nuclear medicine. Departments utilizing molybdenum generators may be able to return the old, partially decayed generator to the manufacturer. As part of the purchase of new long-lived sealed ^{57}Co flood source or dose calibrator constancy checks, the old source may be exchanged if it was purchased from the same manufacturer. Programs may exist where the contaminated ma-terials used with long-lived materials, such as for ^{89}Sr therapy, may be returned. The specific requirements for such returns must be arranged in advance with the manufacturer or supplier, who will also usually supply the appropriate paperwork, copies of which are maintained by the department.

Dry waste. Most of the dry waste generated in nuclear medicine consists of items contaminated with radionuclides with relatively short physical half-lives. Radioactive waste with half-lives of 60 days or less may be stored for extensive decay before disposing of the material. State and federal regulatory authorities permit the disposal of short-lived radionuclides by decay-in-storage programs. The material is held in storage a minimum of 10 half-lives and then is carefully monitored with an appropriate survey instrument of good sensitivity. If the survey indicates that the material has decayed to less than two times background levels, it may then be transferred to the appropriate regular trash for disposal (e.g., needle containers to biohazard waste). Before disposing of the material, all radiation signs and symbols must be obliterated or defaced. This is most easily and safely accomplished as the item is placed in waste, so that it is not necessary to later go through a waste bag. The radionuclides for which decay is used are usually separated by half-lives to minimize the time shorter half-lived material must be stored and therefore the space required for decay in storage.

Long-lived materials, usually found only in research programs, may require the material to be shipped to a federally approved low-level radioactive material land burial site. Waste materials shipped for disposal must be properly packaged and labeled according to U.S. Department of Transportation requirements. A number of commercial companies act as brokers in the handling of radioactive waste material destined for either burial or incineration.

Liquid waste. Small quantities of liquid waste that are either soluble or dispersible in water can be discharged in a designated sink to a sanitary sewer system provided the collective amounts disposed of by this method do not exceed specified concentrations and annual amounts. The maximum permitted concentrations specified by regulatory authorities are based on the total water discharge rates of the licensee (water discharge rate can generally be assumed to be equal to the water consumption rate; hence water bills provide a record of the licensee's water discharge rates) and the released radioactivity. To demonstrate compliance with the concentration limits, the released concentrations can be averaged over extended periods, such as a month. Records of the date of disposal and the type and amount of radioactivity must be maintained by the department.

Gaseous wastes. Certain gases, principally ^{133}Xe, are often disposed of after their utilization by discharging them to the atmosphere. This does not apply to unused xenon, which is held for decay. This method of waste disposal is discussed in the section on Control of Airborne Activity. An important alternative method of disposing of ^{133}Xe is to utilize activated charcoal to trap the gas after its use. The activated charcoal traps containing the ^{133}Xe are periodically placed in storage for an extended period to permit most of the radioactivity to decay before reuse of the filter. Several precautions are important with this method. Other gases, such as CO_2 and water vapor, compete with the xenon for trapping by the charcoal. Thus, the traps can become saturated and ineffective in trapping ^{133}Xe and should be periodically replenished with fresh charcoal.

Part 20 of Title 10 of the Code of Federal Regulations[17] defines a category of waste that can be disposed of without regard to its radioactivity: ^{3}H and ^{14}C in liquid scintillation cocktails or animals that have a concentration less than 185 Bq/g (0.05 μCi/g). This category of waste can be found in many hospitals and universities involved with clinical and biomedical research. It needs only to be treated as hazardous waste and can be incinerated as nonradioactive.

Radiation safety audit. A review of the Radiation Safety Program should be conducted quarterly to ensure that procedures are followed. The review, which is conducted by a medical physicist or other appropriate personnel, should include a visual check of personnel safety practices and camera quality control records. The department policy and procedures and related records must be reviewed annually by a medical physicist. The results should be presented to the Radiation Safety Committee.

PATIENT PRECAUTIONS

The radiation dose that the patient receives is considered acceptable in that the study provides needed medical information, which is a benefit. To ensure that the use of radioactivity is beneficial, procedures must be in place so that the correct patient receives the correct amount of radioactivity for an appropriate study. All studies must be properly requisitioned. When the patient arrives, his/her identity must be clearly ascertained. This may be done in a number of ways, such as by checking an in-patient wrist band or asking for date of birth, which may be checked against the requisition. The radiopharmaceutical to be used must be checked and the proper material must be selected. For example, if kits are prepared in the department, color coding may be used so that a bone agent is not confused with pertechnetate. Before administration, the radionuclide

must be assayed, the radioactivity must be compared with the recommended amount, and the syringe must be properly labeled. Lastly, the correct route of administration must be used and care must be taken to prevent administration of a useless radiation dose to the patient, such as extravasation.

Additional precautions, using a written directive, must be taken for medical procedures that have a higher risk to the patient, for example, using any ^{131}I or ^{125}I procedures greater than 30 μCi, or any other unsealed source therapy procedures such as ^{32}P or ^{89}Sr. For these procedures, a written directive must be completed by the authorized user (i.e., the nuclear medicine physician authorized for unsealed source therapy procedures). The written directive must identify the patient, the procedure, radiopharmaceutical form, and route of administration. The directive must be signed and dated. Before administration, the patient must be identified in two ways. Prior to administration by the authorized user, the material must be assayed and documentation must be provided that the radioactivity is within 10% of the prescribed amount. There must also be documentation that the administration is in accordance with the written directive, for example, by having the physician who administers the material sign the dose slip. The written documentation must be kept on file. The description of how these additional precautions will be addressed and the mechanism for review should be contained in the institution's Quality Management Program (QMP). It is a requirement of the materials license that a QMP be in place. At specified intervals (e.g., quarterly) the paperwork should be reviewed to further evaluate that no problems have occurred. The files of patients who fall into the above categories should be reviewed for accuracy and completeness during inspections by federal or state regulators.

If an error is made in dosing a patient, the incident should be documented. It must then be determined if the event is one that should be reported to the appropriate regulatory agency. Incidents that must be reported are *misadministrations*. A misadministration occurs when (1) a radiopharmaceutical other than ^{131}I or ^{125}I is administered to the wrong patient, the prescribed dose differs by more than 20% from the administered dose, or the wrong radiopharmaceutical is administered AND the dose to the patient is greater than 5 rems effective dose equivalent or 50 rems dose equivalent to any organ and (2) a dose of greater than 30 μCi of ^{131}I or ^{125}I or another therapeutic dose is administered to the wrong patient, by the wrong route of administration, the wrong radiopharmaceutical is used, or there is more than a 20% difference between the prescribed and administered dose. In the case of a misadministration, it is necessary to immediately notify the appropriate regulatory agency. Since it is highly unlikely that a diagnostic study would meet the whole body or organ dose requirement, most misadministrations result from errors in the Quality Management Program. Another category of reporting is the *recordable event*, which is of lower severity and involves errors in the Quality Management Program. A recordable event occurs when there is no written directive for any ^{131}I or ^{125}I or therapeutic administration or when the measured dose differs from the prescribed dose by more than 10%. For these circumstances, a written record describing the event and the steps taken to prevent a reoccurrence must be maintained. Although generally not required, it is good practice to also document any incorrect administration, investigate the cause, and determine possible methods to prevent reoccurrence.

Studies of women of childbearing age also require additional precautions. Before beginning the study, the last menstrual period (LMP) must be ascertained and documented, such as on the requisition. If a woman is pregnant or late in her menstrual cycle, the nuclear medicine physician and the referring physician must decide if the study should be performed. If the study is performed, documentation of the administered radioactivity and type of study should be recorded so that the probable dose to the fetus may be calculated. If the woman is nursing, she should discontinue for a designated time following the study.

Therapeutic Procedures

Specific authorization for therapeutic procedures must be given in the radioactive materials license. Often, smaller institutions are not licensed for therapy administrations, and patients are treated at larger facilities.

Treatments with radioactive iodine typically comprise the greatest percentage of therapeutic use. Treatments under 30 mCi are usually done on an outpatient basis. This would include ^{131}I hyperthyroid treatment and some thyroid carcinoma ablations. For these procedures, few special precautions need to be taken. Since only nuclear medicine personnel are involved, the annual training is adequate. The documentation required for the QMP must be accurate and complete. The iodine is often given as a capsule, minimizing the possibility of volatilization or a spill. The patient may leave immediately with discharge instructions as in Table 7-11. In the event that a patient is treated while hospitalized, the precautions described below should be followed, providing a consistent Radiation Safety Policy.

For treatments of greater than 30 mCi, hospitalization is required for regulatory purposes. Since these treatments often exceed 150 mCi or greater of ^{131}I, precautions must be in place to protect personnel and members of the public from exposure during the treatment and contamination following the treatment. A room that is identified on the license must be used.

Table 7-11 ^{131}I Patient discharge instructions

A time interval (usually 3-7 days) should be specified for each instruction depending on the patient's household.

	Days
Try to keep the time you spend in close contact with others to a minimum.	_____
Minimize the time spent with young children or pregnant women.	_____
Sleep alone if possible.	_____
Discuss with your physician how long after treatment you should wait to become pregnant.	_____
Practice good hygiene habits; wash your hands after each toilet use.	_____
Drink plenty of liquids.	_____
Use separate bath linens; wash these linens and your underclothing separately from other laundry.	_____
Use separate (or disposable) eating utensils.	_____

The room must be designed so that any patient in adjacent areas will not receive greater than 100 mrem/yr. A large room on an outside corner often works best, particularly if a roof is above or the floor-to-floor heights are large. The room must also have a private bathroom. Before the patient is admitted, the room should be prepared so that any contamination can easily be removed. Areas that the patient is likely to touch, such as chairs, the floor, and door knobs, should be covered with plastic or plastic-backed paper. If a phone is present in the room, it should either be covered or replaced with a phone that may be removed for decay. Disposable service should be ordered for meals so that all contaminated materials may be put in the trash.

Instruction of the nursing staff is critical. These instructions must cover radiation safety principles, techniques for reduction of exposure, methods for caring for the patient, and the requirements of the Quality Management Program. For example, emphasis should be placed on the use of time and distance to reduce exposure; lead shielding at the energy of ^{131}I is only effective if approximately 1 inch thick. Most iodine patients who must be hospitalized are self-care patients, so use of distance when talking with the patient is very effective. This instruction must be documented. Personnel caring for the patient must also be issued radiation dosimeters.

Before the patient receives the iodine, it is useful to review the precautions that he or she must take, such as staying in the room and flushing twice after using the toilet. The choice of whether the patient may have visitors is one that must be decided by the institution. It is possible, particularly with larger rooms, to mark the line behind which the exposure rate is 2 mR/hr. If the patient remains at the location for the measurement, visitors may stay behind the marked line without regard to time. Staff and visitors must not use the patient's bathroom or sink.

The iodine may be administered as a capsule(s) or liquid. It is possible to obtain the liquid in a sealed vial, which may be punctured by a long needle with a straw attached. In this way the convenience of drinking the material rather than taking many capsules is possible and the potential for spills is almost eliminated. Any staff in the room at the time of the administration must have a thyroid bioassay. Following administration of the material, an exposure rate measurement is taken 1 meter from the patient. This serves as the baseline measurement for determination of when the radioactivity remaining is below 30 mCi. For example, if the patient receives 100 mCi and has an initial exposure rate of 25 mR/hr, the patient may be discharged when the exposure rate is below 7.5 mR/hr.

$$\frac{30 \text{ mCi}}{100 \text{ mCi}} = \frac{X \text{ mR/hr}}{25 \text{ mR/hr}}$$

Measurements are made once or twice a day to determine when the patient is below the calculated level. The patient may then be discharged, with instructions such as given in Table 7-11.

Following discharge, it is necessary to decontaminate the room. All contaminated items are removed to waste storage. The room is then surveyed with a low-range GM meter. Any area above background level must have a wipe test and must be further decontaminated until wipes result in less than 200 dpm. All patient measurements and room surveys must be documented.

Other therapeutic procedures that may be performed are injection of ^{32}P and ^{89}Sr. These procedures are usually performed on an outpatient basis. The primary precaution during the administration of these injections is to use a thick plastic syringe shield to attenuate the beta particles. Following injection, all personnel and the room used should be surveyed with a GM meter with the end cap off, which makes the meter extremely efficient for detecting beta particles. Since some of the material will end up in the urine, the patient should be instructed to use care when urinating and flush twice. If it is necessary to treat an inpatient, any bandages that are removed following injection should be retained to determine if they are contaminated. In the case of ^{89}Sr for treatment of metastatic bone pain, many institutions only treat on an outpatient basis and further recommend that the patient be continent. For this material, the exposure rate around the patient is minimal and requires no special precautions.

BIOLOGIC EFFECTS OF IONIZING RADIATION

The radiation safety practices that have been described are intended to minimize the dose received (i.e., energy deposited) to the body due to ionizing radiation. This is necessary because biologic effects due to radiation have been observed, either directly, as in the case of high, single exposures, or in some percentage of a population, as in the case of somewhat lower exposures. A knowledge of these biologic effects helps to assess the risks associated with exposure to radiation.

Acute Effects

A high, single radiation exposure to all or most of the body results in acute effects (i.e., those showing rapid onset, severe symptoms, and a short course). At a minimum whole body dose of 2 Sv (200 rem), radiation sickness will be observed. Note that this requires a dose to the whole body delivered in a short time, a situation that would occur only due to a severe radiation accident. Within an hour or two of exposure, nausea, vomiting, and, at higher doses, diarrhea will be observed. Neurologic symptoms including headache, decreased blood pressure, and fatigue are also observed. This is called the *prodromal stage*. Except with the highest doses, a *latent period* follows, during which the victim shows no visible signs and symptoms of radiation injury.

The radiation syndrome (the signs and symptoms) exhibited, depends on the whole body dose received. The dose levels given are approximate in that there is fortunately little human data. At doses of 100 Gy (10,000 rad) *cerebrovascular* damage results in death in a matter of hours. Although the exact cause of death is unknown, it appears that vascular damage results in rapid accumulation of cerebral fluid, resulting in disorientation, diarrhea, convulsions, coma, and death. At doses of a 10 Gy (1000 rad) and higher, the damage that results in death is due to damage of the *gastrointestinal* system. Following a short latent period, the victim will exhibit severe diarrhea, dehydration, loss of weight, and exhaustion. Death occurs in approximately 3 to 10 days. Death of the immature cells of the epithelial lining of the intestine, which are normally sloughed off and replaced, results in inability to absorb necessary nutrients and maintain body fluid balance. At doses of approximately 0.2 to 0.8 Gy (200 to 800 rads), the dose is not high enough to seriously affect the gastrointestinal tract. It is high enough to kill mitotically active precursor blood cells. It will be the *hematopoietic* system, then, that will be affected. In humans, there is a rather long latent period of a few weeks. During this time, as mature blood cells die off naturally, the supply of immature cells is inadequate for replacement. At about 3 weeks, fatigue, petechial hemorrhages, ulceration of the mouth, and bleeding may occur. More seriously, infections and fever from white blood cell depression may occur. If other symptoms are not too severe, infection may be controlled by antibiotics.

One way of expressing the lethality of a dose is the LD_{50}. This means the dose that will result in a specified end-point, in this case death, to 50% of the population. For humans, the LD_{50} is thought to be about 3 to 3.5 Gy (300 to 350 rads) for healthy adults irradiated but with no medical intervention. With medical intervention, particularly prevention and treatment of infection, it may be possible to raise this by a factor of two.[8]

Cataract Induction

The lens of the eye differs from other organs in that dead and injured cells are not removed. Damage to the lens caused by a single dose of approximately 5 Sv (500 rem) will induce opacities that interfere with vision within a year. When the dose occurs over a protracted time, a total dose of 8 Sv (800 rem) or larger is required, and the cataract appears several years after the last exposure.[10] The 1980 BEIR report[2] concludes that cataract induction should not be a concern for the doses currently permitted radiation workers. For example, even if a worker received 0.05 Sv/yr to the eyes, for a working lifetime of 40 years, (both high estimates), the lifetime dose would be 2 Sv, which is still well below the threshold.

Fertility Effects

Doses of a few Sv to the human testes can lead to permanent sterility; smaller doses cause only a temporary reduction in the number of sperm cells. A single dose of 4 Sv(400 rem) to the ovaries is required to produce permanent sterility; at 0.5 Sv (50 rem) temporary amenorrhea (SP) can occur. Occupational exposure levels will not result in fertility effects.[6]

Late Effects

Radiation has also been shown to produce effects that may occur long after the dose is received due to damage to cells that is expressed much later. If this cell is a germ cell (oocyte or sperm), damage may result as a genetic mutation. Damage to all other cells of the body, *somatic cells,* may result in leukemia or cancer in the exposed individual. These are *stochastic* effects, meaning there is a probability of occurrence that has no threshold, increases with increasing doses to the individual, but that does not increase with severity as a function of the dose. For example, both a dose of 0.1 Sv (10 rem) and 1 Sv (100 rem) may cause leukemia to develop later in life, but in both cases the leukemia is the same in severity. The difference is that the probability of occur-

rence will be greater with the higher dose.

Knowledge of somatic late effects of radiation is based on studies of groups of people who were exposed to ionizing radiation. There have been a number of such groups, the largest of which are the survivors of the bombing of Hiroshima and Nagasaki who have been carefully followed. Many other examples exist, often with irradiation to specific areas of the body, such as children irradiated for an enlarged thymus who developed subsequent thyroid cancer and women irradiated for pneumothorax who developed subsequent breast cancer. In all cases the dose received and the time to acquire the dose are estimated and the data plotted (Figure 7-10). Animal studies will also be used to expand the data. The data points in Figure 7-10 demonstrate the difficulty that arises in estimating the risk at low doses. Most of the data available are for high total doses and often, high dose rates, defined as greater than 0.1 Gy/min. The doses of concern are at much lower doses and dose rates. It is necessary to attempt to interpret the data to develop a mathematical model that may be used to predict the response at low doses. Groups such as the National Academy of Sciences Committee on the Biological Effects of Ionizing Radiation (BEIR V) have done extensive reviews and analysis of the data. The two most common models, as shown in Figure 7-11, are the linear model *(curve 1)* and linear-quadratic model *(curve 2)*. There is disagreement, however, about which model should be used for estimating risk. The most current recommendation is to use the linear model, but with the proviso that the risk at low dose rates, as found in most diagnostic situations, is a factor of two or more lower than predicted by that model.

There are two additional difficulties present in estimating late effects. There is a *natural incidence* of the cancers and leukemia observed, often rather large. Also, there is a *latent period* following exposure, before

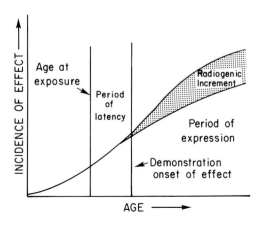

Figure 7-10 Graph illustrating the periods of latency and expression.

the effect is observed. Beyond the latent period, there will be an increase in the incidence of the cancer or leukemia, the *radiogenic increment* (Figure 7-10). This may increase at a constant rate with time or extend for a given number of years beyond exposure, depending on the cancer.

Organs and tissues differ greatly in their susceptibility to cancer induced by radiation. The organs most sensitive to radiation-induced carcinogenesis are the active bone marrow, thyroid, female breasts, and lungs.[13] Risk coefficients of radiation-induced malignancies are listed in Table 7-12. Because of the relatively high susceptibility of female breast and thyroid tissues, women have an overall greater somatic risk than men. Radiation-induced leukemia is better understood than other types of radiocarcinogenesis because of the natural rarity of the disease, the relative ease of its induction, and its short latent period. However, the combined risk of induced solid tumors (such as thyroid, lung, and female breast) exceeds that of leukemia. The

fatal risk from all malignancies is likely to be on the order of 10^{-2}/Sv, that is, the probability of death due to a radiation-induced malignancy is approximately one chance in a hundred per Sv of whole body radiation dose. The ranges of fatal risk estimates are listed in Table 7-13. The risk factors shown in Table 7-13 were derived to apply to acute doses of about 10 rem or more and should not be used for doses comparable to natural background levels or even many occupational exposures. In fact, the 1980 BEIR report refuses to discuss the effects of exposures below 0.1 Sv (10 rem) and states, "Below these doses, the uncertainties of extrapolation of risk were believed by some members of the committee to be too great to justify the calculation." Accordingly, the use of the risk factors for lower doses will yield upper-limit estimates of the fatal cancer risk of radiation exposure. Incidentally, the malignancy will result in death roughly half the time. Thus the risk of cancer induced by radiation is of the order of 2×10^{-2}/Sv.

The risks due to radiation may be compared with other occupational or overall risks. The American Cancer Society[3] has reported that approximately 25% of all adults in the 20- to 65-year age bracket will develop cancer at some time from all possible causes including cigarettes, food, drugs, air pollutants, and naturally occurring background level radiation. Thus, in any group of 10,000 workers not exposed to radiation on the job, about 2500 will develop cancer. If each of this entire group of 10,000 workers were to receive an occupational exposure of 10^{-2} (1 rem), the risk factor of 2×10^{-2}/Sv (2×10^{-4}/rem) would predict an additional two cases of cancer.

An interesting measure of risk is the life expectancy lost on the average due to radiation-induced cancer. It is estimated that the average loss of life expectancy due to radiation exposure is about 1 day/rem of whole body dose equivalent. Table 7-14 lists comparative loss of life expectancy attributed to selected health risks.

Another useful comparison is the relative fatal risk of certain everyday endeavors. For example, an NCRP publication[15] states that a one in a million risk of death has been attributed to each of the following:

400 miles by air
60 miles by car
¾ of a cigarette
20 minutes being a man of age 60
0.1 mSv (10 mrem) of whole body radiation

In conclusion, the only somatic effect thought to occur due at occupationally permitted levels is cancer induction. The probability of death due to radiation-induced cancer is conservatively believed to be less than 10^{-2}/Sv (10^{-4}/rem) when applied to the situation of a few Sv received over several years. This risk, approximately one chance in 100/Sv of whole body dose, is low when compared to the risks of fatality associated with smoking, driving, being overweight, and so on.

| | **Table 7-12** | Risk coefficients for selected organs |

Tissue	Risk coefficient (probability of biologic change per Sv)	
Gonads	40×10^{-4} Sv^{-1}	(40×10^{-6} rem^{-1})
Breast	25×10^{-4} Sv^{-1}	(25×10^{-6} rem^{-1})
Red bone marrow	20×10^{-4} Sv^{-1}	(20×10^{-6} rem^{-1})
Lung	20×10^{-4} Sv^{-1}	(20×10^{-6} rem^{-1})
Thyroid	5×10^{-4} Sv^{-1}	(5×10^{-6} rem^{-1})
Bone surfaces	5×10^{-4} Sv^{-1}	(5×10^{-6} rem^{-1})
Remainder	50×10^{-4} Sv^{-1}	(50×10^{-6} rem^{-1})
TOTAL	165×10^{-4} Sv^{-1}	(165×10^{-6} rem^{-1})

From Recommendations on limits for exposure to ionizing radiation, *National Council of Radiation Protection Report No. 91*, Washington, DC, 1987, The Council.

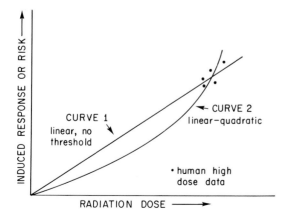

Figure 7-11 Dose response relationships.

Table 7-13 Risk coefficients for selected organs

Tissue or site	Age of exposure (years)	Years at risk*	Absolute risk coefficient†	
			Male	Female
Leukemia	0-9	5-26	1.7	1.1
	10-19	5-26	0.85	0.54
	20-34	5-26	1.1	0.67
	50+	5-26	1.6	0.99
Lungs	10-19	10-33	0.30	0.3
	20-34	10-33	0.56	0.56
	35-49	10-33	0.86	0.86
	50+	10-33	1.2	1.2
Breast	0-9	10-35	—	3.8
	10-19	10-35	—	7.6
	20-29	10-35	—	4.9
	30-39	10-35	—	4.9
	40-49	10-35	—	1.3
	50+	10-35	—	0.8
Thyroid	0-9	10-34	1.5	5.0
	10-19	10-34	1.5	5.0
	20-34	10-34	0.5	1.5
	35-49	10-34	0.5	1.5
	50+	10-34	0.5	1.5

From Rall JE et al: *Report of the National Institutes of Health working group to develop epidemiological tables,* NIH Publication No. 85-2748, Washington, DC, 1985, U.S. Government Printing Office.
*Number of excess cases of cancer per million persons per year per rem of organ dose (low-level, low-LET radiation) averaged over the specified period of expression.
†Following the radiation exposure.

Table 7-14 Estimated loss of life expectancy from selected health risks

Health risk	Estimated days of life expectancy lost, average
Smoking 20 cigarettes per day	2370
Overweight (by 20%)	985
All accidents	435
Auto accidents	200
Alcohol consumption (U.S. average)	130
Home accidents	95
Drowning	41
10 mSv (1 rem)/year for 30 years	30
Natural background radiation	8
All catastrophes (earthquakes, floods, etc.)	3.5
10 mSv (1 rem)/year occupational radiation DE	1

From U.S. Nuclear Regulatory Commission: Instruction concerning risk from occupational radiation exposure, *Draft Regulatory Guide,* Washington, DC, 1980, The Commission.

Genetic Effects

Radiation may also result in a genetic mutation. A mutation is an inherited change in a *gene,* a finite segment of DNA within a chromosome. Mutations are, generally speaking, *dominant* or *recessive.* Dominant genes are expressed in the first generation. Recessive genes are expressed only when matched with similar recessive genes and so may not be expressed for a number of generations. The genetic mutations that occur are not unique. Rather, there may be an increase in the occurrence of mutations that occur naturally or spontaneously in the population.

Radiation genetic risk estimates have been derived primarily from mouse data. Large scale human genetic studies that have been carried out to date show no significant increase in genetic endpoints with increasing dose. In particular, ongoing studies of Japanese bomb survivors have shown no statistically significant increase in five different genetic endpoints. However, based on the mouse data, there is reason to believe that humans receive radiation-induced genetic effects in a somewhat similar fashion. The current estimate of radiation induced genetic effects is that the risk of serious genetic disorders is 6 to 35 first generation cases per 10^6 live born per 10 mSv.

The *doubling dose* is the dose of radiation that will double the spontaneous mutation rate in a biologic system. Data from mouse studies and Japanese survivors have been used by groups such as BEIR V to estimate the doubling dose in humans. The current estimate as given in BEIR V is 1 Sv (100 rem).

Developmental Effects

At high doses of in utero exposure (single exposures greater than approximately 0.25 Sv), effects to the fetus have been observed. These effects include growth and developmental retardation, congenital abnormalities, and prenatal or neonatal death. Below this level, these effects are not observed or are at levels low enough to be indiscernible above the normal incidence of abnormalities, which is approximately 6% of live births. The effects are dose related and are also related to the time in pregnancy. The three periods of concern are *preimplantation,* which extends to roughly 10 days postconception; *organogenesis,* which extends to 7 weeks postconception; and *fetal development* through birth.

During preimplantation, radiation damage results in either death of the fertilized egg or survival with no measurable effect.[1] Outwardly, no effect would be noticed other than a failure to conceive.

Irradiation during organogenesis is the period of most concern. For this reason, it is often noted that radiation should be particularly limited "during the first trimester." The implanted egg multiplies rapidly and differentiation occurs, with development of organ systems. The effect of radiation is to produce congenital abnormalities. In early organogenesis these may be skeletal effects, whereas in late organogenesis neurologic effects are noted. In addition, there may be some form of growth retardation due to loss of cells. Much of the information available, however, is based on studies of mice and rats, which develop at a rate that varies from humans in extent and timing. This makes it difficult to extrapolate to the expected human effect. These effects have not been observed at less than a 0.1 Sv (10 rem) dose delivered to the embryo.

After organogenesis, the fetus continues to grow and develop. Irradiation during this stage but at higher doses may result in growth retardation or damage to organs. There is contradictory evidence that lower doses may result in an increased incidence of leukemia.[8]

In nuclear medicine the possibility for exposure to the embryo or fetus is very small. Of particular concern is that there not be accidental exposure of the fetal thyroid due to administration of radioactive iodine. The fetal thyroid takes up iodine after the tenth week of pregnancy. Since pregnancy may be easily ascertained, any woman of childbearing age who receives radioactive sodium iodide should have the pregnancy status confirmed.

REFERENCES

1. AAMP Report, College Park, MD, American Association of Physicists in Medicine.
2. Advisory Committee on the Biological Effects of Ionizing Radiations: *The effects on populations of exposure to low levels of ionizing radiation,* Washington, DC, 1980, Division of Medical Science, National Academy of Sciences, National Research Council.
3. American Cancer Society: *Cancer facts and figures,* New York, 1978, The Society.
4. Brill A, Adelstein A, Johnston R, et al, eds: *Low-level radiation effects: a fact book,* New York, 1985, Society of Nuclear Medicine.
5. Brodsky A: *Principles and practices for keeping occupational radiation exposures of medical institutions as low as reasonably achievable,* Washington DC, 1977, U.S. Nuclear Regulatory Commission Office of Standards Development.
6. Environmental Protection Agency: *Proposed federal radiation protection guidance for occupational exposure,* Washington, DC, 1981, U.S. Environmental Protection Agency Office of Radiation Programs.
7. Exposure of the population of the United States and Canada from natural background radiation, *National Council of Radiation Protection Report No. 94,* Washington, DC, 1987, National Council of Radiation Protection.
8. Hall EJ: *Radiobiology for the Radiologist,* ed 3, Philadelphia, 1978, JB Lippencott.
9. International Council of Radiation Protection Report 26: *Ann Intern Comm Radiol Protect,* vol 1, No. 3, 1977.
10. International Council of Radiation Protection Report 41: Nonstochastic effects of ionizing radiation, *Ann Intern Comm Radiol Protect,* vol 1, No. 3, 1977.
11. Implementation of the principles of ALARA for medical and dental personnel, *National Council of Radiation Protection Report No. 107,* Washington, DC, 1990, National Council of Radiation Protection.
12. Ionizing radiation exposure of the population of the United States, *National Council of Radiation Protection Report No. 93,* Washington, DC, 1987, National Council of Radiation Protection.
13. Laws P: Evaluation of health detriment from delayed effects of ionizing radiation. In *Proceedings of a symposium on biological effects, imaging techniques and dosimetry of ionizing radiations,* HHS Publication FDA 80-8126, Rockville, Md., 1980, Bureau of Radiological Health.

14. Nishiyama H: Administration of radiopharmaceuticals to patients, In Sodd V, ed: *Radiation safety in nuclear medicine: a practical guide,* HHS Publication FDA 82-8180, Rockville, Md., 1981, Bureau of Radiological Health.

15. Pochin EE: Why be quantitative about radiation risk estimates? *Lauriston S. Taylor Lecture No. 3,* Washington, DC, 1978, National Council of Radiation Protection.

16. Recommendations on limits for exposure to ionizing radiation, *National Council of Radiation Protection Report No. 91,* Washington, DC, 1987, National Council of Radiation Protection.

17. U.S. Nuclear Regulatory Commission Title 10, Code of Federal Regulations, Part 20: *Standards for protection against radiation,* Washington, DC, 1987, The Commission.

18. U.S. Nuclear Regulatory Commission Title 10, Code of Federal Regulations, Part 35: *Human uses of byproduct material,* Washington, DC, 1987, The Commission.

19. U.S. Nuclear Regulatory Commission: Information relevant to insuring that occupational radiation exposures at medical institutions will be as low as reasonably achievable, *Regulatory Guide 8.18,* Washington, DC, 1977, The Commission.

20. U.S. Nuclear Regulatory Commission: Applications of bioassay for I-125 and I-131, *Regulatory Guide 8.20,* Washington, DC, 1978, The Commission.

21. U.S. Nuclear Regulatory Commission: Guide for the preparation of applications for medical programs, *Regulatory Guide 10.8,* Washington, DC, 1980, The Commission.

22. U.S. Nuclear Regulatory Commission Title 10, Code of Federal Regulations, Part 20: Standards for protection against radiation, *Fed Reg* 56(98): 23390-23470, 1991.

chapter 8

Marcia Boyd, Kathy E. Thompson

Patient Care and Quality Improvement

Objectives

List the positive attributes of patient encounters.

Demonstrate the proper techniques for transferring patients from wheelchairs and stretchers.

Demonstrate the proper method of moving patients to obtain imaging positions.

Discuss medications commonly prescribed for patients and medications used in nuclear medicine.

Demonstrate precautions for using and disposing of sharps.

Perform the proper technique in venipuncture and intravenous administration.

Discuss monitoring and care of intravenous lines.

List and discuss sources of infection and methods to prevent disease transfer.

Discuss techniques used in universal precautions.

Demonstrate good hand-washing technique.

Obtain accurate respiration rate, pulse rate, and blood pressure measurements.

Describe actions to be taken in various medical emergencies and how to activate emergency teams in your institution.

Discuss quality improvement programs and their relationship to nuclear medicine services.

Describe methods to provide quality improvement in custom service.

Discuss techniques to obtain and analyze data relative to patient care, including problem solving.

INTRODUCTION

Few nuclear medicine facilities today have the luxury of full-time nursing personnel available at all times to assist with procedures. The nuclear medicine technologist is often the only person available to provide basic nursing care to the patient while performing the nuclear medicine procedure. In competitive markets it is also the responsibility of the nuclear medicine technologist to be accountable for providing excellent customer-oriented, quality services. This chapter will discuss the various responsibilities associated with the first encounter with the patient, patient care, and associated nursing skills and will provide a framework for continuous quality and performance improvement in nuclear medicine.

THE MECHANICS OF GETTING READY

The patient's first encounter with nuclear medicine personnel may be the most important in establishing trust and cooperation. This may be through the clerical support employee, the technologist, or assistant. As jobs are continually redesigned or reengineered in healthcare, the technologist may be the primary contact for patient encounters from scheduling to completion of the procedure.

There are multiple settings for nuclear medicine such as outpatient diagnostic centers, physicians' offices, mobile units, and hospitals. Patient encounters are modified based on the setting, but basic quality controls must be maintained and efforts to continuously improve the process must be investigated.

The first step is usually to review the referring physician's request to correlate the procedure with the history and to determine if there are any contraindications. The format used for requesting a procedure will vary with the setting. A hospitalized patient will have orders written in the hospital chart or entered electronically in the information system. Orders for an outpatient may be electronically transmitted, verbally ordered, or presented upon arrival in hard-copy or written format. There may be restrictions on the method of ordering procedures within the institution or based on legal requirements.

Some nuclear medicine procedures require special standardized patient preparation. Standardized protocols should be established with the scheduling source, for example, nursing units, physician offices, and clinics. A reminder by the nuclear medicine personnel regarding patient preparation at the time of scheduling can help prevent delays later. The scheduling source should also be aware of any conflicting exams, such as barium radiographs, nuclear medicine procedures, or interfering medications.

Basic information included on the request should be patient's name, identification number, referring physician's name, and clinical indications for the procedure. Hospitalized patients will have additional information such as room number and mode of transportation.

Arrangements must be made for the availability of the radiopharmaceutical required for the procedure. Orders must be placed for radiopharmaceuticals not routinely stocked. When radiopharmaceuticals are prepared on site, the timing from preparation to injection must be a consideration. Ample time must be allocated when ordering from an "external" nuclear pharmacy so that arrival of the patient and the radiopharmaceutical dose are synchronized.

A simplified flow chart of the process of scheduling a patient is presented in Figure 8-1. Several preparations must be made including the following:

Quality control measurements must be taken on all equipment, for example, the dose calibrators, camera, and computer.

Personnel must be trained in the technical aspects of procedures and in customer service.

Necessary supplies must be assembled.

Radiopharmaceutical doses must be assayed.

Emergency equipment and supplies must be available.

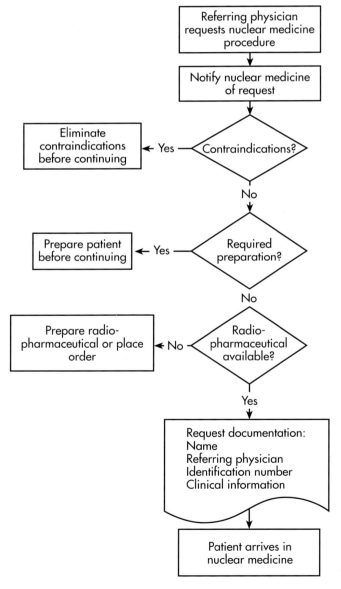

Figure 8-1 Flow chart of scheduling process in nuclear medicine department.

THE PATIENT ENCOUNTER

The first 30 seconds are considered crucial to setting the stage for the perception of excellent customer service. The person greeting the patient, whether it is the transporter, technologist, or clerical personnel, must do so in a friendly, caring manner. It is important to remember that most patients have limited knowledge of the nuclear medicine procedures, and the term *nuclear* alone may initiate unrealistic fears.

The patient must be clearly identified on arrival. The wrist band serves as an identifying tool for the hospitalized patient. An outpatient may be asked for information such as to repeat his or her name, spell the name, and recite the address and social security number. Often billing information must be obtained at the time of arrival; this will provide a means to assist with identification.

When the patient arrives in the nuclear medicine department, further investigation must be made that the correct procedure is scheduled and that there are no contraindications. A brief history is taken on the patient that will give insight if there are any contraindications. Medication or a disease that will interfere with the procedure will call for special precautions or an alteration of the protocol used. For outpatients, minimal information may be available. Hospitalized patients normally arrive with their hospital chart, and the current medical status is easily determined by reviewing the chart. If preparation for the procedure is required, a determination must be made that orders were clearly followed.

Patients expect the courtesy of receiving an explanation of what is expected of them, what the nuclear medicine personnel will be doing, any discomfort they will experience, the required length of time for the procedure, and how and when they will hear about the results. Careful explaining at this point will help ensure cooporation throughout the procedure and beyond. It is important not to use technical terminology that the patient may have difficulty understanding.

The technologist must ascertain the extent of the patient's physical ability. Special care needs may be required for patients who are physically challenged. Assistance must be provided for those patients unable to move on and off imaging tables. The geriatric patient may have a hearing loss, making it difficult to follow instructions. Pediatric cases require special handling techniques, and the psychiatric patient may have special needs.

Information is presented in the next few pages on body mechanics and patient handling, medications and their administration, infection control, basic nursing skills such as vital signs, caring for the patient requiring emergency procedures, and the use of special equipment. Establishing a quality or performance improvement process, which involves strategic planning, process management, customer satisfaction, analysis and management of data, and specific problem-solving

tools and techniques for the individual technologist and nuclear medicine teams, is also discussed.

BODY MECHANICS AND PATIENT HANDLING

The principles of proper body alignment, movement, and balance are referred to as body mechanics. Practicing the concepts of body mechanics is important in terms of the health and wellness of the technologist as well as the safety of the patient.

Concepts of Body Mechanics (Figure 8-2)

Base of support—Provide wide and stable base of support by standing with feet apart shoulder width and one foot slightly advanced.
Center of gravity—Keep objects close rather than reaching out for them. The weight of an object is multiplied by a factor of 10 for every inch it is held away from the body.
Line of gravity—Keep the back straight and avoid twisting the trunk when lifting and carrying. Bend the knees when reaching near the floor.

Lifting Tips

Avoid heavy lifting above shoulder or below hand or knuckle level.
Keep stomach muscles tight when lifting while using leg and abdominal muscles.
Bend at the hips and knees when lifting below the hands or knuckle level.

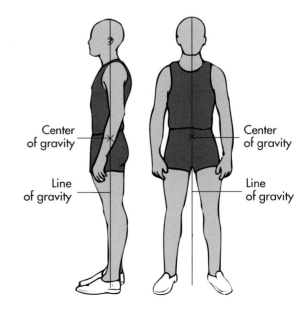

Figure 8-2 Correct body alignment. (From Kowalczyk N, Donnett K: *Integrated patient care for the imaging professional,* St. Louis, 1996, Mosby.)

Pushing/Pulling Tips

Push rather than pull, using leg and abdominal muscles.
If pulling is necessary, do so by walking forward.

Carrying Tips

Hold loads with arms and legs working together.
Avoid bending neck to the side when carrying a load on the shoulder.
Vary carrying techniques and pause for rests when carrying long distances.

Patient Transfers

The first step is to determine that the technologist has the correct patient. The next step is to assess the patient's ability to move and explain to the patient his/her role in the transfer.

Wheelchair Transfers

To transfer a patient from the bed to a wheelchair, start by lowering the bed to the level of the wheelchair seat and elevating the head of the bed. Position the wheelchair parallel to the bed with wheels locked, and remove footrests. Place one arm under the patient's

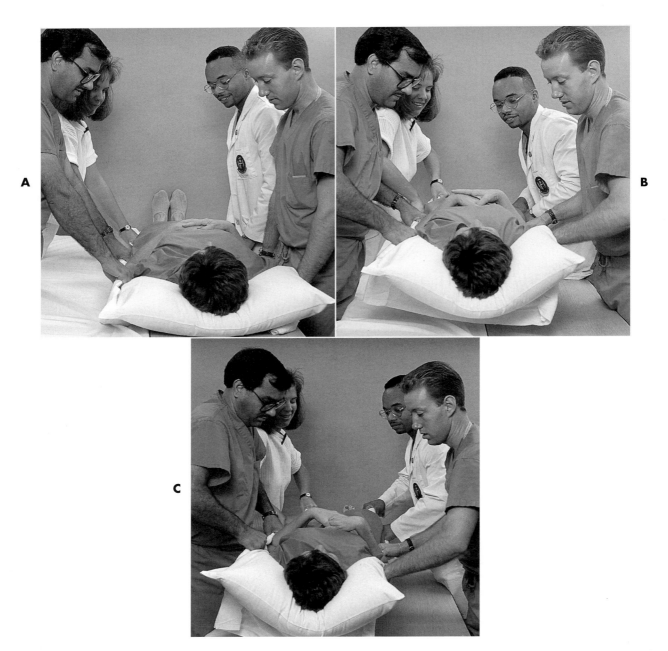

Figure 8-3 Patient transfer using a sheet. (From Kowalczyk N, Donnett K: *Integrated patient care for the imaging professional,* St. Louis, 1996, Mosby.)

shoulders and the other arm under the knees to raise the patient to a sitting position. Take time for the patient to adjust to the upright position. Take precautions to ensure patient safety by supporting the patient. Many patients suffer from orthostatic hypotension after long periods of rest and feel light headed or faint when rising suddenly. After this adjustment period, most patients will be able to move to the wheelchair with only minimal assistance.

Orthopedic or neurologically impaired patients require more assistance. Always position the patient's strongest side toward the area he/she is being transferred to. Stand facing the patient. Reaching around the patient, place hands over scapulae. The patient's hand may rest on the technologist's shoulders. On signal, lift upward. If the patient has an injured leg or foot, the technologist should place his/her feet around the affected foot and using knees block the patient's knee. Pivot the patient toward his/her strong side and into the wheelchair.

To move a patient from the wheelchair to imaging table, place the wheelchair parallel to the table with the patient's strongest side toward the table. Lock the brakes, move footrests, and help the patient stand, using face-to-face assist as described. Have the patient place one hand on the footstool handle and one arm on the technologist's shoulder and step onto stool, with strong side first, pivoting with his/her back to the table. Ease the patient into a sitting position. Place one arm around the patient and the other arm under the patient's knees. With a single motion, place the legs on

the table while lowering the head and shoulders into the supine position.

If a patient is unable to stand, a stretcher should be used. Start with the patient in the supine position with knees flexed and feet flat. Position the stretcher parallel to the imaging table toward the patient's strongest side and lock the wheels. Place one arm under the patient's shoulders and the other arm under the pelvis. Instruct the patient to push with his/her feet and elbows as the technologist lifts and pulls. For the first pull, use only the arm muscles. The maneuver should be repeated. The next pull should be accomplished as the technologist places his/her leg or knee on the stretcher or table to lock the lumbar spine and prevent using the lower back. Repeat as required until the transfer is complete.

Use "draw sheet" lifts or a slide board when a patient is unable to assist. A draw sheet is a sheet folded in half that is placed under the patient. When transferring the patient, the sheet is rolled up close to the patient to provide a handhold for lifting and pulling the patient. A slide board can be used in conjunction with the draw sheet. Roll the patient on his/her side and insert the board under the draw sheet, including the patient's head and torso. The slide board provides a hard surface to make the transfer easier. The use of antistatic spray will prevent the build up of static electricity on the board. Note: these techniques require two or more persons (Figures 8-3 and 8-4).

Safety straps are to be used with all transfer patients from a wheelchair or stretcher. Safety straps should also

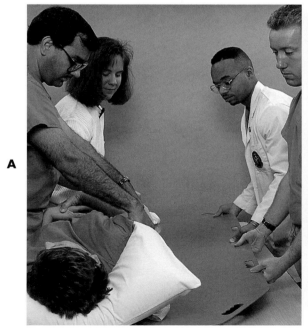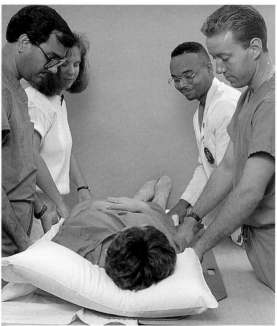

Figure 8-4 Patient transfer using a slide board. **A,** Log roll the patient to one side and position the slide board. **B,** Slide the patient onto the slide board. (From Kowalczyk N, Donnett K: *Integrated patient care for the imaging professional,* St. Louis, 1996, Mosby.)

be used on imaging tables if possible. A patient transferred by stretcher should have side rails in place at all times. The use of restraints may require a physician's order. For more information on the use of immobilizers, see Chapter 18.

MEDICATIONS AND THEIR ADMINISTRATION

Verify the order by checking patient's written records. No medication is given without the order of a physician. The order may be written or oral. The generic name of a medication identifies its chemical family. Different pharmaceutical companies may manufacture the same generic substance under a different proprietary or trade name. A useful resource that lists medications alphabetically according to their generic classes, trade names, or indications is the Physician's Desk Reference (PDR) (Tables 8-1 and 8-2).

Medication Administration

The correct administration of pharmaceuticals include the five rights system as follows:

1. The right dose
2. Of the right medication
3. To the right patient
4. At the right time
5. By the right route

Medications may be administered by several routes: topical, oral, parenteral, and intravenous.

- *Topical Route*—Medication is applied to a limited area for a local effect, for example, germicidal solution used to cleanse the skin. An example of a topical drug used for heart patients is nitroglycerin. Nitroglycerin is administered sublingually and is absorbed directly into the bloodstream, dilating the coronary arteries. This produces a systemic effect to counteract angina pectoris.
- *Oral Route*—Oral medications are supplied in a variety of forms including tablets, capsules, granules, and liquids. Sodium iodine is administered by mouth, usually in capsule or liquid form, for thyroid uptakes, scans, and therapy, for example,

I-123 or I-131. Radioactive vitamin B_{12} is administered in capsule form by mouth.

  Oral medications are administered as follows: Wash hands.

  Read the label and prepare for administration.

  If physician is administering the medication, show him/her the label.

  If the physician requests the technologist to administer the medication, check the patient's identification and read the label again before administering. Stay with the patient while the medication is swallowed, and offer water if permitted.
- *Parenteral route*—These are medications injected directly into the body and may be of several types and are classified according to the depth of the injection (Figure 8-5).

  Subcutaneous (under the skin) medications are injected at a 45-degree angle using a ⅝-in needle with a 23 to 25 gauge. The most common injection sites are the upper arm or outer aspect of the thigh. Injection volume is usually 2 ml or less. Example: allergy injections.

  Intramuscular (into the muscle) medications are given into the deltoid muscle of the upper arm, the upper quadrant of the gluteus maximus muscle in the hip, or the vastus lateralis muscle of the lateral thigh. The injection volume may be up to 5 ml, and the needle size can range from 25 to 22 gauge. Example: vitamin B_{12} injections.

  Intradermal (between the layers of skin) medications are administered using a tuberculin syringe with a very small needle (26 or 27 gauge). Example: tuberculin skin test and lymphoscintigraphy.

  Intravenous administration is the parenteral route most often used in nuclear medicine and will be discussed in more depth later.

Withdrawal of Nonradioactive Medications

Assemble the syringe and needle. Read the label to ascertain the correct medication, concentration, and ex-

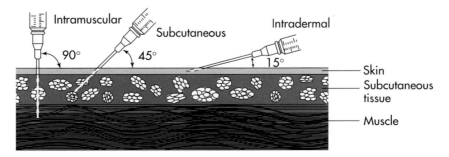

Figure 8-5 Comparison of the angles of needle insertion. (Modified from Potter PA, Perry AG: *Fundamentals of nursing: concepts, process, and practice*, ed 3, St. Louis, 1994, Mosby.)

piration date. If the drug is supplied in ampule form, a small file is needed to nick the neck of ampule. Use a 2 in × 2 in gauze to protect fingers and snap off the top (Figure 8-6). A filter needle may be used to draw up the medication and eliminate the glass particles. If the drug is supplied in a vial, a metal or plastic cap will need to be removed. If the vial is used for multiple doses, after the first puncture, clean the rubber septum with alcohol. Remove the needle cover, taking care not to contaminate the needle. Insert the needle into the rubber septum at a 45-degree angle, straighten the needle when puncturing the septum, and withdraw the desired amount while checking for any air bubbles. Air bubbles may be removed by tapping the sides of the syringe.

Withdrawal of Radioactive Material

Gloves should always be worn when handling radioactivity. Required lead glass syringe shields are available

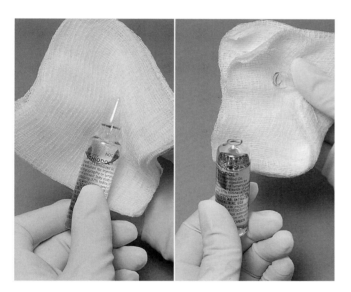

Figure 8-6 Preparing medication from an ampule. (From Kowalczyk N, Donnett K: *Integrated patient care for the imaging professional*, St. Louis, 1996, Mosby.)

in several syringe sizes to decrease the exposure when withdrawing and injecting radioactivity. Assemble the syringe and needle, and lock them securely into the syringe shield. Remove the needle cover, taking care not to contaminate the needle. Clean the rubber septum with alcohol and insert needle at a 45-degree angle, straightening the needle when puncturing the septum. This will prevent breaking off pieces of the rubber septum and introducing them into the vial. Turn the shielded vial upside down and withdraw the desired volume while checking for air bubbles. Do not inject air into vial when withdrawing radiopharmaceuticals (Figure 8-7).

Preparation for Venipuncture

The antecubital or median cubital vein on the anterior surface of the elbow is usually used. The medial basilic or cephalic veins or veins of the anterior wrist and posterior hand may also be used. Dilate the vein by applying the tourniquet 4 to 6 in above the venipuncture site. Ask the patient to hold a tight fist. Apply gloves. Palpate the area, using the first finger to locate a vein by feeling for a rebound sensation. Prepare the site using an alcohol swab, working outward from the site in a circular motion (Figure 8-8).

Intravenous Equipment

Venipuncture may be accomplished with a hypodermic needle, a butterfly set, or an intravenous catheter. A butterfly set is often used for direct injections with a syringe. Before the butterfly needle is inserted into the vein, the tubing is filled with liquid from the syringe to avoid injecting air. To insert a winged steel needle of a butterfly set, remove the cover and turn the bevel of the needle up, grasping the wings of the device between the thumb and index finger. The wings of the device may be taped to the patient's skin after the needle is in place. This prevents movement of the needle in the vein.

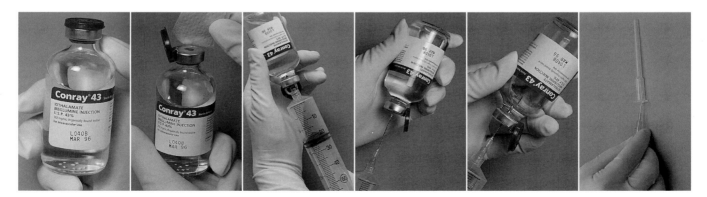

Figure 8-7 Drawing up medication from a vial. (From Kowalczyk N, Donnett K: *Integrated patient care for the imaging professional*, St.Louis, 1996, Mosby.)

Table 8-1 Overview of clinical pharmacology

Class	Why used	Examples (brand names) other uses
Antihistamines		
Allergies	Prevent allergic reactions	Diphenhydramine *(Benadryl)* Astemizole *(Hismanal)*
Antiinfectives		

Antibiotics	Treat/prevent
	 Bacterial infections
		Aminoglycosides (IV)
		    Gentamicin, tobramycin—nephrotoxic
		 Penicillins, cephalosporins
		    Amoxicillin *(Amoxil), Unasyn, Timentin*
		    Cefazolin, cefuroxime, ceftriaxone *(Rocephin)*
		 Quinolones
		    Ciprofloxacin *(Cipro)*, ofloxacin *(Floxin)*
		 Other miscellaneous
		    Clindamycin, erythromycin, metronidazole,
		    Trimethoprim/sulfamethoxazole *(Bactrim)*, vanco-
		    mycin, doxycycline

Antifungals	Treat/prevent Fungal infections	Fluconazole *(Diflucan)* Amphotericin B—nephrotoxic
Antineoplastics		
	Treat cancer	Cyclophosphamide, ifosfamide—nephrotoxic doxorubicin, fluorouracil, methotrexate, cisplatin, carboplatin, vincristine, vinblastine
Autonomic		
Anticholinergics	Inhibit effects of parasympa- thetic nervous system activity	Atropine—preop for salivation; causes dry mouth, constipation Ipratropium *(Atrovent)*—inhaled for COPD
Adrenergics	Bronchodilation Increase HR, BP	Albuterol *(Ventolin)*—inhaled for asthma See cardiac drugs
Coagulation		
Anticoagulants	Treat/prevent blood clots: for DVT/PE, AMI, Afib	Heparin (IV) Warfarin *(Coumadin)*
Thrombolytics	Break up clots for AMI	TPA, streptokinase
Cardiovascular		

Cardiac drugs	Increase heart's contraction	Digoxin *(Lanoxin)*—also for Afib
		 Dobutamine *(Dobutrex)*
		 Dopamine
		    Low dose increases urine output
		    High dose increases heart contractility

	Treat arrythmias	Lidocaine, Bretylium
Antilipemic	Treat elevated cholesterol	Lovastatin *(Mevacor)* Cholestyramine *(Questran)*

Hypotensives	Reduce blood pressure	ACE-inhibitors—also CHF, diabetes
		    Captopril *(Capoten)*, enalapril *(Vasotec)*
		 Beta-blockers—also post MI
		    Atenolol *(Tenormin)*, metoprolol *(Lopressor)*
		 Calcium chanel blockers
		    Diltiazem *(Cardizem)*, verapamil *(Calan)*
		    Nifedipine *(Adalat, Procardia)*
		 Central a_2 agonists
		    Clonidine
		    Methyldopa *(Aldomet)*
		 Peripheral a_1 antagonists
		    Prazosin *(Minipress)*, terazosin *(Hytrin)*

From McEvoy GK, ed: *American Hospital Formulary Service—Drug Information*, Bethesda, Md., 1996, American Society of Health-System Pharmacists. Modified by Ted Morton, PharmD, Baptist Memorial Hospital, Memphis, Tenn.

Table 8-1 Overview of clinical pharmacology—cont'd

Class	Why used	Examples (brand names) other uses
Cardiovascular—cont'd		
Vasodilators	Angina, acute MI	Nitrates
		Nitroglycerin, isosorbide dinitrate *(Isordil)*
CNS-agents		
Analgesics and antipyretics	Pain and fever	Aspirin—also antiplatelet (stroke, MI, angina)
		Acetaminophen *(Tylenol)*
		NSAIDs—Can be nephrotoxic esp w/ ACE-inhibitor
		Ibuprofen *(Motrin)*
		Indomethacin *(Indocin)*—also for gout
Analgesics	Pain	Opiates
		Morphine, meperidine *(Demerol)*
	Reverse opiate-induced sedation and respiratory depression	Opiate antagonist
		Naloxone *(Narcan)* (IV)
Anticonvulsants	Prevent seizures	Phenytoin *(Dilantin)*
		Carbamazepine *(Tegretol)*
		Valproic acid *(Depakene)*
Psychotherapeutics	Depression	Amitriptyline *(Elavil)*
	Psychosis, agitation	Fluoxetine *(Prozac)*
		Haloperidol *(Haldol)*
Anxiolytics	Anxiety, insomnia	Benzodiazepines
		Midazolam *(Versed)*, lorazepam *(Ativan)*
Water/electrolytes		
Diuretics	Remove fluid	Loop—also in CHF
		Furosemide *(Lasix)*
		Thiazide—also in HTN
		Hydrochlorothiazide
Gastrointestinals		
Miscellaneous	Prevent acid secretion	H_2 blockers
		Ranitidine *(Zantac)*, cimetidine *(Tagamet)*
		Proton pump inhibitors
		Omeprazole *(Prilosec)*
Prokinetics	Speed passage of food out of stomach	Metoclopramide *(Reglan)*
		Cisapride *(Propulsid)*
Antiemetics	Prevent/treat nausea/vomiting	Promethazine *(Phenergan)*
		Ondansetron *(Zofran)*
Hormonal		
Adrenals	Supplement, antiinflammatory	Prednisone (PO)
		Methylprednisolone (IV)
		Triamcinolone *(Azmacort)*—inhaled-asthma
Antidiabetics	Replace insulin	Insulin (many kinds)
	Stimulate insulin release	Sulfonylureals
		Glipizide *(Glucotrol)*
		Glyburide *(DiaBeta, Micronase)*
	Increase glucose uptake	Metformin *(Glucophage)*
		Contraindication: Must not give within 2 days of radiological procedures, and then hold metformin until renal function returns
Thyroid	Replace	Levothyroxine *(Synthroid)*
	Suppress	Propylthiouracil
Miscellaneous		
Asthma/COPD	Relax bronchial muscle	Theophylline *(Theo-Dur)*, aminophylline
Gout	Acute	Colchicine
	Chronic	Allopurinol
Parkinson's disease	Restore dopamine/ACh balance	Benztropine *(Cogentin)*
		Carbidopa/levodopa *(Sinemet)*

Table 8-2 Nonradioactive pharmaceuticals used in nuclear medicine

Pharmaceutical	Indication	Dosage	Adverse effects
Acetazolamide (Diamox)	Brain perfusion	1 g in 10 ml sterile water, IV over 2 min	Tingling sensations in extremities and mouth, flushing, lightheadedness, blurred vision, headache
Adenosine (Adenocard)	Cardiac stress imaging	140 μg/kg/min for 6 min, or 50 μg/kg/min increased to 75, 100, and 140 μg/kg/min each min to 7 min	Chest, throat, jaw, or arm pain, headache, flushing, dyspnea, ECG changes
Bethanechol (Urecholine)	Gastric emptying	2.5-5 mg subcutaneously	Abdominal discomfort, salivation, flushing, sweating, nausea, fall in blood pressure
Captopril (Capoten)	Renovascular hypertension evaluation	25-50 mg orally 1 hr before study	Orthostatic hypotension, rash, dizziness, chest pain, tachycardia, loss of taste
Cholecystokinin (Kinevac)	Hepatobiliary imaging	0.02 μg/kg in 10 ml saline, IV over 5 min	Abdominal pain, urge to defecate, nausea, dizziness, and flushing
Cimetidine (Tagamet)	Meckel's diverticulum imaging	Adult: 300 mg/kg Pediatric: 20 mg/kg in 20 ml saline, IV over 2 min with imaging 1 hr later	Diarrhea, headache, dizziness, confusion, and bradychardia
Dipyridamole (Persantine)	Cardiac stress imaging	0.57 mg/kg IV over 4 min (0.142 mg/kg/min)	Chest pain, nausea, headache, dizziness, flushing, tachycardia, shortness of breath, and hypotension
Dobutamine (Dobutrex)	Cardiac function reserve	Incremental dose rate of 15 μg/kg/min up to 15 (child); up to 40 μg/kg/min every 3 min (adult)	Angina, tachyarrhythmia, headache, nausea, and vomiting
Enalaprilat (Vasotec IV)	Renovascular hypertension evaluation	0.04 mg/kg in 10 ml saline, IV over 5 min	Orthostatic hypotension, dizziness, chest pain, headache, vomiting, and diarrhea
Furosemide (Lasix)	Renal imaging	Adult: 20 to 40 mg Pediatric: 0.5 to 1 mg/kg, IV over 1-2 min	Nausea, vomiting, diarrhea, headache, dizziness, and hypotension
Glucagon	Meckel's diverticulum imaging	Adult: 0.5 mg (range 0.25 to 2 mg) Pediatric: 5μg/kg, IV or IM	Nausea, vomiting
Morphine (Astramorph, Duramorph)	Hepatobiliary imaging	0.04 mg/kg, diluted in 10 ml saline, IV over 2 min (range 2-4.5 mg)	Respiratory depression, nausea, sedation, lightheadedness, dizziness, and sweating
Pentagastrin (Peptavlon)	Meckel's diverticulum imaging	6 μg/kg subcutaneously	Abdominal discomfort, urge to defecate, nausea, flushing, headache, dizziness, tachycardia, and drowsiness
Phenobarbital (Luminal)	Hepatobiliary imaging	5 mg/kg/day orally for 5 days	Respiratory depression, nausea, vomiting, dizziness, drowsiness, headache, and paradoxical excitement in children
Vitamin B$_{12}$ (Cyanoject, Cyomin)	Schilling test	1 mg IM 2 hr after radioactive B$_{12}$ dose	None

Modified from Park HM, Duncan K: Non-radioactive pharmaceuticals in nuclear medicine, *J Nucl Med Technol*, vol 22, No. 4, 1994.

The use of hypodermic needles is generally restricted to withdrawing blood samples or for single injections. Hypodermic needles are supplied in various diameters and lengths. The gauge of a needle indicates the diameter, and the gauge increases as the diameter of the bore decreases. The length of the needle is measured in inches, and may vary from ½ in for intradermal use to 4½ in for intrathecal (spinal cord) injections. To insert a hypodermic needle, remove the needle cover and turn the bevel upward.

The technique for venipuncture is the same using a butterfly set or hypodermic needle. Anchor the vein by stretching the vein firmly in the opposite direction of the course of the needle. Hold needle at a 30-degree angle, and penetrate the skin just below the point where the vein is to be entered. Avoid touching the insertion site after cleaning it with alcohol. Advance the needle quickly but cautiously, penetrating the vein with the needle point. Usually there is a sensation of resistance followed by an ease of penetration with a flashback of blood into the tubing, in the case of the butterfly set, or into the needle hub, in the case of the hypodermic needle, as the vein is entered. Carefully advance the needle into the vein while continuing to hold the skin taut and the needle in a direct line with the vein to prevent puncture of the posterior wall of the vein.

To confirm that the needle is in the vein using a hypodermic needle and syringe, withdraw a small amount of blood before injecting the radiopharmaceutical. To confirm placement of needle using a butterfly set, inject sterile water or saline before injecting the radiopharmaceutical. Observe for signs of possible infiltration such as puffiness in the area. If signs are present, discontinue immediately. Release the tourniquet and withdraw the needle. Apply pressure immediately with a dry gauze or cotton ball and maintain pressure for 1 min or until bleeding stops (Figure 8-9).

Intravenous catheters are frequently used when repeated intravenous injections, infusions, or bolus injections will be administered. An over-the-needle catheter is composed of a silicon catheter with a stylet/needle inside the catheter lumen. To insert an over-the-needle catheter, remove the needle cover and turn the bevel of the stylet/needle up. Anchor the vein and insert the needle at a 25- to 30-degree angle, and lower the needle unit until it is almost flush with the skin and enter the

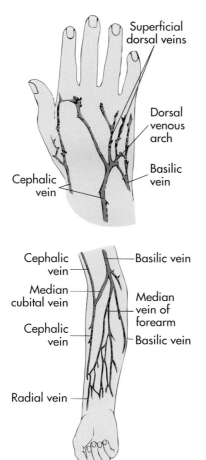

Figure 8-8 Veins easily accessible for venipuncture. (From Kowalczyk N, Donnett K: *Integrated patient care for the imaging professional,* St. Louis, 1996, Mosby.)

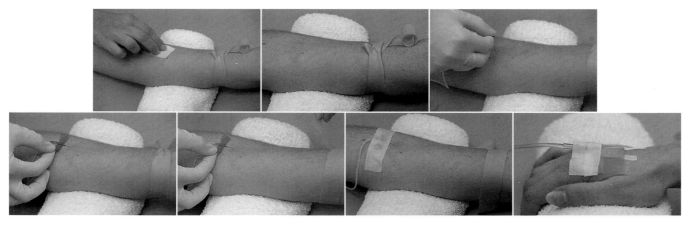

Figure 8-9 Venipuncture. (From Kowalczyk N, Donnett K: *Integrated patient care for the imaging professional,* St.Louis, 1996, Mosby.)

vein. This is to prevent piercing of the posterior wall. Check for vein entry by observing a flashback of blood, and advance the needle ¼ in farther into the vein to establish catheter tip. Holding the stylet/needle hub with one hand, use the thumb and forefinger of the other hand to gently advance the catheter off the stylet/needle and into the vein. Do not reinsert the stylet/needle. Release the tourniquet and relax the tension on the skin. Remove the stylet/needle from the catheter. To prevent excessive flashback of blood, use the index finger to apply digital pressure on the vein above catheter. A 2 in × 2 in sterile gauze pad may be placed under the catheter hub to prevent leakage of blood onto the patient's skin (Figure 8-10).

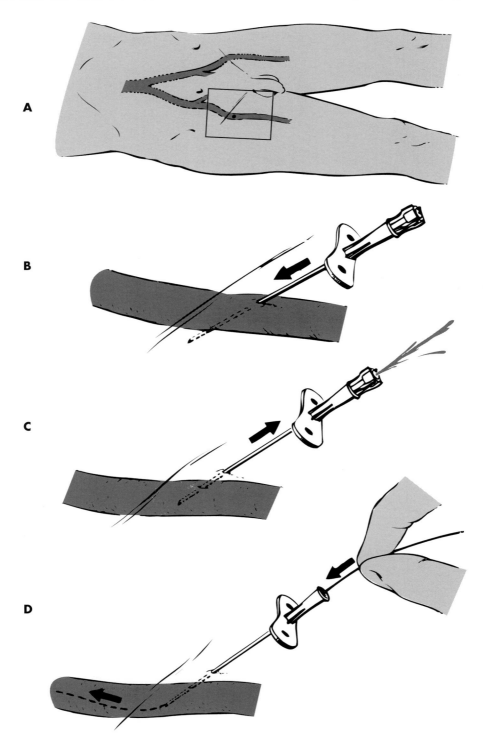

Figure 8-10 Seldinger technique **(A–G)**. (From Kowalczyk N, Donnett K: *Integrated patient care for the imaging professional,* St.Louis, 1996, Mosby.)

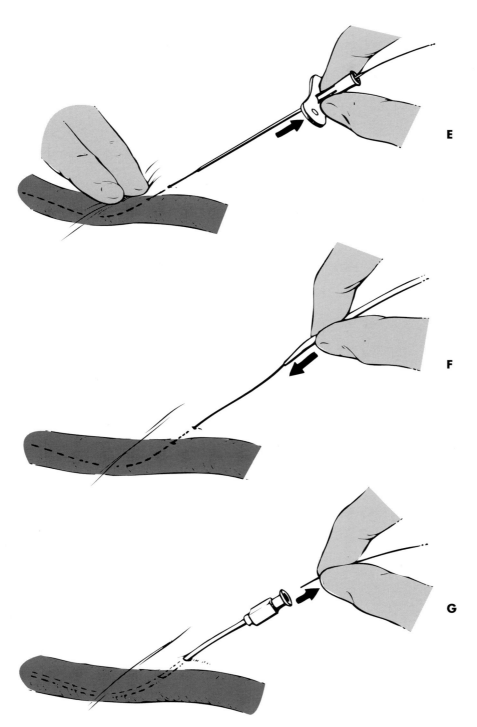

E

F

G

Figure 8-10 cont'd.   For legend see opposite page.

Needleless Systems

Blunt cannulae can be used to draw up medications and to access established intravenous lines for blood draws and medication administration. (Figures 8-11, 8-12, and 8-13).

Extravasation or Infiltration Precautions

Extravasation or infiltration occurs when fluid leaks from the venous system into the tissues. The following precautions should be taken:

1. Check for backflow or flashback to determine needle placement.
2. Immobilize the needle or catheter at the injection site.
3. Stop the injection immediately if the patient complains of discomfort at the injection site, if any resistance to the injection is felt, or if puffiness around the site is observed.

If infiltration does occur, maintain pressure on the vein until bleeding has stopped completely. This procedure may avoid a painful hematoma.

Needle Disposal

Dispose of all syringes and needles directly into a puncture-proof container without recapping. Containers are labeled according to the type of contamination: biohazard and/or radioactive.

Radioactive syringes will sometimes require recapping before disposal to avoid radioactive contamination. If it is necessary to recap a used needle, place the needle cover on a firm surface and insert the needle using one hand only or use a needle cap holder.

Several additional points must be remembered when administering medications:

1. Know the indications and side effects of the medication before administration.
2. Follow the established rules of the aseptic technique.
3. Read the label three times: before and after withdrawal of the medication and before administration. The technologist is responsible for medication that he/she administers, regardless who has prepared it.
4. Check medication for proper concentration and expiration date (Figure 8-14).
5. Check patient identification before administration.
6. Monitor the patient for side effects. Be familiar with any medication that may require an antidote and where the emergency cart is located.
7. A medication error must be reported according to institutional policy. The patient's physician must also be notified.

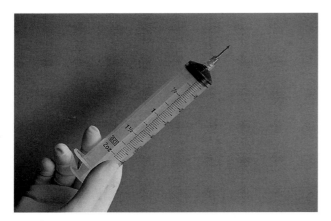

Figure 8-11 Interlink vial access cannula. (Courtesy Baxter Health Care.)

Monitor Intravenous Lines

The drip or flow rate of an intravenous line can be determined by consulting the patient's chart. An infusion

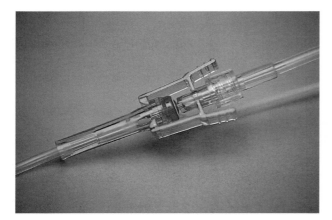

Figure 8-12 Needleless system interlink level lock for intravenous piggyback medication administration. (Courtesy Baxter Health Care.)

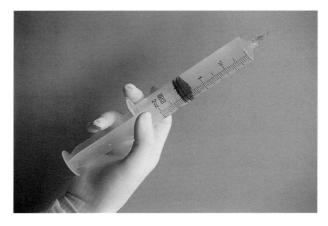

Figure 8-13 Interlink syringe cannula. (Courtesy Baxter Health Care.)

rate of 15-20 drops/min or approximately 60 ml/hr is common. The infusion rate can be controlled by a clamp or medication pump.

Several precautions should be taken when monitoring an IV. Always keep the IV solution 18 to 20 in above the level of the vein. If the solution is inadvertently placed lower than the vein, blood will flow back into the needle or tubing and may clot. An IV solution that is too high may cause fluid to infiltrate into surrounding tissues because of the increased hydrostatic pressure.

Precautions in caring for patients with IV lines include the following:

Call in advance and inform the nurse if the procedure will be lengthy.

Whenever possible, plug the IV pump into an electrical outlet rather than relying on battery power.

Watch IV fluid levels and allow enough time for fluid replacement before the IV fluid is exhausted.

If an IV set does run out or if an alarm sounds despite appropriate trouble shooting, call the nursing service immediately rather than waiting until the patient is returned to the nursing unit.

When performing IV injections through lines, flush with at least 10 cc saline or sterile water.

Have a good understanding of the pumps used in the facility.

Charting Medications

Notation that the study was completed along with any medications given should be recorded in the patient's records. The notation should include the time of day, the name of the drug, the dosage, and the route of administration. The entry must include the identification of the person who charted it. For legal purposes the technologist who charts medications must use the procedure established by the institution.

Infection Control

Medical asepsis is the technique used to prevent the spread of infection or disease by reducing the number of infectious microorganisms or pathogens. Microorganisms include bacteria, viruses, protozoans, and fungi.

The cycle of infection involves a pathogenic organism, reservoir of infection, means of transmission, and a susceptible host (Figure 8-15).

The reservoir of infection can be any place the microorganisms can find nutrients, moisture, and warmth. The human body provides this type of medium. Some microorganisms live on or within the body as part of our normal flora and aid in digestion and skin preservation. These organisms are nonpathogenic as long as they are confined to their usual environment but can assume a pathogenic role outside of their environment. Pathogens can also live in the bodies of healthy individuals without causing apparent disease. These persons are called carriers and may be a reservoir for infection without realizing it.

Although the human body is the most common reservoir of infection, any environment that will support growth of the microorganisms has the potential to be a secondary source. Such sources may include contaminated food or water or any damp, warm place that is not cleaned regularly.

Compromised immune systems of our patients make them susceptible hosts. They may develop a secondary problem or nosocomial (hospital-acquired) infection.

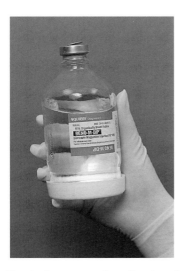

Figure 8-14 Check the name of medication, its strength, and the expiration date. (From Kowalczyk N, Donnett K: *Integrated patient care for the imaging professional,* St. Louis, 1996, Mosby.)

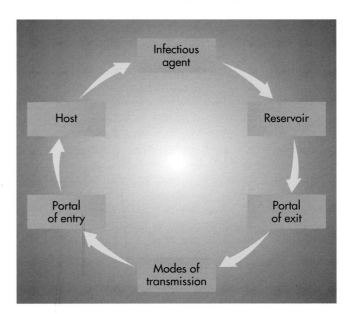

Figure 8-15 The cycle of infection. (From Kowalczyk N, Donnett K: *Integrated patient care for the imaging professional,* St. Louis, 1996, Mosby.)

The incidence rate of nosocomial infections is approximately 5% of patients admitted to hospitals yearly. Most of these infections are not life threatening. The most common nosocomial infection is an urinary tract infection. Statistics indicate that 20,000 patients a year die of hospital-acquired infections and that more than half of these are preventable.

Hospital-acquired infections also pose a threat to healthcare workers. In the United States 8,000 to 12,000 healthcare workers are infected with hepatitis B virus (HBV) each year, resulting in 2,000 deaths. In December of 1991, the Occupational Safety and Health Administration (OSHA) published regulations that require healthcare employers to provide HBV immunizations to employees, as well as procedures and equipment to prevent transmission of human immunodeficiency virus (HIV) and other blood-borne diseases to which employees are exposed.

There are four main routes of transmission of disease as follows:

Direct contact
Fomite
Vector
Airborne contamination

Direct contact occurs when the pathogens are placed in direct contact with a susceptible host. For example, HIV infections may be contracted when infectious organisms from the mucous membrane of one individual are placed in direct contact with the mucous of a susceptible host. Skin infections can also occur from direct contact.

Fomite, vector, and airborne contamination are considered indirect transmissions and involve transport of the pathogen by a secondary source. An object that has been in contact with a pathogen is called a fomite. Examples of a fomite are a contaminated urinary catheter or the surface of the gamma camera.

A vector is an animal in whose body an infectious organism develops or multiplies before becoming infective to a new host. Examples of vectors are mammals or insects that transmit disease through bites.

Airborne contamination can be initiated by a cough or sneeze and is spread by means of droplets and dust. An example of a pathogen transmitted by droplets is the tuberculosis (TB) bacteria.

The most direct way to intervene in the cycle of infection is to prevent transmission of the pathogen from the reservoir to susceptible host. The most effective system to prevent transmission of disease is by practicing universal precautions. Universal precautions or body substance precautions (BSP) are recommended by the Centers for Disease Control and Prevention (CDC). This system is based on the use of barriers for all contacts with all body substances rather than focusing on the isolation of a patient with a particular diagnosis. All patients are treated as potential reservoirs of infection.

Universal Precautions

Use individual judgment in determining when barriers are needed.

- Consider all patient specimens and body fluids as potentially infectious.
- Wear gloves when it is likely that there will be contact with any body fluids, mucous membranes, nonintact skin, or any item or surface contaminated with body fluids (blood, urine, feces, wound drainage, oral scratches, sputum, and vomitus).
- Wear masks and/or protective eyeware when it is likely that there will be exposure of the mucous membranes of the mouth, nose, or eyes with body fluids.
- Wear protective clothing when it is likely that clothing will be soiled with body substances.
- Wash hands before and after patient contact. Wash hands and other skin surfaces immediately and thoroughly after contamination with body fluids.
- Discard uncapped needle/syringe units and "sharps" in puncture-resistant biohazard containers.
- Clean blood and body fluid spills promptly with a 1:10 solution of bleach and water (prepared daily).
- Immediately report all needle sticks or incidents involving contamination by blood, body fluids, or tissues.

Hand-Washing Technique

Hands should always be washed before and after each patient contact. Friction produced by good hand-washing technique is the most effective means of eliminating microorganisms (Figure 8-16).

- If there are no foot or knee levers, use paper towels to turn the faucet on and off.
- Wet hands with continuously running water, keeping hands lower than elbows.
- Apply liquid soap and lather.
- Rub hands front and back and between fingers for at least 10 seconds.
- Rinse and dry thoroughly.

Good Housekeeping

The technologist is responsible for maintaining a clean environment. These responsibilities include changing linen between patients and disinfecting the imaging area on a daily basis. Use a cloth moistened with disinfectant. The CDC recommend sodium hypochlorite bleach (Clorox) as the preferred disinfectant for preventing the spread of HIV and HBV. If bleach is used, it should be prepared daily in a 1:10 solution (1 part

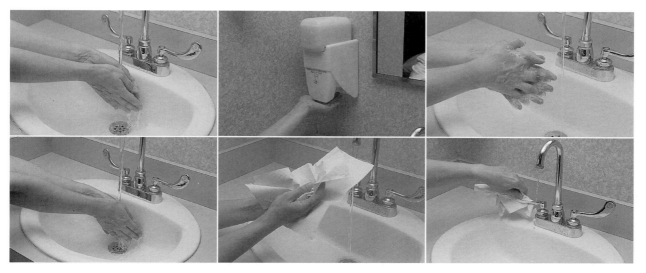

Figure 8-16 Hand-washing technique. (From Kowalczyk N, Donnett K: *Integrated patient care for the imaging professional*, St. Louis, 1996, Mosby.)

bleach to 9 parts water) because its effectiveness declines rapidly after preparation.

HIV infection or acquired immunodeficiency syndrome (AIDS) is not acquired by casual contact (touching or shaking hands; eating food prepared by an infected person; contact with drinking fountains, telephones, toilets, or other surfaces). It is not an airborne disease. The routes of transmission are through sexual contact, from contaminated blood or needles, and to the fetus if the mother is infected. Since AIDS is a condition caused by the suppression of the immune system, opportunistic infections are usually the primary cause of death, such as *Pneumocystis carinii* pneumonia.

VITAL SIGNS—PATIENT ASSESSMENT

Good evaluation skills play a role in meeting the needs of the patient while they are under the care of the technologist. Several aids are available to assist in assessing the patient. Review the chart before starting the procedure and ask how the patient feels. Observe the patient closely while preparing him/her for the procedure. One of the easiest signs to recognize is skin color. Individual complexions vary, but if the patient becomes pale or cyanotic, quickly begin assessing the change. Cyanosis is a term that describes a bluish coloration in the skin and indicates lack of oxygen to the tissues. The patient that becomes cyanotic needs immediate medical attention. Touching the patient allows the technologist to further assess the patient as well as reassure the patient. The acutely ill patient may be pale, cool, and diaphoretic.

If these symptoms are present, ask if the symptoms are new.

Measurements used to assess the patient are called vital signs and consist of the following:

Temperature
Pulse rate
Respiration rate
Blood pressure

A pulse is the advancing pressure wave in any artery caused by expulsion of blood when the left ventricle of the heart contracts. Normal rate is 60-90 beats per minute (bpm). A rapid pulse is called tachycardia. A slow pulse rate is bradycardia.

Normal rate—60-90 bpm
Tachycardia—>100 bpm
Bradycardia—<60 bpm
Common pulse points are as follows (Figure 8-17):
Radial artery
Brachial artery
Femoral artery
Carotid artery

If the pulse is weak distally, then palpate a more proximal pulse. If pulse points are slow or irregular, the apical pulse can be assessed by placing the stethoscope between the fifth and sixth ribs and listening for the heart sound, "lubb-dubb," which equals one beat.

The most convenient site for taking the pulse is the radial artery, located on the thumb side of the wrist. The pulse is felt by gently compressing the artery with the fingertips. The technologist should never feel the pulse with his/her own thumb because it has a pulse of its own that interferes with obtaining an accurate reading. Count the beats of the pulse for at least 30 seconds and multiply by 2 to obtain beats per minute (Figure 8-18).

The normal respiratory rate is 12-16 breaths/min. Notify the physician of any change in the patient's breathing pattern. Difficult or labored respiration is called dyspnea. Rapid breathing is tachypnea or hyperventilation. Oxygen may be needed for some patients but with the physician's order only. It may be difficult for the patient with lung disease to lie flat for even a short period. Many times, a change in position will alleviate the dyspnea.

Count the respirations without the patient being aware and count the breathing sequence (in and out) as one respiration. Count for 30 seconds and multiply by 2 to obtain respirations per minute.

Blood pressure is the lateral pressure exerted on the walls of the arteries by blood flowing through the arteries. It reflects the rhythm of the heartbeat and is a measure of the volume of blood pushed into the vessels by the heart. The pressure of blood within the arteries is highest whenever the heart contracts and is called systolic pressure. Between beats, when the ventricles are at rest, arterial pressure is at its lowest and is called diastolic pressure.

Blood pressure is measured in millimeters of mercury (mm Hg). Normal blood pressure varies, depending on age, weight, and physical status, but blood pressures of 100/60 to 140/90 are considered to be within an acceptable range. The top number, systolic (S for squeezing of the heart muscle) is a measure of the pumping action of the heart muscle itself. The diastolic pressure (D for down or dilatation of the heart muscle) indicates the ability of the arterial system to accept the pulse of blood that is forced into the system by the contraction of the left ventricle. Elevated blood pressure is hypertension; low blood pressure is hypotension and may indicate shock. In a changing or emergency situation, the physician will need accurate readings to be able to make a valid evaluation of the patient's status.

The most common site for taking blood pressure is the brachial artery of the upper arm, but arteries of the lower arm, thigh, and calf may also be used. When the arm is used, the patient should either sit or lie down

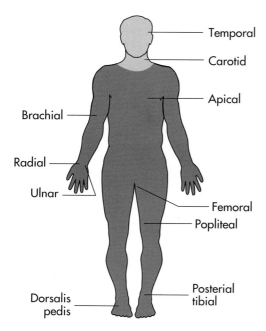

Figure 8-17 Location of peripheral pulses. (From Kowalczyk N, Donnett K: *Integrated patient care for the imaging professional,* St. Louis, 1996, Mosby.)

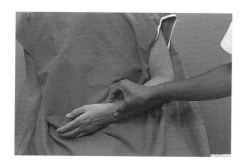

Figure 8-18 Measuring the radial pulse. (From Kowalczyk N, Donnett K: *Integrated patient care for the imaging professional,* St. Louis, 1996, Mosby.)

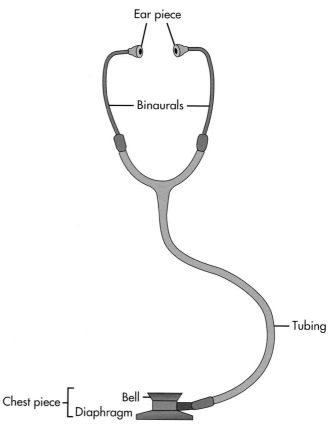

Figure 8-19 Parts of an acoustical stethoscope. (From Kowalczyk N, Donnett K: *Integrated patient care for the imaging professional,* St.Louis, 1996, Mosby.)

with the arm and blood pressure cuff at the level of the heart.

Equipment used to measure blood pressure includes a sphygmomanometer, a cuff, and a stethoscope. The procedure is begun by raising the silver column of mercury to 180-200 mm Hg by inflating the cuff. The cuff contains an inflatable rubber bladder that should be centered over the brachial artery, 1 to 2 in above the elbow. Cuffs should be wrapped snugly but not tightly. If the cuff is too loose, both systolic and diastolic readings will be falsely elevated (Figures 8-19 and 8-20).

A stethoscope with a flat diaphragm is best for taking blood pressures. After locating the brachial artery by palpation, place the diaphragm of the stethoscope over the artery without touching the cuff or patient's clothing. Gentle application of the stethoscope should be used because too much pressure can cause abnormally low diastolic sound (Figure 8-21).

Blood Pressure Procedure

1. Explain the procedure to the patient and make him/her comfortable in a sitting or recumbent position.
2. The patient should be resting for 5 minutes before the blood pressure is taken.

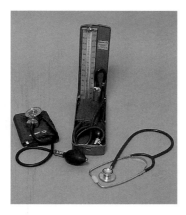

Figure 8-20 Aneroid *(left)* and mercury *(right)* manometers. (From Kowalczyk N, Donnett K: *Integrated patient care for the imaging professional,* St. Louis, 1996, Mosby.)

3. Select the site and use the same site consistently because of variations in blood pressure taken in different locations. Blood pressure should also be taken with the patient in the same position each time.
4. Expose the site and position the patient's arm on a supporting structure at heart level.
5. Place the cuff so that its lower edge is 1 to 2 in above the elbow, leaving space over the brachial artery free.
6. Using the middle and index fingers, palpate the brachial artery, which is located on the medial aspect of the arm at the level of the elbow.
7. Place the diaphragm of the stethoscope directly over the point of strongest pulsation.
8. Holding the rubber bulb in the palm of one hand, close the valve on the bulb with your thumb and finger, then rapidly inflate the cuff by pumping the bulb.
9. Inflate the cuff to about 20-30 mm Hg above the expected systolic reading or approximately 180 mm Hg. Inflation of the cuff should take 7 seconds or less.
10. Slowly open the valve on the bulb, releasing the pressure on the cuff steadily. Listen carefully for sounds of the first heartbeat, and watch the mercury column. Note the mercury level at the first sound heard, which is the systolic pressure.
11. After the first sound the pulsing will get louder as the pressure is released slowly from the cuff (approximately 2-3 mm Hg per heartbeat). Continue deflation until all sound stops or the intensity of the sound suddenly decreases and appears muffled. Note the mercury level as the diastolic pressure.
12. Open the valve to deflate cuff rapidly.
13. Remove the cuff and record values as systolic/diastolic (e.g., 120/80).
14. If you need to repeat a reading, let all the air out of the cuff and wait 15 seconds before inflating the cuff again. Do not reinflate the cuff during the reading.
15. Wipe the eartips and diaphragm of the stethoscope with alcohol before storing.

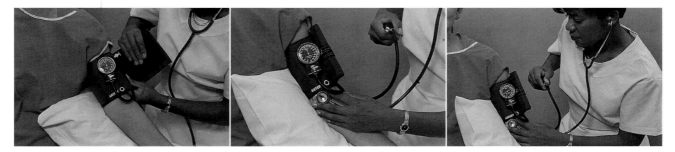

Figure 8-21 Assessing blood pressure. (From Kowalczyk N, Donnett K: *Integrated patient care for the imaging professional,* St. Louis, 1996, Mosby.)

If there is difficulty hearing the diastolic sounds, completely deflate the cuff. Wait 15 seconds, have the patient raise his/her arm for a few seconds, and then retake the blood pressure. The diastolic sounds may become muffled before stopping or may remain muffled down to zero. In this case, record the diastolic pressure at the point the change is distinguished from clear to muffled, as well as when the sound ends completely (e.g., 120/80/62).

EMERGENCY CARE

Patient assessment is critical in determining the action to be taken when a patient experiences difficulty in breathing. Obstructed airways, heart attacks, strokes, seizures, and syncope are common causes of medical emergencies. The universal sign of a choking person is the hand placed around the throat area. If the patient can cough and/or talk, observe the patient and do nothing. If the patient's coughing reflex does not remove the object and the patient loses the ability to cough and/or talk, perform the Heimlich maneuver. The following are skills that should be taught by a qualified instructor. This information should be used for review purposes only and not as a substitute for certification.

Obstructed Airway—Conscious Victim (Figure 8-22)

The Heimlich maneuver can be performed with the person standing, sitting, or lying down as follows:
1. Ask the victim, "Are you choking?"
2. Give quick upward thrusts to the abdomen slightly above the navel, applying pressure upward against the diaphragm just below the ribs.
3. For pregnant women or obese persons, perform a chest thrust. Apply pressure to the middle of the sternum, exerting quick backward pressure to the chest.
4. For infants the technologist should place the child face up on his/her forearm, holding the head lower than the body. Perform 5 chest thrusts using only two fingers, followed by 5 back blows between the scapulae. Perform a finger sweep only if an object is seen.
5. Repeat the thrusts until effective or victim becomes unconscious.
6. If victim becomes unconscious or if the obstructed airway is not relieved after about 1 minute, activate emergency code or EMS system.

Obstructed Airway—Unconscious Victim

1. Open the airway and try to ventilate; if the airway is still obstructed, reposition the head and try to ventilate again.

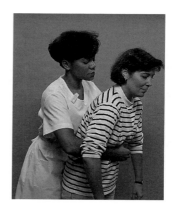

Figure 8-22 Heimlich maneuver. (From Kowalczyk N, Donnett K: *Integrated patient care for the imaging professional,* St. Louis, 1996, Mosby.)

2. If ventilation is unsuccessful, give up to 5 abdominal thrusts.
3. Perform a tongue-jaw lift, followed by a finger sweep to remove the object.
4. For an infant, perform 5 chest thrusts, followed by 5 back blows.
5. For an infant or child, only perform a finger sweep if an object is seen.
6. Repeat steps until effective.

Artificial Respiration

If breathing stops and you cannot get a response from the patient, assess the patient for artificial respiration (Figure 8-23).
1. Tilt the patient's head with the chin pointing upward by placing one hand on the patient's forehead (head tilt) and the other hand on the bony portion of the chin (chin tilt).
2. Immediately look, listen, and feel for air. While maintaining the tilted head position, the technologist should place his/her cheek and ear close to the patient's mouth and nose to hear or feel air exchange. Look for the chest to rise and fall while in this position. Check for 3 to 5 seconds.
3. Check for a carotid pulse using the first three fingers during the 3 to 5 second assessment of the patient's breathing.
4. If there is a pulse but no breathing, give the patient 2 slow breaths, followed by 1 breath every 5 seconds. Maintain the head tilt and with the hand that is on the patient's forehead pinch the patient's nose to prevent air leakage. Using a plastic respirator or mouth seal, give the patient full breaths, watching for the chest to rise.
5. If the air cannot enter, reposition the head and attempt another breath. If air still does not enter, follow the procedure for airway obstruction.

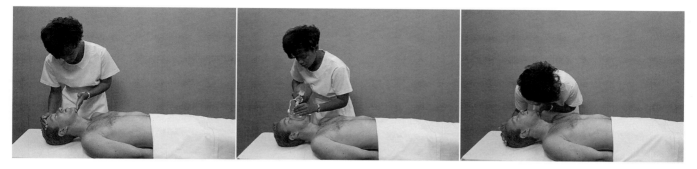

Figure 8-23 Rescue breathing. (From Kowalczyk N, Donnett K: *Integrated patient care for the imaging professional*, St. Louis, 1996, Mosby.)

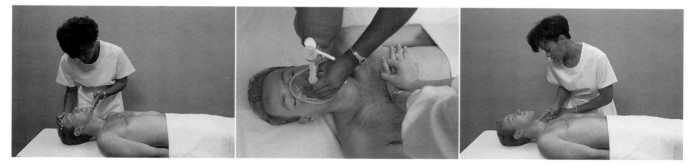

Figure 8-24 Adult CPR. (From Kowalczyk N, Donnett K: *Integrated patient care for the imaging professional*, St. Louis, 1996, Mosby.)

6. For infants use slow, gentle puffs and make a seal over mouth and nose. The breathing rate should be 1 puff every 3 seconds.
7. If there is no pulse, give the patient a breath, initiate emergency code or EMS, and proceed with cardiopulmonary resusitation (CPR).

Cardiopulmonary Arrest

CPR (Figure 8-24) is the basic life support system that is used to ventilate the lungs and circulate the blood in the event of cardiac and respiratory arrest. Part of the professional education of the technologist should include CPR training. Technologists are responsible for updating their certification in basic life support on a regular basis. Do not attempt CPR on infants or children unless your certification specifically includes pediatrics.

Basic Steps for One-Rescue CPR (American Heart Association)
1. If there is no pulse give cycles of 15 chest compressions (80 to 100 compressions/min), followed by 2 slow breaths.
2. After 4 cycles of 15:2 (about 1 minute), check the pulse. If there is no pulse, continue 15:2 cycle, beginning with chest compressions.

Basic Steps for Two-Rescue CPR (American Heart Association)
1. If there is no pulse, give cycles of 5 chest compressions (80 to 100 compressions/min), followed by 1 slow breath by Rescuer 1.

2. After 1 minute of rescue support, check the pulse. If there is no pulse, continue 5:1 cycles.

Syncope

Syncope, or fainting, is a mild form of neurogenic shock. The blood pressure falls as the blood vessels dilate, and the heart rate slows, resulting in a decreased supply of oxygen reaching the brain. The technologist needs to be responsive to any change in the patient's condition. There may be a noticeable change in the patient's coloring, and the skin may feel cool and clammy to the touch. This may be accompanied by weakness or change in thinking. Protecting the patient's head is the primary concern while easing the patient to the floor or any flat surface. Place the patient in the dorsal recumbent position, and elevate the patient's feet (Figure 8-25).

Seizures

The technologist's first duty is to protect the patient from injury. Assist the patient to the floor or any flat surface, remembering to protect the patient's head. Do not attempt to restrain the patient. There are different types of seizures, which may or may not result in loss of consciousness. Intense motor seizures (grand mal) usually result in loss of consciousness, followed by severe muscle spasms. Less intense motor seizures without loss of consciousness may be described as uncontrollable tremors that cause hyperventilation. Another type of seizure is characterized by a brief loss of consciousness during which the patient stares and is nonresponsive. Ask someone to call for a physician immediately, and observe the symptoms of the seizure as accurately as possible. Note when the seizure began and how long it lasted. Were both sides of the body involved equally? Where did the motor contractions begin, and did the contractions progress from one area to another? This information can be very helpful in treating the patient.

Myocardial Infarction (Heart Attack)

Sudden onset of chest pain or angina is assumed to be a myocardial infarction until proven otherwise. The technologist should prevent further damage by limiting the patient's movement and any exertion. The patient may become diaphoretic and pale, and may experience some nausea or heartburn. Assist the patient to a comfortable position, and ask someone to call for a physician. If the patient experiences shortness of breath, raise the head and administer oxygen.

Diabetes

The diabetic patient cannot metabolize glucose due to the lack of insulin production by the pancreas. These patients are usually on some form of insulin, which has the potential to cause problems when they have taken their insulin and can have nothing by mouth (NPO). These patients may develop hypoglycemia (low blood sugar). The onset of symptoms may be sudden and include the following:

General weakness
Sweating, clammy, cold skin

Tremors, nervousness, and irritability
Hunger
Blurred vision
Loss of consciousness

The condition can be quickly remedied by the administration of sugar (candy or fruit juice). Report the occurrence of such symptoms to a physician. Protect the patient from falling by lying the patient down until the sugar takes effect. People can have hypoglycemia without diabetes; the treatment is the same.

Asthma

Bronchospasms cause difficulty in breathing or dyspnea in asthmatic patients. This condition can be precipitated by stress or anxiety, such as having a nuclear medicine procedure. The treatment of choice is to relieve the bronchospasm without the administration of oxygen. If the patient has a nebulizer that contains bronchodilating medication, this usually relieves the symptoms. An injection of epinephrine will relieve the symptoms of an acute episode. This must be ordered by a physician.

Emergency Carts

These carts contain essential items that could be needed during an emergency situation. The carts are located throughout the hospital and should be easily accessible to all areas. The items may vary slightly, but most carts contain artificial ventilation equipment, emergency medications, bags of intravenous solutions, a defibrillator, blood pressure cuff, and stethoscope. These carts are inventoried and locked to keep them ready for use. To be able to assist if needed, the technologist needs to become familiar with the location of the cart and its components (Figure 8-26).

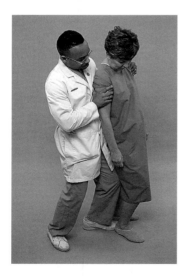

Figure 8-25 Support of a patient who is fainting. (From Kowalczyk N, Donnett K: *Integrated patient care for the imaging professional*, St. Louis, 1996, Mosby.)

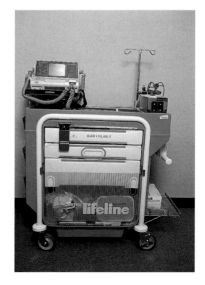

Figure 8-26 Emergency cart with defibrillator. (From Kowalczyk N, Donnett K: *Integrated patient care for the imaging professional*, St. Louis, 1996, Mosby.)

SPECIAL EQUIPMENT

Intravenous Equipment

Computerized infusion pumps are used in most institutions to regulate the drip rate of the prescribed fluids. Unless the technologist is authorized, he/she should not change the rate of flow. The technologist should know how to troubleshoot, as in the case of an occluded line in the system.

Nasogastric (NG) Tubes

This tube is inserted through a nostril and terminates in the stomach. It is used for feeding, to obtain specimens, or to drain fluids. Nasoenteric tubes go farther into the intestinal tract to remove fluid and gas that may cause distention. Precautions should be taken to make sure the tubes are not pulled or tugged on when moving or positioning patients. The technologist needs to report any leakage in the tube or suction system. Suction or feeding can be discontinued if the patient needs to be transferred to the department.

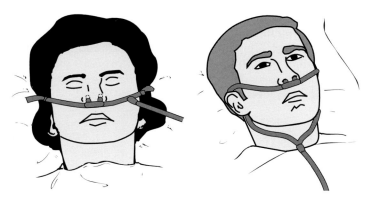

Figure 8-27 Nasal cannula. (Modified from Potter PA, Perry AG: *Fundamentals of nursing: concepts, process, and practice*, ed 3, St. Louis, 1994, Mosby.)

Oxygen Administration

In caring for a patient receiving oxygen, always note the flow rate in the chart or doctor's orders. Oxygen can be administered by high– or low–flow-rate devices. The low–flow-rate devices most often used are the nasal cannula or nasal prongs, nasal catheter, or simple oxygen masks. The nasal prongs are inserted into the patient's nostrils, providing a direct source of oxygen. A nasal catheter is longer than the cannula and is inserted through the nostril into the back of the patient's mouth. This is used when the patient must have oxygen at all times. The simple mask provides total oxygen supply. The transparent mask fits over the mouth, nose, and chin of the patient (Figures 8-27 and 8-28).

During transport, portable oxygen cylinders are used. The cylinder has a on-off valve, with a dial indicating how much gas remains in the tank. The flow meter indicates the rate at which oxygen is administered in units of liters per minute (L/min). Both valves must be on for the patient to receive oxygen. A common oxygen rate is 3 to 5 L/min. Trauma (in shock) patients may require a higher rate of oxygen administration. Patient's with chronic obstructive pulmonary disease (COPD) receive oxygen at a lower rate, usually less than 3 L/min. The respiratory rate in these patients is controlled by the carbon dioxide level, and if too much oxygen is delivered, their respiratory rate may slow down to the extent that ventilation is insufficient (Figure 8-29).

Precautions when using oxygen cylinders include the following:

Secure cylinders in the cylinder cart when transporting. Never use a patient's stretcher to transport cylinders.

Cylinders should be secured at all times and never allowed to stand free.

Care must be taken to prevent fire when oxygen is in use. Never place cylinders near a heat source.

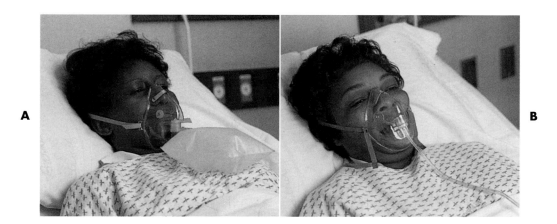

Figure 8-28 Oxygen face masks. **A,** Plastic face mask with reservoir bag. **B,** Simple face mask. (From Kowalczyk N, Donnett K: *Integrated patient care for the imaging professional*, St. Louis, 1996, Mosby.)

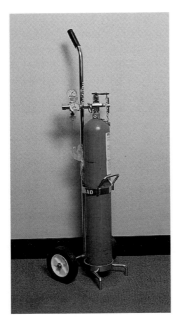

Figure 8-29 Oxygen tank. (From Kowalczyk N, Donnett K: *Integrated patient care for the imaging professional*, St. Louis, 1996, Mosby.)

Catheters

The most common type of catheter is the urinary catheter. Plastic tubing is inserted through the patient's urethra and into the bladder. Urine is drained from the bladder and flows through the tubing into the urine bag. To prevent the backflow of urine, the bag must be kept below the level of the bladder. Catheterization is a sterile technique and needs to remain a closed system to prevent urinary infections. The catheter bag can be attached to the bed, stretcher, or wheelchair but should never be placed directly on the floor.

Wound Drains

Colostomies (surgical opening into the colon) and ileostomies (surgical opening into the ileum) allow for drainage of feces. The opening (stoma) is covered by plastic disposable bags or pouches (appliances), which must be changed frequently. Clean rather than sterile technique is needed when changing these appliances.

Dressings should be maintained, and any signs of fresh bleeding should be reported immediately. If hemorrhaging occurs, apply direct pressure to the site while calling for assistance.

QUALITY IMPROVEMENT

In the present managed care arena, the nuclear medicine facility must maintain reliable quality outcomes, a cost-efficient operation, easy access, and superior customer service to remain competitive in the marketplace.

The words *quality management, quality improvement, continuous improvement, performance improvement, and total quality management (TQM)* are often used interchangeably in present healthcare. These are designs to improve the processes of the work performed. In nuclear medicine there are many different processes that are started and completed within the service, (internal), and others that involve outside parties and, therefore, are external. An example of an internal process is completing the quality control studies on a camera. Obtaining a radiopharmaceutical and its ultimate disposal may involve personnel outside of the nuclear medicine department (external). Sets of tasks in a continuum are referred to as a process. For example, nuclear medicine procedures are a part of the continuum of care of a patient. Case management, care paths, critical paths, and other similar terms are used to describe a process or continuum of care for a patient. Care paths often list nuclear medicine procedures to be obtained at critical times during the patient's care. The Joint Commission on Healthcare Organizations (JCAHO) no longer looks at nuclear medicine as a separate entity to be evaluated but rather how nuclear medicine relates to other functions within the total care of a patient.

To function in a continuous improvement mode, the nuclear medicine technologist, physician, support personnel, and other interactive groups should focus on planning, customer requirements, process management, analysis and management of data, and problem-solving models.

PLANNING

Any quality or performance improvement plan must relate to the overall strategic plan of the nuclear medicine facility. This is a continuation of the institutional plan if nuclear medicine is part of a larger organization. Short-term plans are usually developed for 1 year or less, and long-term planning normally extends to 3 years. Planning should take into account the customer's needs and expectations, fiscal restraints, and the environmental influences.

There are a number of environmental factors to consider in planning. The type of market will have a direct effect on the nuclear medicine facility. In a capitated market with heavy managed care contracts there will be more restrictions on the types of nuclear medicine procedures performed and the amount of reimbursement. A good understanding of the actual case mix is important in any planning. The competition must be considered. This includes other nuclear medicine facilities as well as other modalities. As algorithms are developed for patient care, nuclear medicine may or may not play a role in the diagnostic care of a patient or group of patients.

Fiscal restraints must be considered, especially in the area of human resources and facilities. The most efficient use of staff may mean addressing issues of cross training, productivity measures, and threats of downsizing. Equipment must be operationally sound, and replacement plans must be developed. Routine suppliers must be evaluated and partnerships must be established, when feasible.

CUSTOMER SERVICE

It is imperative that a nuclear medicine facility identify the customers and assess their needs and expectations. A customer is anyone to whom a service, product, or information is provided. Nuclear medicine facilities normally identify the referring physician as an important customer. The referring physician's staff may be direct contacts in scheduling and providing important information about the patient. In many instances nuclear medicine must depend on a unique customer/supplier relationship for patients. As more regions operate in a managed care market, third-party payers, such as insurance companies and health maintenance organizations (HMOs), may actually be the primary customer because they dictate to the patient where he or she will go for services. Clinical outcomes become an important factor in assessing the quality of ancillary services. Third-party payers are interested in clinical outcomes, accessibility, and overall satisfaction of their clients when they select nuclear medicine suppliers.

The patient's needs and expectations must be considered in developing quality and performance improvement plans. The primary type of patient will influence perceptions of good customer service. For example, a geriatric population and a pediatric population will not view exceptional service in exactly the same manner.

Not to be forgotten is the internal customer, both within the department and institution. Many of the deficiencies within a process are produced when accountability moves from one party to the next. There are many times when the nuclear medicine technologist is in contact with other customers or suppliers that can affect the success or failure of the total process, for example, scheduling the patient, ordering or preparing the radiopharmacuetical, performing the procedure, generating the report, and correlating with other modalities.

Understanding the customer's needs and expectations will involve asking the right questions. This is normally done in survey format and focus group settings. Only by asking these questions can the nuclear medicine department provide viable services.

PROCESS MANAGEMENT

The greatest improvements can be seen in a nuclear medicine facility through efficient process management. One of the most effective ways of evaluating a process is to develop a flow chart. By using a flow chart, the technologist can identify those "bottlenecks" that cause delays or confusion. Time becomes an important factor in customer satisfaction, as well as cost effectiveness. When turnaround time is decreased, quality, productivity, and cost effectiveness improve. Once the time deficiencies have been identified, various problem-solving techniques can be used to determine the root cause of the problem.

It may be of value to identify "best practices" through benchmarking. Once a process has been determined and fully understood, it may be necessary to network with other nuclear medicine facilities to determine which facility has the most efficient process management, for example, who has the shortest turnaround time, lowest expense, and most accurate results. Studying another type of business may also be of value when looking at processes. For example, bank billing practices may be related to nuclear medicine billing practices, delivering a package on time may be related to transporting a patient on time, and the patient check-in process may be related to the hotel check-in process.

ANALYSIS AND MANAGEMENT OF DATA

It has been said that we can only manage that which we can measure. Within any system, measurements must be reliable and accurate. The decisions as to what data to collect should be based on the relative importance. Often in nuclear medicine, measurements have been done for accreditation without affecting overall improvements. Measuring must be selective and meaningful and should support process management, planning, and customer satisfaction. Measurement outcomes can benefit patient care.

PROBLEM-SOLVING MODELS

Understanding and properly using problem-solving tools and techniques can help the nuclear medicine technologist to improve a process.

Plan, Do, Check, Act (PDCA)

The Shewhart Cycle, or a similar model, is commonly considered the format for problem solving. It begins with the "Plan" phase—determining the problem or what needs to be changed or improved. The "Do" phase involves data collection and analysis; the root cause of the problem is determined. Based on the data, possible solutions are determined and controls are established. A change is initiated in the "Check" phase. In the "Act" phase, results of the change are reviewed and modified as necessary and continuous monitoring is established. Modifications of the Shewhart Cycle include the Ten-Step JCAHO Model and other methods that use a number of steps but follow the same principle.

PROBLEM-SOLVING TECHNIQUES

Many problem-solving techniques or tools may be used in combination or alone to improve a process. Several options follow.

Brainstorming is a technique used to generate ideas from several people. Specific rules to obtain the most positive outcomes may include the following:

Select a topic.

Record *all* ideas.

Record one idea at a time in the sequence given.

Pass over participants who have no spontaneous ideas.

Do not criticize any of the ideas listed.

Continue brainstorming until all ideas are listed or the time limit is reached.

Clarify all ideas listed.

The *affinity diagram* is another brainstorming method that is effective with large groups. It is most often used with groups who do not work together, when full participation is required, in political environments, or when "group think" should be avoided. It is also an effective method when the topic under consideration is sensitive, there is a need to break from traditional ideas, thinking is chaotic, or many creative ideas are needed. The procedure includes the following steps:

Select a broad topic.

Write each idea on a separate Post-it note or card.

Be clear and concise.

Mix responses together randomly.

Group similar cards together without discussing the ideas.

Select a heading (main topic) for each group of ideas.

Fish bone (also referred to as the "cause and effect" diagram) is a method that is used to determine the causes of a problem. Causes are most commonly grouped under the following categories:

Methods

Machines

People

Materials

Measurements

Force-field analysis is used to identify the forces that drive a situation and those that restrain it. The procedure for using the method is as follows:

Identify the current situation.

Identify the desired (ideal) situation.

Identify the driving forces (those that make the desired situation achievable).

Identify the retraining forces (those that prevent the current situation from becoming the desired situation).

Determine which factors can be altered to achieve the desired situation.

The *flow chart* is one of the most useful tools to identify and improve a process. By listing process steps in a symbolic format, areas that are "bottlenecks" can be more easily identified and removed or changed. Typical symbols are used in Figure 8-1 (the rectangle indicates a step in the process, the diamond indicates a decision point, the curved rectangle indicates a document, and arrows indicate a connector to next step).

The *contingency diagram* is an effective method for looking at the negative parts of a problem and then reversing them to positive action steps. The usual format to complete a contingency diagram is as follows:

Identify the problem.

Brainstorm for ideas to ensure that the problem will continue and possibly worsen.

Review each idea to determine if the opposite can occur.

Develop an action plan.

An *interrelationship digraph* is a method of linking related ideas. It involves the following procedure:

Randomly space the ideas/issues.

Select the first idea and relate it to the nearest idea/issue.

Ask the question: Does this idea/issue cause or influence the idea/issue it is being related to?

If the answer is yes, draw an arrow from the first idea to this idea.

Return to the original idea/issue and relate it to the next idea/issue.

Continue to ask the question and draw arrows.

When the first idea/issue has been related to all of the other ideas/issues, follow the same sequence for each of the other ideas/issues.

Identify the idea/issue that has the greatest influence on the others (the one with the most arrows pointing away from it).

Identify the idea/issue that is most influenced by the others (the one with the most arrows pointing to it).

This method will help determine which ideas/issues to work on that will have the greatest possibilities of altering a situation.

Measurements

Most problem solving involves measurement, which may be in any phase of the PDCA cycle but is most important during the analysis (check) phase. The more common types of measurement include the following:

A *Pareto chart* consists of a bar graph from the highest frequency to the lowest and is used to help determine which area to work on first.

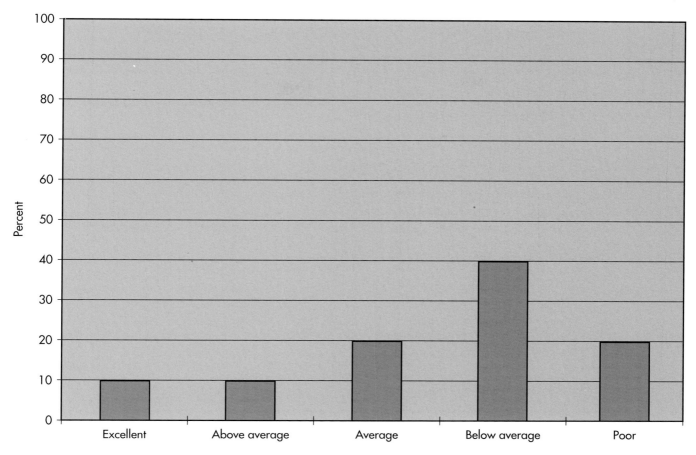

Figure 8-30   Outpatient satisfaction—timeliness of staff.

The *check sheet* is used to collect data to identify patterns.

The *run chart* is used to measure trends.

A *control chart* is a run chart with upper and lower acceptable limits.

The *histogram* is a bar graph of the distribution of data that demonstrates variation.

A *scatter diagram* is used to correlate two variables to look for cause and effect.

Example

The following example is used to illustrate how a team could use several of the problem-solving tools and measurements to improve a process.

SITUATION: Patient waiting time has been identified as the greatest source of dissatisfaction for patients scheduled for nuclear medicine procedures. A team is formed to develop a solution that will ensure the best outcome.

During the planning phase, the team analyzes data already available as in Figures 8-30 and 8-31. Of the patients studied in nuclear medicine, 65% are outpatients and 35% inpatients. The team develops a flow chart of the process of scheduling patients through the depart-

ment and discovers that the "bottleneck" causing longer waiting times for outpatients is during the check-in phase; for inpatients it is waiting for transportation to return to the nursing units after the procedure has been completed. Based on the data the team determines that improving the process of checking in outpatients will have the greatest impact on outpatient satisfaction since they make up the greatest number of patients and are most dissatisfied with patient waiting time.

A number of tools can be used by the team to work on solutions to the problem. The fish bone diagram can be used to brainstorm for root causes (Figure 8-32). Once causes have been identified, the team can develop measures to determine which causes can be changed to bring about the greatest impact on outpatient satisfaction. The contingency diagram can be used to identify those factors that will cause the problem to continue or worsen (Box 8-1). The force-field analysis can be used to identify the desired situation, (i.e., that outpatient waiting time for nuclear medicine procedures be decreased) and then identify the forces that would drive the desired outcome and those that are currently preventing it (Table 8-3).

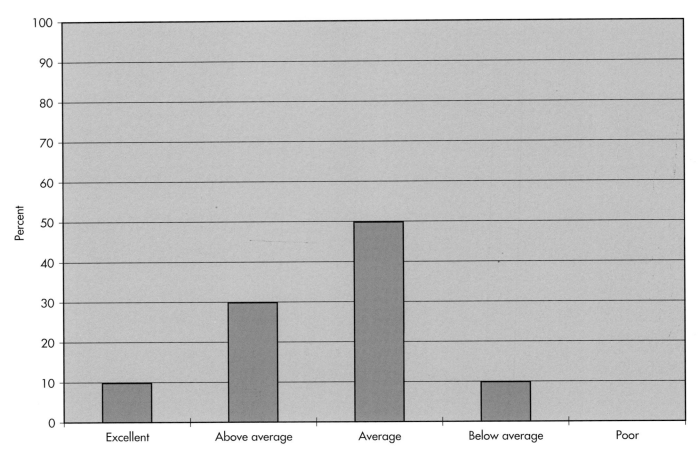

Figure 8-31 Inpatient satisfaction—timeliness of staff.

Box 8-1	Contingency diagram

QUESTION: How can we ensure that outpatient satisfaction for timeliness of staff continues to be low?
- Do not change the current process.
- Wait until patients arrive to tell them what information is needed.
- Schedule all patients for same arrival time.
- Eliminate the job position of nuclear medicine clerk.
- Keep the old, unreliable copier.
- Do not service the copier.
- Increase the information required of patients.
- Do not communicate with HMOs and insurance companies.
- Do not provide information to referring physicians' offices.

Table 8-3	Force-field analysis

CURRENT SITUATION: Waiting time for outpatients is too long during check-in.

DESIRED SITUATION: Decrease waiting time for outpatient check-in to improve patient satisfaction.

Driving forces	Restraining forces
• Require less information on patients.	• Billing department requires too much information.
• Get information before patient's arrival.	• Patient is not told of information needed before arrival.
• Electronically communicate with referring physicians' offices.	• Lack of communication with referring sources.
• Electronically communicate with HMOs and insurance companies.	• Only one person in the nuclear medicine department is trained to obtain information.
• Cross train others to help obtain information.	• Patient's perception that waiting time is too long.
	• Process has too many steps.

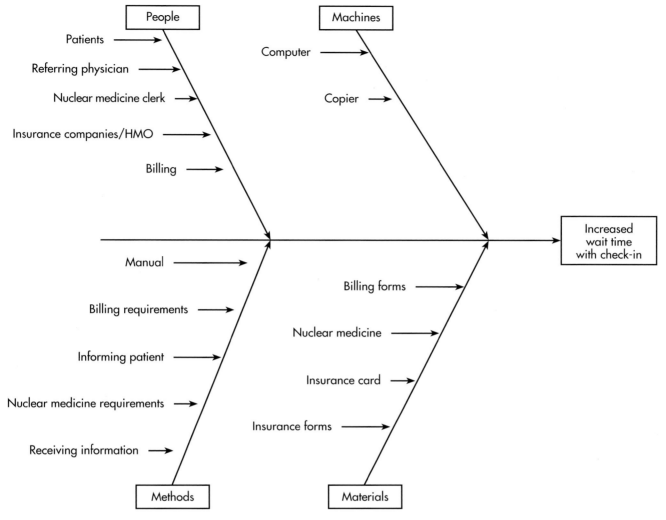

Figure 8-32 Fish bone diagram.

Once the team has determined what they believe to be the major causes of the problem, measurements must be taken to prove the hypothesis. The checklist is commonly used to measure multiple variables. It may be necessary to divide the measurements, such as for different days, times of the day, and source of the patient referral. It is important to determine all the parameters that may be important when solving the problem before measurements begin to prevent having to take additional measurements later. Examples of possible checklists for this particular problem are presented in Tables 8-4 and 8-5.

To analyze the data, the information is usually plotted on a Pareto chart, which identifies the cause having the greatest impact on the problem. This is sometimes referred to as the 80:20 rule, which means that 20% of the factors cause 80% of the problem, and if the 20% are fixed, 80% of the "headaches" will disappear. Unfortunately, the 20% are usually the hardest to fix.

Another chart that is helpful is the run chart, which is used to identify trends over time. If the example presented in Figure 8-33 were analyzed by the team, they would conclude that something was causing greater delays on Wednesday and would look for causes such as the clerk not working and more patients being scheduled from a particular referring physician.

Based on the data analysis, the team might develop the following action plan:

Work with the billing department to evaluate the amount of information required of outpatients and eliminate what is unnecessary.

Develop a checklist of patient demographics and insurance requirements, and distribute this to referring physicians' offices to give to patients before their arrival in the nuclear medicine department.

Determine what information can be provided by the referring physicians' offices before the patient's arrival. Work more closely with referring physicians' offices whose patients were least informed to better educate their staff regarding

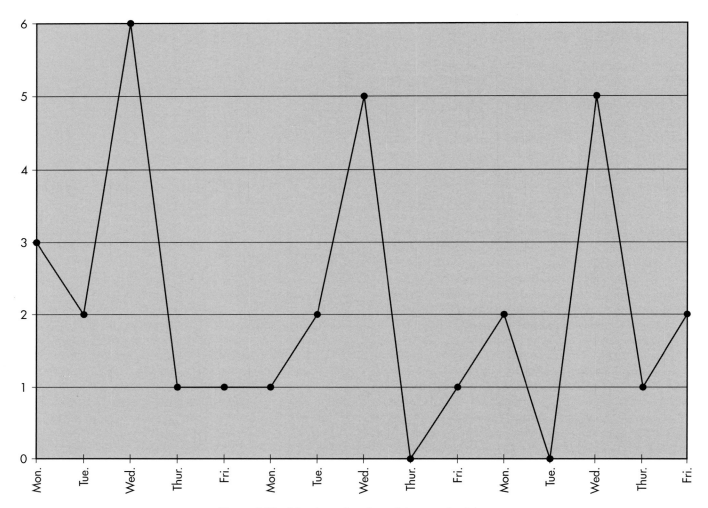

Figure 8-33 Number of patient delays at check-in.

Table 8-4 | Checklist

Reason for wait	Mon	Tue	Wed	Thur	Fri
Copier broken					
Clerk not available					
Patient arrives with no information					
Patient arrives late					
Patient arrives early					
Patient unable to fill out form					
Other					

| Table 8-5 | Checklist | | |

Patients arriving without billing information

Referral source	Week 1	Week 2	Week 3
HMO A			
HMO B			
HMO C			
Dr. Jones			
Dr. Smith			
Dr. Johns			
Neurology group			
Cardiology group			
Pulmonary group			

the information that will be required from patients.

Reschedule the clerk's off time to better cover Wednesday mornings.

When the action plans are in place, the team must continue to monitor for improvements and alter the actions accordingly. Once the outpatient satisfaction starts improving, the team should begin to tackle causes of the "bottleneck" identified for inpatients, using similar techniques.

BIBLIOGRAPHY

Brassard M: *The memory jogger plus*[+], Methuen, Mass, 1989, GOAL/QPC.

Craig C: *Introduction to ultrasonography and patient care,* ed 1, Philadelphia, 1993, WB Saunders.

Ehrlich RA, McCloskey ED: *Patient care in radiography,* ed 4, St. Louis, 1993, Mosby.

Hibbard W: *Laboratory manual for nuclear medicine technology,* New York, 1984, Society of Nuclear Medicine.

Keefer BS: Back to basics: the ABCs of back injury prevention, *RT Image* October, 1991.

Leathers D: Oh, my aching back! *RT Image* December, 1993.

Scholtes PR: *The team handbook,* Madison, Wisc, 1988, Joiner Associates.

chapter *9*

Central Nervous System

Henry N. Wagner, Jr., Jay K. Rhine, Julia W. Buchanan

Objectives

Diagram and describe the anatomy of the central nervous system.

Describe intercellular communication and neurotransmitters.

Diagram and describe the circulation of cerebrospinal fluid.

Discuss the properties of radiopharmaceuticals used in SPECT brain imaging.

Describe the technical parameters and instrumentation used for CSF studies.

Describe the use, dose, administration, and procedures for SPECT brain studies.

Describe the radionuclides used in PET imaging procedures.

Discuss PET imaging techniques of the brain.

INTRODUCTION

All living systems require properly functioning communication and control processes. The information necessary for cells to function is stored and transferred by means of molecules, beginning with DNA and extending up through hormones, neurotransmitters, and other specific molecules. The DNA molecule contains 8000 bits of information, whereas the average protein molecule contains 4000 bits. A single cell contains about 10^{12} bits of information, which is equivalent to the information in 1000 volumes of the Encyclopedia Britannica.

Neurons, the fundamental units of the nervous system, talk to each other in two ways: by means of electrical action potentials and by molecular messengers that carry information and modulate the electrical activity. Many of these molecules serve as receptors of molecular messages secreted into the synapses connecting dendrites and axons. They are involved in the movement of sodium, calcium, and potassium ions across cell membranes. Molecules such as adenosine triphosphate (ATP) provide energy that influences the overall activity of neurons. Neuroreceptors are polymers that recognize specific messenger molecules that are released locally or circulate through the body until they encounter the appropriate biopolymer on the surface of neurons or other cells that fit their specific configuration. Molecular neurotransmitters, including amines, amino acids, and peptides, have the right shape, charge, and other physiochemical properties to bind to the receptor biopolymers. The patterns and quantities of these recognition sites integrate individual cells of the body to make the person a unique, whole individual. Disintegration results in disease or death.

The maintenance of life in all organisms, including human beings, requires intercellular communication, which in turn requires energy to generate the ion gradients that produce electrical action potentials and to synthesize transmitters and receptors. The rate of consumption of the principal source of energy of the brain—glucose—can be measured by means of positron emission tomography (PET) (Figure 9-1). Regional blood flow and intracellular communication within the brain can be examined with both PET and single photon emission computed tomography (SPECT) (Figure 9-2). Since the 1950s more than 100 neurotransmitters, or chemical messengers, such as serotonin and dopamine, have been discovered. Acetylcholine stimulates skeletal muscle cells to contract but causes heart muscles to relax. Thus, muscarinic acetylcholine receptors are excitatory; nicotinic acetylcholine receptors are inhibitory.

Enzymes within the cells of the body control the innumerable energy-transforming processes within cells, whereas membrane receptors control much of the transfer of information from one cell to another. The most highly specialized system for information transfer within the body is the brain and nervous system. One neuron may interact with between 1000 and 10,000 other neurons. Molecular messengers, called neurotransmitters, include amines, amino acids, and peptides.

Neuronal membrane receptors respond to specific neurotransmitters and ignore other molecules that continually come in contact with them as they circulate through the body. Neurotransmitters secreted at the terminals of presynaptic neurons interact with receptors on postsynaptic neurons, which results in translation of information by means of changes in the state of ion channels or by formation of "second messenger" molecules. The most widely studied neurotransmission systems have been those involving dopamine, serotonin, norepinephrine, and acetylcholine.

Neurotransmitters are stored in vesicles at the terminal axonal branches of presynaptic neurons. When a sufficiently large number of impulses arrives at the nerve terminal, the molecules of the neurotransmitters are released in a burst and diffuse into the synaptic cleft, where they are bound to the specific molecular configuration of the receptor on the membranes of the postsynaptic neuron. Drugs may mimic the transmitter and bind to the receptor to produce the same action as the naturally occurring transmitter. Antibodies can block receptors, as in myasthenia gravis, and recent evidence suggests that abnormal metabolites can also block neuroreceptors.

Drugs, both licit and illicit, affect intercellular communication. These include amines such as norepineph-

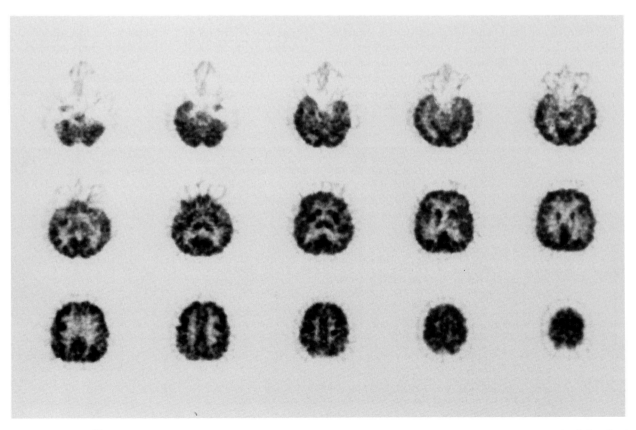

Figure 9-1 Normal ^{18}F-fluorodeoxyglucose (FDG) PET scan. (Courtesy Frost JJ, MD, Johns Hopkins University School of Medicine, Baltimore.)

rine, dopamine, and serotonin; amino acids such as gamma-aminobutyric acid (GABA), glutamic acid, aspartic acid, and glycine; and peptides such as endogenous enkephalins. Neurotransmitters are secreted in varying amounts depending on the number and rate of electrical impulses traveling down the axon of the presynaptic neuron from which the neurotransmitter is secreted.

In addition to involvement in neuron-to-neuron information transfer, neurotransmitters, including enkephalins, act as modulators of regional neuronal activity. Some chemical messengers act within fractions of a second, whereas others have an effect over hours or even days. Thousands of synapses, connecting with a single postsynaptic neuron, are integrated and determine whether the postsynaptic neuron fires an action potential. The availability of 20 different messenger amino acids means that a vast number of different combinations are possible and can encode a tremendous quantity of information.

Radioactive tracers make it possible to detect and quantify molecular abnormalities, including those involved in intercellular communication. Positron-emitting radionuclides, particularly ^{11}C and ^{18}F, have been used to carry out studies with many receptor systems. Radioligands labeled with the single photon emitting radionuclides, such as ^{123}I and ^{99m}Tc, have been developed, making it possible to perform these studies with SPECT systems.

In the care of patients with diseases of the central and peripheral nervous system, nuclear medicine techniques can be used to assess the effectiveness of surgery or radiation therapy, can document the extent of involvement of the brain by tumors, and can determine progression or regression of the lesions in response to different forms of treatment. Such data permit modifications of the treatment plan sooner than can be determined by the clinical response of the patients or by changes in the size of the lesions. Thus, treatment no longer needs to be based solely on clinical response, gross morphology of the lesions, and histopathologic examination of biopsies.

In addition to measuring blood flow to tumors, blood volume, glucose or amino acid incorporation into tumors, and DNA synthesis, PET and SPECT can be used to measure the number and affinity of hormone receptors that characterize certain tumors. Estrogen receptors are increased in many breast tumors, in both the primary and metastatic sites. ^{18}F estradiol accumulation as determined by PET makes it possible to tailor the treatment of a specific patient on the basis of the number of estrogen receptors in a metastatic lesion from carcinoma of the breast. A brain metastasis containing estrogen receptors is more likely to be treated successfully with estrogen-receptor blocking drugs, such as tamoxifen, than cancers that do not contain estrogen receptors. The presence of progesterone receptors as well as estrogen receptors is the best prognostic sign. Histopathology alone is no longer the only criterion for diagnosis, prognosis, and therapy.

Receptors are also found on pituitary tumors. Using the dopamine-receptor binding agent ^{11}C N-methylspiperone (NMSP), it is possible to classify pituitary adenomas according to whether they possess dopamine receptors. If the tumors contain such receptors, they can be treated chemically rather than surgically, that is, by administering the dopamine receptor agonist bromocryptine. If a tumor contains somatostatin receptors, it can be treated with somatostatin analogues.

After treatment, measurement of the metabolic ac-

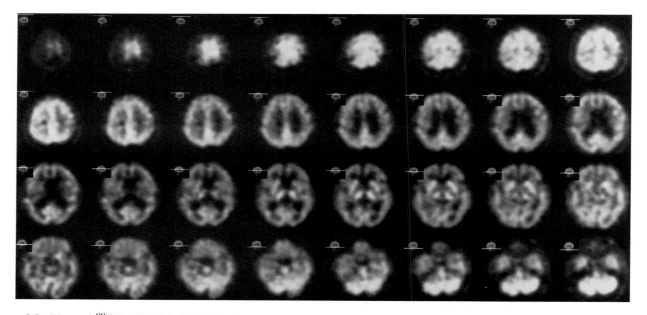

Figure 9-2   Normal ^{99m}Tc HMPAO SPECT brain scan. (Courtesy Trionix Corp and Middleheim General Hospital, Antwerp, Belgium.)

tivity of the tumor makes it possible to detect persistence or recurrence of the tumor and damage to normal brain tissue, such as that resulting from radiation. For example, ^{11}C methionine is useful for delineating the boundaries of brain tumors, providing information of value in the planning and performance of brain surgery, by permitting differentiation of the metabolizing brain tumor from simple disruption of the blood-brain barrier.[1]

ANATOMY AND PHYSIOLOGY

The central nervous system (CNS) consists of the brain and spinal cord. One of the body's largest organs, the brain is divided into four major parts: the cerebrum, the cerebellum, the diencephalon (thalamus and hypothalamus), and the brain stem (Figure 9-3).

Cerebrum

The surface of the cerebrum is composed of gray matter (cerebral cortex), which contains primarily neurons, with an underlying layer of white matter, which contains primarily nerve tracts. The two hemispheres of the cortex are connected by the corpus callosum. The cortex (Figure 9-4) is subdivided into four lobes that are named for the cranial bones that overlie them: the frontal lobe, the temporal lobe, the parietal lobe, and the occipital lobe. The frontal lobe extends from the forehead posteriorly to the central sulcus and inferiorly to the lateral fissure. It is involved in higher mental activities such as planning, judgment, and personality. The prerolandic gyrus is involved in motor function, including speech. The temporal lobe is located below the lateral fissure

and extends posteriorly along the sides of the brain. It is involved in hearing, language, memory, and learning. The parietal lobe is separated from the frontal lobe by the central sulcus and from the temporal lobe by the lateral sulcus. The postrolandic region involves sensory function. The occipital lobe is located posteriorly and forms boundaries with the parietal and temporal lobes. It contains the principal cortical areas involving vision.

Deep within each cerebral hemisphere are paired structures of gray matter called the basal ganglia, which are responsible for the control of muscle tone and tremor, the initiation of movement, and emotions. Fibers extend from the basal ganglia to other parts of the cerebral cortex.

Cerebellum

The cerebellum is located in the inferior and posterior portion of the cranial cavity beneath the occipital lobes of the cerebrum. It is involved in the coordination of movement of skeletal muscle, or proprioception, but other functions such as memory can also involve the cerebellum.

Diencephalon (Thalamus and Hypothalamus)

The diencephalon consists primarily of the thalamus and the hypothalamus. The thalamus is composed of two ovoid masses of gray matter, which are involved in the relay of sensory impulses from other parts of the central nervous system. The thalamus also aids in the sensations of pain and temperature. The hypothalamus, also composed of gray matter, is located beneath the thalamus. It is involved in autonomic functions

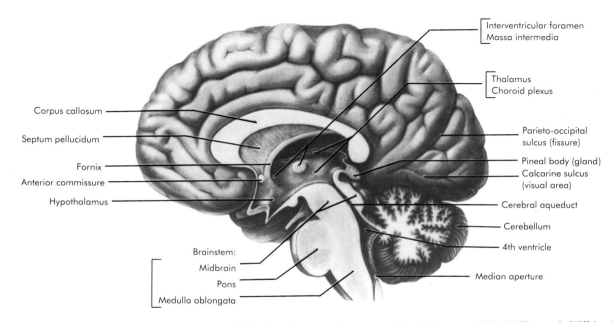

Figure 9-3   Brain anatomy. (From Agur AMR: *Grant's atlas of anatomy,* ed 9, Baltimore, 1991, Williams & Wilkins.)

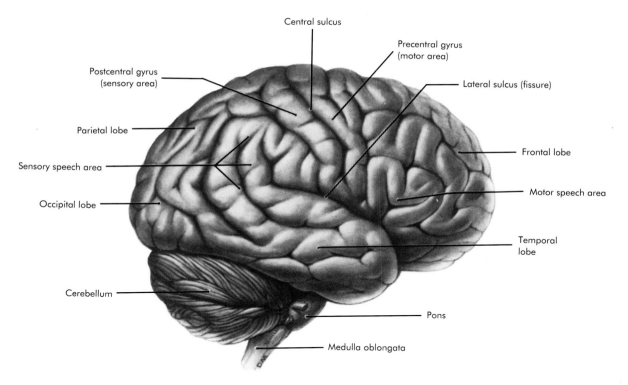

Figure 9-4 Topographic anatomy of major cortical regions. (From Agur AMR: *Grant's atlas of anatomy,* ed 9, Baltimore, 1991, Williams & Wilkins.)

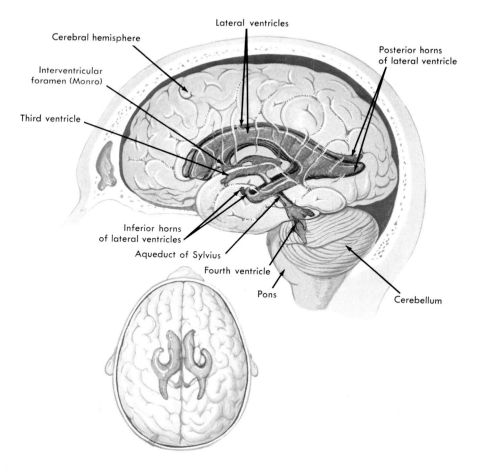

Figure 9-5 Cerebral ventricles projected on lateral surface of cerebrum. *Smaller drawing,* Ventricles from above. (From Anthony CP, Thibodeau GA: *Textbook of anatomy and physiology,* ed 10, St. Louis, 1979, Mosby.)

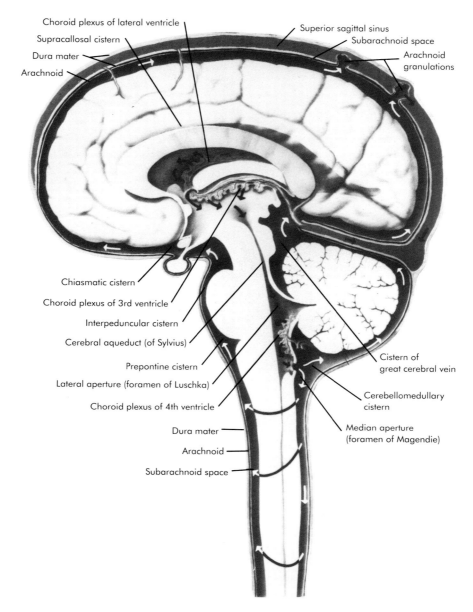

Choroid plexus of lateral ventricle

Supracallosal cistern

Dura mater

Arachnoid

Superior sagittal sinus

Subarachnoid space

Arachnoid granulations

Chiasmatic cistern

Choroid plexus of 3rd ventricle

Interpeduncular cistern

Cerebral aqueduct (of Sylvius)

Prepontine cistern

Lateral aperture (foramen of Luschka)

Choroid plexus of 4th ventricle

Dura mater

Arachnoid

Subarachnoid space

Cistern of great cerebral vein

Cerebellomedullary cistern

Median aperture (foramen of Magendie)

Figure 9-6   Circulation of cerebrospinal fluid. (From Netter FH: *The CIBA collection—nervous system,* vol 1, West Caldwell, NJ, 1983, CIBA Pharmaceutical.)

such as regulating body temperature, water balance, pituitary function, hunger, and emotional expression.

Brain Stem

The brain stem consists of the medulla, the pons, and the midbrain. Cardiac and respiratory centers necessary for survival are located here, as are pathways connecting the cerebrum, the cerebellum, and the spinal cord.

Spinal Cord

The spinal cord, composed of both gray and white matter, is a cylindrical structure that extends from the medulla and brain stem to the second lumbar vertebra.

The spinal cord and its spinal tracts convey sensory impulses to the brain and motor impulses from the brain to the periphery. The spinal cord also contains reflex neuronal circuits.

Ventricular System

Cavities within the brain, called ventricles, are filled with cerebrospinal fluid (CSF), a transudate of blood formed by the secretion from the choroid plexus located in the lateral, third, and fourth ventricles of the brain (Figure 9-5). CSF is a clear, colorless liquid that protects the brain from shocks, delivers nutritive substances, and removes waste from the brain and spinal cord. The dynamics of CSF flow are demonstrated in Figure 9-6.

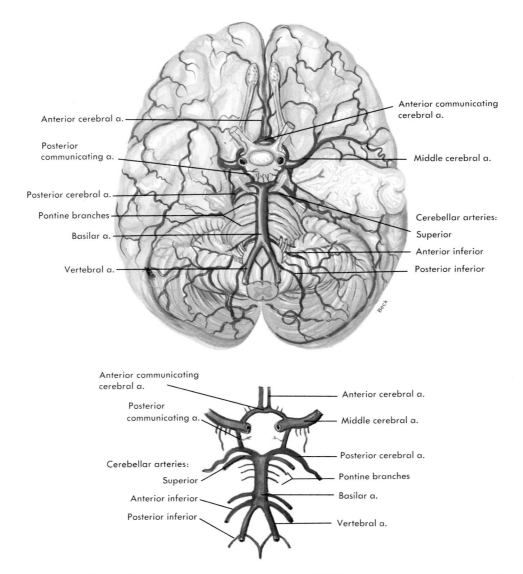

Figure 9-7 Arteries at base of brain. The arteries that comprise circle of Willis are the two anterior cerebral arteries joined to each other by anterior communicating cerebral artery and to posterior communicating arteries. (From Anthony CP, Thibodeau GA: *Textbook of anatomy and physiology,* ed 10, St. Louis, 1979, Mosby.)

Blood Supply

The brain is metabolically very active and requires a continual supply of oxygen and glucose. About 20% of the oxygen utilized by the entire body is consumed by the brain. If deprived of oxygen for more than several minutes, the brain can suffer permanent damage. Glucose is the principal source of energy for the brain. In fact, measurement of regional glucose utilization is used to reflect neuronal activity of groups of neurons. Those areas of the brain involved in mental functions show an increase in the utilization of glucose, as is demonstrated with PET.

The right common carotid artery originates from the right subclavian artery, and the left common carotid artery originates from the aorta. At the level of the larynx these arteries divide into internal and external ca-

rotid arteries. Inside the cranium the right and left internal carotid arteries come together and with the basilar artery form the circle of Willis. From this circle of blood vessels arise the anterior and posterior cerebral arteries (Figure 9-7). These arteries are connected with the internal carotid arteries by the anterior and posterior communicating arteries, respectively. The circle of Willis tends to equalize blood pressure to the brain and provides collateral blood flow. Large dural sinuses (superior and inferior sagittal, straight, and transverse) drain blood into the internal jugular veins that descend on either side of the neck and join with the right and left subclavian veins. The joining of the internal jugular with the subclavian vein forms the right and left brachiocephalic veins, which deliver blood to the superior vena cava (Figure 9-8).

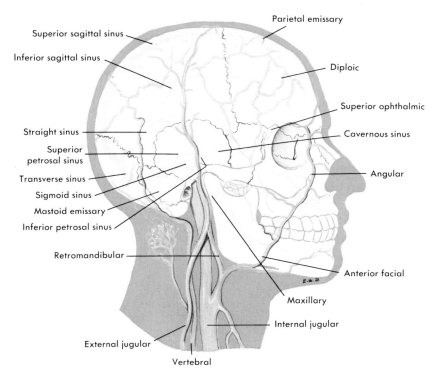

Figure 9-8   Semischematic projections of large veins of head. Deep veins and dural sinuses are projected on skull. Note connections (emissary veins) between superficial and deep veins. (From Anthony CP, Thibodeau GA: *Textbook of anatomy and physiology,* ed 10, St. Louis, 1979, Mosby.)

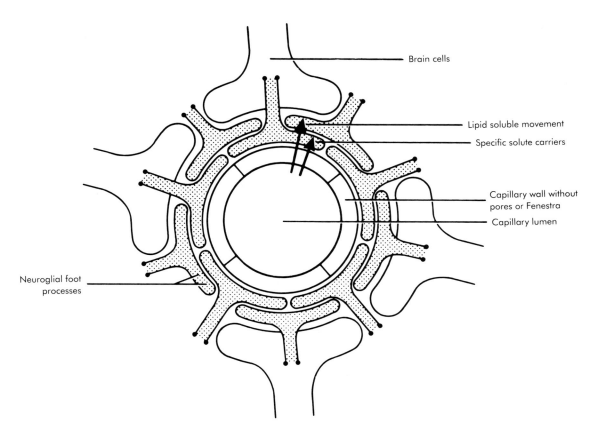

Figure 9-9   Blood-brain barrier (BBB). (From Maisey M, Britton KE, Gilday DL, eds: *Clinical nuclear medicine,* ed 2, London, 1992, Chapman & Hall.)

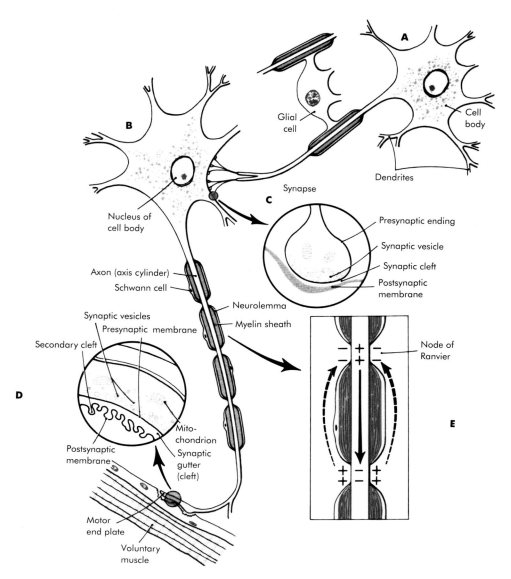

Figure 9-10 Neurons of the central nervous system (CNS). Neuron *A* is confined to the CNS and terminates on neuron *B* at a typical chemical synapse *(C)*. Neuron *B* is a ventral horn cell; its axon extends to a peripheral nerve and innervates a voluntary muscle at the myoneural junction *(D)*. In *E* the action potential is moving in the direction of the solid arrow inside the axon; the dashed arrows indicate the direction of flow of the action current. (From Gilman S, Newman SW: *Manter and Gatz's essentials of clinical neuroanatomy and neurophysiology,* ed 7, Philadelphia, 1987, FA Davis.)

Blood-Brain Barrier

The blood-brain barrier (Figure 9-9) serves to protect the brain from potentially toxic substances from the diet or metabolic processes. The barrier exists because the brain's capillaries have tight endothelial junctions and continuous basement membranes, which prevent the exit of large molecules. The close approximation of the astrocyte foot processes also restricts the entry of material. Movement of substances across the blood-brain barrier is controlled by either active transport or the degree of lipophilicity of the substance, which makes it possible for them to cross the cells.

Injury to the brain related to disease, trauma, or tox-ins often causes the blood-brain barrier to lose its integrity, and normally restricted substances can enter the brain. Many radiopharmaceuticals used to examine the brain depend on lipophilicity or specific transport processes.

Neurons and Neuroglia

The nervous system consists of two major cell types: neurons and neuroglia. Neurons are highly specialized cells that carry either sensory impulses to the brain (afferent) or motor response impulses to the body with an appropriate response (efferent). There are millions of sensory neurons, tens of millions of motor neurons, and tens of billions of interneurons that connect the two and make complex human mental functioning possible.

Neurons consist of three major parts: the cell body, the dendrite, and the axon (Figure 9-10). Dendrites conduct nerve impulses (action potentials) toward the cell body, which contains the cell nucleus. Axons conduct the nerve impulses away from the cell body to other neurons or tissue. The interface between one neuron and another is called a *synapse.* At the synapse, chemicals called neurotransmitters are secreted from membrane-enclosed sacs, called *vesicles,* at the distal end of each axon. The actions of neurotransmitters impinging on a postsynaptic neuron are integrated to determine whether the postsynaptic electrical action potential will be passed to another neuron. Acetylcholine and the catecholamines norepinephrine and dopamine are examples of neurotransmitters. Each of these substances has a characteristic inhibitory or excitatory effect on the neurons. The effect of acetylcholine is excitatory in the brain and inhibitory in the heart. The repolarization of neurons after transmission of action potentials consumes much of the energy of the brain and accounts for about half of the glucose utilization.

Neuroglial cells do not transmit electrical impulses but instead are supportive and protective of neurons. Some contain neuroreceptors, such as benzodiazepine receptors of a type not found on neurons.

CLINICAL STUDIES

Cerebrovascular Disease

Clinical symptoms and signs often suggest the sites of cortical or subcortical injury in patients who have acute stroke. However, lesions are not always at the site suggested by clinical manifestations. The clinical picture may be the result of secondary effects resulting from lesions in other locations caused by deafferentation or other effects. The degree of mental dysfunction may be far greater than that suggested by the anatomic lesions seen in computed tomography (CT) or magnetic resonance imaging (MRI). Subcortical lesions, such as lacunar infarctions, can result in extensive cortical dysfunction on the affected side. The neurologic examination cannot effectively predict what the patient's eventual neurologic deficiency will be. CT often will not reveal the extent of involvement until structural changes have developed several days after the onset of symptoms and signs. Arteriography can reveal the status of large vessels but does not provide information about cerebral perfusion through the microcirculation. SPECT and PET make it possible to delineate the severity and extent of the perfusion defects from the time of onset of the stroke (Figure 9-11).

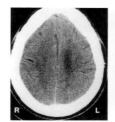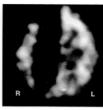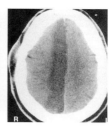

Figure 9-11   The CT scan performed 2 hr after the patient had a seizure is normal *(left).* The ^{99m}Tc HMPAO brain SPECT scan performed immediately after the CT scan *(center)* shows a large area of decreased perfusion involving the territory of the right anterior cerebral artery. A subsequent CT scan performed 3 days later shows a well-defined region of hypodensity in the territory of the right anterior cerebral artery, which correlated well with the defect observed on the first SPECT scan. (From Mountz J, Deutsch G, Khan S: *Clinical nuclear medicine,* Philadelphia, 1993, JB Lippincott.)

PET makes it possible to measure cerebral blood flow, glucose and oxygen metabolism, blood volume, and pH, thus providing a more complete understanding of the severity of the patient's illness. The area of lowest regional blood flow or metabolism usually predicts the region that will eventually develop radiolucency on CT, although the perfusion and metabolic lesions are often larger. The blood flow or metabolic abnormalities seen with PET or SPECT correlate better with the neurologic defects than do those seen with CT or MRI. The nuclear medicine images reflect function, whereas CT and MRI images reflect structure. Thus, studies of the cerebral circulation are helpful in establishing prognosis following acute cerebral ischemia. In stroke, metabolic abnormalities seen on PET frequently are more extensive than the corresponding CT findings. The pattern of metabolic abnormalities in PET correlate with the clinical syndrome and with the degree of eventual recovery.[11,7]

Tumors

Tumors involving the central nervous system are a treatable cause of neuropsychiatric dysfunction. Glioblastoma multiforme occurs in 15% to 20% of all intracranial neoplasms. Treatment includes surgical resection, external radiotherapy, and chemotherapy. At times, radiation necrosis of the brain results in patients who have received 5000-6000 rad of external radiation therapy. The use of nuclear medicine technology can define the precise localization of the extent of the tumor better than CT or MRI, which often reveal the response of the body to tumor, such as edema. The nuclear studies can help distinguish between the tumor and the effect of radiation (Figure 9-12).

When neurologic symptoms recur or change in patients treated with radiation, it is virtually impossible to distinguish radiation necrosis and gliosis from tumor

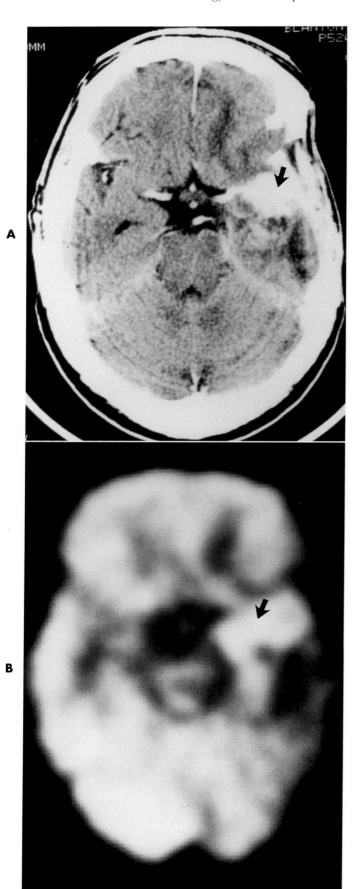

recurrence by anatomic imaging techniques or clinical examination. Nuclear procedures often eliminate the need for a second craniotomy and tissue biopsy.[1,10,19] Cerebral blood flow and blood volume are not well correlated with the degree of malignancy, therefore metabolic studies are preferred.

Epilepsy

Epilepsy is one of the most common diseases of the brain. Approximately 800,000 Americans have focal seizures that do not progress to grand mal seizures (partial complex epilepsy). For most patients with partial epilepsy, diagnosis and classification are based on the use of surface electroencephalography (EEG), which records electrical activity associated with neuronal activity. However, for the approximately 20% of patients who are uncontrolled by medication, additional information about localization of the epileptic focus is required if surgical therapy is anticipated. Radiologic techniques such as CT scanning usually show no abnormalities in these patients. Special localizing measures including intraoperative electrocorticography and direct recordings from stereotaxically implanted depth electrodes are valuable for improved localization, but these techniques can give rise to conflicting results and are accompanied by certain risks. In such a setting the PET scan can provide independent, confirmatory information about the site of the epileptogenic lesion (Figure 9-13).

During focal seizures, brain metabolism and blood flow are increased at the site of onset of the seizures and in regions to which the seizure activity is propagated. Between seizures (interictal state), both metabolism and blood flow are reduced at the site of onset. When PET was first applied in epilepsy, it was anticipated and subsequently confirmed that PET imaging would localize these focal changes in cerebral metabolism and perfusion and thus provide unique diagnostic information useful in the management of patients with epilepsy.[16] PET techniques most useful in the study of epilepsy include determinations of glucose utilization (^{18}F fluorodeoxyglucose, FDG), oxygen utilization (^{15}O oxygen), and cerebral perfusion (^{13}N ammonia and [15]O water).

Figure 9-12 Contrast enhanced CT and PET metabolic FDG images in a patient with a recurrent glioma. The CT scan **(A)** shows an area of contrast enhancement in the left temporal lobe *(reader's right)* following surgery and radiation therapy. The area of increased metabolic activity seen with FDG-PET **(B)** and the area of contrast enhancement seen with CT were found to be recurrent tumor following reoperation and biopsy *(arrows)*. Conversely, when glucose metabolism is reduced in regions of contrast enhancement on x-ray CT, radiation necrosis is the diagnosis. (Courtesy R. Edward Coleman, MD, Duke University, Durham, NC.)

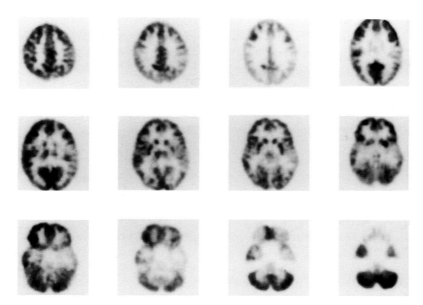

Figure 9-13 Images of regional glucose metabolism in a patient with a left temporal lobe seizure focus. There is reduced glucose utilization in the left lateral and medial temporal cortex (readers right). The region of hypometabolism extends to the frontal and parietal cortices, seen on the higher slices, although these regions were normal by EEG. This case demonstrates that, although FDG metabolic PET is useful for localizing seizure foci, it tends to overestimate the size of the focus as shown by EEG. (Courtesy Frost JJ, MD, Johns Hopkins University School of Medicine, Baltimore.)

PET scans obtained during partial seizures have shown marked increases in local brain metabolism and perfusion at the site of seizure onset, but because of propagated neuronal activity, the ictal scans are less useful in predicting epileptic origin than those made during the interictal state.[3,4,5] PET scans made during nonfocal seizures show generalized increase in brain metabolism and perfusion. Unlike the typical PET scans found in partial epilepsy, no focal changes are found during interictal or ictal scans of patients with petit mal seizures. A diffuse increase of metabolism is seen at the time of the petit mal seizure.

PET scans obtained during the interictal state are most valuable in the management of the patient with partial epilepsy. The results of interictal PET scans in patients with partial epilepsy have been compared with the results of CT and EEG in multiple reports.[9,15,22] The results have been essentially the same in the 50-patient series reported from the University of Southern California, Los Angeles, the 20-patient series from the National Institutes of Health, and the 24-patient series from Montreal Neurological Institute. PET data have been compared with interictal EEG findings, depth electrode measurements, and pathologic evaluations from resected specimens. Approximately 70% of these patients demonstrate zones of hypometabolism on interictal FDG scans or decreased cerebral blood flow in the involved regions. PET and EEG are complementary methods of localizing areas in the brain causing epileptic activity. Focal abnormalities can be identified with PET even if EEG data are unable to reveal the focus. The combined use of surface EEG and PET has elimi-

nated the need for depth electrodes in some surgical candidates. PET can aid in the localization of the site when the EEG findings are inconsistent. EEG can verify the epileptogenic nature of a zone of hypometabolism determined by PET. Furthermore, an excellent correlation has been obtained between the site of hypometabolism as determined by PET and the presence of a pathologic abnormality in the surgical specimen.

In patients with epilepsy PET imaging provides information about local brain function that is quite different from the results of electrical measurements with EEG or structural assessments with CT. The combination of PET and EEG has been useful in presurgical evaluation for determining the site of seizure onset in patients with partial epilepsy who have become refractory to medical treatment. The interictal PET scan effectively detects hypometabolic brain zones considered most likely to be responsible for seizures in these patients, even though these zones usually appear normal on CT scans. A good correlation exists between metabolic and combined electrophysiologic techniques with respect to localization of the epileptogenic focus. Either technique can give false-positive or false-negative results, but when used in combination they yield more reliable localizing information.

The EEG is useful for confirming if a hypometabolic zone is epileptogenic. The PET scan helps determine whether an abnormal EEG focus is likely to represent a primary epileptogenic region or propagation from a distance and serves as an independent confirmation of the epileptogenic site.[9]

The advantage of SPECT is that one can measure regional cerebral blood flow immediately after the onset of the seizure. The ^{99m}Tc blood-flow tracers can be prepared rapidly and kept near the patient being monitored by EEG so that the injection can be made as soon as there is evidence of seizure activity. This is not possible with PET tracers, which are more difficult to prepare. It is important that the injection be made before seizure activity has spread to other parts of the brain.

Parkinson's Disease

Many dopamine neurons have their cell bodies in the substantia nigra, from which axons project into the caudate nucleus and putamen, where dopamine is released to bind to dopamine receptors. These neurons are involved in Parkinson's disease, which develops when dopamine levels in the caudate and putamen fall to less than 20% of normal levels. The discovery of dopamine deficiency in the caudate nucleus and putamen of patients with Parkinson's disease whose brains were examined at autopsy was a major discovery in neurobiology and paved the way for the development of an effective means of treating this debilitating disease: the administration of L-dopa to increase the synthesis of dopamine.

One of the best examples of the use of in vivo biochemical assessment of neuroreceptors is in Parkinson's disease. The ability to quantify the status of presynaptic and postsynaptic dopaminergic neurons can be related to neuropsychologic and clinical assessment.

Parkinson's disease is characterized by degeneration of dopaminergic neurons that pass from the substantia nigra region of the brain into the region of the caudate nuclei. Studies of postsynaptic D1 and D2 dopamine receptors have demonstrated preservation or even an increase in these postsynaptic receptors. In contrast, early in Parkinson's disease there is a decrease in the number of presynaptic dopamine transport sites. Measurement of these sites with either a positron or single photon emitting radiotracer makes it possible to identify the chemical abnormalities in the brains of patients with Parkinson's disease even before symptoms occur.

Recently, a ^{99m}Tc-labeled compound that crosses the human blood-brain barrier and binds to the dopamine presynaptic transporter was reported.[13,18] This milestone marks the first time a ^{99m}Tc tracer was used to image a recognition site within the brain. Previously, the commercially available ^{99m}Tc tracers were only able to measure cerebral blood flow, or trace hepatic or renal clearance, that is, excretory processes.

Dementia

The number of persons suffering from dementia has increased with the increasing age of the population. In the United States this represents 10% of all persons over age 65, half of whom will eventually require institutional care. Approximately 1 million persons in United States hospitals at any given time are suffering from dementia.

Dementias fall broadly into two categories: those treatable by specific medical means and those for whom the only treatment consists of supportive care. About 30% of demented elderly patients suffer from impairment of brain blood flow from cerebrovascular disease. Another 20% of dementias are caused by diseases for which there are specific treatments, one of the most common being drug intoxication. Older people often take many medications, which singly or in combination can cause dementia. Depression is also common in the elderly and can be associated with increased forgetfulness and confusion. If diagnosed correctly, depression is often treatable.

Hyperthyroidism, hypothyroidism, and vitamin B_{12} deficiency are other causes of treatable dementia. Subdural hematomas can lead to dementia and can be the result of unrecognized or minor trauma.

The diagnosis of Alzheimer's disease is usually made by exclusion of the other causes. Since the disease is so progressive, the diagnosis needs to be made in the early stages and can be 90% accurate on the basis of clinical and psychologic testing in about 50% of the patients who first come to medical attention because of memory loss. Usually, the diagnosis is not made before thousands of dollars have been spent on tests.

Alzheimer's disease accounts for approximately 50% of demented patients. The disease is characterized by abnormally accelerated neuronal death, especially pronounced in the hippocampus, parietal, temporal, and to a lesser degree frontal lobes. As a result of the neuronal degeneration a secondary decrease of blood flow and oxygen and glucose metabolism occurs in the involved regions.

Both PET and SPECT have revealed a characteristic pattern of distribution of regional cerebral blood flow in patients with Alzheimer's disease.[6,8] The disease involves the parietal lobes in a symmetric fashion, often with extension into the adjacent temporal and occipital lobes. Frontal lobe involvement occurs to a lesser degree, and no abnormality is noted in the cingulate gyrus, basal ganglia, sensory-motor cortex, visual cortex, and cerebellum. The distribution of disease is more symmetric in the transaxial plane than that observed in patients with multi-infarct dementia, in which the defects are multifocal and show a high contrast between normal and abnormal areas of brain. Often the defects correspond to the distribution of a major cerebral artery such as the middle cerebral artery. The sensory-motor cortex, basal ganglia, and cerebellum are often involved, with the changes in the cerebellum being secondary to motor abnormalities. The diagnosis of dementia is complicated by the coexistence of Alzheimer's disease and multi-infarct dementia, which is

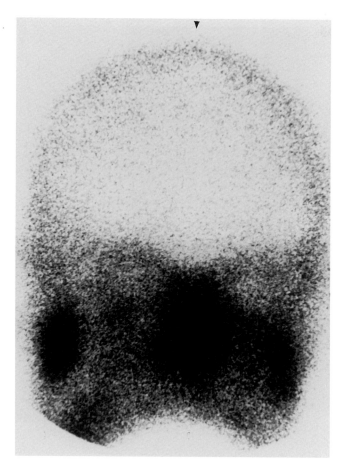

Figure 9-14 Brain death: early flow images demonstrated no intracranial blood flow. This image obtained 1 min after injection reveals an absence of tracer activity in the longitudinal sinus, indicating a complete absence of cerebral perfusion.

found in about 30% of patients who come to autopsy. An advantage of PET compared with SPECT is that one can measure glucose metabolism and oxygen metabolism as well as regional cerebral blood flow. The CT or MRI scan has an important role in detecting focal cerebral disease such as tumor or infarction, in determining ventricular size, or in detecting caudate atrophy in Huntington's disease. In depressed patients with dementia the PET studies are normal. The CT scan may show old infarctions in patients with dementia from multiple infarctions, but the PET metabolic study reveals more prominent defects throughout the brain. The FDG scan is more sensitive than the CT scan for detecting these focal zones of brain dysfunction.

Patients with Alzheimer's disease have diffuse cortical hypometabolism, which is most prominent in the temporal and parietal cortex, but have preservation of metabolism in subcortical structures. These findings are distinctively different from the FDG-scan results in Huntington's disease, which has markedly abnormal metabolism and blood flow in the caudate and putamen, even in the presence of normal CT scans. Thus, both PET and SPECT studies play an important role in the evaluation of patients with unexplained dementia.

Brain Death Assessment

Although there are clear-cut clinical criteria for establishing death, patients on cardiopulmonary support systems may be brain dead, although the circulation and respiratory systems continue to function. Measurement of regional cerebral blood flow by means of planar, SPECT, or PET imaging is able to document the absence of blood flow through the distribution of the internal carotid arteries, which occurs when there is insufficient neuronal activity to sustain life. The characteristic pattern is shown in Figure 9-14, where one can see blood flow through the external cerebral circulation but no blood flow through the cerebral cortex and no filling of the sagittal and transverse sinuses.

CSF Dynamics

The normal cisternography procedure (Figure 9-15) shows activity in the basal cisterns by 3 hr after injection with flow over the convexities by 24 hr. No reflux into the ventricles is seen. In communicating hydrocephalus (Figure 9-16), reflux into the ventricles is seen with a delayed flow over the convexities.

Noncommunicating hydrocephalus shows a lack of ventricular reflux with slow or normal flow over the convexities. Normal pressure hydrocephalus shows a ventricular reflux that persists 24 to 72 hr. The flow over the convexities is significantly delayed or absent.

RADIOPHARMACEUTICALS

Single photon emitting radiopharmaceuticals (Table 9-1), based on detecting a compromised blood-brain barrier, include ^{99m}Tc pertechnetate, ^{99m}Tc diethylenetriamine pentaacetic acid (DTPA), ^{99m}Tc glucoheptonate (GH), and ^{201}Tl chloride. GH and DTPA are more rapidly cleared from the blood than pertechnetate, provide better signal-to-noise ratios, and do not require any patient preparation. ^{99m}Tc administered as sodium pertechnetate concentrates in the choroid plexus and therefore requires the blockage of this accumulation by oral administration of potassium perchlorate (0.75-1.0 g) within 1 hr of radiopharmaceutical administration. The average adult dose of these ^{99m}Tc chelates is 20 mCi.

In assessing regional cerebral blood flow, imaging is begun immediately after radiopharmaceutical administration. Subsequent images are obtained 2 to 3 hr after injection when using ^{99m}Tc pertechnetate and 30

| | Anterior | Left lateral | Right lateral |

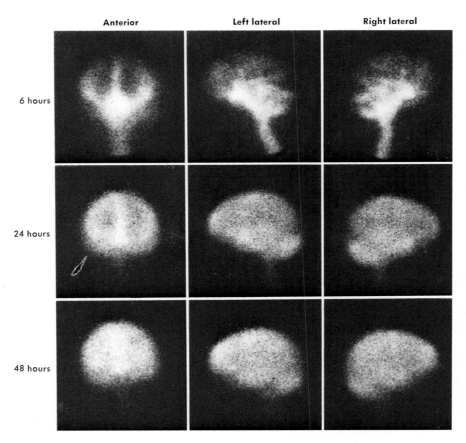

Figure 9-15   Normal cisternogram showing anterior and both lateral views at 6, 24, and 48 hr after intrathecal administration.

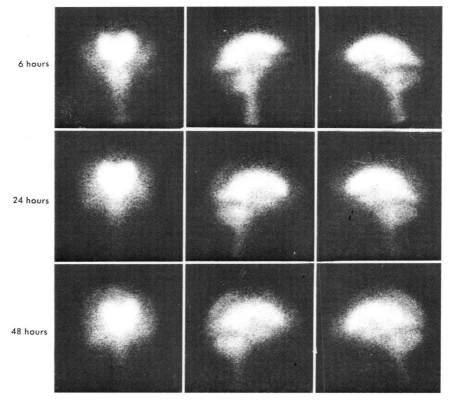

Figure 9-16   Communicating hydrocephalus (normal pressure hydrocephalus) with lateral ventricular reflux on 6-hr images and no significant ventricular clearing on the 24- and 48-hr images.

Table 9-1 Single photon radiopharmaceuticals for brain imaging

Radiopharmaceutical	Photon energy (keV)	Physical half-life	Usual dose	Optimum imaging time	Comments
Imaging agents that do not penetrate intact BBB					
^{99m}Tc pertechnetate	140	6 hr	15-20 mCi	2-4 hr	KC10$_4$ or atropine
^{99m}Tc diethylenetri-amine pentaacetic acid (DTPA)	140	6 hr	15-20 mCi	0.5-1 hr	rapid uptake
^{99m}Tc glucohepto-nate (GHA)	140	6 hr	15-20 mCi	1-4 hr	—
^{67}Ga citrate	92, 187, 296, 388	78 hr	3-6 mCi	24-72 hr	Inflammation
^{201}Tl chloride	80, 135, 167	73 hr	2-3 mCi	Immediate	Metastases
^{99m}Tc phosphonates (MDP, HDP)	140	6 hr	15-20 mCi	2-4 hr	Infarctions
^{99m}Tc red cells (in vivo)	140	6 hr	15-20 mCi	0.5-1 hr	Blood pool
Imaging agents that penetrate intact BBB					
^{133}Xe (xenon gas)	81	127 hr	0.5-10 mCi	Immediate	rCBF
^{123}I iodoamphet-amine (IMP) or ^{123}I HIPDM	159	13.3 hr	3-5 mCi	0.5-1 hr	rCBF
^{99m}Tc d, 1-hexamethyl-propyleneamine oxime (HMPAO)	140	6 hr	20 mCi	0.25-3 hr	rCBF
^{99m}Tc-N,N′−1,2-ethylenediylbis-L-cysteine diethylester (ECD)	140	6 hr	30 mCi	0.25-3 hr	rCBF

BBB, Blood-brain barrier; *rCBF*, regional cerebral blow flow.

to 120 min after injection when using either ^{99m}Tc DTPA or ^{99m}Tc GH. These later images are used to detect compromise of the blood-brain barrier.

^{201}Tl, like many radiopharmaceuticals, does not cross the blood-brain barrier in normal individuals, but it diffuses rapidly across an altered BBB. Thallium and SPECT have been used to diagnose brain tumors, clarify the nature of lesions found at CT or MRI, and detect tumor recurrence. The positive predictive value is much better than the negative predictive value, and thallium is usually not very helpful in determining tumor type or predicting clinical outcome. A dose of 2 mCi is used and images may be obtained as soon as 10 min after injection.

Other single photon radiopharmaceuticals used for the evaluation of regional brain perfusion include ^{133}Xe gas, the ^{123}I-labeled amines, ^{99m}Tc-labeled hexamethylpropylene amine oxime (HMPAO), and ^{99m}Tc-N,N′-1,2-ethylenediylbis-L-cysteine diethylester (ECD). ^{133}Xe is a chemically inert, readily diffusable radio-

active gas that, when injected, rapidly passes into the brain and then washes out at a rate proportional to the regional brain blood flow. Although ^{133}Xe gas is widely available and relatively inexpensive, it presents technical problems related to detection of its low gamma photon energy (80 keV). An advantage is that repeat studies can be carried out within a relatively short time.

^{123}I iodoamphetamine was the first lipophilic gamma photon emitting radiopharmaceutical to cross the intact blood-brain barrier and distribute itself throughout the brain in proportion to regional cerebral blood flow. It is no longer available commercially.

^{99m}Tc HMPAO is a neutral lipid-soluble radiopharmaceutical that crosses the blood-brain barrier and remains trapped in the brain in a manner proportional to the cerebral blood flow. It can be used to reflect regional cerebral blood flow in a manner analogous to the use of microspheres that are trapped in cerebral capillaries. The relatively long retention time (24 hr) combined with the availability and superior imaging characteristics of ^{99m}Tc are attractive features. The average adult dose of ^{99m}Tc HMPAO is 20 mCi.[21,22]

^{99m}Tc ECD, which is more stable than ^{99m}Tc HMPAO, is also used to measure cerebral blood flow. It has a high first-pass extraction, and the in vivo conversion of this lipophilic agent into nondiffusable metabolites is slower than it is for HMPAO.

PET extends the technology to include biologically important radiotracers that can be synthesized using radioactive forms of carbon (^{11}C), oxygen (^{15}O), nitrogen (^{13}N), and fluorine (^{18}F, a hydrogen substitute). Many of the radiotracers are identical to substances normally found in the body. These radionuclides are cyclotron produced and have short half-lives, so they require rapid synthesis and quality assurance methods. Radiopharmaceutical doses range from 5-10 mCi for ^{18}F FDG to 20 mCi for ^{11}C compounds (^{11}C NMSP or carfentanil).

The development of regional pharmacies to distribute PET radiopharmaceuticals to hospitals and clinics unable to obtain and support a cyclotron will extend the benefits of PET to more patients. We have seen this happen as many radiopharmaceuticals first developed for PET subsequently have been successfully labeled with ^{99m}Tc, ^{123}I, or ^{111}In and translated into SPECT studies. The new SPECT camera systems that are capable of imaging positron emitting isotopes will also extend the use of PET, particularly FDG. As more and more "outcome" studies are published, it will become increasingly convincing that PET is no longer just a research tool limited to large academic centers. In many clinical situations patients' problems cannot be answered completely with anatomic imaging studies, laboratory data and physical examination, or a combination of these. PET is expensive to install and maintain, but the results it produces are saving the healthcare system lots of money by avoiding unnecessary, unfruitful diagnostic tests and operative procedures and prolonged hospitalizations.

^{111}In DTPA is an ideal radiopharmaceutical for the assessment of CSF dynamics. It satisfies the following criteria: (1) it is physiologically governed by CSF flow; (2) it has an adequate physical half-life of 2.8 days for the desired study; (3) it has a desired photon emission for imaging (173 and 247 keV); (4) it has a relatively low radiation dose to the patient; (5) it has the least probable chemical toxicity; and (6) it has a controlled radiopharmaceutical quality.

A physician performing a lumbar puncture administers 500 μCi of ^{111}In DTPA intrathecally to the patient. A 21- to 22-gauge spinal needle connected to a three-way stopcock is often used to monitor CSF pressure, sample the CSF for routine cell and chemical tests, and to administer the radiopharmaceutical flush. The patient is kept in a horizontal position for 2 hr after injection to minimize headaches due to CSF leakage.

RELATIONSHIP OF PLANAR, PET, AND SPECT IMAGING

Many problems can be solved by planar imaging alone, but the value of tomography in all types of medical imaging is now well established. For all imaging modalities, whether anatomic in orientation as in CT, or physiologic and biochemical as in nuclear medicine, viewing the body from a ring of viewpoints surrounding it increases contrast between lesions and normal tissues, which is then translated into improved diagnostic information.[2,14] In clinical problems requiring a high degree of spatial resolution for their solution, such as locating the point of origin of an epileptic seizure, PET or SPECT will always be better than planar imaging.[17]

The most important difference between PET and SPECT lies in the radiotracers used with each. PET is based chiefly on the use of ^{11}C, ^{18}F, ^{15}O, and ^{13}N, the first two being the most commonly used.[12] The workhorses of SPECT are ^{99m}Tc and ^{123}I. Other differences include the greater sensitivity of PET and the more accurate quantification, which results from the better ability to correct for attenuation. Generally, most laboratories purchasing new equipment select SPECT rather than planar imaging systems. If a given clinical problem can be solved with SPECT, it is preferable to PET because the shorter half-lives of the radiotracers (20 min for ^{11}C and 110 min for ^{18}F) always make the PET studies more complicated. The localization of epileptic foci can be taken as an example. With FDG the studies can be carried out only between seizures because it is difficult to have the tracer on hand at the time of the seizure. It is not easy, but it is possible with SPECT to prepare a ^{99m}Tc tracer so that the injection can be made immediately after the start of the seizure. On the other hand, the FDG study helps determine how much brain tissue can be removed at surgery without inducing neurologic defects. SPECT studies can be used to differentiate senile dementia such as Alzheimer's disease from less serious and more treatable brain disease such as depression.

IMAGE ACQUISITION TECHNIQUES

Planar Imaging

Blood-brain barrier. To detect regions in which there is absence or breakdown of the blood-brain barrier as a result of disease, imaging of regional perfusion is performed immediately after IV injection of the tracer. When using ^{99m}Tc pertechnetate, 0.75-1.0 g of potassium perchlorate is administered orally within 1 hr of radiopharmaceutical administration. Giving the patient water or other fluids to drink will increase urinary output with a subsequent decrease in radiation exposure. No patient preparation is required when using [99mTc] DTPA or [99mTc] GH.

As in the case of all [99mTc] tracers, a low-energy parallel-hole collimator is used. A general-purpose, rather than a high-resolution, collimator is usually employed, since count rates are low because of the short time frames obtained during the perfusion study. Later images (equilibrium images) are obtained using a low-energy, high-resolution collimator, because longer imaging times per frame can be obtained. The energy calibration is a 20% window centered on the 140 keV gamma emission of [99mTc].

To examine regional cerebral blood flow, the anterior projection is performed with the patient either supine (brain death evaluation) or seated (Figure 9-17). Depending on the clinical problem, other positions can be selected. When the anterior view is used, the head should be flexed with the canthomeatal line perpendicular to the surface of the detector. A Velcro strap or adhesive tape should be used to prevent movement of the patient's head.

A vertex projection can be obtained with the patient supine and the head extended off the imaging table and resting on the detector such that the canthomeatal line is parallel to the surface of the crystal detector (Figure 9-18). In the vertex projection it is essential to shield the body from the camera to prevent photons from the body reaching the detector. This is accomplished by patient positioning and the use of a lead apron or cape placed over the patient's shoulders. The injected volume of the radiopharmaceutical dose should be less than 1 ml and should be injected rapidly through an indwelling catheter into an antecubital vein, followed by a 20-30 ml saline flush. Immediately after injection, serial 1- or 2-sec images are obtained. Sequential images are obtained for 40 sec or until the radiotracer can be seen in the sagittal sinus and the great veins. A blood pool image is routinely obtained after the flow phase of the study. When the clinical question involves brain death, identification of these venous structures without evidence of cerebral perfusion is the basis of the diagnosis. Quantification is obtained by placement of regions of interest over the left and right cerebral hemispheres for the generation of time-activity curves.[20]

Two hours after the rapid sequence of images used to reflect regional perfusion, anterior, posterior, right and left lateral, and vertex images are obtained after the tracer has diffused into the extracellular fluid (equi-

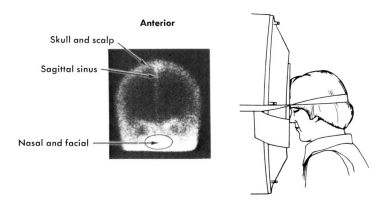

Figure 9-17 Anterior view of normal planar brain image. Patient position for anterior (seated) view.

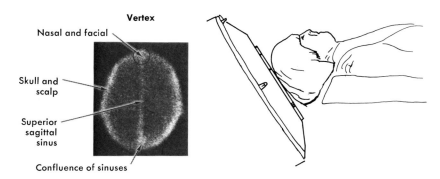

Figure 9-18 Vertex view of normal planar brain image (equilibrium view). Patient position for vertex flow and equilibrium images.

At the later times, 500,000-count images are obtained. Images can be obtained 4 hr after injection if the presence of a subdural hematoma is suspected.

CSF Imaging

The injection site is imaged immediately after radiopharmaceutical administration to rule out extravasation of the injected dose outside of the subarachnoid space. If a wide, segmental appearance is seen initially with no activity in the basal cisterns at 2 to 3 hr, reinjection will be required.

Imaging is routinely performed at 2, 6, 24, and 48 hr after injection. Anterior and one or both lateral projections of the head and an anterior image of the abdomen are obtained 2 hr after injection for 200,000 counts. Positioning of these projections is the same as that used in planar brain imaging. Additional views of the head or spine may be indicated. No data processing is required unless assessing CSF rhinorrhea.

The quantitative diagnosis of CSF rhinorrhea can begin 2 hr after the intrathecal administration of ^{111}In DTPA. Cotton pledgets (1 cm^2) are placed in each nostril by an otorhinolaryngologist in locations of suspected CSF leakage. A string is attached to the pledget to allow for retrieval and the labeling of the anatomic location. A 5 ml heparinized blood sample is obtained from the patient at the time of the placement of the pledgets. The pledgets are removed 6 hr after injection. A second 5 ml heparinized blood sample is obtained. Following centrifugation of both blood samples, 0.5 ml of plasma is withdrawn from each sample. A scintillation well counter employing a 150-250 keV window is used to count each pledget and each blood sample. The results are expressed as the ratio of pledget activity (cpm) divided by the average plasma activity (cpm). Normal pledget to plasma ratios are 1:1.3. Anterior, posterior, and lateral images are obtained for 200,000 counts. Images should be obtained with the patient in a position that would optimize the visualization of CSF leakage. Radiation safety and contamination precautions should be observed.

A variety of shunts are used to remove excess CSF from patients with hydrocephalus. A lumboperitoneal shunt consists of a tubing system placed in the lumbar subarachnoid space and extending into the abdominal cavity. A ventriculoperitoneal shunt consists of a ventricular catheter extending from the ventricles to a valve and distal tubing that drains into the peritoneal cavity. The Ommaya shunt is a system consisting of a reservoir and tubing used to deliver chemotherapeutic agents to the ventricles and the subarachnoid space. Nuclear medicine procedures are performed to evaluate the patency of the shunt and, in the case of the Ommaya shunt, to evaluate the distribution pattern of the radiotracer in the CSF to predict the distribution of chemotherapeutic agents.

Single Photon Emission Computed Tomography (SPECT)

Recently, there has been a renewed interest in nuclear brain imaging due to the availability for a new generation of FDA-approved radiopharmaceuticals for cerebral perfusion and the current generation of gamma cameras that allow for high-resolution (6-8 mm full width at half maximum [FWHM]) single photon emission computed tomography (SPECT) imaging of the brain. SPECT brain images can be obtained with a single-head, rotating gamma camera. Multihead rotating cameras and multicrystal cameras are also in current use.

The time required for a SPECT brain procedure, including patient preparation, is approximately 1 hr. The imaging room should be quiet and dimly lit to minimize the environmental effect on the distribution of the radiotracer. An IV line should be placed before the injection of the radiotracer so that the patient does not experience pain when the radiotracer is injected. The patient is placed in a comfortable supine position with the head in a head holder and immobilized with a Velcro strap. Custom-fitted face masks are also available. Care must be taken to monitor the patient for motion during the imaging procedure. Often patients with certain neurologic disorders find it difficult to maintain a fixed position during the scanning procedure. The sagittal plane of the patient's head should be perpendicular to the table. The head is flexed so that the cerebellum is included in the field of view. The detector must be positioned as close as possible to the patient's head to ensure the acquisition of high-quality images.

The rotating gamma camera is equipped with a low-energy, high-resolution, parallel-hole collimator. Fan-beam collimators are currently in use to improve the resolution of the images. A computer with SPECT capabilities is required for the acquisition and processing of the imaging procedure.

The acquisition begins approximately 20 min after injection of the radiopharmaceutical. A general guideline for acquisition should include 64 images acquired for 20 to 40 sec each through a range of 360 degrees. The ability of the patient to endure the acquisition should be considered when selecting the acquisition time. When choosing the acquisition matrix, the theory that each pixel should approximate half of the extrinsic FWHM provides a general rule. A 128 × 128 matrix, although providing good resolution, might not contain a statistically valid number of counts per pixel and will require longer reconstruction times and a greater need for computer disk space. Magnification can be used to keep both the matrix and pixel size small. A 64 × 64 matrix with a magnification factor (2.0) applied will ap-

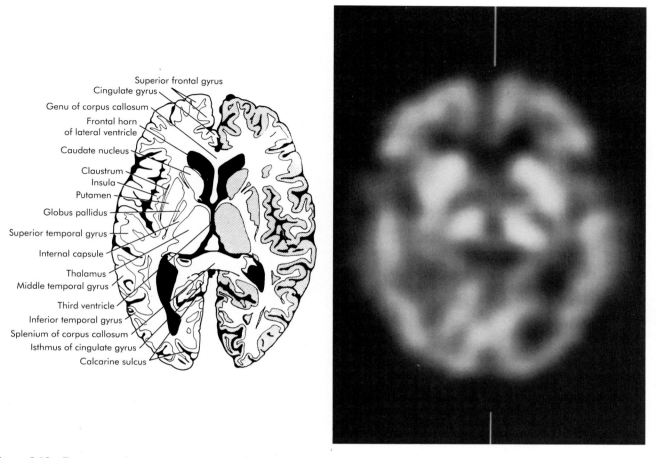

Superior frontal gyrus
Cingulate gyrus
Genu of corpus callosum
Frontal horn
of lateral ventricle
Caudate nucleus
Claustrum
Insula
Putamen
Globus pallidus
Superior temporal gyrus
Internal capsule
Thalamus
Middle temporal gyrus
Third ventricle
Inferior temporal gyrus
Splenium of corpus callosum
Isthmus of cingulate gyrus
Calcarine sulcus

Figure 9-19   Representative anatomic cross sections of the brain and a PET study obtained at the same level. (Drawing from Stark D, Bradley W: *Magnetic resonance imaging*, ed 2, St. Louis, 1992, Mosby.)

Table 9-2   SPECT acquisition parameters*

	Number of images per detector	Time per image	Matrix size	Collimator
One detector	60	30 sec	64 × 64	High resolution
Two detectors	60	30 sec	128 × 128	High resolution/fan beam
Three detectors	40	45 sec	64 × 64	High resolution/fan beam

*30-min acquisition.

proximate a 128 × 128 matrix. This saves both reconstruction time and decreases the amount of computer disk space used. Table 9-2 provides guidelines for brain SPECT acquisition on single-, dual-, and triple-head gamma cameras.

SPECT brain images are obtained using a filtered back-projection technique. To produce high-resolution, low-noise images, a combination of preprocessing, back-projection, and postprocessing filters is employed (Table 9-3). The selection of an appropriate SPECT

processing protocol depends on the radiopharmaceutical, the imaging instrumentation, and the computer software being used. A knowledge of cross-sectional anatomy is essential to process data for the subsequent interpretation by the nuclear medicine physician (Figure 9-19).

Center-of-rotation and field-uniformity corrections should be performed during reconstruction to improve the overall quality of the SPECT images. Attenuation correction is accomplished using a computer-generated

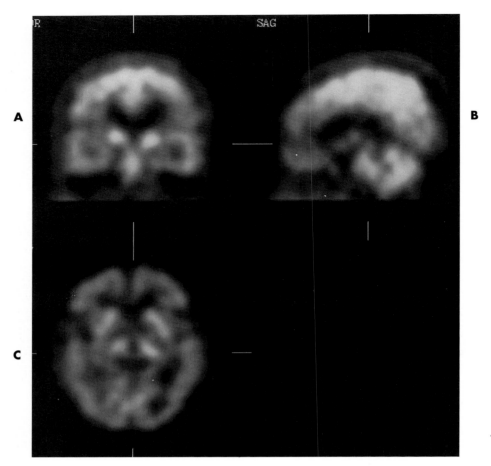

Figure 9-20 Three-view display of a ^{99m}Tc HMPAO brain scan in the **(A)** coronal, **(B)** sagittal planes, and **(C)** transverse planes.

Table 9-3	Processing filters
Preprocessing	Two-dimensional filter applied to planar views before reconstruction with resulting smoothing effect
Reconstruction	Simple back-projection technique of the ramp filter; range of filters used (high-frequency noise contribution to filters, which drastically smooth image)
Postprocessing	Apply filter in all three dimensions of reconstructed image; smoothing

ellipse fitted to the brain image. Using existing calculations, the correction is performed within the ellipse. Failure to perform these corrections can result in the loss of detail of smaller structures located within the brain.

SPECT brain images can be reoriented along either the x, y, or z axes or in a specific oblique plane. This allows for the correction of positioning errors as well. The images can be quantitated using either left-to-right hemisphere ratio programs or by placing individual regions of interest over specific structures located in the brain.

A common method of display of SPECT brain images allows the sagittal, coronal, and transverse planes to be displayed simultaneously (Figure 9-20). This allows the physician to correlate images on one view with the other two tomographic planes. Volume and surface rendering programs allow the three-dimensional display of brain SPECT images, which can be useful in localizing and determining the extent of disease.

Positron Emission Tomography (PET)

A radiopharmaceutical undergoing positron decay emits a positron with a range of energies characteristic of the radionuclide. Once emitted, a positron is an antimatter electron that travels several millimeters in tissue and encounters a free electron in the tissue, resulting in annihilation and the subsequent release of two511 keV photons at 180 degrees to each other. The detection of these photons is accomplished by a ring of opposing detectors surrounding the patient. When two 511 keV photons are detected by these electronically coupled detectors, an annihilation event is assumed to have occurred along the line joining the two detectors. The direction of travel of the photons is electronically determined without the need for a collimator.[12]

Four positron radionuclides (^{11}C, ^{13}N, ^{15}O, and ^{18}F) are used in most PET imaging procedures. All are short lived and require the rapid radiosynthesis into compounds used to evaluate various physiologic functions. These radiotracers are often identical to compounds naturally found in the body. Radiopharmaceutical doses range from 5-10 mCi for ^{18}F FDG to 20 mCi for ^{11}C compounds (NMSP or carfentanil).

The patient is imaged in a supine position. CT or MRI provides techniques to aid in the selection of specific brain structures with respect to the tomographic slice. Once the slice of interest is identified with these techniques, its position can be recorded by use of a custom-fitted mask. This mask allows for slice location on the PET scan as well as immobilization of the patient's head during the imaging procedure. Upon injection of the radiotracer, imaging can continue for up to 2 hr. Arterial and venous blood sampling is often performed throughout the imaging period to provide additional physiologic information.

Upon acquisition of the raw data, the first step in image processing in PET is reconstruction. The coincidence data are reoriented into a set of parallel projections. A standard back-filtered projection algorithm is employed to reconstruct transverse slices. The final image obtained depends on the filter selected in the reconstruction process and the reconstruction algorithm. Once an image is obtained, further processing can be performed, depending on the purpose of the procedure.

Attenuation correction is routinely performed in PET and is accomplished by a calculated correction employing an ellipse or a measured correction employing a transmission scan. Due to the short half-life of PET radiotracers, decay correction can also be performed. PET brain images can be quantitated by placing individual regions of interest over specific structures located in the brain.

REFERENCES

1. Conti PS: Brain and spinal cord. In Wagner HN Jr, Szabo Z, Buchanan JW, eds: *Principles of nuclear medicine,* ed 2, Philadelphia, 1995, WB Saunders.
2. Datz F: *Handbooks in radiology—nuclear medicine,* Chicago, 1988, Year Book Medical.
3. Engel J Jr, Ackermann RF, Kuhl DE, et al: Brain imaging of glucose utilization in convulsive disorders. In Sokoloff L, ed: *Brain imaging and brain function: association for research in nervous and mental disease,* vol 63, New York, 1985, Raven Press.
4. Engel J Jr, Kuhl DE, Phelps ME: Regional brain metabolism during seizures in humans, *Adv Neurol* 34:141-148, 1983.
5. Engel J Jr, Lubens P, Kuhl DE, et al: Local cerebral metabolic rate for glucose during petit mal absences, *Ann Neurol* 17:121-128, 1985.
6. Foster NL, Chase TN, Mansi L, et al: Cortical abnormalities in Alzheimer's disease, *Ann Neurol* 16:649-654, 1984.
7. Frackowiak RSF: Pathophysiology of human cerebral ischemia: studies with positron tomography and ^{15}oxygen. In Sokoloff L, ed: *Brain imaging and brain function,* New York, 1985, Raven Press.
8. Friedland RP, Budinger TF, Ganz E, et al: Regional cerebral metabolic alterations in dementia of the Alzheimer type: positron emission tomography with [^{18}F] fluorodeoxyglucose, *J Comput Assist Tomogr* 7:590-598, 1983.
9. Frost JJ, Mayberg HS: Epilesy. In Wagner HN Jr, Szabo Z, Buchanan JW, eds: *Principles of nuclear medicine,* ed 2, Philadelphia, 1995, WB Saunders.
10. Glantz MJ, Hoffman JM, Coleman RE, et al: Identification of early recurrance of primary central nervous system tumors by [^{18}F]fluorodeoxyglucose positron emission tomography, *Ann Neurol* 29:347-355, 1991.
11. Heiss W-D, Podreka I: Cerebrovascular disease. In Wagner HN Jr, Szabo Z, Buchanan JW eds: *Principles of nuclear medicine,* ed 2, Philadelphia, 1995, WB Saunders.
12. Hubner K, Collmann J, Buonocore E, et al: *Clinical positron emission tomography,* St. Louis, 1992, Mosby.
13. Jones AG, Meltzer PC, Blundell P, et al: Technepine: a technetium-99m SPECT agent for labeling the dopamine transporter in brain, *J Nucl Med* 37(suppl)17P, 1996.
14. Klingensmith W, Eshima D, Goddard J: *Nuclear medicine procedure manual,* Engelwood, Colo, 1991, Oxford Medical.
15. Kuhl DE, Engel J Jr, Phelps ME: Emission computed tomography in the study of human epilepsy. In Ward AA Jr, Penry JK, Purpura D, eds: *Epilepsy,* New York, 1983, Raven Press.
16. Kuhl DE, Engel J Jr, Phelps ME, et al: Epileptic patterns of local cerebral metabolism and perfusion in humans determined by emission computed tomography of FDG and NH, *Ann Neurol* 8:348-360, 1980.

17. Links JM: Nuclear medicine physics, instrumentation, and data processing in pharmaceutical research. In Burns HD, Gibson RE, Dannals RF, Siegl PKS, eds: *Nuclear imaging in drug discovery, development, and approval*, Boston, 1993, Brikhäuser.

18. Meegalla SK, Plössl K, Kung M-P, et al: Tc-99m labeled tropanes as dopamine transporter imaging agents, *J Nucl Med* 37(suppl)17P, 1996.

19. Patronas NJ, Di Chiro G, Kufta C, et al: Prediction of survival in glioma patients by means of PET, *J Neurosurg* 62:816-822, 1985.

20. Rowell K, Harkness B, Christian P: *Clinical computers in nuclear medicine*, New York, 1992, The Society of Nuclear Medicine—Technologist Section.

21. *SPECT brain imaging with Ceretec: a clinician's guide*, Arlington Heights, Ill, 1989, Amersham.

22. Theodore WH, Dorwart R, Holmes M, et al: Neuroimaging in refractory partial seizures: comparison of PET, CT, and MRI, *Neurology* 36:60-64, 1986.

23. Tortora G, Anagnostakos N: *Principles of anatomy and physiology*, New York, 1990, Harper & Row.

SUGGESTED READINGS

Sandler MP, Coleman RE, Wackers FJ Th, et al, eds: *Diagnostic nuclear medicine*, ed 3, Baltimore, Md, 1996, Williams & Wilkins.

Wagner HN: Chemical neurotransmission in man, *Curr Conc Diagn Nucl Med* 3:14-18, 1986.

Wagner HN Jr, Szabo Z, Buchanan JW, eds: *Principles of nuclear medicine*, ed 2, Philadelphia, 1995, WB Saunders.

Stanley J. Goldsmith

chapter *10*

Endocrine System

Objectives

List the organs that comprise the endocrine system, and explain the anatomy, physiology, and the relationships of their hormonal functions.

List and discuss the advantages and disadvantages of radionuclides for thyroid uptake studies.

Discuss the choice of radionuclides that may be used for thyroid uptake and imaging procedures relative to their advantages and disadvantages for imaging.

Discuss the role of radioiodine uptake, thyroid scan, and whole-body imaging in the planning of radioiodine therapy.

Discuss radionuclide therapy for the treatment of hyperthyroidism.

Describe procedures for treating thyroid carcinoma using radioiodine.

Explain procedures for parathyroid imaging using thallium-technetium subtraction techniques and Sestamibi.

Discuss the role of somatostatin-receptor imaging.

Describe the use of radiopharmaceuticals for imaging the adrenal glands.

*T*he endocrine system consists of specialized tissue in various locations throughout the body that share a common mechanism by which they participate in body function: the secretion into the bloodstream of substances known as *hormones*. Hormones have profound effects on overall body function and metabolism. The phenomenon by which secretions from one organ or tissue influence the function of other organs is a basic mechanism of physiologic control and communication between organs.

The term *endocrine system* applies to the small group of organs whose principal function is the elaboration of internal secretions: the pituitary gland (anterior and posterior), the thyroid gland, the parathyroid glands, the islet cells of the pancreas, the adrenal glands (cortex and medulla), and the gonads (ovaries and testes). Recent advances in cell biology, with the recognition that biologically active substances are secreted by many cells and that many cells and tissues have specific receptors for these secreted ligands, have extended the scope of classic endocrinology into tumor and vascular biology. For the purposes of this review, the definition of the endocrine system will be broadened from the classical list of individual organs to include the so-called neuroendocrine tissues, which are distributed throughout the organs and evolve from the primitive foregut, midgut, and hindgut, and the chromaffin autonomic nervous system tissue.

In vivo nuclear medicine, both imaging and nonimaging applications, has played a significant role in the current understanding of the function of the endocrine glands and their disorders. Moreover, nuclear medicine techniques are useful to monitor treatment of the disorders affecting these organs. Radionuclide therapy is used in the management of patients with disorders of the thyroid gland, hyperthyroidism, and thyroid carcinoma.

This chapter provides an overview of the endocrine system and describes the in vivo and imaging techniques used in clinical nuclear medicine departments and their current role in diagnosis and management of patients with disorders of the organs and tissues whose principal function is the secretion of compounds that regulate the function of other organs and tissues.

PITUITARY GLAND

Anatomy and Physiology

The pituitary gland is a small (0.5 g), pea-sized gland located at the base of the midbrain, just behind the optic chiasm. It is encased in its own bony vault at the base of the skull, the sella turcica. The pituitary has two distinctive portions, the anterior pituitary and the posterior pituitary, with the para intermedias, a small zone of specialized tissue, between the anterior and posterior secretory tissue (Figure 10-1). The anterior pituitary has a rich vascular network including the hypothalamic-hypophyseal portal venous system, which provides a means of communication with specialized neurosecretory tissue in the hypothalamus. The hypothalamic tissue elaborates several peptides that specifi-

cally stimulate the synthesis and release of the anterior pituitary trophic hormones, which in turn affect distal organ function. This includes thyrotropin-releasing hormone (TRH), corticotropin-releasing hormone (CRH), and corresponding releasing hormones for the other anterior pituitary polypeptides. Growth hormone release is modulated also by somatostatin, a 14-amino-acid cyclic peptide that inhibits growth hormone synthesis, release, and action.

The anterior pituitary consists of two cell types, acidophils and basophils, based on their staining in histologic preparations (Table 10-1). The acidophils secrete growth hormone in response to the hypothalamic growth hormone–releasing hormone (GRH), or somatotropin, and prolactin in response to prolactin-releasing factor. Prolactin secretion is controlled also by a specific inhibitory factor. Growth hormone has a widespread effect on body and organ growth and utilization of nutrients. Prolactin has known effects on breast secretory gland function and on the corpus luteum.

The basophil cells of the anterior pituitary elaborate several polypeptide hormones: thyrotropin (thyroid-stimulating hormone, TSH); adrenocorticotropin (adrenal cortex-stimulating hormone, ACTH); and the gonadotropins, follicle-stimulating hormone (FSH) and luteinizing hormone or interstitial cell-stimulating hormone (LH or ICSH), which exert their effects by stimulating other endocrine organs (the thyroid, adrenal cortex, and ovaries or testes, respectively). In turn, the hormones secreted by the thyroid, adrenals, and go-

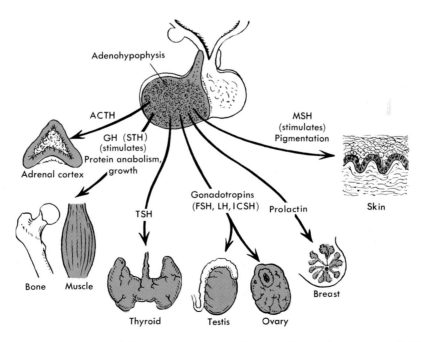

Figure 10-1 Anterior pituitary hormones and their target organs: adrenocorticotropic hormone (ACTH), thyroid-stimulating hormone (TSH), follicle-stimulating hormone (FSH), luteinizing hormone (LH), male analog of LH (ICSH), and melanocyte-stimulating hormone (MSH). (From Thibodeau GA: *Anthony's textbook of anatomy and physiology*, ed 13, St. Louis, 1990, Mosby.)

Table 10-1	Production, control, and effects of pituitary hormones			
Pituitary gland (hypophysis cerebri)	**Hormone**	**Source (cell type or location)**	**Control mechanism**	**Effect**
Anterior pituitary gland (adeno-hypophysis)	Growth hormone (GH); somatotropin (STH)	Acidophils	GRH (growth hormone–releasing hormone) from hypothalamus	Promotes body growth, protein anabolism, and mobilization and catabolism of fats; decreases glucose catabolism; increases blood glucose levels
Pars anterior	Prolactin (lactogenic or luteotropic hormone [LTH])	Acidophils	Prolactin-inhibitory factor (PIF); prolactin-releasing factor (PRF) from hypothalamus and high blood levels of oxytocin	Stimulates milk secretion and development of secretory alveoli; helps maintain corpus luteum
	Thyrotropin (TH); thyroid-stimulating hormone (TSH)	Basophils	Thyrotropin-releasing hormone (TRH) from hypothalamus	Growth and maintenance of thyroid gland and stimulation of thyroid hormone secretion
	Adrenocorticotropin (ACTH)	Basophils	Corticotropin-releasing factor (CRF) from hypothalamus	Growth and maintenance of adrenal cortex and stimulation of cortisol and other glucocorticoid secretions
	Follicle-stimulating hormone (FSH)	Basophils	Follicle-stimulating hormone-releasing hormone (FSH-RH) from hypothalamus	In female stimulates follicle growth and maturation and estrogen secretion. In male stimulates development of seminiferous tubules and maintains spermatogenesis
	Luteinizing hormone (LH in female, ICSH in male)	Basophils	Luteinizing hormone–releasing hormone (LHRH) from hypothalamus	In female (LH) induces ovulation and stimulates formation of corpus luteum and progesterone secretion. In male (ICSH) stimulates interstitial cell secretion of testosterone

Continued

Table 10-1	Production, control, and effects of pituitary hormones—cont'd			
Pituitary gland (hypophysis cerebri)	**Hormone**	**Source (cell type or location)**	**Control mechanism**	**Effect**
Pars intermedia	Melanocyte-stimulating hormone (MSH); intermedin	Basophils	Unknown in humans	May cause darkening of skin by increasing melanin production
Posterior pituitary gland (neurohypophysis)	ADH (vasopressin)	Hypothalamus, mainly supraoptic nucleus	Osmoreceptors in hypothalamus stimulated by increase in blood osmotic pressure, decrease in extracellular fluid volume, and stress	Decreased urine output
	Oxytocin	Hypothalamus, paraventricular nucleus	Nervous stimulation of hypothalamus caused by stimulation of nipples (nursing)	Contraction of uterine smooth muscle and ejection of milk into lactiferous ducts

From Thibodeau GA: *Anthony's textbook of anatomy and physiology,* ed 13, St. Louis, 1990, Mosby.

nads have a negative feedback on the secretion of the hypothalamic-releasing hormones, so at elevated levels of the distal target gland hormone, the hypothalamus and subsequently the pituitary secretion of stimulating hormones are suppressed.

When the distal target gland is absent or ineffective in hormone synthesis resulting in low levels of circulating hormone, the hypothalamus is stimulated (not inhibited) to secrete the specific releasing hormone that stimulates the pituitary production and secretion of the appropriate stimulating hormone. End organ failure, therefore, can be primary (i.e., due to some inherent defect in the gland), in which case the pituitary-stimulating hormone concentration in the plasma is high, or secondary, as a result of failure of the hypothalamus or pituitary to adequately secrete one or more stimulating hormones. Provocative and suppressive tests of pituitary hormone function have been described utilizing radioimmunoassay methods to measure the pituitary polypeptide concentration in plasma in response to known physiologic or pharmacologic stimuli.

The posterior pituitary communicates directly with hypothalamic nuclei and elaborates vasopressin (or antidiuretic hormone, ADH), which has a role in salt and water homeostasis, and oxytocin, which has a role in lactation and labor in response to stimulation of appropriate hypothalamic receptors.

Nuclear Medicine Procedures

Given the close proximity of the pituitary gland to the skull and soft tissues of the face, it is not surprising that nonspecific techniques such as ^{67}Ga, ^{201}Tl, or ^{99m}Tc MIBI imaging have not been demonstrated to be of value in the detection or management of pituitary tumors. Since cells of the anterior pituitary gland express increased amounts of somatostatin receptors, however, the availability of ^{111}In DTPA pentetreotide, a radiolabeled somatostatin-receptor ligand, makes possible the imaging of the pituitary gland and tumors arising from it. [111]In DTPA pentetreotide (*Octreoscan*, Mallinckrodt) agent became available in the United States in 1994.

Anterior pituitary tumors may be functional or nonfunctional. Functioning tumors secrete hormones in excess amounts and also fail to respond to the usual negative feedback signals to turn off hormone synthesis and release. Nonfunctioning tumors cause symptoms as a result of the tumor mass or invasion and compromise of other pituitary function. Somatostatin-receptor scintigraphy would be most useful in detecting viable residual tissue in postoperative or postirradiation patients with nonfunctional tumors. Unfortunately, however, nonfunctional tumors may have reduced somatostatin receptors, which decreases the utility of the technique to monitor residual tumor or recurrence.

Somatostatin-receptor scintigraphy of the pituitary is performed with the usual dose of ^{111}In DTPA pentetreotide (adult dose: 6.0 mCi). Patients may be imaged within hours after administration, but better contrast between the pituitary and background activity is achieved at 24 hr. When there is specific interest in the pituitary, SPECT imaging should be performed. If a high-resolution neuroSPECT system is available, it should be used.

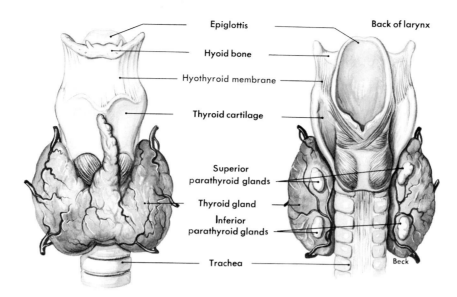

Epiglottis

Hyoid bone

Hyothyroid membrane

Thyroid cartilage

Superior parathyroid glands

Thyroid gland

Inferior parathyroid glands

Trachea

Back of larynx

Beck

Figure 10-2 Thyroid and parathyroid glands in "normal" anatomic configuration. The thyroid is represented as a butterfly-shaped structure with a lobe of tissue on each side of the inferior portion of the thyroid cartilage. A prominent pyramidal lobe of the thyroid is depicted in the midline. Four parathyroid glands are illustrated in the classic superior and inferior symmetric distribution. In clinical nuclear medicine imaging of both the thyroid and parathyroid glands considerable anatomic variation is encountered. (From Thibodeau GA: *Anthony's textbook of anatomy and physiology,* ed 13, St. Louis, 1990, Mosby.)

On whole-body somatostatin-receptor scintigraphy with ^{111}In pentetreotide, variable but small amounts of tracer activity are seen in the region of the pituitary gland. Quantitative analysis of transverse SPECT images through the pituitary region shows that normal subjects may vary fivefold in terms of the amount of activity accumulated.[34] The ratio of pituitary to background activity (an ROI selected in the midline, posterior to the pituitary activity) continues to increase after administration of the diagnostic tracer. At 24 hr, the ratio may be as high as 30:1 in normal subjects. Although patients with adenoma tend to have higher values than patients without pituitary disease or normal subjects, there is some overlap among these populations.[34]

Provided that the patient has not been referred for the purpose of evaluating the pituitary gland, this variability is usually of passing interest. It is not clear what an appropriate clinical indication for somatostatin-receptor imaging of the pituitary might be since hormone-secreting active tumors can be detected with sensitive radioimmunoassays. Furthermore, nonsecreting pituitary tumors frequently have a paucity of somatostatin receptors. When a patient is referred specifically to evaluate whether a lesion, which has probably been visualized on MRI or CT, is likely to be functionally significant or to evaluate if a residual tumor is present or if it is likely that it will respond to octreotide therapy, it becomes necessary to know what degree of tracer uptake is acceptable as a normal variation. In a quantitative study of ^{111}In pentetreotide uptake in normal subjects and patients without pituitary disease, a fivefold variation in counts was observed in the anterior pituitary region on SPECT imaging at 24 hr. Nev-ertheless, although there is some overlap, patients with pituitary tumors have greater activity in the pituitary region than normal patients.

THYROID GLAND

Anatomy

The thyroid gland is located in the neck. It is somewhat butterfly shaped, with a lobe of tissue on each side of the thyroid cartilage joined to a variable degree in the lower portion by an isthmus of tissue (Figure 10-2). In the adult each lobe weighs approximately 10 g. The embryonic origins of the thyroid gland involve evagination of tissue from the midline primordial gut, the base of the tongue, which then migrates caudally (downward) into the neck. Occasionally remnants of tissue remain along the migration path and are an incidental finding during imaging. Asymmetry of the gland can also be observed. The most common evidence of the embryologic descent is a small amount of midline tissue arising from the isthmus, the pyramidal lobe. The thyroid gland tissue can even develop as a lingual thyroid at the base of the tongue without migrating into the usual location astride the thyroid cartilage. Another common but less frequently observed remnant of thyroid gland origin is the thyroglossal duct cyst, a midline cyst found superior to the thyroid, which evolves from a remnant of the embryonic duct that normally atrophies during fetal development. Most often, functioning thyroid tissue is not associated with the thyroglossal duct cyst. The diagnosis is made clinically;

scanning is performed to confirm the absence of functioning tissue before excision.

Physiology

The thyroid gland secretes the thyroid hormones thyroxine (T_4) and triiodothyronine (T_3). These hormones regulate tissue metabolism and are essential for normal body development and maintenance of function. Thyroid hormone synthesis depends on the trapping and organification of iodine (Figure 10-3). Iodine is ingested in food and water. It is reduced to neutral iodine or iodide and is actively trapped by the thyroid gland. This intrathyroidal iodine pool is in equilibrium with plasma iodine, but a gradient of 6:1 (intrathyroidal iodine/plasma iodine) is maintained in the euthyroid state and as much as 10-11:1 in the hyperthyroid state. The net flux of iodine into the thyroid is continuous in the normal (unblocked) state because it is from this intrathyroidal pool that iodine is organified, that is, bound to tyrosine to form monoiodotyrosine (MIT) and diiodotyrosine (DIT). As tyrosine-bound iodine, the iodine no longer participates in the equilibrium gradient, allowing more iodine to be trapped (to main-

tain the gradient). Following organification of the iodine (or iodination of tyrosine), the iodinated MIT and DIT molecules undergo an enzymatic step known as coupling in which MIT and DIT, or DIT molecules, combine to form T_3 or T_4. As organified molecules MIT, DIT, T_3, and T_4 are bound to an intrathyroidal binding protein, thyroglobulin, which also serves as the storage site for the T_3 and T_4. In response to TSH stimulation in the normal subject, or whatever other stimuli if any that are involved in the various forms of hypersecretion, the thyroid hormones T_3 and T_4 are proteolytically cleaved from the thyroglobulin and released into the circulation.

In the circulation T_3 and T_4 are bound to the circulating, specific binding protein, thyroxine-binding globulin (TBG). T_4 is bound with high affinity, whereas T_3 is more loosely bound. At the tissue level T_4 is converted to T_3. T_3 has a direct effect on cellular metabolism, stimulating oxidation. Metabolic status is determined by the dissociated or free fraction of T_4 and T_3, which can be measured by the determination of the so-called free T_4 and T_3. Alterations in the total TBG available, the fraction of TBG-binding sites available, or the affinity of binding of the T_4 and T_3 influence measured

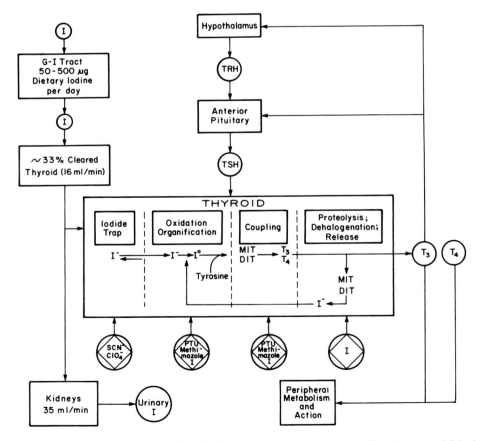

Figure 10-3 Schematic of iodine metabolism and thyroid hormone regulation, synthesis, release, and biochemical site of pharmacologic effect of antithyroid drugs. (From Goldsmith SJ: Thyroid: in vivo tests of function and imaging. In Rothfeld B: *Nuclear medicine: endocrinology,* Philadelphia, 1978, JB Lippincott.)

T_4 and the relationship between T_4, T_3 measurements, and the patient's metabolic state. In hyperthyroidism there are increased T_4 and T_3 syntheses and secretions as well as increased levels of TBG, resulting in increased plasma levels of total T_4 and T_3, as well as free fraction of T_4 and T_3. Likewise, in hypothyroidism there is a decrease in thyroid hormone secretion and in the absolute amount of TBG, and the T_4 or T_3 levels are low.

In the usual in vitro tests of thyroid function, plasma or serum total T_4 (or T_3) is measured, and these values are sufficient for diagnosis. Occasionally, there are abnormalities in the amount of TBG-binding sites available, either due to an alteration in the concentration of TBG or in the available binding sites. Drugs such as estrogens increase the amount of TBG, whereas androgens decrease TBG levels. Salicylates and the anticonvulsant drug phenylhydantoin (Dilantin) occupy binding sites on the TBG molecules, leaving fewer available for T_4 (or T_3) occupancy. Consequently, in the in vitro tests of T_4 and T_3 concentration the measured T_4 value is artifactually increased or decreased and the test result is incompatible with the clinical impression. The free fraction of T_4 and T_3 that determines the body metabolic level remains consistent with the clinical status despite aberrant serum total T_4 or T_3 levels.

A pharmacologic block at the organification step of iodine metabolism provides the basis for therapy of hyperthyroidism with the so-called antithyroid drugs, the sulfonylureas methimazole and propylthiouracil. These drugs also interfere with proteolysis and release of the thyroid hormone. Defects of this enzymatic organification step also occur on a congenital basis (goitrous cretinism) and after radiation and inflammation. The existence of a defect in organification of iodine can be demonstrated by either one of two in vivo radionuclide procedures, the perchlorate discharge test and the thiocyanate washout test. These techniques can be used also to demonstrate the degree of pharmacologic block produced by therapy with the antithyroid drugs.

Usually thyroid hormone secretion is regulated by the pituitary hormone TSH, which in turn is regulated by thyrotropin-releasing hormone (TRH), which is regulated via negative feedback by the thyroid hormones. If the thyroid is unable to synthesize sufficient T_4 or T_3, TSH levels rise if the hypothalamic-pituitary axis is intact. Direct measurement of TSH, therefore, discriminates between physiologic variations in T_4 concentration or variations in T_4 concentration due to decreased or increased concentration of the binding protein TBG and pathologic low levels of T_4, which would result in elevation of serum TSH. Conversely, interpretation of borderline high T_4 or T_3 levels versus pathologic elevation in an individual is also augmented by knowledge of the serum TSH concentration, since abnormal elevation of T_4 or T_3 suppresses TSH levels. The use of serum TSH levels to determine or confirm clinical status has been augmented in recent years by the availability of highly sensitive TSH radioimmunoassays, with assay sensitivity down to 0.01 mU/L. This assay permits differentiation of low levels from thoroughly suppressed values. Benign tumors (functioning adenomas) and malignant tumors (differentiated carcinoma) maintain the ability to synthesize thyroid hormones even without TSH stimulation. In Graves disease thyroid growth and hormone synthesis are stimulated by an immune globulin. Excessive production of thyroid hormone, which continues despite suppression of TRH or TSH, results in the clinical syndrome of hyperthyroidism.

Nuclear Medicine Procedures

In vitro procedures. Radioimmunoassay is the most widely used procedure for the measurement of circulating serum T_4 and T_3 and provides the most direct estimate of thyroid function. Radioimmunoassay also provides direct measurement of TBG concentration to assess if variations in this binding protein account for alterations in serum T_4 or T_3. TSH levels, also measured by radioimmunoassay, provide information about the thyroid status (elevated in secondary hypothyroidism and undetectable in hyperthyroidism). The currently available third-generation sensitive TSH assays performed either by the double-sandwich radioimmunoassay or enzyme-linked immunosorbent assay (ELISA) methods are sensitive to the 0.01 mU/L range. Sensitivity in this range permits differentiation of low values in the euthyroid population from patients with hyperthyroidism even if T_4, free T_4, or T_3 values are in the borderline range. Indeed, measurement of serum TSH by the sensitive immunoassay method serves as the most sensitive and specific indicator of the biologic effect of circulating thyroid hormone.[21,30]

Assays are also available to measure thyroglobulin, the intrathyroidal binding protein. Thyroglobulin is normally not detected in the plasma. Detection of thyroglobulin provides a measure of abnormal vascular access to the glandular protein. This occurs in differentiated carcinoma; serum thyroglobulin levels thus provide an index of tumor presence.

In vivo function tests and imaging. Thyroid in vivo function tests and imaging are based on the unique avidity of the thyroid gland for iodine and the availability, from the very beginning of the era of artificial radioactivity, of radioactive isotopes of iodine. For many years these procedures utilized ^{131}I, an isotope of iodine that decays by beta decay and that is readily available as a product of nuclear fission, as well as the neutron bombardment of suitable target material in nuclear reactors. With a physical half-life of 8.1 days, ^{131}I was widely used for in vivo thyroid studies and became a mainstay of nuclear medicine in the 1960s. At present, the procedures are used in clinical practice.

In vivo tests to evaluate thyroid function are based on the usual association of the degree of iodine uptake and overall thyroid function. The most common of these in vivo procedures is the thyroid uptake test. Uptake can be measured at any time after administration of radioiodine, but it is most convenient for both the department and the clinical community to identify and use a consistent interval. For a variety of reasons the 24-hr interval has evolved to be the most practical and reliable, providing better discrimination between hyperthyroid, euthyroid, and hypothyroid populations than earlier time points. It is long enough after oral administration to reduce the significance of small variations in the rate of gastrointestinal absorption. Nuclear medicine personnel should bear in mind that uptake values can vary with the type of radioiodine preparation used (e.g., liquid is absorbed more rapidly than capsules) and there are variations in the degree of digestion and rate of absorption of capsules from different manufacturers. Furthermore, the uptake is usually complete at 18 to 20 hr and stable for several hours thereafter. Thyroid gland imaging is used to determine the size, location, and function of the thyroid gland and to evaluate palpable findings near, on, or within the thyroid gland (Figures 10-4 to 10-9).

Choice of radionuclide. The historic radionuclide of choice for thyroid studies was ^{131}I. With the convenient 8.1-day physical half-life, it could be transported and stored in departments, providing an economic source of a thyroid-avid radionuclide that could be detected readily outside the body because of the principal 364 keV gamma emission. In microcurie doses ^{131}I laid the foundation for contemporary nuclear medicine, leading to the development of reproducible techniques for the quantification of in vivo thyroid function (thyroid clearance and the 24-hr thyroid uptake) and thyroid imaging (Table 10-2).

With the beta emission, ^{131}I also provided a therapeutic potential, which was exploited for treatment of hyperthyroidism (Graves disease, multinodular toxic goiter, and toxic solitary nodule or adenoma) and thyroid carcinoma with local or distal metastases.

In 1965 Andros and colleagues[2] noted that the thyroid concentrated the newly available ^{99m}Tc pertechnetate (TcO$_4$). With the widespread use of the ^{99}Mo-^{99m}Tc generator in the 1970s (as well as distribution of unit dose ^{99m}Tc pertechnetate), this radionuclide became available for thyroid imaging. Atkins and Richards[3] developed a method to quantify the uptake, but the method was too variable or too difficult for routine

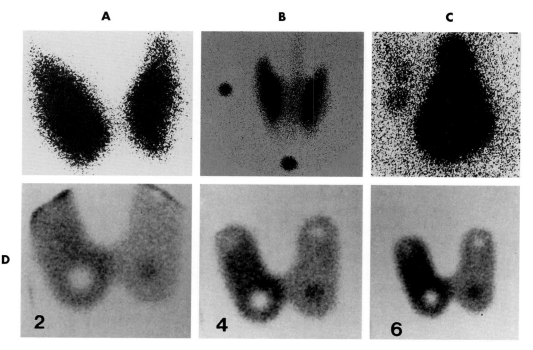

Figure 10-4 Thyroid gland scintigraphy (pinhole collimator technique). **A,** Normal, virtually symmetric thyroid gland, right and left lobes. No isthmus or pyramidal lobe activity. (4 mCi ^{99m}Tc pertechnetate.) **B,** Normal thyroid gland with isthmus and prominent pyramidal lobe. (400 µCi ^{123}I sodium iodide.) **C,** Marked asymmetry of thyroid gland following near total thyroidectomy and compensatory enlargement of the left lobe. Asymmetry is secondary to surgical resection, but similar patterns are seen in congenital hemiagenesis of the thyroid. Interpretation requires correlation of scan findings with history and physical examination. (4 mCi ^{99m}Tc pertechnetate.) **D,** Effect of distance of pinhole collimator on scintigraphic thyroid gland size: images are shown at 2, 4, and 6 cm from surface of thyroid phantom. As the pinhole collimator comes closer to the imaged object, the recorded image is larger. Accordingly, conclusions about gland size require simultaneous imaging of a source of known size or correlation with findings on palpation.

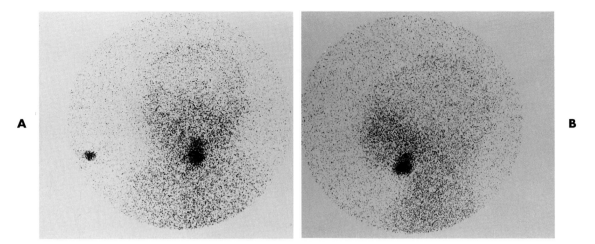

Figure 10-5 Lingual thyroid demonstrated in a 9-year-old child. (2 mCi ^{99m}Tc pertechnetate.) Anterior **(A)** and left lateral **(B)** views demonstrate outline of skull, facial activity, and neck. A solitary focus of radiotracer uptake is seen in the midline of the neck near the base of the tongue. No uptake is seen in the thyroid bed.

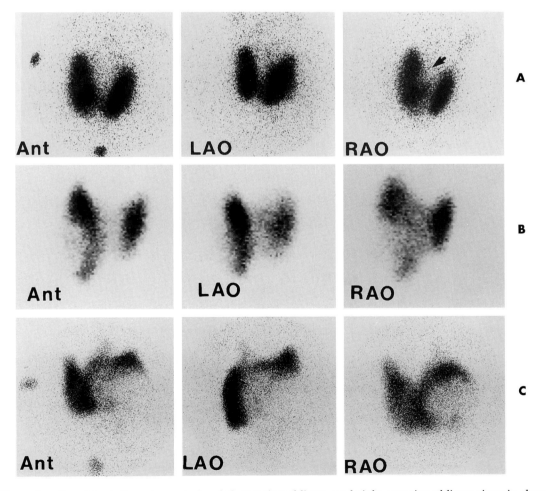

Figure 10-6 Three-view thyroid scintigraphy: anterior, left anterior oblique, and right anterior oblique views in three different patients demonstrating a solitary cold nodule of various sizes. (400 μCi ^{123}I sodium iodide.) **A,** Small defect (cold nodule) corresponding to a palpable nodule *(arrow)* is seen on the medial aspect of the right thyroid lobe in the RAO view. Oblique views increase the sensitivity of thyroid scintigraphy in the anterior view for the detection of small cold nodules, which might not be seen *en face*. **B,** Moderately large (3 × 1 cm) cold nodule in the lower portion of the right lobe. **C,** Large (5 × 4 cm) cold nodule replacing most of the left thyroid lobe.

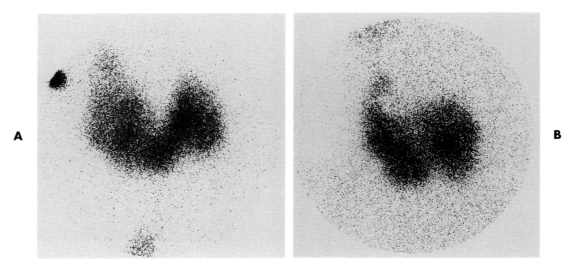

Figure 10-7 Multinodular goiter in a patient with Hashimoto disease. Pinhole collimator, anterior views in the same patient, 9 months apart. Occasionally discrepancies are seen in areas that trap pertechnetate but do not organify iodine. **A,** 400 μCi ^{123}I. **B,** 4 mCi ^{99m}Tc pertechnetate.

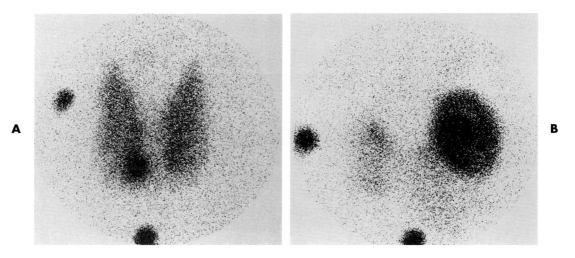

Figure 10-8 Thyroid imaging: hot nodule. **A,** Nonsuppressed thyroid and an area of hyperfunction seen overlying the medial aspect of the right thyroid lobe. The symmetric right and left thyroid lobes are readily seen. (400 μCi ^{123}I sodium iodide.) **B,** Large, somewhat heterogeneous area of activity is seen on the left, representing the dominant functioning thyroid nodule, with only faint activity representing the suppressed thyroid gland seen. (400 μCi ^{123}I sodium iodide.)

use and never became widely used. Nevertheless, ^{99m}Tc pertechnetate was used commonly for thyroid imaging, and small doses of ^{131}I continued to be used for thyroid-uptake measurements. ^{99m}Tc pertechnetate has several advantages over ^{131}I. The 140 keV gamma emission of ^{99m}Tc is more efficiently detected by the ⅜- to ½-in scintillation camera crystal, which is comparatively inefficient for the 364 keV photon of ^{131}I. The short physical half-life and isomeric transition mode of decay of ^{99m}Tc resulted in a more favorable patient absorbed radiation dose than ^{131}I and permitted the routine use of millicurie quantities of ^{99m}Tc pertechnetate for diagnostic studies, providing better image information content. A typical scanning dose of ^{131}I resulted

in an absorbed dose to the adult thyroid of 20 rad (assuming a 20% uptake and typical turnover rate) and a 1 rad whole-body dose, whereas a 4 mCi dose of ^{99m}Tc pertechnetate yielded an absorbed dose of less than 1 rad to the thyroid and a whole-body absorbed dose of 0.1 rad.

With an increase in accelerator production of radionuclides in the 1970s and 1980s, ^{123}I became available for clinical use. Despite the relatively short 13.3-hr half-life, improved distribution networks can provide ^{123}I at least 4 days/week throughout most of the United States, Canada, and western Europe. Early methods to produce ^{123}I employed the p,2n reaction, which resulted in a product of variable radiochemical quality

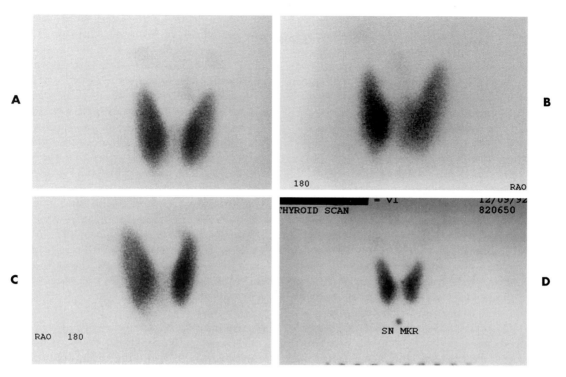

Figure 10-9 Thyroid imaging: normal thyroid gland, parallel-hole collimator, electronic zoom technique. (10 mCi ^{99m}Tc pertechnetate.) **A,** Anterior. **B,** LAO. **C,** RAO. **D,** Anterior view with sternal notch markers (SNMKR) and size bar.

Table 10-2	Physical characteristics and absorbed doses of radionuclides used in thyroid imaging and diagnostic studies

| Nuclide | Dose administered | $t_{1/2}$ | Emission | Energy (keV) | Rad | |
					Whole body	Thyroid
^{131}I	5-10 μCi	8.1 d	Gamma, beta	364	1.2*	0.05-0.10
	100 μCi				20*	1
^{123}I	200 μCi	13 hr	Gamma	159	0.5-2.0	0.06
	400 μCi				1.0-4.0	0.12
^{99m}Tc	4 mCi	6 hr	Gamma	140	<1	<0.1

*Assumes average body and thyroid weight, thyroid turnover, and 20% uptake.

with significant amounts of long-lived ^{125}I and ^{124}I as contaminants. These radiochemical impurities resulted in poorer image quality due to septal penetration of the high-energy gamma emissions from ^{124}I and loss of some of the dosimetry advantage of ^{123}I. Increased availability of higher energy accelerators now makes possible the convenient production of ^{123}I by the p,5n reaction with a high degree of radiochemical purity.

^{123}I has a gamma emission of 159 keV and is well suited for gamma camera imaging. A typical adult scanning dose is 300-400 μCi, resulting in a thyroid absorbed dose of 1-4 rad and a whole-body absorbed dose of 0.12 rad. Imaging is best performed 2 to 4 hr after oral administration. Quantification of uptake can

also be performed at that time, but this application is less satisfactory because there is less differentiation between the euthyroid, hyperthyroid, and hypothyroid values at this earlier point. Thyroidal iodine-uptake measurements at 24 hr after ingestion of ^{123}I can be obtained because there are still sufficient counts. This latter exercise involves preparation of a suitable standard and counting in a geometric configuration approximating the patient's neck to provide corrections for attenuation and scatter. Imaging can also be postponed. Kusic and colleagues[19] have reported that 100,000-count images can be obtained at 20 hr after ^{123}I administration in less than 10 min.

At one time there was concern about whether images obtained 2 to 4 hr after ^{123}I administration allowed sufficient time to differentiate between nodules that simply trapped iodine but lacked the capacity to organify and nodules that had intact mechanisms for organification. It has been demonstrated that images obtained with [123]I 2 to 4 hr after administration of the tracer are satisfactory to demonstrate the capacity to organify iodine and are equivalent to ^{131}I images at 24 hr. At present, there is no justification to use ^{131}I in diagnostic imaging of the thyroid except in patients with known thyroid carcinoma, when whole-body ^{131}I imaging is performed to locate distal metastases and activity is seen in the neck. It is appropriate in this circumstance to obtain high-resolution (pinhole) images of the cervical area to better define the number, size, and location of these foci.

Because the gamma emission energy of ^{123}I is less than that of ^{131}I, there is greater attenuation of activity and therefore a slight difference between the activity recorded in a phantom at a given distance and the activity recorded in a patient at a greater distance. There may also be slight differences in the rate of absorption of ^{123}I capsules and ^{131}I capsules, but this should not have an observable effect on the 4-hr measurement.

In comparison studies blinded observers regularly prefer ^{123}I images, probably because of the better thyroid-to-background contrast.[19] The physical properties of ^{123}I provide excellent images and low radiation absorbed dose, and its localization is more specific than pertechnetate for functioning thyroid tissue. The only significant limitations are its availability and expense: the 13.3-hr physical half-life makes storage prohibitive, and doses have to be ordered as a patient is scheduled. Nevertheless, ^{99m}Tc pertechnetate provides excellent quality images at great convenience to the nuclear medicine service and the patient. When it is not feasible to schedule a patient and wait for an ^{123}I dose to be delivered, or if ^{123}I is otherwise unavailable, ^{99m}Tc pertechnetate is a satisfactory substitute to provide size and location of probable thyroid tissue. Images are obtained 15 to 20 min after intravenous injection of 4-10 mCi ^{99m}Tc pertechnetate.

The greatest limitation of ^{99m}Tc pertechnetate for thyroid imaging is that, although it is trapped by functioning thyroid tissue, it is not organified and hence is of debatable value in evaluating the function of a palpable thyroid nodule. Cystic lesions, hemorrhages, and granulomas are "cold" with ^{99m}Tc pertechnetate as well as with radioiodine, whereas nodules with organification defects (adenomas or adenocarcinomas) are not identified as cold if they are perfused and trap pertechnetate as well as surrounding areas.

Identification of solitary cold nodules is one of the principal uses of the thyroid scan, since 20% to 35% of these cold nodules are malignant and require further therapy. Based on the high incidence of malignancy in cold nodules, the usual response to this finding is surgical removal. A warm, functioning nodule has a low incidence of malignancy and can be treated with exogenous thyroid hormone to suppress TSH and remove stimulation of the nodule. The nodule is evaluated clinically at intervals, whereas suppression of the plasma TSH is monitored.

Significant discrepancies between pertechnetate and radioiodine images have been observed in Hashimoto thyroiditis. Figure 10-7 shows nodules in a patient with Hashimoto thyroiditis. Some nodules are perfused and trap pertechnetate and therefore are warm on ^{99m}Tc images but fail to organify iodine and hence are cold on delayed imaging with radioiodine. The traditional view that ^{99m}Tc pertechnetate can fail to properly identify cold nodules is not consistent with a recent report by Kusic and co-workers,[19] which compared the findings on blind readings of ^{99m}Tc and ^{123}I scans in 316 patients and found agreement in 92% to 95%. No discrepancy in images was found among the 12 patients with thyroid carcinoma.

Thyroid uptake. In the 1960s specific and rapid in vitro tests of thyroid function were not yet available, and the 24-hr thyroid-iodine uptake was the principal and certainly the most readily available test of thyroid function. The thyroid uptake of iodine is somewhat nonspecific as a measure of thyroid function, since the handling of the tracer iodine dose is influenced by total dietary iodine and alterations of intrathyroidal iodine metabolism. In areas of iodine deficiency the 24-hr uptake is greater than normal, whereas in patients with abundant dietary iodine (or iodine ingested in medication or contrast material) the 24-hr thyroid uptake is decreased. Furthermore, disorders of organification of iodine result in increased uptake as a result of the failure of the intrathyroidal iodine utilization, impaired hormone synthesis, and subsequent increased TSH stimulation in an effort to synthesize sufficient thyroid hormone for body homeostasis.

Since 1960 ingestion of dietary iodine in the United States has increased in many areas as a result of the use of iodized salt, the improved availability and increased preference for saltwater fish, the use of iodinated preservatives in food (such as white bread), and widespread use of iodinated compounds in food dyes and medication. This has resulted in a decrease in mean 24-hr thyroid-iodine uptake values. In 1960 the mean value reported from a large institution in New York was $25 \pm 7\%$, whereas in 1975 the mean value was $16 \pm 8\%$.[15]

The wide regional variation in dietary iodine observed throughout the United States would seem to suggest that no single published figure or range can be accepted for the normal 24-hr thyroid-iodine uptake. Nuclear medicine departments should establish their own physiologic range. Nevertheless, if there is no history of exposure to excess dietary iodine (kelp, mineral supplements) or iodinated organic compounds (contrast media), the thyroid-iodine uptake will be increased in hyperthyroidism, reflecting increased thyroid function, and decreased in hypothyroidism, reflecting decreased thyroid function. In general, values below 12% are considered low at this time and require explanation. Any 24-hr thyroid uptake values in excess of 25% represent greater iodine uptake than usually encountered in a normal population with normal iodine uptake. Of course, in the hyperthyroid population, values of 35% to 95% are frequently observed.

As indicated, the thyroid-iodine uptake can be performed at any time after the administration of radioiodine, but it is important to compare patient readings with normative data obtained at comparable intervals and under comparable conditions.

A 1- to 2-in sodium-iodide crystal with appropriate collimation is used. Standards should be counted in an appropriate phantom. With the modern use of pulse height analysis, the influence of backscatter related to geometry is eliminated, but it is best to approximate the cervical anatomy to provide some element of correction for attenuation by tissue even though the precise depth of the thyroid gland might not be reproduced in all cases (Table 10-3). The Society of Nuclear Medicine has published consensus procedure guidelines on the issues involved in performing this procedure.[8]

Perchlorate discharge and thiocyanate washout tests.
These procedures are based on the rapid organification of iodine in normal thyroid tissue (see also thyroid gland physiology). Tracer radioactive iodine does not discharge or wash out of the thyroid in the normal subject when further iodine trapping is competitively inhibited by the administration of relatively large amounts of anionic perchlorate or thiocyanate.

The test is performed after the administration of radioactive iodine (5-20 μCi ^{131}I) orally or intravenously (sterile, pyrogen-free preparation) and is recorded over the thyroid bed with a probe type of scintillation detector. When the radioiodine is administered by mouth, counts should be taken every 15 to 30 min (or more often) for approximately 2 hr. When sterile pyrogen-free material is available for intravenous administration, more frequent counting (every minute if an automatic recording device is available or at 5-min intervals if manual counting is performed) for at least 30 min. At these intervals, plasma activity falls because of thyroid trapping and renal clearance. A dose of 600-1000 mg of potassium perchlorate is administered orally. In normal subjects the count rate remains stable over the next measured period (1 hr for oral perchlorate, 10 to 20 min for intravenous thiocyanate). If an organification defect is present, a significant fall (10% to 50% or more) in the count rate occurs. If a decrease in count rate is detected, it is interpreted that the perchlorate has discharged the radioactive iodine; hence the procedure is called the *perchlorate discharge test.*

Since the procedure is infrequently performed, there has not been a published description using ^{123}I.

Certainly 50-200 μCi of ^{123}I could be used as a tracer for this procedure. The remainder of the procedure would be unchanged.

Thyroid stimulation and suppression tests. With the ready availability of sensitive plasma TSH immunoassay measurements, the in vivo TSH and T_3 suppression tests are no longer performed. Autonomy (lack of suppressibility) of the pituitary thyroid axis can be made directly by assay of plasma TSH. Measurable TSH excludes hyperthyroidism.

The TSH stimulation test in which the patient received serial injections of bovine TSH was also performed before the availability of sensitive TSH assays. With the ability to directly measure TSH, there is no longer any need to evaluate if the absence of thyroid function is due to thyroid gland failure or the lack of endogenous TSH, which was inferred if the patient responded to exogenous TSH administration. Genetically engineered human TSH has been produced and evaluated in clinical trials. In published reports it is an effective method to stimulate thyroid tissue uptake of radioiodine. It has not yet been approved by the FDA for clinical use in the United States.

Thyroid imaging. Thyroid imaging began in the era of the rectilinear scanner. Even after the widespread use of the gamma camera, some departments continued to use a rectilinear scanner for thyroid imaging. Rectilinear scanners have the advantage of providing life-size images with 1:1 representation of thyroid gland size and functional distribution.

The Society of Nuclear Medicine has published a consensus guideline on the technical details recommended in thyroid scintigraphy.[7] A gamma camera with a pinhole collimator provides an image that is more esthetically pleasing, generally with better resolution, and oblique views can be readily obtained. There are a variety of pinhole inserts available. The diameter of the aperture of the insert determines the spatial resolution of the system. As usual, there is a tradeoff between sensitivity and resolution, with sensitivity decreasing as the aperture diameter decreases and the resolution improves. Since image size varies with distance, the pinhole collimator should be used at a fixed distance from the surface so that some uniformity is established within a department (see Figure 10-4, *D*). Physicians and technologists become accustomed to images of usual size and recognize enlarged lobes or glands. It is possible also to take an additional image with a marker of known dimension within the field of view. Regardless of the specific distance of the camera crystal surface to the thyroid, the marker provides an internal calibration by which estimates of organ dimensions and a calculation of area (or volume) can be made.

In addition to inconsistent size representation, there are two other technical artifacts involved in imaging of the thyroid with a pinhole collimator: parallax spatial distortion and the pin-cushion effect. The parallax distortion occurs because objects in the center of the field appear in the center of the image regardless of the depth from the collimator, whereas sources or defects displaced from the center project away from the central ray. The projection in the image varies with the distance from the aperture. If a marker is placed on the neck surface overlying a nodule, it projects away from the nodule unless the marker and the nodule are centered in the field. The pincushion artifact is a concentric expression of the parallax effect, that is, there is no uniform sensitivity across the field because the activity at the periphery (of a flat field) is at a greater distance from the crystal surface than the center of the field.

A recent advance in gamma scintillation camera imaging involves electronic zoom. With improved electronics and collimator manufacturing techniques, magnified images with good resolution using a parallel-hole collimator can be obtained (see Figure 10-9). Systems have been described with a resolution of 8 mm at a 10 cm distance from the collimator surface in air at 140 keV. This resolution is apparently due in part to improved (more precise) collimator bore alignment, which is reportedly less than 1 degree. These images can be calibrated to obtain size information. They should not be used to assess thyroid nodule function in clinical practice, however, as the system (despite the above specifications) does not produce images with sufficient resolution for this purpose.

The two-lobed thyroid is just medial to the sternocleidomastoid muscle, 3-5 cm above the sternal notch. It is customary to obtain an anterior image and both right and left anterior (45-degree) oblique views, the latter views particularly if there is suspicion of palpable findings (see Figure 10-6). The sternal notch should be identified, usually by obtaining an additional image with a marker at the notch. In addition, right-left orientation should be identified routinely. This is accomplished by regularly placing an additional marker on the right side.

Although usually symmetric, various degrees of asymmetry in size between the two lobes can be observed. Asymmetry can represent a simple developmental anomaly and is probably not significant if there are no corresponding palpable findings.

The scan findings are ideally correlated with palpable findings. Activity in palpable nodules can be uniform (similar to the remainder of the gland), increased (warm or hot), or decreased (cold) in activity (see Figures 10-6 to 10-8). Solitary, cold nodules carry an increased potential (20% to 35% incidence) for malignancy, usually differentiated thyroid carcinoma. Although it is well to remember therefore that at least two thirds of the cold nodules are not malignant, aggressive pursuit of histology (biopsy or resection) is the most accepted course when a solitary cold nodule is

identified. In some settings it may be desirable to observe these nodules, in which case the patient should receive exogenous thyroid hormone to therapeutically suppress the gland. This course can be chosen in chronic thyroiditis (if thyroid antibodies are found) on the premise that the finding might represent a focal area of organification defect secondary to Hashimoto involvement as opposed to malignancy. Multiple nodules can be uniformly active or vary in activity one from the other. In the euthyroid patient this usually represents a post–Hashimoto thyroiditis and is associated with elevated TSH (a compensatory response to the inefficient handling of iodine and thyroid hormone synthesis). A solitary warm nodule is likely to represent a functioning adenoma. If the remainder of the thyroid gland is imaged, the patient is likely to be euthyroid, whereas if the patient were hyperthyroid as a result of excessive thyroid hormone production by the functioning adenoma, TSH would be suppressed, resulting in lack of stimulation of the remainder of the gland.

Occasionally a euthyroid patient is seen with only a solitary focus of thyroid activity. This finding can represent a euthyroid phase of an autonomous adenoma with sufficient hormone production to suppress TSH but not yet hyperthyroid (see Figure 10-8, *B*). Alternatively this can represent an anatomic variant in which only one lobe or a portion of a lobe developed congenitally. If there is a history of surgical resection, the area of activity can represent residual thyroid tissue, which also can hypertrophy and present as a mass even if the previous surgery was for benign thyroid disease (see Figure 10-4, *C*). Finally, the solitary focus can represent residual malignant tissue. Patient history contributes to the scan interpretation and differential diagnosis. In the event there is no history of prior surgery in a euthyroid patient, it is possible to differentiate between the autonomous adenoma and congenital anomalous development by performing the T_3 suppression test, with imaging before and after suppression. In the case of an autonomous nodule, there will be no suppression of the focus of functioning tissue, whereas the congenital anomalous focus under TSH control will suppress.

Thyroid carcinoma. Carcinoma of the thyroid is a common disease found in 3% to 10% of all autopsied patients. Mortality from thyroid carcinoma exceeds the mortality from all other malignant endocrine tumors (except ovarian carcinoma) but accounts for less than 1% of all deaths from malignancy. The challenge for nuclear medicine is to detect this relatively common neoplasm and any evidence of metastases, to provide effective therapy, and to minimize morbidity so that neither the knowledge of the diagnosis nor the effect of therapy is more destructive than the disease itself.

Several types of malignant tumors are found in the thyroid gland: differentiated carcinoma such as papillary carcinoma, follicular variant of papillary carcinoma (the so-called mixed or papillary-follicular), follicular carcinoma, and medullary carcinoma; undifferentiated carcinoma; lymphoma of the thyroid; and metastases to the thyroid. These tumors can present as a palpable nodule of the thyroid, in which case the patient should be referred for a thyroid scan with ^{131}I or ^{99m}Tc. These malignancies appear as cold (nonfunctioning) areas within the thyroid gland (see Figure 10-6). Of course, the finding of a cold area does not differentiate between a malignant basis and one of the more frequent benign findings: benign adenomas, cysts, focal thyroiditis, and focal bleeding. Accordingly, a nonfunctioning (cold) solitary nodule is an indication for needle biopsy.[27] If this procedure is unavailable or if the results are indeterminate, an excisional biopsy should be performed. In various series 20% to 35% of the solitary cold nodules are malignant (usually differentiated carcinoma of the thyroid). A number of additional noninvasive procedures are available or are being evaluated. This includes ultrasound, CT, MRI, and additional radionuclide imaging procedures with ^{201}Tl or ^{99m}Tc MIBI. Although these procedures are of interest, none of them has an established place at this time in the clinical management of the patient with a thyroid nodule. Some patients present directly to a surgeon who will proceed to obtain a biopsy specimen or remove the palpable mass. The advantage of presurgical evaluation of a palpable thyroid finding is to prepare the surgeon (and the patient) for a definitive procedure. In an alternative clinical scenario, thyroid carcinoma is found serendipitously, presenting as a metastatic lesion in a lymph node or some distant organ. In either case optimal treatment involves a near total thyroidectomy, with examination of the lymph nodes on the involved side and removal if tumor is suspected or found.

Following the histopathologic diagnosis of papillary, papillary-follicular (mixed), or follicular carcinoma and surgical treatment, the patient is referred to the nuclear medicine service for diagnostic imaging to determine the amount and location of residual thyroid tissue or tumor based on the ability of this tissue to concentrate radioiodine.

Evaluation of patients with thyroid carcinoma begins with discontinuing exogenous thyroid hormone, which had been given as replacement therapy in patients who have had a total thyroidectomy but is also given to patients who have had less surgery. The goal of replacement thyroid therapy is not simply to render the patient clinically euthyroid but also to suppress endogenous TSH to ensure that there is no stimulation of residual thyroid tumor cells. Some modification of thyroxine dosage may have to be made depending on the patient's cardiac status, but generally replacement thyroxine is given in an amount sufficient to ensure TSH suppression. There are various approaches to preparing the patient for diagnostic radioiodine imaging and dosimetry studies.

Replacement thyroid hormone should be discontinued and the patient should be given a low-iodine diet. The patient should not have studies with iodinated contrast material during this interval. Several weeks can elapse before radioiodine imaging is performed to allow TSH levels to rise, as is expected if sufficient thyroid tissue has been removed surgically. The patient gradually develops symptoms and signs of hypothyroidism, including lethargy, soft tissue swelling, weight gain, constipation, coarsening of the skin, and bradycardia as well as intolerance to cold. Serum T_4 and T_3 levels fall to the hypothyroid range. The serum TSH level can be assayed before a diagnostic radioiodine dose is administered. Failure of the TSH to rise might indicate that a significant functioning remnant remains. If TSH has not risen and the patient has not developed signs of thyroid deficiency, the amount of residual tissue can be evaluated with a traditional thyroid uptake and scan or alternatively with a ^{99m}Tc-pertechnetate scan.

At this point the patient is found either to have had a thorough surgical excision of the thyroid to permit whole-body scanning or to have a significant functioning remnant that must be excised surgically or ablated with radioactive iodine to evaluate if local or distal metastases are present. ^{131}I is administered in doses from 1-10 mCi. Tumor foci are identifiable on gamma camera imaging when less than 10 μCi of ^{131}I are accumulated in the focus. This represents 1% of a 1 mCi dose. Accordingly, administration of larger diagnostic doses (i.e., 10 mCi) permits identification of foci with a fractional uptake in the 0.1% range. In general, we have taken the approach of using a lower dose when there is reason to suspect that there is residual thyroid tissue or tumor. Doses even less than 1 mCi may be used to complete dosimetry if it has already been determined that the patient will be treated subsequently with a dose of 29 mCi or more. After the total body radiation burden has decreased to a level to permit removal of isolation procedures, the patient is imaged to assess the distribution of the therapeutic dose. If, however, the patient has no known thyroid tissue and is being evaluated to determine if any therapy is needed, a large dose is recommended. A number of centers use as much as 10 mCi for this purpose. Clearly the diagnostic yield increases with the imaging dose. The argument has been made that if a focus can only be identified with a 10 mCi dose, representing perhaps a 0.1% uptake, can it be treated effectively? (See thyroid carcinoma treatment, p. 286.) The recently published "Procedure Guideline for Extended Scintigraphy for Differentiated Thyroid Cancer" developed by the Society of Nuclear Medicine provides for a 5.0 mCi dose of ^{131}I.[9]

Cervical and whole-body images can be obtained at 24-hr intervals. Images obtained at 48 or 72 hr have been found to be optimal, since imaging at these intervals allows sufficient time for reduction of background activity via renal excretion.[35] There is a recent report that imaging beyond 48 hr increases the identification of metastases. Since radioiodine is secreted into the saliva and gastric fluids, activity in the gastrointestinal tract can be seen at 48 hr and can even be the source of background and bladder activity for several days as the intestinal activity undergoes absorption and redistribution.

The patient should be imaged from head to toe with sufficient image accumulation time to allow visualization of even small amounts of localized activity. The head, neck, thorax, abdomen, and pelvis should be imaged in both the anterior and posterior projection. If suitable collimation is available, whole-body scanning cameras provide excellent images. Alternatively, a gamma camera with a high-energy collimator, that is, with septa appropriate for the relatively energetic 364 keV gamma emission of ^{131}I, can be used (Figures 10-10 to 10-12).

Recently, we have reviewed the characteristics of two different manufacturers of 364 keV collimators. (These had been called "high energy" but with the introduction of collimators for 511 keV SPECT imaging, it is necessary to specify which energy range is intended.) In the case of the two manufacturers evaluated, there is considerable difference in the sensitivity and resolution of the collimators available for ^{131}I imaging (Table 10-3). Collimator "A" provides excellent images when larger diagnostic doses are used or when the patient is imaged after the therapeutic dose. There is minimal septal penetration. When a 1 or 2 mCi dose of ^{131}I is used, it is insufficiently sensitive (Figure 10-13), whereas collimator "B" produces satisfactory images of the radioiodine distribution. At high doses, collimator "B" produces images with considerably more evidence of septal penetration. There has been less attention to collimation for ^{131}I imaging than to "low-energy" collimators, probably because the volume of patients imaged is relatively small in most institutions. It is important to appreciate that there is considerable variability in the response of ^{131}I collimators from manufacturer to manufacturer and that this variability will influence the diagnostic performance.

Each imaging field is recorded for 10 min. Radioactive markers are placed to identify anatomic landmarks, such as top of the skull, axillae, umbilicus, iliac crests, and knees. If the sternal notch is to be marked, a repeat image without the marker should be obtained so as not to obscure a thyroid remnant or local tumor focus. By definition, radioiodine identifies only tumor tissue capable of concentrating radioiodine. Nevertheless, the degree of uptake is apt to be insufficient to identify by traditional techniques as described. In addition to the practice of employing a larger "diagnostic" dose,

it has been observed that additional metastatic foci are observed on scans obtained at a suitable interval (72 hr or more) after the therapeutic dose, which can be several hundred mCi of ^{131}I. In addition, several other techniques have appeared in recent years that provide

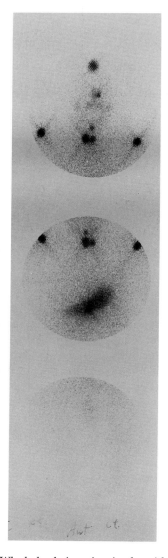

Figure 10-10 Whole-body imaging in thyroid carcinoma. 1-10 mCi ^{131}I are used as the "diagnostic" tracer with high-energy collimation. This figure illustrates anterior images using gamma camera technique at 24 hr after tracer administration. Markers are placed at the top of the head and shoulders. Background activity is seen throughout the soft tissue with secretion in the nasal and oral cavities, the parotid and submaxillary glands, and the salivary glands. Residual thyroid tissue is seen in the bed of both the right and left thyroid lobes. A small midline focus cephalad to the thyroid remnants is also seen, representing metastasis to a paratracheal lymph node. Prominent activity is seen in the stomach. There is no activity seen in the bladder, although bladder activity is quite common, particularly at 24 hr after tracer administration. Posterior images are also obtained to evaluate possible osseous metastases.

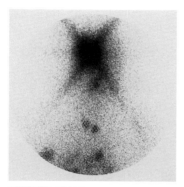
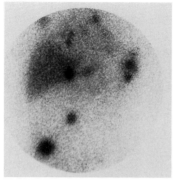
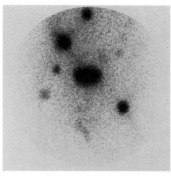

Figure 10-11 Whole-body imaging in thyroid carcinoma. Gamma camera images at 72 hr after ^{131}I therapy (134 mCi); 30 sec/frame. Metastases are seen in the brain (with a star artifact due to septal penetration, readily observed because of the large amount of activity concentrated in a brain metastasis). Additional metastases are seen in the cervical, mediastinal, hepatic, and femoral lymph nodes. Diffuse activity is seen in the liver parenchyma representing hepatic excretion of radiolabeled thyroid hormone synthesized in the functioning metastases.

greater sensitivity for the detection of thyroid tumor. This includes the in vitro assay for thyroglobulin, the intrathyroidal binding protein, in the plasma. Any detectable amount of this marker of thyroid-derived tissue is indicative of thyroid tissue. In patients previously demonstrated to be athyrotic, this finding suggests viable tumor, presenting a challenge to nuclear imaging to identify the source of the thyroglobulin. Greater success in identifying the source of thyroglobulin is achieved with larger doses of ^{131}I. Administered doses as large as 10 mCi are used. In some instances foci that had not been identified after a diagnostic dose are seen when the patient is imaged after several days following a therapeutic dose of radioiodine.

Radionuclide therapy. The efficient localization of iodine by thyroid tissue provides a basis for the use of radioactive iodine, specifically ^{131}I, to deliver a radiation dose sufficient to reduce the functioning mass of thyroid tissue. The significant radiobiologic effect of ^{131}I is a product of the beta particle emissions.

Hyperthyroidism. ^{131}I has been used therapeutically for many years to treat hyperthyroidism due to either diffuse toxic goiter (Graves disease), toxic multinodular goiter, or toxic nodule (toxic adenoma). In the 1950s and 1960s there was some use of ^{131}I to render euthyroid patients with severe coronary artery disease hypothyroid to reduce the metabolic needs of the myocardium. With the availability of adrenergic blockers and other pharmacologic agents, this role no longer exists. Although treatment of hyperthyroidism with ^{131}I has many advantages (it is simple, safe, effective, relatively inexpensive, with minimal if any morbidity), this disorder can also be treated with antithyroid drugs or surgery. Generally, the physician explains the benefits and disadvantages of each therapeutic option to the patient and makes a recommendation. Radioiodine therapy is the most frequent choice of therapy for adults with Graves disease, and surgery is rarely used at present.[5,6] A great deal has been written about the appropriate dose of radioactive iodine to achieve the desired effect—control of the hyperthyroid state with a minimal incidence of early hypothyroidism. In general, the greater the amount of radioactivity administered,

Table 10-3 Comparison of ^{131}I (364 keV) collimators from two different manufacturers. "Relative" compares count rate for an equivalent source against a specific (but randomly designated reference), low-energy, all-purpose collimator.

	Septal penetration (%)	FWHM (mm)	Sensitivity in cpm/μCi	Air at 10 cm relative
Manufacturer A	6	19.0	260	0.77
Manufacturer B	3.5	12.6	106	0.31

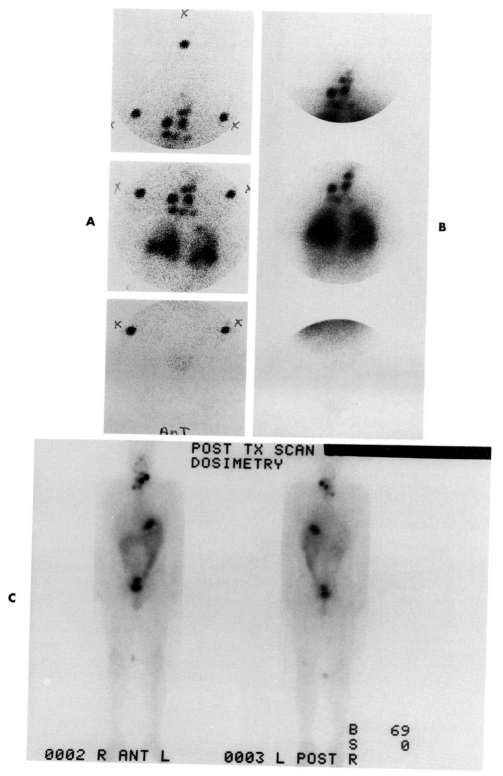

Figure 10-12 Whole-body imaging in thyroid carcinoma. Gamma camera technique **(A)** 48 hr after 10 mCi ^{131}I and **(B)** 72 hr after 200 mCi ^{131}I (therapeutic dose). In **A** markers are seen on the top of the skull, at the shoulders, and at the iliac crests. Focal metastases are seen at multiple sites in the neck, superior mediastinum, and diffusely throughout the lungs. **C,** Scanning in a different patient at 72 hr after 200 mCi ^{131}I (therapeutic dose). Prominent activity is seen in the left thyroid lobe remnant, a cervical lymph node lateral to the left lobe, and in two small foci in the superior mediastinum. Excreted activity is seen in the stomach, bowel, and bladder. A standard source has been placed between the knees.

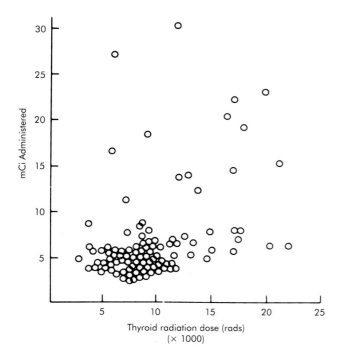

Figure 10-13 Relationship of radiation absorbed dose to the thyroid and the amount of ^{131}I administered in 92 hyperthyroid patients. (Reprinted with permission from Becker DV, Hurley JR: Current status of radioiodine (^{131}I) treatment of hyperthyroidism. In Freeman L, Weissman HS, eds: *Nuclear medicine annual 1982*, New York, 1982, Raven Press.)

range to achieve this effect, however, is great. As long as the therapist is also seeking to minimize the incidence, or delay the onset, of hypothyroidism, some balance is necessary between a dose that controls as many patients as possible and a dose that produces hypothyroidism in as few patients as possible.

Hypothyroidism occurs as a late sequela of hyperthyroidism regardless of the treatment (radioiodine, surgery, and drugs) used.[5,6] There is no doubt that the immediate or short-term incidence is greater after radioiodine than other forms of therapy in many published series. This has resulted in the approach that accepts hypothyroidism as inevitable, and perhaps even desirable. Hypothyroidism is certainly readily treatable with thyroid hormone replacement, but effectiveness of this therapy depends on long-term patient compliance. The ease of replacement therapy and the suggestion that the thyroid remnant can act as a continuous source of antigenic stimuli for, and possibly the site of synthesis of, thyroid-stimulating antibodies has encouraged some thyroidologists to recommend ablative doses of radioiodine.

There are three basic approaches to selecting the dose of radioactive iodine (^{131}I) to be administered: (1) fixed dose, in which all patients receive 3-7 mCi of ^{131}I with some slight variation for a number of factors per-

ceived by the treating physician; (2) delivered microcuries per gram, in which the estimated weight of the thyroid gland is taken into account as well as the 24-hr thyroid uptake—a choice is made as to whether a moderate amount of activity (50-80 $\mu Ci/g$) or a more vigorous amount (160-200 $\mu Ci/g$) is administered based on age, presence of nodules, and severity of hyperthyroidism; or (3) a delivered rad dose, in which the turnover rate of the radioactive iodine is estimated or determined to calculate an amount of radioactivity to be administered that will deliver a known rad (or Gray) dose.

There is a great deal of literature that discusses the merits of each approach.[5,6] The simplest approach (a more or less fixed dose) points out that there is a significant and indeterminable amount of variation in the biologic sensitivity to radiation, and even the best efforts fail to accurately determine an ideal dose in all patients. Moreover, since hypothyroidism is perhaps inevitable, certainly not catastrophic, and readily treatable, the goal is simply to control the hyperthyroid state. As previously stated, some have suggested intentional overtreatment to remove the thyroid as a source of immunoglobulins, which provokes persistence of the Graves pathophysiology, specifically progression of exophthalmos and other ocular manifestations even if the patient is rendered euthyroid. The virtue of this approach is that no additional studies are required, and the patient can be treated immediately with 10-20 mCi of ^{131}I, if available.

Nevertheless, it is a relatively simple matter to make an effort to individualize the therapeutic dose to determine thyroid gland mass, either by palpation or by estimate from scans, or by specific calculation based on measuring areas of functioning tissue. A formula correlating mass and area has been reported in which mass (in grams) = 0.86 area (cm^2). All patients should have a 24-hr radioactive iodine uptake before radioiodine therapy, so this value is always available. The formula to determine a somewhat individualized therapeutic dose therefore is as follows:

Dose to be administered

$$(\mu Ci) = \frac{\mu Ci/g \text{ desired} \times \text{Gland weight (g)} \times 100}{24\text{-hr uptake (\%)}}$$

The $\mu Ci/g$ *desired* term leaves a great deal of flexibility, and the value used has evolved by experience within the thyroid nuclear medicine community. In the early 1960s it was common practice to administer an amount of ^{131}I so that the residual therapeutic dose was in the order of 120-160 $\mu Ci/g$. Current empirical practice has reduced the $\mu Ci/g$ desired to about 60 $\mu Ci/g$ based on anecdotal evidence.

For many years I have practiced and encouraged the use of a slightly more individualized dose calculation, incorporating the measurement of thyroidal iodine turnover (effective half-life [$t_{1/2e}$]), which can vary from 1.5 to 6.0 days. Many patients' effective half-life values fall within a narrower range (3.5 to 5.0 days), particularly if they have not been treated previously. Nevertheless, an individualized measurement should be made. This is readily accomplished by repeating the 24-hr uptake technique at 48 and 72 or 96 hr; the effective half-life is determined from a semilogarithmic plot of the thyroid counts versus time. In determination of the effective half-life these counts should not be corrected for decay. If decay-corrected values are determined at 24, 48, 72, and 96 hr, the half-value interval is the biologic half-life ($t_{1/2b}$). The effective half-life value can be determined by combining the value for biologic half-life with the value for physical half-life ($t_{1/2p}$) (8.04 days):

$$t_{1/2e} = \frac{(t_{1/2b})(t_{1/2p})}{(t_{1/2b})(t_{1/2p})}$$

The formula to determine the prescribed dose of radioactive material to be administered to achieve a specified rad dose has been simplified by adapting the classic Quimby-Marinelli-Hine formula to the geometry of the thyroid and combining constants[5]:

Dose to administered (in μCi) =
$$\frac{\text{Rad desired} \times \text{Thyroid mass (g)} \times 6.67}{t_{1/2e} \text{ (days)} \times \% \text{ 24-hr uptake}}$$

The merit of calculating a rad dose versus a simplistic, fixed millicurie dose to be administered[5] can be illustrated. A 5 mCi ^{131}I administered dose can result in a thyroid radiation dose of 3000-15,000 rad, a fivefold range depending on the percent uptake, the effective half-life, and the thyroid gland weight. Furthermore, 7000 rad (a frequently recommended absorbed dose) can be achieved with doses from 3-27 mCi.

It is acknowledged that there is no documentation that the additional effort and calculation has a demonstrable clinical advantage. For many patients (those in the usual range for effective half-life values), the individualized calculated dose to be administered would be similar to the simpler calculation or even to the fixed dose. Nevertheless, it is our belief that the minimal additional effort creates an opportunity to relate a radiation dose (rad) to a therapeutic effect as opposed to the practice of comparing administered radioactivity (mCi) to the biologic response. Despite the current enthusiasm for cost-effectiveness, it seems archaic to be performing radiation therapy without a concept of the radiation absorbed dose administered. Becker and colleagues[5,6] have elucidated their enthusiasm for determination of the rad dose in several excellent, extensive reviews.

Thyroid carcinoma treatment. The treatment of thyroid carcinoma with ^{131}I has evolved from the earliest days of nuclear medicine. In 1938 when Hertz, Roberts, and Evans[16] reported their initial observations on the distribution of ^{128}I (28 min $t_{1/2}$) in rabbits, they noted: "It is therefore logical to suppose that when strongly active materials are available, the concentrating power of hyperplastic and neoplastic thyroid for radioactive iodine may be of clinical or therapeutic significance." The short half-life of ^{128}I was unsatisfactory for clinical studies, but ^{131}I was "synthesized" by Seaborg shortly thereafter. Clinical observations began immediately, but publication of the diagnostic findings and results of therapy with radioactive material were suppressed because of the war. In 1946 Seidlin[30] reported the complete disappearance of multiple functioning metastases in a patient with thyroid carcinoma treated with ^{131}I. This report captured the imagination of the public and the press, leading to political support for a civilian nuclear industry in the United States.

Radioiodine treatment using ^{131}I is involved at several points in the management of patients with thyroid carcinoma. This includes the ablation of the residual thyroid remnant (after variable degrees of surgical thyroidectomy) and the treatment of local and distal metastases (see Figures 10-10 to 10-12). Despite the 50-year experience with ^{131}I as a therapeutic agent for thyroid carcinoma, the issue of appropriate dose remains unresolved. For the most part the therapeutic recommendations are generalizations from observations on a small number of patients: 30-75 mCi of ^{131}I to ablate remnants, 75-150 mCi to treat local (cervical) metastases, and doses of 150-300 mCi to treat distal metastases.

The incidence of thyroid carcinoma is less than 1:100,000/year in the United States. One of the difficulties in the evolution of a more scientific method to determine a therapeutic dose is the relatively low frequency of thyroid carcinoma. The natural history of the disease is variable: many patients do well for long periods regardless of the therapeutic regimen, but a small subgroup of patients seem to have an accelerated course with an unsatisfactory result despite aggressive therapy. Although several uncertainties remain, there is a growing amount of literature in support of a more rational, scientific determination of the therapeutic administered dose based on individualized determination of the variables involved in the delivery, retention, and distribution of the administered dose. Preliminary investigations have demonstrated that the radiotherapeutic effectiveness of radionuclide therapy is consistent with the substantial body of radiotherapy literature when confounding variables such as dose rate and distribution are considered.[20-22]

Individualized dosimetric calculation of the radiation absorbed dose to the functioning tissue and to other appropriate radiosensitive organs, specifically the bone marrow, is part of the training of nuclear medicine physicians and scientists who have received training in radiation biology and dosimetry. This involves the use of the medical internal radiation dose (MIRD) formulation

$$\text{Dose(rad)} = [\mathring{A}/m]\,1.44\,t_{1/2e}\,\Sigma\Delta_i\Phi_i$$

for the calculation of the radiation absorbed dose. This equation permits determination of the amount of radioactive material (^{131}I) to be administered that will deliver a predictable amount of absorbed radiation in individual patients by accounting for patient specific variables such as the mass of tissue exposed, the amount of the administered dose to which the tissue will be exposed, the geometric relationship between the radiation source and the so-called target tissue, and physical factors specific for the radionuclide. Before development and dissemination of the MIRD approach, the Quimby-Marinelli equations for determination of the absorbed dose from the beta and gamma components were used.[20] The currently used MIRD formulation simplifies the calculation, and lookup tables are available for a "standard man" as well as modifications for a woman, a newborn, and children at intervals between infancy and adolescence. Although clinical dosimetry makes many assumptions, even an approximation of the absorbed dose by this method provides a more quantitative approach than the simple selection of amounts of radioactive material based on undefined variables.

Patients receiving radioiodine treatment should, of course, have been evaluated with whole-body imaging and dosimetry before administration of treatment doses. Accordingly, these patients will have been demonstrated to have had elevated TSH levels so as to stimulate radioiodine uptake in residual tissue or tumor. Once again, it is likely that recombinant human TSH will soon be available for administration before radioiodine treatment. Such an approach would appear to be preferable as patients will not have to undergo the prolonged period of thyroid deficiency to permit elevation of endogenous TSH.

Thyroid remnant ablation. Thyroid ablation is limited to patients with thyroid carcinoma who have had surgical removal of a significant portion of the thyroid gland. Although there is a range of surgical practice and skill in performing a "total" thyroidectomy in these patients, it is well established that a large fraction of the patients have residual thyroid tissue in the region of the thyroid bed (see Figure 10-10). Thyroid ablation refers to elimination of this tissue. It had been the practice to administer 75-100 mCi of ^{131}I for this purpose.[11,31] Successful ablation in 87% of patients studied is reported. In 1983 Snyder and colleagues[31] at the Mayo Clinic reopened the controversy of dose selection by reporting the effectiveness of 30 mCi doses of ^{131}I in remnant ablation. They observed complete ablation in 42 of 69 patients (61%) with a single dose of 29 mCi and minimal residual thyroid tissue in another 14

(81%). Four more patients responded to a second 29 mCi dose. Analysis of patient response compared with a calculated delivered absorbed dose (based on several assumptions including an assigned 5-day effective half-life) failed to identify a relationship between dose and response. Patients receiving greater than 30 mCi of ^{131}I are classified as radiation sources by the Nuclear Regulatory Commission (NRC), and the practice had evolved to hospitalize these patients until their body burden (radioactivity) fell to less than 30 mCi. Although the economic advantage of the Mayo approach is appealing, it is not an effective solution for that 12% of patients with persistent functioning remnants or for those patients in whom functioning metastases are identified when imaged after the 29 mCi dose.

Recently Maxon and colleagues at the University of Cincinnati Medical Center have reported the results of quantitative dosimetry.[21] They report ablation with ^{131}I in 122 of 142 thyroid remnants (86%) in 57 of 70 patients (81%) by delivering 30,000 rad. The range of activity administered was 26-246 mCi. Twenty-six of 70 patients (37%) received less than 30 mCi of [131]I. This impressive study speaks forcefully for individualized dosimetric determinations in patients undergoing radionuclide thyroid remnant ablation. Not only are the results as good as those achieved in the high-dose protocols, but they also make it possible to identify those patients "likely to respond to outpatient therapy with a higher chance of success" and "those who will require greater administered activities and inpatient treatment."

Local and distal metastases. There is general agreement that metastases to local lymph nodes or more distal sites such as mediastinal lymph nodes, pulmonary parenchyma, and bone require larger administered doses, usually 150-300 mCi (see Figures 10-11 and 10-12). There is little documentation about the precise determination of the administered dose except that the greater the number and area (volume) of metastases, the greater the likelihood that a larger dose would be administered (i.e., 300 mCi), with the proviso that the accumulated activity in the lungs not be greater than 80 mCi, since radiation pneumonitis or pulmonary fibrosis, a frequently fatal complication, was observed in patients with sufficient metastatic tissue to retain this level of radioactivity. Leeper,[20] Beierwaltes,[12] et al.[21,28] have reported satisfactory resolution of lymph node metastases in patients receiving 150 mCi of [131]I. These patients, of course, are followed with radioiodine scans and retreated with similar doses if necessary. Beierwaltes and co-workers[12] reported 80%, 97%, and 100% ablation of cervical lymph node metastases in patients receiving 150-174, 175-199, and 200 mCi or more in a series of 35, 37, and 9 patients, respectively, at each level of administered activity. As metastases became more distant, ablation of the functioning tissue was somewhat less successful, but results as good as 75% total ablation of mediastinal nodes were observed in patients receiving less than 200 mCi of ^{131}I. It is interesting to note that patients receiving 175-199 mCi had an 89% ablation success rate. It seems likely that the larger administered dose was selected for patients with greater tumor burdens, but this is not documented in the report. It does support the contention, however, that any single variable (e.g., tumor mass, percent uptake of administered dose) is an insufficient basis for dose selection.

In a small number of patients reported by Beierwaltes and colleagues,[12] patients with lung metastases had a 67% success rate when greater than 200 mCi were administered (3 patients) versus a 20% response in patients receiving 175-199 mCi (5 patients) and a 60% response in patients receiving 150-174 mCi (5 patients). In patients with bone metastases there was a 60% response in patients receiving 150-174 mCi (5 patients), a 71% response in patients receiving 175-199 mCi (7 patients), and an 80% response in patients receiving greater than 200 mCi (5 patients).

Two decades ago Leeper and co-workers[20] at the Memorial Sloan-Kettering Cancer Center in New York proposed using a maximal permissible dose for patients with metastases beyond the cervical lymph nodes based on limiting pulmonary parenchymal exposure to less than 80 mCi and bone marrow exposure to less than 200 rad per administered dose, which was limited to one therapeutic dose per year. By dosimetric determination of the bone marrow exposure, bone marrow depression was avoided despite the administration of doses in excess of 300 mCi. One patient is reported who was free from disease 3 years after a 320 mCi administered dose.

Recently Maxon and colleagues[21] reported the results of a larger series of thyroid cancer patients who underwent quantitative radiation dosimetry. This group had previously reported successful ablation of thyroid remnants at 30,000 rad and of nodal metastases at 8000 rad.[22] When the radiation dose to the involved nodes was greater than 8000 rad, 98% of patients responded to treatment, whereas only 20% responded at less than this radiation absorbed dose. In the recent series they observed a success rate of 86% of patients and 90% of involved nodes in situations in which 14,000 rad or more was administered.

In summary, therefore, an extensive argument exists for the use of quantitative dosimetry for the selection of a therapeutic dose of ^{131}I. Bone marrow exposure is determined as a worst-case calculation, assuming that the exposure is equivalent to the blood exposure. This is determined by measuring the blood disappearance rate of a tracer dose and assuming a blood volume of 20% of the body mass. A maximal "safe" dose is determined that will limit the calculated marrow exposure to 200 rad. Administered doses that result in less than

200 rad exposure to the marrow can be used if it is determined that an effective absorbed dose can be delivered to a remnant, nodal, or distal metastasis. For remnants this calculation indicates if an effective dose can be administered on an outpatient basis or if hospitalization is required. Optimal therapeutic doses to metastases might not be possible, but in general, calculation of the maximal safe dose provides a basis to administer doses greater than 150 mCi of ^{131}I.

An additional category of patients to consider for therapy are those without demonstrable foci of ^{131}I uptake but with elevated serum thyroglobulin levels (>10 ng/ml). The generally accepted approach would be to continue to evaluate or observe these patients and not to treat them with radioactive iodine unless iodine-concentrating tissue is identified. Moreover, it is not possible to determine a desired radiation absorbed dose, since neither tumor mass nor turnover can be evaluated by current methodology. Nevertheless, there are two carefully studied groups of patients who have been treated based on a previous diagnosis of thyroid carcinoma, total removal of the thyroid gland, and the finding of elevated serum thyroglobulin and negative-body ^{131}I scans. Of 83 patients treated at the University of Pisa, Italy, one third had positive scans after a therapeutic dose of 100 mCi of ^{131}I.[26] Many of the patients had a significant lowering of serum thyroglobulin after radioiodine treatment. At the National Institutes of Health (NIH), nine of ten patients with similar diagnostic results (elevated thyroglobulin levels and negative ^{131}I diagnostic scans) had abnormal scans when imaged after a therapeutic dose.[1] It is not clear at this time if this therapeutic approach is effective long term.

PARATHYROID GLANDS

Anatomy and Physiology

The parathyroid glands are located in the neck. As the name implies, they are multifocal and found alongside the thyroid gland, lying either adjacent, beneath, or within the substance of the thyroid (see Figure 10-2). As the parathyroids migrate from their embryologic origins in the branchial clefts into the neck, considerable variation occurs in their ultimate location. At times the glands are at some distance from their usual location alongside the thyroid. They can be found within the thyroid gland, within the thymus, among the great vessels (within the carotid sheath above the level of the thyroid to the area around the subclavian and innominate vessels in the thorax), and within the mediastinum.

The parathyroid glands elaborate parathyroid hormone, a polypeptide hormone that regulates calcium and phosphorus metabolism via action on the bone, kidney, and gastrointestinal tract. In bone, parathyroid hormone directly stimulates osteoclastic activity, increasing bone resorption and making calcium (and phosphorus) available to the plasma and tissues. In the kidney, parathyroid hormone increases urinary excretion of phosphorus (as phosphate) by inhibiting tubular reabsorption. Finally, there is a direct effect on the gastrointestinal tract by enhancing the absorption of calcium from the bowel lumen.

The synthesis and secretion of parathyroid hormone are regulated by the plasma-ionized calcium level, so the ionized calcium level is maintained in a physiologic range via a negative feedback loop: lowering of plasma (or serum) calcium stimulates parathyroid hormone release, which acts as described to make the calcium ion available. Failure of the parathyroid tissue to respond to lowered calcium, as in hypoparathyroidism, results in hypocalcemia, with eventual clinical manifestations associated with depolarization of cell membrane electrical potential—muscle spasm and irritability, as well as conduction disturbance in the heart.

Excessive parathyroid hormone secretion (inappropriate secretion despite normal or elevated calcium levels) results in elevated serum calcium (hypercalcemia). This is associated with increased urinary excretion of calcium and can cause renal stones and calcinosis, as well as calcification of other soft tissue. Since the source of the calcium is the bones, orthopedic complications can arise from bone mineral loss. This condition, known as *primary hyperparathyroidism*, is most frequently (80% to 90%) associated with a functioning parathyroid adenoma arising from one of the parathyroid glands. In the remaining cases it can occur as a result of hyperplasia of the parathyroid glands. The underlying mechanism for diffuse hyperplasia with loss of normal feedback suppression is not understood.

In chronic renal disease the kidneys fail to excrete the phosphate ion adequately, and serum phosphate levels rise. Since there is an upper limit on the product of serum calcium and phosphate ion concentration, calcium is deposited in soft tissues or excreted. The lowering of serum calcium in this manner stimulates parathyroid hormone secretion and parathyroid gland growth, leading to a pathophysiologic clinical condition known as *secondary hyperparathyroidism*. The clinical picture is a mixed one, expressing the underlying primary disorder (chronic renal disease) and the consequences of secondary hyperparathyroidism, including hypocalcemia and the consequences of increased bone resorption. Although therapy is directed to the underlying renal disease, the hyperparathyroidism is occasionally so severe that a transplanted kidney is threatened and surgical removal of the excess parathyroid tissue is necessary. In addition, even though the excessive parathyroid hormone synthesis and secretion in chronic renal disease may have begun as a homeostatic response to the hypocalcemia (secondary to the hyperphosphatemia), occasionally the hyperactivity persists and is associated with a functioning parathyroid adenoma. It is unclear if this represents an additional pathologic entity (so-called tertiary hyperparathyroidism, in which the glands that are initially hyperplastic in response to hypocalcemia become autonomous) or if this represents simply the coincident occurrence of primary hyperparathyroidism in a patient who initially had secondary hyperparathyroidism.

In the last several decades the availability of serum calcium determinations in routine blood chemistry screening has led to earlier recognition of patients with asymptomatic hypercalcemia, which may represent an early sign of hyperparathyroidism. This finding, as well as the other clinical situations reflecting disturbance of calcium homeostasis, demands further evaluation of the parathyroid gland.

Nuclear Medicine Procedures

In clinical situations in which abnormalities of parathyroid gland function are suspected, direct measurement of serum parathyroid hormone is indicated and provides the basis for the diagnosis. The measurement is made using radioimmunoassay techniques.

The nuclear medicine service has an active role in the management of patients with hyperparathyroidism by identifying the site of excess parathyroid hormone production, that is, the localization of a probable parathyroid adenoma in a patient with hyperparathyroidism. Because parathyroid adenomas are found in diverse locations alongside, behind, and within the thyroid, as well as in areas somewhat distant from the thyroid such as high or low in the neck or the mediastinum (see Figure 10-2), there is a significant need for a method to accurately and noninvasively identify the location of excess parathyroid hormone production.

In the past few years a highly successful, relatively convenient technique of parathyroid imaging using ^{99m}Tc MIBI has emerged as the method of choice for the localization of parathyroid adenomata.[24,33]

^{99m}Tc MIBI was introduced in 1989 as an alternative to ^{201}Tl for myocardial imaging and has also been used with ^{99m}Tc subtraction in parathyroid imaging.[25,32] It is efficiently extracted and proportional to blood flow. Although the extraction efficiency is slightly less than ^{201}Tl, the washout rate is slower. It appears to be retained in tissue in proportion to the metabolic rate. It appears to be bound more intensely in tissue rich in mitochondria.

Shortly after introduction for myocardial perfusion imaging, it was noted that ^{99m}Tc MIBI was taken up in tumors also. Although ^{99m}Tc MIBI is retained in some tumors, it is eliminated from the cell in drug resistant tumors by the multiple drug resistance p50 protein pump mechanism. This does not occur in parathyroid adenomata. In fact, the increased cellular metabolism of these tumors compared with the thyroid and surrounding soft tissues of the neck makes it possible to frequently identify parathyroid adenomata with a delayed image acquired at 2 hr after injection, at which time the adenoma has retained the tracer while the surrounding tissue washes out to varying degrees. Some protocols favor a two-phase study in which the patient is imaged at 20 min after injection and subsequently at 2 hr (Figure 10-14).

The use of ^{99m}Tc MIBI has supplanted the use of ^{201}Tl with ^{99m}Tc pertechnetate or ^{123}I subtraction of thyroid tissue. Nevertheless, some departments still use a protocol that involves subtraction of thyroid tissue activity by subtracting a ^{99m}Tc pertechnetate or ^{123}I image from the ^{99m}Tc MIBI image.

Recently, a number of other ^{99m}Tc tracers for myocardial perfusion imaging have become available from radiopharmaceutical developers. These compounds have slightly different extraction efficiencies and efflux rates. These compounds (e.g., ^{99m}Tc tetrofosmin) have been evaluated in small groups of patients for parathyroid adenoma identification. Although satisfactory images have been obtained in many instances, the few comparison studies available suggest that at present ^{99m}Tc MIBI is superior to its competitors for the localization of parathyroid adenoma.

There is a long history of efforts to image the parathyroid gland. Early efforts involved the use of ^{57}Co cyanocobalamine and ^{75}Se selenomethionine. Of these the latter, introduced in 1962, found some use in more experienced facilities. ^{75}Se selenomethionine was taken up preferentially by parathyroid tissue in contrast to the tissue surrounding it. This was probably based on its role as a marker of protein synthesis.

Initial results with ^{99m}Tc pertechnetate and ^{201}Tl subtraction imaging report surgically confirmed positive scintigraphic findings in 24 of 26 patients. There were two false-negative studies, which at surgery were found to be small foci, $0.5 \times 0.2 \times 0.2$ cm and $0.4 \times 0.4 \times 0.2$ cm. Adenomas or hyperplastic glands larger than these dimensions were regularly identified. The technique employed a gamma camera, pinhole collimator, and computer. Okerland[25] and colleagues proposed increasing the ^{201}Tl dose to 2-3 mCi, imaging sequentially for 15 min, finally selecting a 45,000-count image, followed by injection of 5-10 mCi of ^{99m}Tc pertechnetate and acquisition of a 50,000-count image at 4 to 6 min. Forty-four of 50 parathyroid adenomas (88%) were detected with this technique, with an additional three cases detected with the use of a color display. All adenomas greater than 690 mg were detected; the undetected false-negative lesions were 100-580 mg. There were no false-positive images.

In 1983 a group at the Mount Sinai Medical Center in New York reported a sensitivity of 93% (13 of 14 patients) and a specificity of 73% (8 of 11 patients).[31] False-positive studies were seen in patients who were found to have thyroid adenomas. Thallium-pertechnetate subtraction was, therefore, a very sensitive technique for the localization of parathyroid adenomas, certainly above a size threshold in the 500- to 600-mg range. Smaller lesions were detectable, but there is a decrease in sensitivity with a decrease in size. The determination of specificity probably has little meaning, since the technique regularly identifies other lesions such as thyroid adenomas. The incidence of detection of this abnormality depends on its frequency in the population studied. Since thyroid nodules are more common than parathyroid adenomas, thallium-avid palpable nodules are a frequent finding.

The thallium-pertechnetate subtraction technique had been extolled in the surgical literature.[4] Even though experienced neck surgeons have very high success rates in finding and removing parathyroid adenomas, operative time can be significantly reduced if a site is identified by a noninvasive imaging technique in advance. A limitation of this technique, however, was the lack of information about the mediastinum, an occasional site of ectopic parathyroid adenoma.

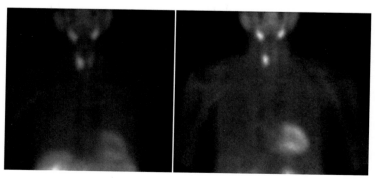

Figure 10-14 Anterior neck and upper thorax region images at 10 min and 2 hr after 20 mCi ^{99m}Tc MIBI. In the early images, activity is seen throughout both thyroid lobes. The delayed image shows prominent activity in the lower pole of the right thyroid lobe. This focus of persistant activity is characteristic of a parathyroid adenoma and has a high degree of accuracy in predicting the location of this lesion in an appropriate at-risk population (patients with hyperparathyroidism). False-positives may be associated with thyroid abnormalities.

As stated ^{99m}Tc MIBI imaging has emerged as the method of choice for the detection of parathyroid adenomata. The sensitivity (and specificity) of this technique appears to exceed that of the results obtained with ^{201}Tl. This is due in part to the superior imaging characteristics (lower energy) and greater photon flux (larger dose, shorter half-life) and also to the pharmacology-biochemistry of the ^{99m}Tc MIBI itself. Because it binds efficiently to mitochondrial proteins, washout from the mitochondrial-rich parathyroid adenoma is decreased. This results in a greater parathyroid-to-thyroid and parathyroid-to-background ratio than was observed with ^{201}Tl. In some cases this allows differentiation from thyroid adenoma. It might be expected, however, that with increased experience exceptions to this generalization will be observed. In the initial report comparing Tc-Tl subtraction technique with ^{99m}Tc MIBI scintigraphy, O'Doherty et al. reported that 37 of 40 adenomas were detected with ^{201}Tl and 39 of 40 were detected with ^{99m}Tc MIBI.[24] In 15 patients with hyperplastic glands, ^{99m}Tc MIBI identified 32 glands, whereas ^{201}Tl localized 29 hyperplastic glands. In late 1992 Taillefer et al. reported a so-called "Double Phase Study" in which anterior cervical images are obtained at 15 to 20 min after injection of 20-25 mCi of ^{99m}Tc MIBI and again at 2 to 3 hr after injection. Ten-minute acquisition was obtained using a parallel-hole, low-energy, high-resolution collimator with a 1.5 zoom factor. The differential washout of the ^{99m}Tc MIBI (with retention by the parathyroid tissue) resulted in preferential visualization of parathyroid in 19 of 21 instances[33] (see Figure 10-14). Another advantage of the Taillefer technique is the convenient acquisition of mediastinal images at both the early and late acquisition sessions, since the patient is already positioned under a camera with a parallel-hole collimator.

PANCREAS

Anatomy and Physiology

The pancreas is a somewhat serpentine organ nestled between the inferior (greater) curvature of the stomach and loops of small bowel. Most of the organ secretes digestive enzymes into the proximal small bowel. The endocrine elements of the pancreas are the islets of Langerhans, so-called because they are easily identified on histologic preparations as distinct islands of tissue, differentiated from the surrounding acinar (secretory) tissue by their cellular arrangement and staining characteristics. The islet cells are further classified histologically as alpha, beta, and delta. Alpha cells secrete glucagon, a polypeptide with a major role in glucose homeostasis, principally by its action in physiologic concentration on hepatic glycogen, glycogenolysis, or the conversion of glycogen to glucose.

Insulin is the principal product of the beta cells. It is the major regulator of glucose homeostasis, principally by promoting the active transport of glucose at the cell membrane. Many other metabolic effects occur as a consequence of this biochemical action, such as preferential utilization of glucose with preservation of stored glycogen, adipose tissue, and protein. In the normal subject, blood glucose is regulated and body energy metabolism is efficiently maintained. By contrast, in insulin-dependent diabetes mellitus there is an atrophy of the beta cells and failure to secrete sufficient insulin to maintain the homeostatic mechanisms just described. Blood glucose rises, but it is not used effectively by the tissues. The amount of glucose that appears in the glomerular filtrate exceeds the capacity for reabsorption, resulting in loss of glucose (and water) in the urine. Glycogen stores are depleted and adipose tissue is mobilized for energy. All of these metabolic consequences produce the dramatic clinical picture of insulin deficiency, culminating in diabetic ketoacidosis, hyperglycemia, dehydration, and death if insulin, fluids, electrolytes, and glucose are not replaced.

By contrast, both benign and malignant tumors of the beta cells (insulinomas) secrete insulin in excess of the amount needed for glucose regulation and frequently produce hypoglycemia (low blood glucose) and the clinical state associated with it—mental confusion, the metabolic and cardiovascular responses to stress, and eventual loss of consciousness.

The islet cells are also capable of producing a variety of active peptide hormones, such as gastrin and other small molecules that affect water regulation. Their role in normal physiology is not well understood. They are of clinical significance when overproduced by an islet cell tumor, resulting in a complex clinical picture associated with the action of the secretory product. The most common example is a gastrin-producing tumor (gastrinoma).

Nuclear Medicine Procedures

The technique of radioimmunoassay evolved from the study of insulin by Berson and Yalow.[13,14] With this powerful tool, capable of quantifying the amount of insulin in small volumes of plasma, these and subsequently other investigators revolutionized the modern understanding of insulin physiology. As indicated earlier, the technique can be used generically. With appropriate choice of reagents, radioimmunoassay provides a method to quantify glucagon, gastrin, and the other less commonly studied peptides.

Imaging of the islet cells, or at least imaging of tumors elaborating excessive amounts of these metabolically powerful substances, has been recognized as a worthwhile endeavor for a long time, since even a small tumor not readily detectable by other means, including surgical exploration, can have profound clinical effects. In the past, nonspecific nuclear imaging techniques with ^{75}Se selenomethionine and ^{67}Ga gallium citrate were not effective because of a failure to differentiate the tumor from background tissue activity. This entire area has been changed with the availability of ^{111}In DTPA pentetreotide, a diagnostic tracer that binds to somatostatin receptors.

SOMATOSTATIN-RECEPTOR IMAGING

Anatomy and Physiology

Somatostatin is a 14-amino-acid regulatory neuropeptide initially identified as a hypothalamic hormone that inhibited the release of the growth hormone from the anterior pituitary. Subsequently, it was demonstrated that somatostatin has effects on many tissues, most specifically secretory cells distributed throughout the gastrointestinal tract and respiratory passages. Somatostatin inhibits the release of the islet cell hormones insulin and glucagon, the release of gastrin and other internal secretions that regulate bowel function, and the secretion of digestive enzymes in response to other localized regulatory secretions. It also has complex effects on the immune system and generally seems to inhibit cell proliferation.

The inhibiting effects of somatostatin on tissues throughout the body are modulated via specific somatostatin receptors. Rather than reflecting the classic "endocrine" relationship implying the influence of a secretory product of one organ or a remote organ or tissue, this relationship actually reflects a role for somatostatin as a common but local ("paracrine") regulator of tissue function. Nevertheless, since labeled somatostatin and its analogues specifically bind these distributed cell types, it will be considered here as a distributed endocrine axis. Somatostatin-receptor imaging is useful in identifying the presence and extent of tumors including pituitary tumors; medullary carcinoma of the thyroid; pancreatic islet cell tumors; carcinoid tumors; and tumors of the chromaffin tissue, pheochromocytomas, neuroblastomas, and paragangliomas. Because of the distributive nature of the cell types from which these tumors arise, the tumors themselves may have an idiosyncratic distribution. These tumors may present as a result of symptoms related to the mass effect, as primary or metastatic involvement discovered during a surgical procedure or CT, or as a result of the excessive secretion of a physiologically active product.

Carcinoid tumors arise from the Kulchitzsky or chromaffin cells found in the gastrointestinal tract. They are found in the appendix (38%), the ileum of the small intestine (23%), the rectum (13%), the bronchus (11.5%), at sites throughout the gastrointestinal tract, and rarely in other organs.

The technique has been particularly useful also in identifying functional and nonfunctional islet cell carcinomas. The frequency of increased receptor density seems to vary somewhat with the type of islet cell tumor. This is reflected clinically in the frequency of positive detection of these relatively rare tumors. Gastrin-secreting tumors (gastrinomas) have virtually 100% detectability, whereas insulin-producing tumors (insulinomas) have a 50% detection sensitivity. Of course, identification of the tumor is not tumor type specific. [111]In pentetretide scintigraphy will also detect somatostatin-positive, nonfunctional islet cell tumors. The presence of somatostatin receptors has anecdotally been reported to be a more reliable means of differentiating nonfunctioning islet cell tumors from adenocarcinoma of the pancreas than histopathologic examination of the tumor. Surgical tissue from patients who have had a prolonged survival despite a pathologic diagnosis of adenocarcinoma of the pancreas was reevaluated for somatostatin receptors. All of the prolonged survivors had somatostatin receptors, which demonstrates immunohistology. Since adenocarcinoma of the pancreas is known not to have somatostatin receptors, it is concluded that the classic microscopic examination (with immunohistology or radioautographic identification of somatostatin receptors) was inaccurate or at least not capable of differentiating between islet cell tumors and adenocarcinoma of the pancreas.

[111]In DTPA pentetreotide is also useful for the detection and localization of pheochromocytoma and neuroblastoma.

Medullary carcinoma of the thyroid may also be identified with ^{111}In DTPA pentetreotide. The frequency of somatostatin receptors of radioautograhic examination is reported to be about 33%, which is less than ideal. In small series, tumors have been identified in 50% to 70% of the instances. Results are probably better in the de novo patient, but the more frequent instance is when the nuclear medicine facility is asked to identify the source of the recurrent elevation of thyrocalcitonin in a patient who has undergone total thyroidectomy for medullary carcinoma. In this instance the tumor may have decreased receptor expression, saturation of the receptors as a result of synthesis of somatostatin by the tumor. A technique that has been of value in several instances when the question is not "Does the patient have disease?" but rather "We know that the patient has recurrent medullary carcinoma of the thyroid because of the elevated thyrocalcitonin levels. Now, where is it? Is it resectable?" is the 10-min image. Ten-minute images are acquired and stored in a 128×128 or 256×256 matrix followed by SPECT imaging of the likely area of involvement (thorax and/or liver). By increasing the intensity on the digital planar or coronal projection image, multiple foci representing mediastinal lymph node involvement has been demonstrated.

Nuclear Medicine Procedures

Somatostatin-receptor scintigraphy is performed with ^{111}In DTPA pentetreotide, a radiolabeled derivative of octreotide.[17] It has been useful in the identification of benign or malignant tumors that arise from the widely distributed specialized secretory cells with somatostatin receptors, the so-called *neuroendocrine tumors.*

Octreotide (*Sandostatin,* Sandoz) is an 8-amino-acid analogue of somatostatin. It retains an affinity for somatostatin receptors and has a longer plasma and biologic half-life than native somatostatin. It is approved by the FDA as a therapeutic agent and is used to control the excessive secretion of the growth hormone in patients with acromegaly who, for one reason or another, are inoperable and in patients with syndromes associated with excessive secretion of metabolically active substances such as in the malignant carcinoid syndrome, in which a carcinoid tumor is secreting serotonin, catecholamines, and other active products into the posthepatic circulation.

Much of the early clinical evaluation of somatostatin-receptor scintigraphy was performed by Krenning, Lamberts, et al. in Rotterdam, The Netherlands who first evaluated an ^{123}I tyrosyl derivative of octreotide.[18] Although much was learned about the clinical potential for this type of imaging, the utility of ^{123}I tyrosyl octreotide was handicapped by the cost of ^{123}I, deiodination of the product, and the significant fraction of the administered dose, which was secreted into the bile and appeared as intestinal activity.

Somatostatin-receptor scintigraphy can be either a gratifying, relatively easy technique or an exceedingly frustrating, challenging procedure. In many instances the tumor is readily identifiable. This should not lead to a false degree of confidence. To achieve the greatest possible diagnostic yield, the nuclear medicine department should be prepared to perform a full set of images of the highest quality and to modify the protocol to suit the particular clinical and scintigraphic setting.

The adult dose of ^{111}In DTPA pentetreotide (*Octreoscan,* Mallinckrodt) is 6.0 mCi. The usual approach to pediatric dosage can be employed. Despite the cost of the radiotracer and the excellent results frequently obtained, the dose should not be reduced in adult patients because receptor affinity for this agent varies from tumor type to tumor type and from patient to patient.

[111]In pentetreotide should be slowly injected intravenously. Although the amount of octreotide injected is a fraction of the pharmacologic dose, instances of blood pressure drop and other consequences have been observed in patients whose clinical state is dominated by the secretory products of their neuroendocrine tumor.

Since plasma is rapidly cleared of ^{111}In pentetreotide, one would expect that imaging at 4 hr would be sufficient. Although lesions are frequently identified at this time, many lesions are better identified at 24 hr, probably due to further enhancement of the tumor/background ratio since there is very little plasma activity available for further uptake between 4 and 24 hr. Nevertheless, we have found it advisable to continue to image the potentially involved areas of interest at 4 hr also since it is frequently valuable to have these early images to decide whether clearly identifiable abdominal lesions represents bowel contents (often seen at 24 hr despite bowel preparation) or bowel wall activity, indicating tumors (Figures 10-15 and 10-16).

Since approximately 10% of the ^{111}In DTPA pentetreotide administered is cleared through the hepatobiliary system, a gentle laxative should be administered on the evening after the injection. Although we have not performed a critical comparison of a 1-day versus 2-day laxative protocol, we have the impression that even better results are obtained by pretreating the patient with a laxative before injection of the tracer and again on the evening after the injection but before the 24-hr images.

Dual energy acquisition is performed with 20% windows centered on the 179 and 267 keV photopeaks. In most instances (excepting pituitary or other cranial tumors), high-count static acquisitions should be ob-

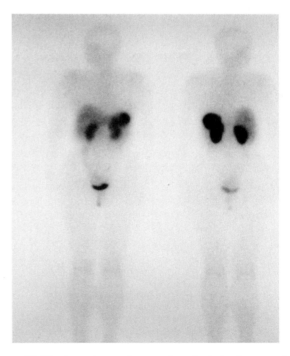

Figure 10-15 Anterior and posterior whole-body scan obtained 4 hr after IV injection of 6.0 mCi ^{111}In pentetreotide. Although patient was referred to locate residual medullary carcinoma of the thyroid, this figure was interpreted as normal. Scan speed 10 cm/min; at 24 hr, scan speed is reduced to 8 cm/min. Normal distribution includes mild hepatic uptake, marked spleen, and renal uptake. At 4 hr, excretion into the bladder is also seen.

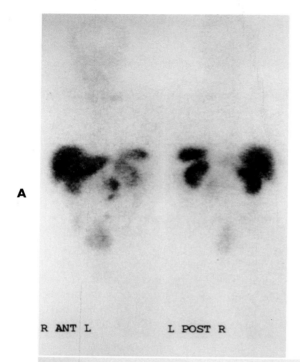

A

R ANT L   L POST R

Figure 10-16 **A,** Anterior and posterior scanning gamma camera images obtained at 24 hr after ^{111}In pentetreotide administration. Acquisition was stopped below the pelvis. Uptake in liver, spleen, and kidneys is seen. There is minimal bladder activity at 24 hr. In addition to the usual organ distribution, there are two foci in the abdomen slightly to the left of the midline. These represent a primary carcinoid tumor in the wall of the small bowel and a regional nodal metastasis. Neither lesion was identified on abdominal CT or contrast studies. The image is too dark to reveal several metastatic foci in the liver. **B,** Transverse, coronal, and sagittal slices after SPECT acquisition of same patient. Three distinct foci are seen within the hepatic parenchyma. The bowel and lymph node focus are confirmed.

B

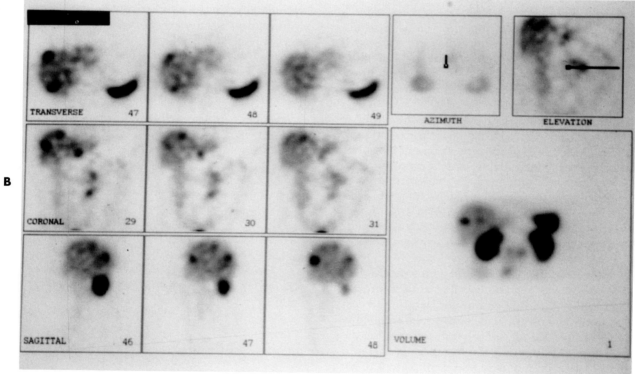

tained of the thorax and abdomen in the anterior and posterior projections for at least 10 min each. These images should be stored digitally for further manipulation if necessary. In recent years, scanning gamma cameras have been increasingly available that produce good quality whole-body images. Although these instruments may produce diagnostic images, neither the nuclear medicine technologist nor physician should conclude

that a negative study excludes disease or provides complete identification of disease involvement. In patients suspected of having functioning or nonfunctioning carcinoid or islet cell tumors, as well as pheochromocytomas or other chromaffin tissue tumors, complete evaluation should include SPECT imaging of the abdomen. Scintigraphy of patients with Ectopic ACTH syndrome should include SPECT of the thorax also unless the somatostatin-receptor positive focus has been identified in the abdomen.

After intravenous administration of ^{111}In DTPA pentetreotide, the material is cleared rapidly from the plasma with a plasma half-time of 20 min. On whole-body images obtained at 4 hr, activity is seen in the liver, spleen, kidneys, and bladder.

Approximately 50% is cleared by the kidneys and appears in the urine. On 24-hr images, the bladder is usually clear and a variable amount of activity, depending upon patient variability and the effort involved in bowel preparation, is seen in the bowel (see Figures 10-15 and 10-16).

The nuclear medicine physician should not assume activity that appears to be due to gall bladder activity or bowel or bladder activity is in fact explained on that basis. Although the conclusion may be frequently correct, many surprising and rewarding diagnoses have been made based on the skeptical requirement that the impression be confirmed. The 4- and 24-hr images provide a good deal of assistance in this regard. Bowel activity does not appear at 4 hrs. Even if a lesion is not clearly identified until the 24-hr images, it usually can be seen in retrospect on the earlier images. This is particularly helpful in evaluating activity in the cecum, which is the most frequent site of carcinoid tumors. Gall bladder activity may be seen at 4 hr but should not be present at 24 hr. Similarly, urinary excretion should not be prominent at 24 hr. Activity in the midline pelvis should be considered suspect particularly in a patient under evaluation for pheochromocytoma.

Activity in the kidneys remains an obstacle because they occupy a large portion of the coronal plane of the abdomen. The right kidney obscures part of the right hepatic lobe and may interfere with the identification of metastases in that region as well as confuse the identification of right adrenal masses and lesions in the head of the pancreas. Tumors in the tail of the pancreas may be obscured by the left kidney. SPECT imaging provides an opportunity to identify lesions that would otherwise be obscured, but there is a limit to the ability of this technique to reconstruct the distribution of activity found in small lesions near the kidneys, which are relatively large and contain a considerable fraction of the administered dose of radioactivity.

Knowledge of the underlying disorder is helpful in directing the search for somatostatin-receptor positive tumors. Since ectopic ACTH syndrome may be due to a bronchial carcinoid, SPECT imaging of the thorax and manipulation of the image intensity and contrast should be performed. Similarly, medullary carcinoma of the thyroid may involve mediastinal lymph nodes that are not visible on standard displays. When there are plasma markers indicating the presence of tumor, the nuclear medicine physician and technologist would be remiss in accepting a negative study without resorting to these manipulations of the patient and acquired images in an effort to identify the site and extent of disease so as to afford the patient every opportunity for a therapeutic decision.

In addition to the technical factors considered above, there are a number of biologic features of somatostatin-receptor imaging that may contribute to false-negative and false-positive findings. Our understanding of somatostatin-receptor biology is still evolving. It is now appreciated that in humans, there are at least five receptor subtypes. These subtypes have different degrees of affinity for the indium-labeled octreotide analogue. Receptors may decrease in affinity or number per cell; indeed, a tumor may de-differentiate to a point where it no longer expresses this receptor. This biologic alteration may account for an accelerated clinical course as the tumor cells would no longer be receptive to the inhibiting effect of somatostatin. Certain drugs may down regulate or cross-react with the receptor so that it can no longer be occupied by the labeled octreotide. It is currently controversial, for example, if a patient who is receiving octreotide therapeutically should have this medication discontinued before therapy. It has been shown that it is possible to identify tumors in patients who receive such treatment and that, in fact, octreotide therapy up regulates the receptors in various cell lines. It is believed that if it is desirable to evaluate the extent and location of disease involvement, octreotide therapy should be discontinued. This belief is based on the conclusive demonstration that the uptake of the labeled agent is specific and readily blocked by unlabeled peptide administered before the labeled form.

False-positive image interpretation is a result of either misreading normal distribution of activity as lesions, for example, interpreting gall bladder, bowel, or bladder activity as lesions, or due to the increased expression of somatostatin receptors on other tissue. Activated lymphocytes express somatostatin receptors. Consequently, positive foci of activity are seen in a variety of disorders with lymphocytic responses such as Graves' orbitopathy, tuberculosis or other pulmonary granulomatous disorders, pulmonary and nonpulmonary sarcoid, changes in the pleura after radiation, activation of respiratory tract lymph nodes during viral upper respiratory infections, and rheumatoid arthritis or tumors expressing somatostatin receptors other than neuroendocrine tumors (lymphomas, breast carcinoma).

ADRENAL GLANDS

The adrenals are located in the retroperitoneum at the superior pole of the kidneys (suprarenal), lying approximately below the eleventh rib. The right adrenal is higher and more posterior than the left (even though the left kidney is frequently higher than the right); the right adrenal is triangular, sitting astride the upper pole of the right kidney. The left adrenal is more crescent shaped and lies anteromedial to the upper pole of the left kidney. The adrenal cortex contains 6% cholesterol by weight, the highest fraction per organ in the body. This cholesterol is the principal metabolic precursor in the synthesis of the adrenal corticosteroids. These organs consist of the adrenal cortex and an interior, neurosecretory adrenal medulla.

ADRENAL CORTEX

Anatomy and Physiology

The adrenal cortex is further classified on histologic section into three zones: glomerulosa, intermedia, and fasciculata, each with specific secretory products. The zona glomerulosa is the site of synthesis of the glucocorticoid cortisone and hydroxycortisone. These corticosteroids have profound effects on body function, metabolism, and the inflammatory and immune responses. Although these compounds have salt-retaining properties, another steroid, aldosterone, with more potent effects on sodium retention and potassium loss, is synthesized in and secreted from the zona intermedia. The zona fasciculata is the site of adrenal androgen synthesis in both men and women.

Destruction of the adrenal glands by tumor, inflammation, or spontaneous atrophy results in adrenal insufficiency with profound sodium loss, inability to respond to external stresses, hypotension, and death. Excessive production of one or more steroid species is a result of adrenal hyperplasia, adenoma, or carcinoma, resulting in a number of well-characterized and dramatic syndromes. Cushing syndrome is a result of excess glucosteroids, Conn syndrome is due to excess aldosterone, and hyperandrogenic syndromes are secondary to excess adrenal elaboration of androgens. In addition to the benign gross adenomas just cited as a pathologic basis for oversecretion, the adrenals can also exhibit a focal or diffuse microadenomatous or even macroadenomatous histologic configuration. The significance of this observation is that it complicates the diagnostic workup, since bilateral hyperplasia is secondary to pituitary stimulation and leads to intense evaluation of the pituitary and hypothalamus for a lesion, whereas bilateral macroadenomas direct therapeutic removal of the functioning adrenal adenoma.

It is ironic that the availability of alternative diagnostic imaging modalities have confounded rather than simplified the differential diagnosis and management decision. Abdominal CT and MRI regularly identify adrenal (benign) masses. It becomes necessary to define the functional significance of these masses. These findings have earned the name *incidentalomas,* since they might *not* be responsible for the observed state of steroid excess. This defines an even greater role for a functional imaging technique.

Nuclear Medicine Procedures

Adrenal cortical imaging is indicated in clinical situations characterized by increased cortisolism, increased aldosteronism, and increased virilization when the source of the hypersecretion of the appropriate hormone is not clear. Identification of the site of adrenal hormone synthesis initiates adrenal cortical imaging with radiotracers. The unique dependence on cholesterol as the biochemical precursor of the steroid hormones provides the tool to accomplish this task. Since it had been demonstrated that ^{14}C cholesterol injected intravenously in animals is incorporated into newly synthesized steroids, as early as 1969 Sarkar, Beierwaltes, and colleagues[29] evaluated the utility of ^{131}I iodocholesterol as a marker of the site of cholesterol synthesis. This compound resulted in ratios of adrenal/liver of 168:1 and adrenal/kidney of 300:1. Subsequently, it was identified that a number of analogs were produced during the labeling process and that one of these, ^{131}I-6-beta-iodomethyl-19-norcholesterol (^{131}I NP-59) had even greater avidity for adrenal cortical functioning tissue as well as greater in vivo stability and less deiodination than the original iodocholesterol compound.[10]

Since the total demand for an adrenal cortical imaging agent is assumed to be rather limited, no commercial source of this agent is available. In addition, the costs associated with premarket evaluation and the FDA approval process are prohibitive. Since the late 1970s, however, the Radiochemistry Section of the Nuclear Medicine Department at the University of Michigan has supplied ^{131}I NP-59 as a radiochemical to investigators with appropriate radionuclide possession licenses. Human use in the United States requires physician-sponsored investigational new drug (IND) status and institutional human use committee approval for use as an investigational agent. Via this mechanism a number of reports have appeared in the literature demonstrating clinical utility in the differential diagnosis of adrenal hyperplasia, adenoma, or carcinoma in patients with syndromes of suspected adrenal corticoid excess.

[131]I NP-59 is available in 3 mCi batches and is administered as a 1-mCi dose to the average adult patient (1.7 m²), correcting for size if necessary on a weight or body-surface basis. The ^{131}I NP-59 is a cholesterol derivative, insoluble in aqueous solutions, and therefore prepared in an alcohol-saline solution with the solubilizing agent Tween-80, a polyoxyethylene sorbital fatty acid ester. The material should be used as soon as possible after receipt to minimize aliquot volume. It should be injected slowly (2 to 5 min recommended), since the Tween-80 can release endogenous histamine, resulting in characteristic manifestations—shortness of breath, chest tightness, palpitations, vasodilatation, nausea,

and dizziness for 5 to 20 min after injection. In susceptible patients pretreatment with oral benadryl might be indicated.

Clinical sites are expected to confirm radiochemical purity with a simple, thin-layer chromatography (TLC) procedure using silica gel and chloroform. The ratio of solute migration to solvent flow, for example, relative flow (R_f) of ^{131}I NP-59 in this system is 0.4 and the R_f of free iodide ion is 0.0, indicates no elution with chloroform. Preparations with more than 10% free iodide should be rejected. Nevertheless, some elution of iodine bound to ^{131}I NP-59 occurs, and patients should be pretreated with Lugol solution: 3 drops daily for 2 days before tracer administration. Lugol solution should be administered daily for 6 days throughout the study.

The role of pretreatment with dexamethasone depends on the patient's degree of hypercortisolism and the clinical indication for ^{131}I NP-59 imaging. Patients with clinical Cushing syndrome need not receive additional corticosteroids once hypercortisolism is documented, since the elevated level of endogenous cortisol provides the appropriate physiologic setting to identify nonsuppressible tissue. Other patients who are being evaluated for the site of excess production of aldosterone or adrenal androgens should receive steroid suppression in the form of dexamethasone: 1 mg four times a day for 7 days before ^{131}I NP-59 administration and throughout the study.

Patients should be injected in a fasting state (overnight) or at least have avoided fatty food ingestion, since elevated serum cholesterol in excess of 400 mg/dl interferes with tracer transport by lipoproteins and uptake by the lipoprotein receptors.

Patients are imaged at 72 hr with appropriate instrumentation (i.e., gamma camera, high-energy collimator, and 20% energy window centered at 364 keV). At this interval there is usually sufficient plasma clearance to provide good quality images with 75,000-150,000 counts in 10 to 15 min (Figures 10-17 to 10-19). If the right adrenal location is obscured by gallbladder or colonic activity, additional images can be obtained at 96 hr or later. A lateral view can be obtained to assist in evaluating if the asymmetric activity between the left and right adrenals is due to the more anterior location of the left adrenal and in correcting for depth if the images are digitized and quantitative analysis is performed. Asymmetry of greater than 2:1 is indicative of adenoma. Adrenal uptake greater than 0.3% injected dose is abnormal.

The normal distribution of ^{131}I NP-59 reflects lipoprotein-receptor uptake, with a significant fraction being removed by the liver, excreted into the bile, and subsequently appearing in the bowel. In the presence of elevated cortisol levels, normal adrenal tissue is not visualized. The appearance of activity bilaterally usually indicates or confirms bilateral adrenal hyperplasia. This is usually associated with elevated plasma ACTH levels,

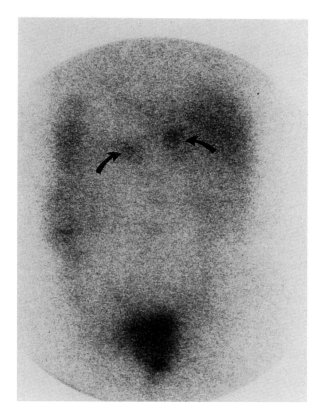

Figure 10-17 Adrenal cortical imaging. Bilateral adrenal activity 72 hr after 1 mCi ^{131}I NP-59 in a 63-year-old woman with clinical Cushing syndrome and normal CT of the adrenals. A CT of the brain and skull revealed a small intrapituitary adenoma, producing bilateral adrenal hyperplasia. Excreted radiotracer is also seen in the liver, large bowel, and rectum.

but ACTH radioimmunoassay might not be available. Bilateral functioning adrenal tissue in the absence of elevated ACTH suggests bilateral adrenal microadenomas or macroadenomas. Unilateral uptake identifies the site of a functioning adenoma, whereas the failure to identify functioning adrenal tissue despite proper technique in a hypercortisol patient increases the likelihood of functioning adrenal carcinoma as the underlying pathologic lesion. These tumors are capable of enormous rates of steroid synthesis even though they may be below the sensitivity of this procedure. Benign adenomas weighing less than 1 g have been identified. In patients evaluated for aldosteronism, low-renin hypertension, and virilization syndromes, uptake in a dexamethasone-suppressed patient identifies the site or sites of excess steroid synthesis. Although adenomas are typically unilateral, bilateral uptake suggests either hyperplasia or a bilaterally adenomatous process. ^{131}I NP-59 imaging has been particularly useful in providing direction to the surgeon as to whether a unilateral or bilateral approach is necessary because the usual anatomic modalities might not identify microadenomas or macroadenomas (see Figure 10-19).

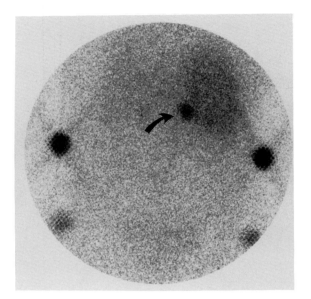

Figure 10-18   Adrenal cortical imaging with 1 mCi ^{131}I NP-59. Posterior abdominal view in a 67-year-old woman who received oral dexamethasone, 1 mg daily for 7 days before radiotracer administration and throughout the study. Intense activity is seen in the right adrenal bed *(arrow)*. At surgery an adrenal adenoma was resected. No increased activity is seen in the region of the left adrenal. A faint outline of hepatic parenchyma is seen. The other foci represent markers at the lower margin of the rib cage and superior iliac crests.

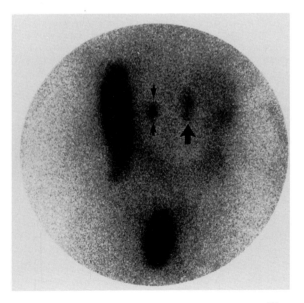

Figure 10-19   Adrenal cortical imaging with 1 mCi ^{131}I NP-59. Posterior abdominal view in a 55-year-old woman with Cushing syndrome. The patient had a mass in the right adrenal cortex on CT. The scintigraphic study demonstrates a large area of uptake in the right adrenal and a second area in the left adrenal *(arrows)*. These findings suggested a bilateral surgical exploration. At surgery a 1.7 cm^2 macroadenoma was found on the right adrenal and a 0.67 cm^2 macroadenoma was found in the left adrenal. A significant amount of excreted radiotracer is seen in the ascending, transverse, and (most prominent) descending colon and rectum (midline).

For the identification of adrenal hyperplasia and adenoma in Cushing disease, the technique has been reported to be 81% to 100% accurate. In patients with aldosterone-producing lesions the specificity for lateralization is high, but the overall sensitivity is relatively low (approximately 50%). The failure to detect an adenoma in a patient suspected of hyperaldosteronism does not exclude the possibility of such disease. In one series of 37 patients evaluated because of excessive androgen production, 15 had bilateral uptake identified in less than 5 days. All were confirmed to have bilateral adrenal hyperplasia. Five of the 37 had unilateral uptake and 4 had adenoma. The remaining 17 patients had only minimal uptake, which was not clearly apparent until at least 5 days after injection; all had normal adrenals.

The radiation absorbed dose per mCi ^{131}I NP-59 administered is whole body 1.2, adrenals 25, ovaries 8, testes 2.3, and liver 2.4 rad.

ADRENAL MEDULLA

Anatomy and Physiology

The adrenal medulla is typically located within the adrenal gland surrounded by the adrenal cortex. The medullary tissue is quite small; on sectioning the area of the adrenal cortex/adrenal medulla is approximately 10:1. The adrenal medullary tissue synthesizes and secretes the catecholamines epinephrine and norepinephrine, hormones that maintain (or increase) smooth muscle tone, heart rate and force of contraction, and other physiologic responses associated with stress. Benign or malignant functioning tumors of this tissue are known as *pheochromocytomas,* which are hyperplastic nodules 1 cm in diameter or larger. Below this size the entity is defined as macronodular hyperplasia. These tumors elaborate excessive amounts of epinephrine or norepinephrine, producing a classic picture of undesirable symptoms, particularly hypertension and other consequences of excessive catecholamine product. Pheochromocytoma occurs as an apparently spontaneous benign or malignant tumor of the adrenal medulla and is a frequent component of the hereditary syndrome multiple endocrine neoplasia (MEN) types IIa and IIb. Despite advances in clinical chemistry that make direct assay of catecholamines, and even specific assays of plasma and urinary epinephrine and norepinephrine, more readily available, the disease is often a clinical enigma, frequently not diagnosed until postmortem examination. The small size of the adrenal medullary tissue and a propensity for ectopic sites make diagnosis even by CT and MRI unreliable. The potential for aberrant distribution is documented in Figure 10-20, in which 24 of 107 pheochromocytomas were found outside of the adrenal glands.[23]

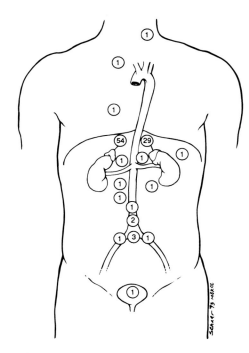

Figure 10-20 In a large surgical series pheochromocytoma was found in the adrenal bed in 83 of 100 patients (3 patients had bilateral pheochromocytoma) and in extraadrenal sites in 17 patients. These sites were distributed principally along the paraaortic tissue as far caudally as the bifurcation and iliac vessels and cephalad above the aortic arch. In one patient a pheochromocytoma was found in the bladder wall. (Redrawn from data reported by Melicow MM: *Cancer* 40:1987-2004, 1977.)

Nuclear Medicine Procedures

The role of nuclear medicine is to provide a physiologic imaging technique that identifies the site or sites of excessive neurosecretory activity. Since the last edition of this text, the FDA has approved the use of ^{131}I methyliodobenzylguanidine (^{131}I MIBG) for clinical use as a diagnostic imaging agent to identify normal, ectopic, or hyperfunctioning adrenal medullary tissue. This material is the product of many years of dedicated research by chemists in that department under the leadership of William Beierwaltes. The saga is documented in several recent reviews[7,8] which demonstrate the clinical utility of this technique. More recently, a group at the University of Michigan has described also the synthesis of ^{123}I MIBG, but the short half-life of ^{123}I precludes availability of this material except at institutions prepared to synthesize the radiotracer themselves, provide evidence of sterility and pyrogenicity, and seek approval from institutional approval committees and local regulatory agencies.

MIBG has some structural similarities to norepinephrine. Norepinephrine is usually secreted by adrenergic tissue, and a portion is reabsorbed by that special tissue and stored in adrenergic granules. Although MIBG has little or no pharmacologic effect and does not bind significantly at postsynaptic receptors, it is incorporated into the adrenergic storage granules.

Whereas ^{123}I MIBG would seem to be advantageous in terms of increased photon and hence information flux, the short half-life limits delayed imaging to 24 hr after the injection, whereas it is possible to image patients with ^{131}I MIBG at 3 to 5 days after radiopharmaceutical administration. The longer interval provides for an improved target-to-background ratio and hence images of potentially greater diagnostic accuracy. Since the blood flow to the adrenal medulla is only a small fraction of the circulation, a considerable interval is necessary for sufficient material to be taken up and for plasma and soft tissue activity to fall sufficiently to identify localization.

Labeling with ^{131}I, therefore, provides a tracer with a physical half-life that makes patient imaging several days after tracer administration possible.

Lugol solution is given to the patient to block thyroid uptake of released iodine at least 1 day before ^{131}I MIBG (or ^{123}I MIBG) administration; Lugol solution is continued for 7 days thereafter. The adult dose of ^{131}I MIBG is 0.5 mCi, slowly injected intravenously over 15 sec. Patients less than 18 years of age receive a reduced dose based on body weight, but the dose is calculated based on a full adult dose of 1.0 mCi, that is, 1.0 mCi/70 Kg with a maximum dose of 0.5 mCi. Patients are imaged with a gamma camera fitted with a collimator suitable for the 364 keV gamma emission from [131]I. There is considerable difference in the sensitivity and resolution of collimators designed to image in the 364 keV range. If a choice is available, the nuclear medicine department should opt for greater count rate. In fact, given the small dose of ^{131}I available, certain ^{131}I collimators, which are ideal to image after high doses of ^{131}I, actually produce uninterpretable images and should not be used. If the department elects to use this newly available agent, evaluation of collimator response is essential before its use for patient studies. A 15% to 20% energy window centered at 364 keV is used. For detection of pheochromocytoma the entire thorax, abdomen, and pelvis should be imaged anteriorly and posteriorly with ^{131}I capsules (approximately 5 μCi) used as markers at the axillae, lower rib markings, and iliac crests. The patient should be encouraged to void before imaging. Since total counts per view depends on many factors, acquisitions for a reasonable time interval (i.e., 20 min/view) are appropriate. The images should be digitized in at least a 128 × 128 matrix to allow subsequent optimization of images. Imaging should be performed on day 1 (24 hr after injection of the tracer), day 3, and day 7 if necessary. The normal distribution of ^{131}I MIBG includes the heart because of the rich neural innervation, the liver, spleen, salivary glands, and bladder; the latter two sites are due to excretion of free iodine eluted from the tracer. In normal subjects the adrenal medulla is either not visualized or seen only transiently on the first day of imag-

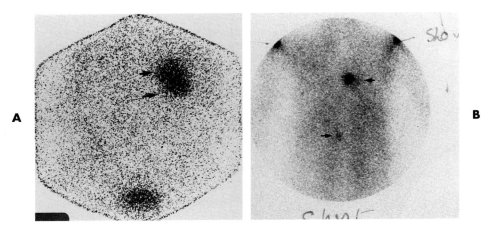

Figure 10-21 Imaging at 72 hr after 500 μCi ^{131}I MIBG. **A,** Gamma camera view of the anterior abdomen in a patient with a pheochromocytoma arising from the left adrenal medulla *(arrows)*. **B,** Gamma camera view of the posterior thoracolumbar region in another patient with a recurrent malignant pheochromocytoma. A small residual focus is seen in the left adrenal bed region, and a prominent intense focus is seen in the right thoracic paraspinal region *(arrows)*.

ing. Significant (abnormal) uptake persists on subsequent images, and the contrast improves with time. Day 3 (72 hr) usually provides the most useful images with maximal contrast between foci of activity and background. Intense tracer uptake is seen in pheochromocytoma, which can be identified in the adrenal bed or elsewhere in the abdomen or thorax (see Figures 10-20 and 10-21). Persistent or increased uptake bilaterally suggests bilateral pheochromocytoma, although this should not be considered if only faint uptake is seen at 24 hr, which does not increase in activity or contrast. In malignant pheochromocytoma, uptake is seen in metastases in the liver, bone, lymph nodes, heart, lungs, and mediastinum, as well as other sites. At the University of Michigan, analysis of a 400-patient series with malignant pheochromocytoma demonstrated a sensitivity of 92.4% and a 100% specificity.[7,8] ^{131}I MIBG is also useful to determine the extent of involvement of neuroblastoma, a malignant tumor of childhood that can be widely disseminated.

^{111}In DTPA pentetreotide (*Octreoscan*, Mallinckrodt) has also been used to image pheochromocytoma. In limited series, it is reported to be equally sensitive for the detection of this tissue based on the presence of somatostatin receptors on the cell surface. Since the emitted gamma energy of ^{111}In is less than the emission from ^{131}I, it should be used first if both agents are going to be used. Imaging is complete in 24 hr, whereas ^{131}I MIBG imaging may require images 5 days after tracer administration. If a study is positive in identifying ectopic or recurrent pheochromocytoma, it is probably correct. A negative study, however, should be followed with ^{131}I MIBG imaging before it can be concluded that the case is truly negative. Assuming that the Octreoscan procedure is performed well, it is still possible to have a false-negative result because pheochromocytma frequently expresses somatostatin-receptor subtypes other than subtype 2, which recognizes Octreotide. Other pitfalls include interpretation errors as the pheochromocytoma, initial or malignant recurrences, may be localized in unusual sites (see Figure 10-20).

GONADS

Anatomy and Physiology

The gonads are the principal source of sex hormones, accounting for the differentiation of male and female sexual characteristics. In the female the ovaries are found in the pelvis, one on each side, near the termination of the fallopian tubes. As a result of complex endocrine orchestration, an ovum matures and is released from one of the ovaries to the opening of the fallopian tube each month during a 35- to 40-year interval after sexual maturity. The ovaries produce estrogens, several structurally related steroid hormones that control and maintain secondary sexual characteristics and other metabolic effects such as skeletal osteoid. In the adult male the testes produce sperm and elaborate testosterone, which produces the male secondary characteristics. The testes are normally found in the scrotum, but one or both can fail to descend adequately from the pelvis.

Scrotal imaging using ^{99m}Tc pertechnetate to demonstrate perfusion of the testes is useful to identify torsion of the testes and missed torsion and to differentiate these situations from orchitis or epididymitis (see Chapters 12 and 18).

SUMMARY

In this chapter the elements of endocrine organ anatomy and physiology and the nuclear medicine techniques available for the evaluation of these organs have been reviewed. Imaging and in vivo function tests have been dealt with primarily, as well as radioiodine therapy of thyroid diseases. These procedures are based on nuclear medicine, a medical discipline and technology that requires particular training and expertise of the technologists and physicians involved in the use of these procedures for patient care. The physiologic basis for the technology has been elaborated, as well as the technologic aspects of the nuclear medicine procedures presently in use to characterize human physiology in health and disease.

REFERENCES

1. Ain KB: Thyroid cancer: a lethal endocrine neoplasm: biology and management of differentiated thyroid carcinoma of the follicular cells, *Ann Intern Med* 115:133-147, 1991.
2. Andros G, Harper PV, Lathrop KA, et al: Pertechnetate-99m localization in man with applications to thyroid scanning and the study of thyroid physiology, *J Clin Endocrinol Metab* 35:250-256, 1972.
3. Atkins HL, Richards P: Assessment of thyroid function and anatomy with ^{99m}Tc-pertechnetate, *J Nucl Med* 9:7-9, 1968.
4. Attie JN, Kahn A, Rumancik WM, et al: Preoperative localization of parathyroid adenomas, *Am J Surg* 156:323-326, 1988.
5. Becker DV, Charkes ND, Dworkin H, et al: Procedure guideline for thyroid scintigraphy: 1.0, *J Nucl Med* 37:1264-1266, 1996.
6. Becker DV, Charkes ND, Dworkin H, et al: Procedure guideline for thyroid uptake measurement: 1.0, *J Nucl Med* 37:1266-1268, 1996.
7. Becker DV, Charkes ND, Dworkin H, et al: Procedure guideline for extended scintigraphy for differentiated thyroid cancer: 1.0, *J Nucl Med* 37:1269-1271, 1996.
8. Becker DV, Hurley JR: Current status of radioiodine (^{131}I) treatment of hyperthyroidism. In Freeman L, Weissmann HS, eds: *Nuclear medicine annual 1982,* New York, 1982, Raven Press.
9. Becker DV, Hurley JR: Radioiodine treatment of hyperthyroidism. In Gottschalk A, Hoffer PB, Potchen EJ, eds: *Diagnostic nuclear medicine, vol 2,* Baltimore, 1988, Williams & Wilkins.
10. Beierwaltes WH: Clinical applications of 131-I labeled metaiodobenzylguanidine. In Hoffer PB, ed: *1987 Year Book of nuclear medicine,* Chicago, 1987, Year Book Medical.
11. Beierwaltes WH: Endocrine imaging: parathyroid, adrenal cortex and medulla, and other endocrine tumors, part II, *J Nucl Med* 32:1627-1639, 1991.
12. Beierwaltes WH, Nishiyama RH, Thompson NW, et al: Survival time and "cure" in papillary and follicular carcinoma with distant metastases: statistics following University of Michigan therapy, *J Nucl Med* 23:561-568, 1982.
13. Berson SA, Yalow RS: Immunoassay of endogenous plasma insulin in man, *J Clin Invest* 35:170-177, 1960.
14. Berson SA, Yalow RS, Glick SA, et al: Immunoassay of protein and peptide hormones, *Metabolism* 13:1135-1140, 1964.
15. Goldsmith SJ: Thyroid: in vivo tests of function and imaging. In Rothfield B, ed: *Nuclear medicine: endocrinology,* Philadelphia, 1978, JB Lippincott.
16. Hertz S, Roberts A, Evans RD: Radioactive iodine as an indicator in the study of thyroid physiology, *Proc Soc Exp Biol Med* 38:510-514, 1938.
17. Krenning EP, Bakker WH, Kooij PPM, et al: Somatostatin receptor scintigraphy with Indium-111 DTPA-D-phe-1-octreotide in man: metabolism, dosimetry and comparison with iodine-123-tyr-3-octreotide, *J Nucl Med* 33:652-658, 1992.
18. Krenning EP, Kwekkeboom DJ, Bakker WH, et al: Somatostatin receptor scintigraphy with [In-111 DTPA-D-Phe-1]- and [I-123-Tyr3] octreotide: the Rotterdam experience with more than 1000 patients, *Eur J Nucl Med* 20:716-731, 1993.
19. Kusic Z, Becker DV, Saenger EL, et al: Comparison of technetium-99m and iodine-123 imaging of thyroid nodules: correlation with pathologic findings, *J Nucl Med* 31:393-399, 1990.
20. Leeper RD, Shimaoka K: Treatment of metastatic thyroid cancer, *J Clin Endocrinol Metab* 9:383-404, 1980.
21. Maxon HR, Englaro EE, Thomas SR, et al: Radioiodine-131 therapy for well-differentiated thyroid cancer—a quantitative radiation dosimetric approach: outcome and validation in 85 patients, *J Nucl Med* 33:1132-1137, 1992.
22. Maxon HR, Thomas SR, Hertzberg VS, et al: Relation between radiation dose and outcome of radioiodine therapy for thyroid cancer, *N Engl J Med* 309:937-941, 1938.
23. Melicow MM: One hundred cases of pheochromocytoma (107 tumors) at the Columbia-Presbyterian Medical Center, *Cancer* 40:1987-2004, 1977.
24. O'Doherty MJ, Kettle AG, Wells P, et al: Parathyroid imaging with technetium-99m-sestamibi: preoperative localization and tissue uptake studies, *J Nucl Med* 33:313-318, 1992.
25. Okerland MD, Sheldon K, Corpuz S, et al: A new method with high sensitivity and specificity for localization of abnormal parathyroid glands, *Ann Surg* 200:381-383, 1984.

26. Pacini F, Lippi L, Formica N, et al: Therapeutic doses of iodine-131 reveal undiagnosed metastases in thyroid cancer patients with detectable serum-thyroglobin levels, *J Nucl Med* 28:1888-1891, 1987.

27. Ridgeway EC: Clinician's evaluation of a solitary thyroid nodule, *J Clin Endocrinol Metab* 74:231-235, 1992.

28. Samaan NA, Schultz PN, Haynie TP, et al: Pulmonary metastases of differentiated thyroid carcinoma: treatment results in 101 patients, *J Clin Endocrinol Metab* 60:376-381, 1985.

29. Sarkar SD, Beierwaltes WH, Ice RD, et al: A new and superior adrenal scanning agent, NP-59, *J Nucl Med* 16:1038-1042, 1975.

30. Seidlin SM, Marinelli LD, Oshry E: Radioactive iodine therapy: effect on functioning metastases of adenocarcinoma of the thyroid, *JAMA* 132:838-841, 1946.

31. Snyder J, Gorman C, Scanlon P: Thyroid remnant ablation: questionable pursuit of an ill-defined goal, *J Nucl Med* 24:659-665, 1983.

32. Strashun A, Vaquer RA, Goldsmith SJ: Localization of parathyroid adenomata by thallium-201 and technetium-99m subtraction scintigraphy, *Mt Sinai J Med* 55:171-175, 1988.

33. Taillefer R, Boucher Y, Potvin C, et al: Detection and localization of parathyroid adenomas in patients with hyperparathyroidism using a single radionuclide imaging procedure with technetium-99m sestimibi (double phase study), *J Nucl Med* 33:1801-1807, 1992.

34. van Royen EA, Verhoeff NPLG, Meylaerts SAE, et al: Indium-111 DTPA octretide uptake measured in normal and abnormal pituitary glands, *J Nucl Med* 37:1449-1451, 1996.

35. Waxman A, Ramanna L, Chapman N, et al: The significance of I-131 scan dose in patients with thyroid cancer: determination of ablation: concise communication, *J Nucl Med* 22:861-865, 1981.

David J. Phegley, Roger H. Secker-Walker

chapter *11*

Respiratory System

Objectives

Possess a general understanding of normal lung anatomy and physiology.

Understand how the blood flow within the lung is altered by pathology.

Understand the mechanism of perfusion imaging.

Be aware of the special care needed for perfusion imaging of patients with severe pulmonary hypertension.

Understand the patient preparation requirements for lung imaging.

Know the importance of the number of particles administered for perfusion imaging.

Understand the effect of time and decay on particle count.

Be aware of the effects of gravity on particle distribution in the lung.

Know the importance of communicating the method of injection to the interpreting physician.

Be aware of the various techniques for ventilation studies.

Understand the limitations and advantages of the various ventilation radiopharmaceuticals.

Possess an understanding of the advantages of the combined diagnostic information of ventilation and perfusion imaging studies.

Understand how lung imaging studies are used to diagnose disease.

Possess a knowledge of the general applications of lung imaging.

Be aware of the various references on the subject of lung imaging.

*R*egional ventilation was first studied by Knipping and colleagues using radioactive xenon almost 40 years ago.[29] Much of our present understanding of regional lung function, both in health and in disease, is based on the use of this gas and other radionuclides by respiratory physiologists working in London and Montreal.[6,46] During this time considerable advances were also made in understanding the detailed anatomy of the lung[50] and in appreciating the mechanical interrelationships of airways, alveoli, and the thoracic cage.[32] Nonrespiratory functions have also been studied, particularly those dealing with lung defense mechanisms[18] and the metabolic activity of the lung.[15]

The development of macroaggregated albumin, at first labeled with iodine-131[44] and later with technetium-99m, led to the widespread use of perfusion scanning for the diagnosis of pulmonary embolism. The use of radioactive xenon to study regional ventilation has spread from the research laboratory to routine use in the last 20 years. This combined insight into regional ventilation and regional blood flow allows more accurate assessment of the disturbed physiology and, at the same time, increases both the diagnostic sensitivity and specificity of the procedure.[3,33]

NORMAL ANATOMY AND PHYSIOLOGY

The lungs, shown diagramatically in Figure 11-1 and schematically in Figure 11-2, lie within the thorax, protected by the rib cage. The ribs offer support to the intercostal muscles and the diaphragm. It is the action of these muscles that enlarges the chest during normal breathing. Air enters the lungs, first passing through the nose or mouth and then the pharynx, larynx, and trachea. It is warmed, moistened, and filtered during this time. The trachea divides into right and left mainstem bronchi, and these in turn divide into lobar bronchi (upper, middle, and lower on the right, and upper and lower on the left). The airways continue to divide in a somewhat irregular fashion, about 16 times from

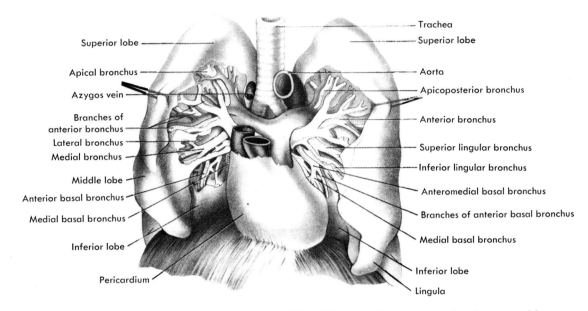

Figure 11-1 Anatomic diagram showing relationships of heart, pulmonary vessels, airways, and lungs.

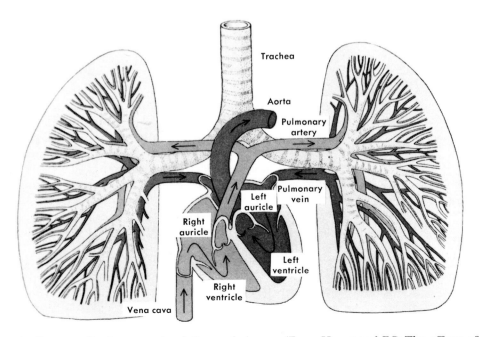

Figure 11-2 Schematic diagram of pulmonary circulation and airways. (From Hammond EC: The effects of smoking, *Sci Am* 39:207, 1962. Copyright 1962 by Scientific American, Inc. All rights reserved.)

the trachea to the terminal bronchioles and a further four to seven times, as respiratory bronchioles, alveolar ducts, and alveolar sacs (Figure 11-3). Bronchi have cartilage in their walls, which distinguishes them from bronchioles. Smooth muscle, collagen, and elastic fibers encircle the airways from the trachea to the alveolar ducts. The collagen and elastic fibers continue to the periphery of the lung as a three-dimensional latticework in the walls of the alveoli. Alveoli first appear in the respiratory bronchioles but are most numerous around the alveolar sacs.

The alveoli are packed together like the cells of a honeycomb (Figure 11-4). Each alveolus offers some support to its neighbors, as well as through the collagen and elastic fibers to the airways. This structural arrangement and the surfactant, which lines the surface of the alveoli, are responsible for the elastic properties of the lungs and provide the main force for expiration during normal breathing.

The bronchial epithelium is lined by ciliated cells interspersed with a few goblet cells and the openings of bronchial glands.[9] The alveoli, where oxygen and carbon dioxide are exchanged, are lined by alveolar type I cells. These are very thin and spread over the surface of the alveoli. Pulmonary capillaries lie in contact with these cells (see Figure 11-4). Two other important cells are found in the alveoli—alveolar type II cells, which make surfactant, and alveolar macrophages, which remove particulate matter that reaches the alveoli.

The pulmonary artery divides to form the right and left pulmonary arteries. These vessels follow the bronchi and bronchioles, dividing with them until they reach the alveoli (see Figure 11-2). Each alveolus, and there are about 250 to 300 million in an adult, is supplied by a terminal pulmonary arteriole, which has a diameter of about 35 μm and which gives rise to about 1000 capillaries per alveolus. The capillaries are 7 to 10 μm in diameter. The distance between the alveolar surface and the capillaries is only about 0.05 to 0.1 μm. The pulmonary capillaries drain into the pulmonary veins and from there into the left atrium.[50]

The lungs also receive blood from the aorta, through the bronchial arteries. These are small but also follow the bronchial tree as far as the respiratory bronchioles. They supply nourishment to the bronchi, surrounding blood vessels, nerves, and lymphatics. Anastomoses are formed between the bronchial and pulmonary circulations at the capillary level around the respiratory bronchioles. Most of the blood from the bronchial circulation drains into the left atrium through the pulmonary veins.[13]

The lungs are richly supplied with lymphatics. Some course over the pleura and pass into the lungs, whereas others arise in the interstitial spaces of the lungs. Lymphatic vessels travel toward the hilum of the lung, with airways and blood vessels, reaching lymph nodes there and then continuing into the mediastinum.

The volume of air breathed out in a normal breath is called the *tidal volume,* and the volume of air in the lungs at the end of a normal breath is called *functional residual capacity. Total lung capacity* is the volume of air in the lungs when as much air has been inhaled as possible, whereas *residual volume* is the volume of air left in the lungs after a complete exhalation. These volumes are measured by standard pulmonary function tests.[49]

During tidal breathing only a small proportion (about 10% to 15%) of the air within the lungs is exchanged with each breath. More is exchanged with deeper breaths or a faster rate of breathing. About one third of each breath is wasted because the air in the bronchial tubes at the end of the breath does not reach the alveoli. This is called *anatomic dead space* because it takes no part in gas exchange.

The structure of the lung is well suited to its chief function of gas exchange, that is, delivering oxygen to the bloodstream and removing carbon dioxide so that the body's cellular metabolism can continue. Despite the numerous divisions of the bronchial tree, the resistance to air flow is low. Most of this resistance (80% to

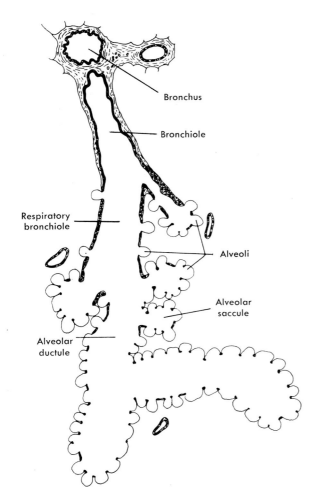

Figure 11-3 Schematic cross section of branching of airways from terminal bronchiole to alveolar ductules, saccules, and alveoli.

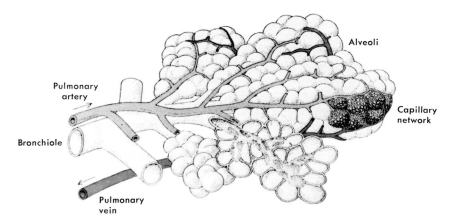

Figure 11-4 Schematic drawing of peripheral airways and alveoli and their accompanying blood vessels. (From Hammond EC: The effects of smoking, *Sci Am* 39:207, 1962. Copyright 1962. Copyright by Scientific American, Inc. All rights reserved.)

90%) is found in the larger bronchial tubes, where air flow is turbulent. It requires only small pressure changes within the chest for normal breathing. The change in volume for a change in pressure is called *compliance,* which is a measurement of the ease with which air enters or leaves the lungs. The pressure in the pulmonary artery is considerably lower than that in the systemic circulation, and there is very little resistance to blood flow. The entire cardiac output passes through the pulmonary capillaries, in an almost continuous sheet, in the alveolar walls.

These thin walls, which have a surface area of 70 to 80 m², offer an almost negligible barrier to the diffusion of gases from alveoli to blood or vice versa.

As the lung ages, its elastic properties diminish and the smaller bronchial tubes tend to collapse during a full expiration. The volume of air in the lungs when closure begins is the *closing capacity.* Both radioactive xenon and nonradioactive tracer gases, for example, nitrogen, helium, and argon, have been used to measure this volume. Early damage to the small airways from any cause increases this volume, an increase that is therefore a sensitive but nonspecific indication of small-airways disease.[4,10]

In the 1960s it was shown that both ventilation and blood flow are not evenly distributed within the lungs. Posture and the direction of gravity or of acceleration play an important part in healthy lungs.

In the upright position ventilation of the upper parts of the lung increases about 1.5 to 2.0 times from the upper third of the lung to the lower third.[6,28,48] In the supine position the distribution is more uniform from top to bottom, but there is then a gradient from front to back. If a person lies on one side, more air is exchanged in the lower part of the lungs compared with the upper part. The distribution is modified by exercise, the rate of breathing, and diseases affecting the bronchial tubes or the lung parenchyma.

In the upright position blood flow increases threefold to fivefold from the upper parts of the lung to the base. In fact, the upper one fourth of the lungs gets very little blood flow at rest while sitting upright.[5,48] In the supine position blood flow is more uniform from apex to base, but then a gradient exists from front to back. Lying on one side will cause more blood to flow to the lowermost part of the lung. Apart from the disease states that usually alter blood flow within the lung, exercise will cause a more even distribution. Lowering the oxygen tension in the bronchial tubes also alters blood flow by causing local constriction of the pulmonary arterioles and diverting blood flow away from this region.

The distribution of blood flow within the upright lung shows the largest gradient from top to bottom when the measurements are made at total lung capacity. At functional residual capacity, blood flow increases from the apex to about the level of the fourth or fifth rib and then decreases a little toward the base. If the distribution of blood flow is measured at residual volume, it is almost even throughout the lungs.[24]

The ratio in which ventilation and blood flow are mixed is not uniform from top to bottom in the upright position. Ventilation exceeds blood flow by about 2:1 to 3:1 in the upper zones. In the midzones they are more closely matched, whereas in the lower parts of the lung blood flow exceeds ventilation. The closer the matching of ventilation and blood flow, the better the oxygenation of the blood. Whenever ventilation is reduced in comparison to blood flow, the oxygenation of the blood is also reduced. If ventilation exceeds blood flow, the red cells quickly take up their maximum load of oxygen (4 molecules per hemoglobin molecule, or 1.34 ml of O_2 per gram of hemoglobin), and the excess ventilation is then wasted.[49]

PATHOPHYSIOLOGY

The distribution of blood flow within the lungs is altered by many disease processes affecting either the

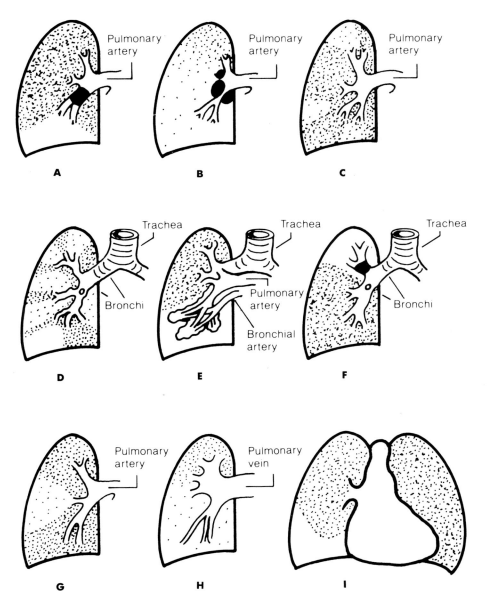

Figure 11-5 Schematic representation of major mechanisms of abnormal perfusion scans **(A-I)**. *Spotted areas,* blood flow; *clear areas,* regions with absent blood flow.

lungs, the heart, the chest wall, or the diaphragm. The mechanisms underlying these disturbances are outlined schematically in Figure 11-5. Figure 11-5, *A* to *C,* represents disease processes affecting the pulmonary vasculature. The most obvious cause, represented by *A,* is pulmonary embolism, in which the embolus (usually a small blood clot) blocks one of the branches of the pulmonary artery so that no blood can flow past this obstruction. The defect produced on the perfusion scan corresponds to the anatomic segment or lobe of the lung involved.

Other causes of defects in blood flow from disease processes affecting the pulmonary vessels are shown in Figure 11-5, *B* and *C. B* represents enlarged lymph nodes at the hilum of the lung, as might be seen in

advanced lung cancer, causing compression of the pulmonary vessels and hence alterations in blood flow. *C* represents disease processes involving the smaller pulmonary arterioles, for example, a vasculitis or multiple small pulmonary emboli.

D to *F* in Figure 11-5 represent diseases in which the initial problem is in the airways (or bronchial tubes) and blood flow is reduced as a result of the diminution in ventilation. *D* is a composite diagram to represent the changes seen in chronic bronchitis, emphysema, and asthma. *E* represents bronchiectasis in which there is dilatation of the peripheral bronchi and surrounding inflammation. The bronchial arteries to the affected region are often greatly enlarged. There is virtually no blood flow through the pulmonary artery and very little exchange of air in the bronchiectatic segment. *F* represents obstruction of a bronchus by tumor or foreign body. Blood flow is reduced in part by the local hypoxia.

G to *I* in Figure 11-5 represent miscellaneous conditions. In *G* the lung parenchyma is filled with inflammatory exudate, as is seen in pneumonia, or blood, as is seen in a pulmonary infarction. Blood flow is greatly reduced and there is no ventilation of the affected region. *H* represents the interesting phenomenon of a reversal of the normal gradient of blood flow. This is seen when there is elevation of the pressure in the left atrium, for example, in mitral stenosis or left ventricular failure. *I* represents the situation when there is a pleural effusion or a large heart compressing lung tissue and hence reducing blood flow in that region.

The mechanisms responsible for the disturbances in ventilation are shown in Figure 11-6. Figure 11-6, *A*, represents diseases that cause obstruction to air flow by narrowing or distorting the airways. In chronic bronchitis there is excess mucus production and some inflammatory swelling of the bronchial walls. Both processes narrow the lumen of the airways, usually in an irregular fashion, producing variable patterns of airway obstruction. In emphysema the main damage is in the alveoli, which are steadily destroyed, losing surface area and capillaries. The small airways are not properly supported, become kinked and distorted, and collapse readily on expiration, which leads to inefficient exchange of air. Chronic bronchitis and emphysema are usually found together because both diseases are caused, for the most part, by cigarette smoking.

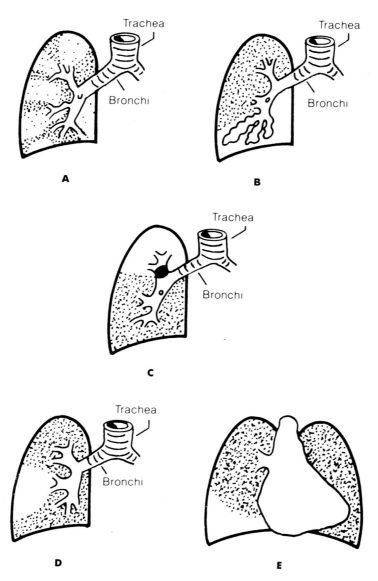

Figure 11-6 Schematic representation of major mechanisms of abnormal ventilation studies **(A-E).** *Spotted areas,* ventilation; *clear areas,* regions of abnormal ventilation.

In bronchial asthma there is spasm of the bronchial smooth muscle, which causes narrowing of the airways and increased mucus production and edema of the bronchial mucosa. Severe abnormalities of ventilation and blood flow may be seen.

Figure 11-6, *B,* represents bronchiectasis. Little or no air exchange takes place in the dilatated bronchi, which are often the seat of chronic infection. Figure 11-6, *C,* represents narrowing or complete obstruction of a bronchus because of a tumor or foreign body. The worse the obstruction, the more obvious the abnormality in ventilation. If the obstruction is in a lobar bronchus, the affected lobe of the lung collapses as its lumen closes off. If the obstruction is in a segmental or smaller bronchus, collateral ventilation through the pores of Kohn can prevent complete collapse by allowing air to enter the segment from a neighboring segment.

Figure 11-6, *D,* represents the condition in pneumonia or pulmonary infarction, when the alveoli are filled with exudate or blood and hence will not exchange any air.

Figure 11-6, *E,* represents pleural fluid or a large heart, both of which occupy lung volume and hence reduce ventilation.

PERFUSION IMAGING

The distribution of pulmonary arterial blood flow is usually demonstrated by the intravenous injection of radioactive particles. The method was shown to be effective by Haynie and his colleagues, who injected labeled ceramic microspheres into dogs.[21] The development of macroaggregated albumin (MAA), labeled with ^{131}I, by Taplin and colleagues[44] and Wagner and colleagues[47] in 1964 led to the first successful lung scans in human beings. After intravenous injection the particles, which measure 30 to 40 μm in diameter, pass through the right atrium and right ventricle, where they are well mixed with blood, and then into the pulmonary artery. They pass into the blood vessels of the lung until they become impacted in the terminal arterioles and capillaries because they are too large to pass through them. The usual diameter of human albumin microspheres corresponds to the size of the smallest pulmonary arterioles. The distribution of particles has been shown experimentally to be closely related to the distribution of pulmonary arterial blood flow,[37] by comparison of their relative distribution to the uptake of oxygen by each lung and also by comparison of the distribution of particles to that of labeled red blood cells.[46] A normal perfusion scan is shown in Figure 11-7.

It is to be understood that the distribution is that which exists at the time of injection.

Macroaggregated albumin, human albumin microspheres, and other particles break up and pass through the pulmonary capillaries and are removed from the circulation in the liver and spleen. These particles have variable biologic half-lives in the lung, which depend not only on the nature of the particles but also, to some extent, on the underlying disease processes. Clearance is delayed in chronic lung disease and heart failure.

With the usual dose of particulate material of the appropriate size, fewer than 1 in 1000 pulmonary arterioles is blocked.[19,44] No abnormalities of pulmonary function can be demonstrated after such an injection.[16,38] Perfusion scanning has a reputation for great safety, but special care should be taken in patients known to have severe pulmonary hypertension because their available vascular bed is reduced in diameter.[12] Special care should also be taken in patients with right-to-left shunts[36] because the particles pass through to the systemic circulation and embolize to the brain, kidneys, heart, and other organs. Half the usual dose should be given to patients who have had a pneumonectomy.

Radioactive xenon dissolved in saline solution is occasionally used to demonstrate the distribution of blood flow. It is given intravenously, and because the gas is relatively insoluble, it comes out of solution as it reaches the air contained in the alveoli. Its distribution can be measured during breath holding and corresponds to pulmonary capillary blood flow. Regions of the lung that are collapsed or consolidated, as in pneumonia, appear to have no blood flow because the alveoli contain no air.

Preparation

No special patient preparation is required for either ventilation or perfusion lung imaging. There are, however, a few things that should be done in advance of the examination. A recent chest radiograph (within 4 hr) should accompany the patient to the nuclear medicine facility. The radiograph allows the physician to be more specific when interpreting the images. Many physicians also require that a blood gases report accompany the patient. Again, this additional information can provide another clue to the correct diagnosis of the patient. It is not the technologist's responsibility to set laboratory policy with regard to this type of advance information. It is however, generally the technologist's responsibility to enforce it.

Dosage

In addition to the amount of radioactivity given, the number of particles and the amount of albumin injected are of special importance. Since, as previously discussed, a small percentage of the capillary bed is being obstructed so that the perfusion image can be performed, care must be taken to ensure that the patient's respiratory ability is not further impaired by a test in-

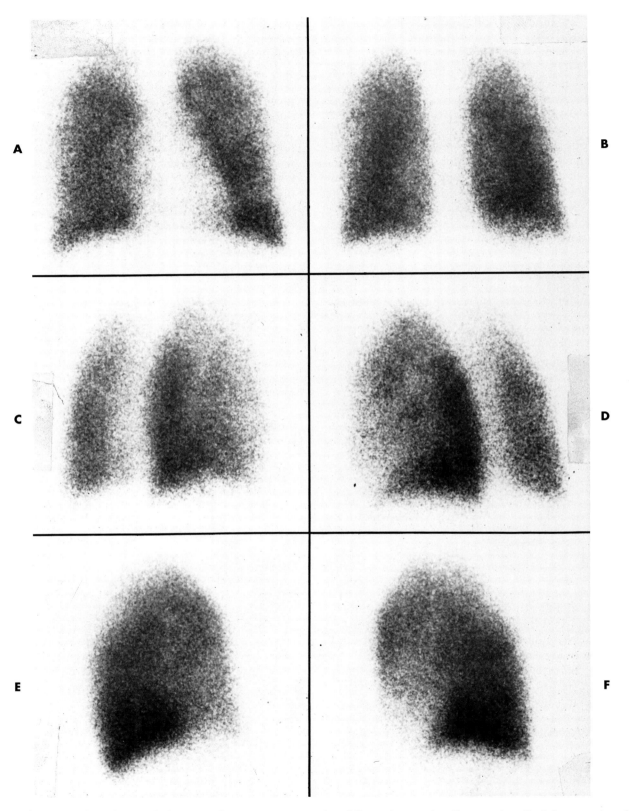

Figure 11-7   Normal six-view perfusion scan. Images are arranged as follows: **A,** anterior; **B,** posterior; **C,** right posterior oblique; **D,** left posterior oblique; **E,** right lateral; **F,** left lateral.

tended to help him.[19] A satisfactory perfusion image can be obtained with anywhere between 60,000 and 150,000 particles in a normal patient.[22] An appropriate reduction in the number of particles should be applied for pediatric patients, those with pulmonary hypertension, and those who have had a pneumonectomy. To help control the number of particles used in perfusion imaging, one should prepare aggregated albumin kits to the same volume every day and schedule patients as close as possible to the preparation time. Every technologist in the laboratory should know the total number of particles in whichever kit the laboratory uses.

If too few particles are given, the scans have an obvious blotchy appearance. An even more blotchy appearance is seen if small blood clots or incompletely separated particles are inadvertently injected.

Method of Injection

There is a difference in the patterns of perfusion depending on whether the particles are injected with the patient in the upright or supine position. As indicated earlier, gravity plays an important role in the pressure relationships within the lungs. Patients injected when upright tend to have a larger proportion of the particles distributed toward the bases. Patients injected when supine demonstrate a more homogeneous distribution of particles from the bases to the apices. There are arguments and situations favoring each position for injection. As long as both technologist and physician are aware of the difference, either method is satisfactory. The method of

injection should be noted somewhere on the film or film jacket. Albumin appears to have an affinity for the plastic tubing of intravenous sets, catheters, and syringes. If these avenues of administration are used, a variable proportion of the dose never reaches the patient. We recommend a saline syringe, three-way stopcock, and dose syringe setup (Figure 11-8) for aggregated albumin injections. This arrangement also eliminates drawing blood back into the dose and prevents the possible formation of small thrombi as a result of the mixing of whole blood and MAA.

Always inject labeled particles slowly over 30 sec or more. Some physicians recommend having the patient take a few deep breaths during the injection to assist the homogeneous distribution of the particles.

Positioning

Standard perfusion imaging includes the six basic views: posterior, anterior, right and left laterals, and right and left posterior obliques.[11,34,40] We recommend doing the posterior view first, for 500,000 counts, and then each of the other views for the same time that it takes to do the posterior view. The lateral views can then be compared more easily. About one third of the counts from the contralateral lung are included during lateral imaging.

Unlike many radiographic procedures the radionuclide images provide the physician with very few landmarks that indicate rotation or distance from the collimator face.[42] The responsibility for good positioning in the nuclear medicine area is basically in the hands of the technologist.

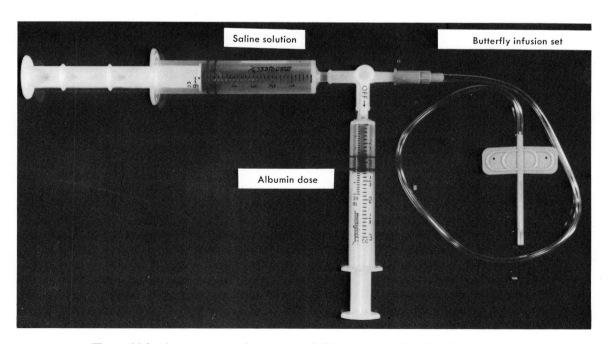

Figure 11-8 Arrangement of recommended injection set for albumin particles.

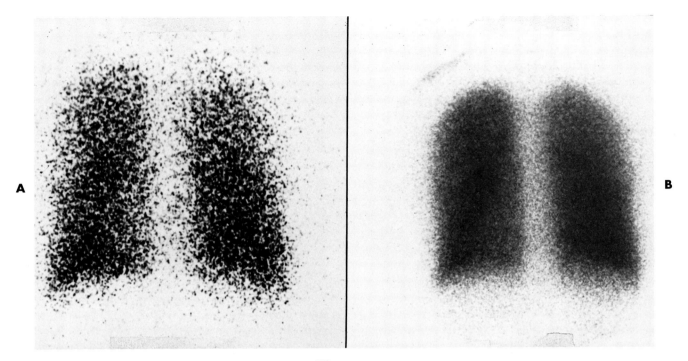

Figure 11-9   A, Normal distribution of a single breath of ^{133}Xe in the posterior projection. **B,** Wash-in equilibrium image of the same patient.

Table 11-1	Radiopharmaceuticals used for ventilation lung imaging		
	Agent		
	^{99m}Tc DTPA aerosol	^{133}Xe	^{81m}Kr
Physical half-life	6.0 hr	5.3 days	13 sec
Principal gamma energy	140 keV	80 keV	190 keV
Radiation absorbed dose per millicurie in lungs	112.5* mrad	12 mrad†	7.5 mrad†

*Actual dose delivered to lung is approximately one fifth as lung deposition is on the order of 200 μCi.
†Radiation absorbed dose has been estimated with a rebreathing time of 3 min.

VENTILATION IMAGING

Table 11-1 shows some of the radiopharmaceuticals used to study regional ventilation. Xenon-133 has been used for quasistatic measurements of regional ventilation and blood flow, for dynamic measurements of regional ventilation, for measurements of regional lung volumes, for closing volume, and for studying factors that influence the distribution of a single breath. Clinical studies of regional ventilation are usually done with ^{133}Xe. Techniques for ventilation studies are not yet standardized, but three aspects of ventilation are often examined: (1) the distribution of a single breath, (2) the distribution of lung volume, and (3) the distribution of the efficiency of ventilation from the clearance of radioactive xenon. Single-breath studies show the

distribution of a bolus of radioactive xenon inhaled, with air, to total lung capacity—a somewhat unphysiologic situation (Figure 11-9, *A*). If the tracer gas is rebreathed to equilibrium, that is, until the concentration of xenon in the lungs and in the rebreathing system is constant, the distribution of xenon within the lungs corresponds to lung volume (Figure 11-9, *B*). Measurements made during a wash-in of xenon to equilibrium reflect the efficiency of ventilation—the faster a region reaches equilibrium, the better its ventilation and vice versa. When air is breathed after a wash-in, the subsequent wash-out provides excellent evidence of the regional variations in ventilation (Figure 11-10). The best ventilated regions clear fastest, and the poorly ventilated ones stand out by contrast, as regions where the clearance of radioactivity is delayed.[1]

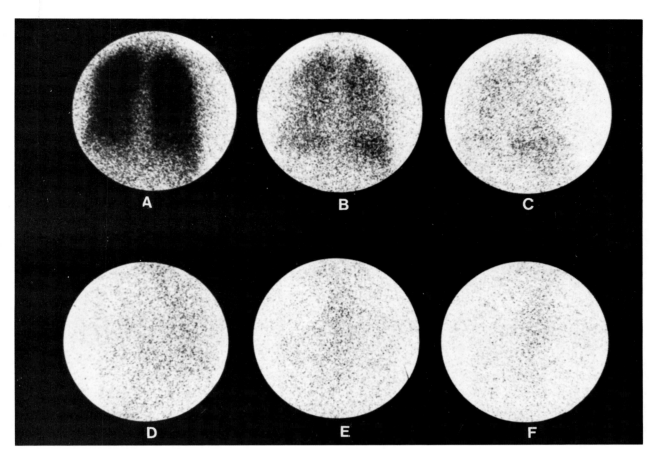

Figure 11-10 Posterior projection of wash-out of xenon from the lungs. **A,** Equilibrium image. **B** through **F,** Wash-out images of 1, 2, 3, 4, and 5 min.

^{133}Xe Ventilation Imaging

At present the most readily available nuclide for performing ventilation studies is ^{133}Xe. Although it is not an ideal nuclide for this study because of its low energy, beta emission, and solubility in fat and blood, its price and ready availability have forced it into prominence. The energy, 80 keV, is not optimal for the Anger camera because so much scattered activity is included in the window. Ideally, the perfusion study should be done first so that, if a ventilation study is necessary, the patient can be positioned for it on the basis of the perfusion scan. Several institutions do the perfusion image first, using only 1 mCi of ^{99m}Tc-labeled particles and then proceed with a ventilation study using 20 to 30 mCi of ^{133}Xe or more. However, because the energy of ^{133}Xe is lower than that of ^{99m}Tc and because of the importance of the wash-out phase, it is technically more satisfactory to perform the ventilation study before the perfusion exam. A number of commercial gas delivery and rebreathing units are available for ventilation studies, but with a little imagination and some engineering skill you can build your own[41] (Figure 11-11). An additional problem with xenon ventilation studies is disposal of the xenon when the study is finished. Many laboratories, if suitably located, simply

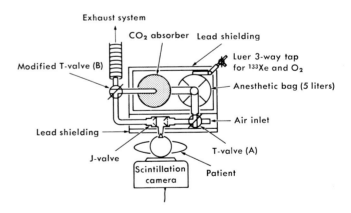

Figure 11-11 Diagram of simple rebreathing apparatus that can be constructed from commercially available parts.

vent the diluted xenon (half-life 5.27 days) into the atmosphere. The Nuclear Regulatory Commission (NRC) requires that the average yearly concentration must be less than 3×10^{-7} µCi/ml. There are some arguments against this practice, but from a pragmatic standpoint this is the simplest solution. An alternative is to trap the xenon. Several commercial units are available for this purpose, most of which use activated charcoal.[31]

There are several methods for doing a ventilation study. Some laboratories use the single-breath technique, which is to have the patient inhale a bolus of 10 to 20 mCi of ^{133}Xe and hold his breath for 10 to 20 sec while a static image is taken. Serial wash-out images are then made at 30 to 60 sec intervals as the xenon clears from the lungs. This method works well but requires a good deal of patient cooperation in taking a deep breath and then holding it for 10 to 20 sec.

We favor the more straightforward wash-in-wash-out method, which can be used even on comatose patients. In this method 10 to 20 mCi of ^{133}Xe diluted in 2 L of oxygen are rebreathed from a simple rebreathing apparatus for approximately 3 min while a static wash-in image is taken. Air is then breathed and serial images are taken at 30 to 60 sec intervals as the xenon clears from the lungs. With the variety of mouthpieces, respiratory masks, and harnesses available it is possible for a technologist to perform a ventilation study without assistance from the patient. We have successfully completed this type of examination on many patients and feel confident in saying that if the patient is breathing, a ventilation study can be done. Such studies can also be done on patients using mechanical ventilation.

The ventilation study may be done in any position. Routinely we use the posterior view in the upright position because this provides the best view of the greatest area of lung. The patient should be seated comfortably with his back to the scintillation camera and should be encouraged to keep as still as possible during the study. The first few breaths of xenon, which are seen on the monitor, can be used to adjust the position of the camera before the wash-in images are started.

^{81m}Kr Ventilation Imaging

Krypton-81m is being used in some centers. This gas has such a short half-life that when inhaled continuously during normal breathing, an equilibrium count rate that is proportional to ventilation is reached. This means that images can be made in the same projections used for perfusion imaging and are directly comparable. Images made in this way show the distribution of regional ventilation, whereas images made with ^{99m}Tc human albumin microspheres show the distribution of regional blood flow. Therefore visual comparisons of the matching of ventilation and blood flow are considerably easier with ^{81m}Kr than with radioactive xenon[14,17] (Figure 11-12).

This gas is obtained by elution of a rubidium-81 generator with a stream of moist air. ^{81m}Kr generators are delivered containing 5 mCi of ^{81}Rb at the time of calibration and possess a useful life of approximately 6 hr. ^{81m}Kr has a 13 sec half-life and an energy of 190 keV so that the examinations can be performed in the preferred order. Its 13 sec half-life also eliminates any

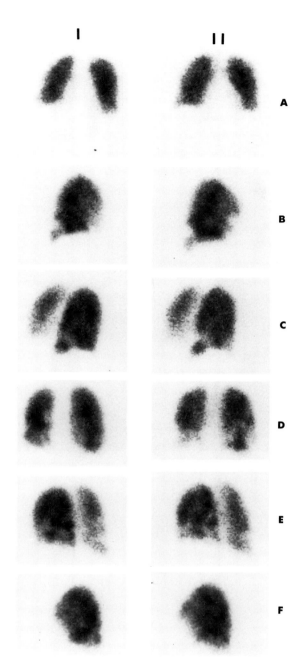

Figure 11-12 Side-by-side comparison of blood flow with ^{99m}Tc MAA *(column I)* and ventilation utilizing ^{81m}Kr *(column II)*. Images are arranged as follows: **A,** anterior; **B,** right lateral; **C,** right posterior oblique; **D,** posterior; **E,** left posterior oblique; **F,** left lateral.

problems of trapping, venting, or contamination. Since ^{81m}Kr decays almost immediately, four- or six-view ventilation studies to match the perfusion images can be done routinely.[14,17]

Aerosol Ventilation Imaging

Aerosols are deposited in the bronchial tree in relation to particle size, air flow rates, and turbulence. The de-

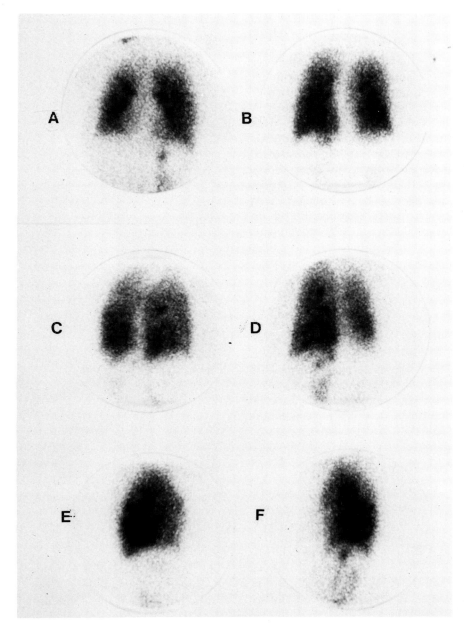

Figure 11-13   Six views of aerosol ventilation scan using ^{99m}Tc DTPA. Images are arranged as follows: **A,** anterior; **B,** posterior; **C,** right posterior oblique; **D,** left posterior oblique; **E,** right lateral; **F,** left lateral.

livery tubing effectively filters out larger particles, 10 to 15 μm in diameter. Smaller ones are deposited in the larger airways during both inspiration and expiration. Particles less than 2 μm can reach the alveoli and be deposited there, whereas even smaller particles, less than 0.1 μm, probably escape in the expired air. Radioactive aerosols have been used for more than two decades to study the patency of the airways. It is important that aerosol particle size be well controlled for reproducible studies. Many radionuclides have been used, specifically ^{99m}Tc DTPA, ^{99m}TcO$_4^-$, ^{99m}Tc sulfur colloid, ^{99m}Tc HSA, and ^{113m}In Cl$_2$.

The aerosol is generated from an ultrasound nebulizer or a positive-pressure nebulizer. It is inhaled through a mouthpiece or a face mask. If older systems are used, exhaled material must be collected and the procedure is best done near a fume hood with an extraction fan. This is not necessary, however, with the newer systems that incorporate a bacterial filter at the outlet. Three to five ml of fluid containing up to 35 mCi of the nuclear pharmaceutical are inhaled. Only 10% to 15% actually reaches the lungs. Images can then be made in the six standard views (Figure 11-13). Normal aerosol scans look much like perfusion scans, except that the trachea and mainstem bronchi can usually be seen, as well as the esophagus and stomach from swallowed material.

In the presence of obstructive disease of the airways there may be central deposition in the larger bronchial tubes with little or no peripheral filling—a pattern seen in severe bronchial asthma and emphysema. Less central, but definitely patchy, peripheral filling tends to be seen in chronic bronchitis, cystic fibrosis, and mild bronchial asthma. Delayed views, 4 to 6 hr after the initial images, can help resolve some central deposition. This is cleared by mucociliary transport in otherwise normal subjects, leaving normal delayed images. Aerosol scans are almost as sensitive as xenon studies in detecting early disease of small airways. Sequential images for several hours after aerosol inhalation have been used to measure mucociliary clearance rates in smokers, nonsmokers, and children with cystic fibrosis.[39]

The development of small, disposable nebulizers has renewed interest in the use of aerosols for lung imaging.[20] These light and portable units are greatly improved over the cumbersome systems designed during the development of this technique. Bedside procedures are possible with a cooperative patient. Even with these improvements the aerosol technique remains one of the more difficult nuclear medicine procedures. It requires detailed attention to variables such as tubing length and diameter, air flow, and pressure.

Technegas and Pertechnegas

Technegas is an ultrafine or gaslike microaerosol of a graphite coated technetium atom that was developed at the Australian National University. Technegas is a derivative of the "buckyball" family with a cross section of 5 to 30 nm and thickness of 3 nm. The particle is a hexagonal crystal of native ^{99m}Tc metal within a "shrink-wrap" of graphite completely enclosing it. Technegas is produced by placing 7 to 10 mCi of sodium pertechnetate (USP) into a pure graphite crucible within a 6 liter lead-shielded chamber (Figure 11-14). The crucible is warmed to evaporate all the liquid as the chamber air is replaced with pure argon. After 6 min, the unit is ready to create Technegas. The patient rehearses the ventilation procedure during this preparation phase, preferably in a supine position on the imaging table with the camera set for a posterior view. The "start" button on the machine is pressed and the crucible in its argon atmosphere heats to 2550° C in less than 0.5 sec and holds that temperature for 15 sec before switching off. The machine is then wheeled into the camera room, and the Technegas is administered to the patient via a self-contained breathing apparatus. Usually only two or three breaths are needed to deliver a suitable dose (1 mCi) for ventilation imaging (Figure 11-15).

Technegas microaerosol images are performed from several projections before lung perfusion images from

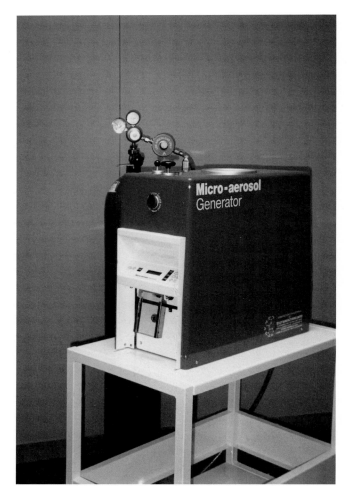

Figure 11-14 The Technegas crucible device, which is labeled as a "Micro-aerosol Generator" for its FDA trials in the United States, with a standard tank of argon behind it. (Courtesy William M. Burch, PhD.)

the same views. The Technegas particle is hydrophobic and chemically inert. Thus, once it lodges in the alveoli, it remains there indefinitely. As a consequence, it is becoming more common for SPECT studies to be routinely performed, particularly as the newer multihead cameras are used. Technegas imaging has become a common ventilation agent outside the United States.

Pertechnegas is a derivative of Technegas formed by the simple expedient of using 3% to 5% oxygen in the argon within the 6 liter chamber of the generator during the main 15-sec heating cycle of the machine. Addition of oxygen to the blanket gas prevents the formation of the graphite "shrink-wrap" leaving Tc oxides only in the chamber. On inhalation, these oxides hydrolyse rapidly in the high water vapor of the lung's airways, reverting to TcO_4^- immediately.

Clinically, Pertechnegas is identical to an inhaled pertechnetate aerosol but with the significant advantage that it is delivered in one or two breaths, even in patients with severe respiratory distress. Again, the administration may be controlled by the technologist

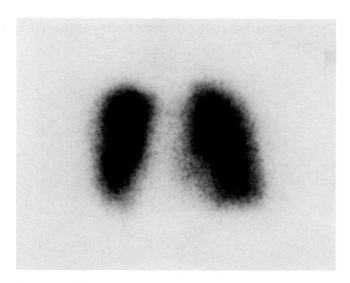

Figure 11-15 Anterior lung microaerosol scan with Technegas. (Courtesy William M. Burch, PhD.)

loading more activity into the crucible and only allowing a predefined level of activity to enter the patient's lungs. Trials in various parts of the world have established that it provides an ideal measure of the permeability of the gas-exchange membrane of the lungs, and so far it has proven useful for diagnosis and management of pneumocystis pneumonia (PCP), radiation pneumonitis, and fibrosing alveolitis, as well as an alternative to Technegas for pulmonary embolism; it is currently under trial in the United States as part of a Food and Drug Administration submission process.

VENTILATION-PERFUSION STUDIES

By combining studies of ventilation and perfusion one can determine whether defects in blood flow are associated with defects in ventilation. The pulmonary diseases commonly seen in clinical nuclear medicine tend to fall into two categories: (1) those with abnormal regional pulmonary blood flow but normal (or almost normal) regional ventilation (pulmonary embolism is by far the most important of these, but early heart failure, interstitial lung diseases, some lung cancers, and other abnormalities of the pulmonary vasculature may show this pattern) and (2) those with abnormal ventilation and abnormal blood flow. The most common conditions are chronic bronchitis, emphysema, and asthma; however, cystic fibrosis and bronchiectasis cause similar patterns. Cancers of the bronchus, other bronchial tumors, or foreign bodies obstructing a bronchus can all produce localized abnormalities of ventilation and blood flow. In general, the disturbance of ventilation is more pronounced than that of blood flow and is detected as a regional delay in the clearance of xenon. When this delay is great, a corresponding de-

fect is usually visible on the wash-in image as an area of diminished activity, where this part of the lung has not reached equilibrium with the tracer gas.

Pneumonias, pulmonary infarctions, and severe pulmonary edema are all associated with defects in the equilibrium images, which correspond to the infiltrates seen on the chest radiograph. No retention of radioactive xenon is seen during the wash-out because no radioactive xenon can enter the fluid-filled alveoli.

Normal perfusion scans show an even gradation of activity, with more activity visible in the lower lobes than in the upper lobes, if the injection is given with the patient in the upright posture. The outline of the lungs and mediastinum corresponds closely to that seen on the chest radiograph. A normal wash-in image shows an even distribution of activity throughout the lungs, and a normal wash-out is usually complete within 3 to 4 min of breathing air. Occasionally the bases can clear a little faster than the upper zones.

Computer Processing of Ventilation-Perfusion Images

The ready access to digital computer processing of image data has led to several different ways of processing the information from ventilation-perfusion imaging. The partitioning of ventilation, lung volume, and blood flow between the lungs can be obtained with considerable ease; however, measurements of regional ventilation and regional ventilation-perfusion ratios are less readily obtained. In most instances the numeric values obtained do not correspond to how much air is exchanged or to the physiologic ventilation-perfusion ratios.[42]

Pulmonary Embolism

In pulmonary embolism the defects in blood flow correspond to anatomic subdivisions of the lung, such as segments or lobes, in 75% of patients. The remaining 25% have ill-defined nonsegmental defects. If the patient had previously healthy lungs, ventilation is usually well maintained to the affected parts of the lung because their bronchial tubes are patent (Figures 11-16 and 11-17). Only a small proportion (10% to 15%) of patients with emboli develop pulmonary infarction with its associated infiltrates as seen on the chest radiograph.

Interpretation is more difficult, and less reliable, when the patients already have chronic obstructive pulmonary disease (COPD), such as chronic bronchitis, emphysema, or asthma.[2]

Retrospective studies from the 1970s suggested that the true positive rate, or sensitivity, and the true negative rate, or specificity, of ventilation-perfusion scanning were more than 90%.[3,33] Subsequent studies have not shown this to be true.[2,7,8]

Two recent prospective studies of the accuracy of ventilation-perfusion scanning in comparison to pul-

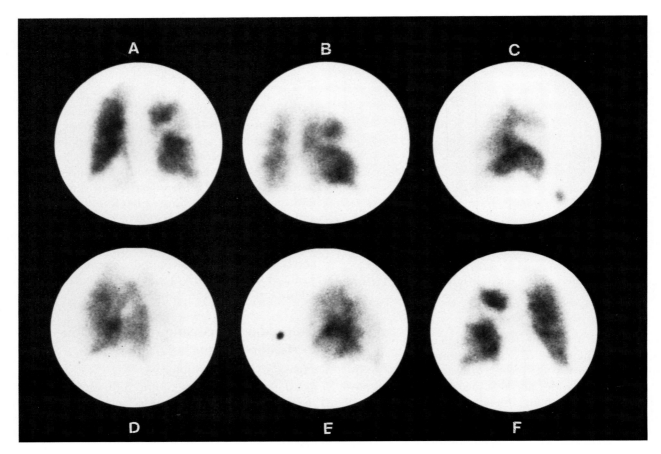

Figure 11-16 Markedly abnormal perfusion scan of the lungs demonstrating multiple segmental defects. Images are arranged as follows: **A,** posterior; **B,** right posterior oblique; **C,** right lateral; **D,** left posterior oblique; **E,** left lateral; **F,** anterior.

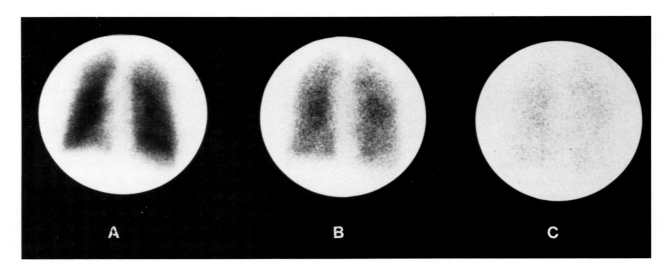

Figure 11-17 Essentially normal ^{133}Xe ventilation scan. Images are arranged as follows: **A,** equilibrium image; **B,** 1 min wash-out; **C,** 3 min wash-out.

monary angiography showed pulmonary embolism to be present in about 90% of patients with high probability lung scan interpretations.[24,35] But for other interpretations, such as intermediate, indeterminate, or low probability, the proportion of patients with angio-graphically proven pulmonary emboli ranged from 40% to 14%. When the perfusion scan was completely normal, pulmonary emboli were rarely found.[24,27]

For patients with ventilation-perfusion scans that are neither high probability nor normal, further diagnos-

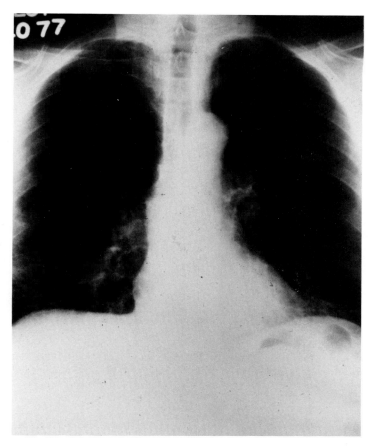

Figure 11-18   Chest radiograph of a 64-year-old man with severe emphysema. He has large lungs and bullous areas in the upper lobes.

tic studies are indicated. Noninvasive tests for proximal vein thrombosis, such as B-mode ultrasound or impedance plethysmography, should be considered, or even the more invasive venography if these noninvasive tests are not available.[26,30] Finding evidence of venous thrombosis would lead to treatment for venous thromboembolism.[26] If there is still doubt as to the diagnosis, pulmonary angiography, if available, may be needed to resolve the problem.[7,8,25] Most, but not all, pulmonary emboli are eventually lysed by the body's own fibrinolytic systems, so that defects in blood flow tend to disappear with time. Most improvement is seen in the first few days. Further improvement occurs more slowly over the following 3 to 4 weeks and can continue for several months.[43] Anticoagulant treatment is important and prevents the formation of new blood clots and the extension of those already present in the lungs.

Chronic Obstructive Pulmonary Disease

Radioactive ventilation studies provide one of the most sensitive ways of detecting damage to the small airways.[45] Patients with chronic bronchitis and emphysema show an endless variety of defects in blood flow and ventilation. Eighty percent of the time the defects

in blood flow cannot be strictly related to anatomic subdivisions of the lung. In general, both lungs tend to be affected to a similar, though rarely identical, degree. In some patients most of the damage is in the lower zones, in others in the upper zones, and in yet others the damage is scattered throughout both lungs. It is by no means rare for one lung to be distinctly more severely affected than the other (Figures 11-18 and 11-19).

In chronic bronchitis, ventilation tends to be more severely affected than blood flow, and some changes in the pattern of ventilation and blood flow can be seen with exacerbations of this disease. In emphysema the defects in ventilation and blood flow correspond more closely and tend to be more stable from year to year.

Patients with bronchial asthma also show considerable changes in both ventilation and blood flow, with ventilation being more severely affected. If just a perfusion scan is done, often the defects are recognizably segmental, or even lobar, leading to a false diagnosis of pulmonary embolism.

In cystic fibrosis the upper lobes are usually the more severely affected, and fissure signs are often seen on the lateral views. The sign is attributable to a defect in blood flow along the greater fissure. It is also seen in

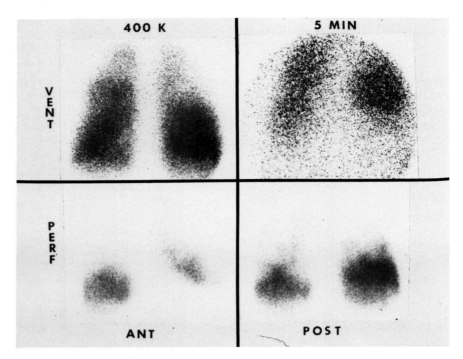

Figure 11-19 Selected ventilation and perfusion images of the patient in Figure 11-18. Perfusion images show decreased perfusion in the upper half of both lung fields. There is diminished filling of both upper lung fields on equilibrium (wash-in) images *(upper left)* and delayed clearance from both lungs during wash-out *(upper right).*

other obstructive airway diseases, as well as in pulmonary edema with pleural fluid and occasionally in pulmonary embolism. The segments or lobes of lung involved with bronchiectasis are clearly outlined by lack of ventilation and absent pulmonary arterial blood flow.

Lung Cancer

In cancer of the bronchus ventilation-perfusion studies can be used to determine individual lung function when a pneumonectomy is planned. The relative distribution of blood flow calculated from an upright perfusion scan enables postoperative lung function to be predicted with considerable accuracy. A successful resection of the tumor tissue is less likely if the affected lung receives less than about 25% to 30% of the total pulmonary blood flow. Occasionally the site of a tumor can be identified by ventilation-perfusion scanning when it cannot be found by conventional means. After radiation treatment for lung cancer, ventilation will usually improve, but blood flow is restored in a much smaller proportion of such patients.

The most important indication for ventilation-perfusion scanning is in the differential diagnosis of pulmonary embolism. Lesser indications are for the follow-up of this condition and for the assessment of regional and individual lung function in the preoperative assessment of patients with lung cancer or other conditions in which lung tissue may be resected.

Ventilation-perfusion scans can sometimes be helpful in the management of patients with COPD. They may also play some part in the follow-up of patients who have had surgical correction of certain congenital heart defects.

REFERENCES

1. Alderson PO, Biello DR, Khan AR, et al: Comparison of ^{133}Xe single-breath and washout imaging in the scintigraphic diagnosis of pulmonary embolism, *Radiology* 137:481-486, 1980.
2. Alderson PO, Biello DR, Sachariah KG, et al: Scintigraphic detection of pulmonary embolism in patients with obstructive pulmonary disease, *Radiology* 138:661-666, 1981.
3. Alderson PO, Rujanavech N, Secker-Walker RH, et al: The role of ^{133}Xe ventilation studies in the scintigraphic detection of pulmonary embolism, *Radiology* 120:633, 1976.
4. Anthonisen NR, Danson J, Roberson PC, et al: Airway closure as a function of age, *Respir Physiol* 8:58, 1969.
5. Anthonisen NR, Milic-Emili J: Distribution of pulmonary perfusion in erect man, *J Appl Physiol* 21:760, 1966.
6. Ball WC Jr, Stewart PB, Newham IGS, et al: Regional pulmonary studies with xenon 133, *J Clin Invest* 41:519, 1962.

7. Biello DR, Mattar AG, McKnight RC, et al: Ventilation-perfusion studies in suspected pulmonary embolism, *Am J Roentgenol* 138:661-666, 1981.

8. Biello DR, Mattar AG, Osei-Wusu A, et al: Interpretation of indeterminate lung scintigrams, *Radiology* 133:189-194, 1979.

9. Breeze RG, Wheeldon EB: The cells of the pulmonary airways, *Am Rev Respir Dis* 116:705, 1977.

10. Buist AS, Van Fleet DL, Ross BB: A comparison of conventional spirometric tests and the test of closing volume in an emphysema screening center, *Am Rev Respir Dis* 107:735, 1973.

11. Burdine JA, Murphy PH: Clinical efficacy of a large-field-of-view scintillation camera, *J Nucl Med* 16:1158, 1975.

12. Child JS, Wolfe JD, Tashkin D, et al: Fatal lung scan in a case of pulmonary hypertension due to obliterative pulmonary vascular disease, *Chest* 67:308, 1975.

13. Daly I de B, Hebb C: *Pulmonary and bronchial vascular systems,* Baltimore, 1966, Williams & Wilkins.

14. Fazio F, Jones T: Assessment of regional ventilation by continuous inhalation of radioactive krypton-81m, *Br Med J* 3:673, 1975.

15. Fishman AP, Pietra G: Handling of bioactive materials by the lung, *N Engl J Med* 281:884 and 953, 1974.

16. Gold WM, McCormack KR: Pulmonary function response to radioisotope scanning of the lungs, *JAMA* 197:146, 1966.

17. Goris ML, Daspit SG, Walter JP, et al: Applications of ventilation lung imaging with [81m]krypton, *Radiology* 122:399, 1977.

18. Green GM: The Amberson Lecture: in defense of the lung, *Am Rev Respir Dis* 102:691, 1970.

19. Harding LK, Horsfield K, Singhal SS, et al: The proportion of lung vessels blocked by albumin microspheres, *J Nucl Med* 14:579, 1973.

20. Hayes M, Taplin GV, Chopra SK, et al: Improved radioaerosol administration system for routine inhalation lung imaging, *Radiology* 131:256-258, 1979.

21. Haynie TP, Calhoon JH, Nasjleti CE, et al: Visualization of pulmonary artery occlusion by photoscanning, *JAMA* 185:306, 1963.

22. Heck LL, Duley JW: Statistical considerations in lung imaging with Tc-99m albumin particles, *Radiology* 113:657, 1974.

23. Hughes JMB, Glazier JB, Maloney JE, et al: Effect of lung volume on the distribution of pulmonary blood flow in man, *Respir Physiol* 4:78, 1968.

24. Hull RD, Hirsh J, Carter CJ, et al: Diagnostic value of ventilation-perfusion lung scanning in patients with suspected pulmonary embolism, *Chest* 88:819-828, 1985.

25. Hull RD, Hirsch J, Carter CJ, et al.: Pulmonary angiography, ventilation lung scanning, and venography for clinically suspected pulmonary embolism with abnormal perfusion lung scan, *Ann Intern Med* 98:891-899, 1983.

26. Hull RD, Raskob GE, Coates G, et al: A new noninvasive management strategy for patients with suspected pulmonary embolism, *Arch Intern Med* 149:2549-2555, 1989.

27. Hull RD, Raskob GE, Coates G, et al: Clinical validity of a normal perfusion lung scan in patients with suspected pulmonary embolism, *Chest* 97:23-26, 1990.

28. Kaneko K, Milic-Emili J, Dolovich MB, et al: Regional distribution of ventilation and perfusion as a function of body position, *J Appl Physiol* 21:767, 1966.

29. Knipping HW, Bolt W, Vanrath H, et al: Eine neue Methode zur Prüfung der Herz- und Lungenfunktion, *Deutsch Med Wochenschr* 80:1146, 1955.

30. Lensing AWA, Prandoni P, Brandjes D, et al: Detection of deep-vein thrombosis by real-time b-mode ultrasonography, *N Engl J Med* 320:342-345, 1989.

31. Luizzi A, Keaney J, Freedman G: Use of activated charcoal for the collection and containment of Xe-133 exhaled during pulmonary studies, *J Nucl Med* 13:673, 1972.

32. Mead J, Takishima T, Leith D: Stress distribution in lungs: a model of pulmonary elasticity, *J Appl Physiol* 28:596, 1970.

33. McNeil BJ: A diagnostic strategy using ventilation-perfusion studies in patients suspect for pulmonary embolism, *J Nucl Med* 17:613, 1976.

34. Nielsen PE, Kirchner PT, Gerber FH: Oblique views in lung perfusion scanning: clinical utility and limitations, *J Nucl Med* 18:967, 1977.

35. The PIOPED Investigators: Value of the ventilation/perfusion scan in acute pulmonary embolism: results of the prospective investigation of pulmonary embolism diagnosis, *JAMA* 263:2753-2759, 1990.

36. Rhodes BA, Stem HS, Buchanan JA, et al: Lung scanning with Tc-99m microspheres, *Radiology* 99:613, 1971.

37. Rogers RM, Kuhl DE, Hyde RW, et al: Measurement of the vital capacity and perfusion of each lung by fluoroscopy and macroaggregated albumin lung scanning, *Ann Intern Med* 67:947, 1967.

38. Rootwelt K, Vale JR: Pulmonary gas exchange after intravenous injection of ^{99m}Tc sulphur colloid albumin macroaggregates for lung perfusion scintigraphy, *Scand J Clin Lab Invest* 30:17, 1972.

39. Sanchis J, Dolovich M, Rossman C, et al: Pulmonary mucociliary clearance in cystic fibrosis, *N Engl J Med* 288:651, 1973.

40. Sasahara AA, Belko JS, Simpson RC: Multiple view lung scanning, *J Nucl Med* 9:187, 1968.

41. Secker-Walker RH, Barbier J, Weiner SN, et al: A simple ^{133}Xe delivery system for studies of regional ventilation, *J Nucl Med* 15:288, 1974.

42. Secker-Walker RH, Evens RG: The clinical application of computers in ventilation perfusion studies, *Progr Nucl Med* 3:166, 1973.

43. Secker-Walker RH, Jackson JA, Goodwin J: Resolution of pulmonary embolism, *Br Med J* 4:135, 1970.

44. Taplin GV, Johnson DE, Dore EK, et al: Lung photoscans with macroaggregates of human serum radioalbumin: experimental basis and initial clinical trials, *Health Phys* 10:1219, 1964.

45. Taplin GV, Tashkin DP, Chopra SK, et al: Early detection of chronic obstructive pulmonary disease using radionuclide lung imaging procedures, *Chest* 71:567, 1977.

46. Tow DE, Wagner HN, Lopez-Majano V, et al: Validity of measuring regional pulmonary arterial blood flow with macroaggregates of human serum albumin, *Am J Roentgenol Radium Ther Nucl Med* 96:664, 1966.

47. Wagner HM, Sabiston DC, McAfee JG, et al: Diagnosis of massive pulmonary embolism in man by radioisotope scanning, *N Engl J Med* 271:377, 1964.

48. West JB: Pulmonary function studies with radioactive gases, *Ann Rev Med* 18:459, 1967.

49. West JB: *Respiratory physiology—the essentials*, Baltimore, 1975, Williams & Wilkins.

50. Weibel ER: *Morphometry of the human lungs*, New York, 1963, Academic Press.

H. William Strauss, Landis K. Griffeth, Farrokh Dehdashti
Shahrokh, Robert J. Gropler

chapter *12*

Cardiovascular System

Objectives

Diagram the structures of the heart.

Describe the mechanical and electrical activity of the heart.

List the acquired abnormalities of the cardiovascular system that can be evaluated with radionuclide techniques.

State the preparation, dosage, and injection technique for radionuclide evaluation of ventricular function.

Discuss the tracer requirements for first-pass studies.

Explain how an ejection fraction is calculated.

Describe an exercise and pharmacologic stress test and when they are used.

Discuss radiopharmaceuticals used for myocardial perfusion imaging.

Describe the imaging techniques for planar and SPECT myocardial perfusion imaging.

Discuss the advantage of PET radionuclides for cardiac imaging.

INTRODUCTION

Radionuclide studies of the cardiovascular system are primarily employed for the detection and characterization of acquired diseases, such as coronary artery disease and congestive heart failure. Although nuclear procedures can be used to characterize congenital diseases and quantitate shunts, those assessments are generally made by a combination of echocardiography and magnetic resonance imaging. This chapter will focus on the primary clinical applications in general use and will refer the reader to other sources for procedures of historic importance.

Most nuclear medicine laboratories utilize single-photon radiopharmaceuticals and single- or multiple-detector gamma cameras to record clinical data. Positron tomographs generally have higher spatial resolution than single-photon systems and can be used to make a similar repertoire of measurements as single-photon devices. Advances in multidetector gamma camera design suggest that hybrid cameras, capable of recording both single-photon images and coincidence images, will be manufactured, making positron imaging techniques available to users who do not have dedicated positron tomographs. Should this occur, there will be greater use of positron-emitting radiopharmaceuticals in the practice of nuclear cardiology. Since the majority of imaging is carried out with single-photon techniques, we will first devote our attention to these techniques.

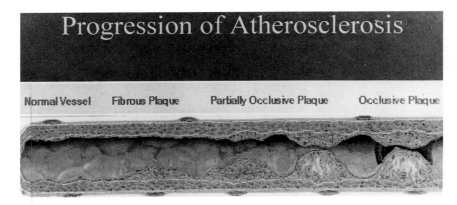

Figure 12-1 Progression of atherosclerosis. Due to factors that are not well defined but are associated with hyperlipidemia and probably injury to vessels, lipids, such as cholesterol and fatty acids, accumulate in the area beneath the endothelium. These lipids are irritating, leading to invasion by monocytes and macrophages, which, over many years, make the lesion larger. The lesion may then break through the endothelial cells, resulting in the formation of a clot at the site of rupture and often myocardial infarction.

The Clinical Problem

Approximately 65 million people in the United States have one or more forms of acquired heart or blood vessel disease. Hypertension occurs in 50 million adults; coronary artery disease occurs in 13.5 million (3 million have angina); rheumatic heart disease occurs in 1.3 million; and stroke occurs in 3.8 million. Coronary heart disease caused about half a million deaths in the United States in 1993. About 1.5 million people will suffer a new or recurrent heart attack this year. As the population ages, heart failure is becoming increasingly prevalent. There are about 2,500,000 patients with heart failure in the United States (about 1% of the population), with about 400,000 new cases occurring each year. This disorder is often the final phase of other heart diseases, including severe coronary disease, valvular heart disease, and cardiomyopathy. An important feature of heart failure is the fact that a significant fraction of patients have coronary artery disease and myocardial ischemia as the cause of their left ventricular dysfunction. Restoring blood flow with either angioplasty or bypass surgery often results in improved function in these patients. Detection of myocardial ischemia in these patients is difficult on clinical grounds and usually requires radionuclide imaging for evaluation.

The following acquired abnormalities can be evaluated with radionuclide techniques:

Myocardial ischemia is a *reversible* condition caused by a temporary deficiency in the supply of oxygen to the myocardium due to atherosclerotic narrowing of the vessel.

Myocardial infarction is an *irreversible* condition leading to death of a portion of the myocardium caused by total occlusion of a coronary artery by a clot usually formed at the site of a severe coronary artery atherosclerotic narrowing.

Cardiomyopathy is a category of diseases associated with either abnormal enlargement of the myocardium (hypertrophic myopathy) or inability to contract effectively in spite of an adequate blood supply, resulting in thinning of the muscle and dilation of the chambers (dilated myopathy), which causes altered function.

Heart failure is often an end-stage condition defined by diminished heart function. Heart failure is usually due to a preexisting condition that results in impaired contractile performance.

Although myocardial infarction can occur with no warning and cause sudden death, the underlying disease of the coronary arteries has evolved over decades. The arterial lesions progress from small lipid deposits in the wall of the vessel that begin around puberty, called *fatty streaks,* to raised lesions that intrude on the arterial lumen over about 20 to 30 years (Figure 12-1). The rate of progression can be controlled to some degree by the patient's diet, cholesterol, genetic heritage, and life style. Atheromatous narrowings that occupy more than 50% of the lumen diameter restrict the maximum amount of blood that can flow through a vessel. These lesions may not be associated with any symptoms.

When patients exercise or certain drugs are administered, the demand for blood flow (oxygen) through the coronary arteries is increased. If the increased demand for oxygen cannot be met, the myocardium becomes *ischemic*. Ischemia is associated with decreased tissue perfusion and decreased contraction in the affected area. These changes can be readily detected by radionuclide imaging studies.

ANATOMY

The adult heart (Figure 12-2) weighs about 300 g and holds approximately 500 ml of blood. The heart is located in the lower portion of the thoracic cavity between the lungs. It is covered by a clear fibrous sac,

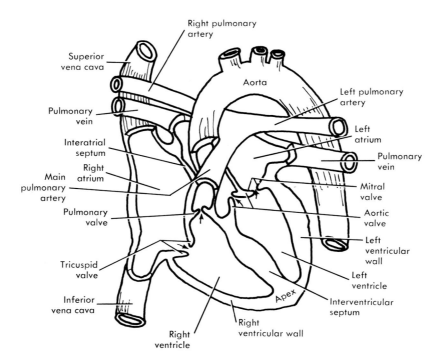

Figure 12-2   Gross anatomy of the heart.

the pericardium, which contains a minimal amount of fluid that acts as a lubricant between the moving surface of heart muscle (myocardium) and the other structures in the chest. It is easiest to think of the heart as two pumps (the right heart and left heart) operating in parallel to eject the same amount of blood each beat. The right heart accepts blood from the body and pumps this blood to the lungs where it is oxygenated. The left heart accepts blood returning from the lungs and pumps it to the body. There is no direct communication of blood between the left and right sides of the heart. Each side has two chambers, a thin-walled atrium and a more muscular ventricle. The atria serve as temporary reservoirs for blood being returned to the heart, whereas the ventricles do the major work of pumping the blood away from the heart. The atria are separated by a thin muscular wall, the interatrial septum, and the ventricles are separated by the thicker, muscular interventricular septum. Valves separate the atria from the ventricles and the ventricles from the arteries. The purpose of the valves is to prevent the backflow of blood from the ventricles to the atria during ventricular contraction or from the arteries to the ventricles during ventricular relaxation.

Venous blood returning from the superior and inferior venae cavae is received in the right atrium. Blood traverses the tricuspid valve (named for its three leaflets or cusps) to enter the right ventricle. The right ventricle is a pyramid-shaped chamber, with the tricuspid valve as its floor. It contracts with a plungerlike motion to expel blood through the pulmonic valve into the pulmonary artery and lungs for oxygenation. The right ventricular myocardium is about 5 mm thick and develops a systolic pressure of 25 mm Hg. Oxygenated blood returning from the lungs via the pulmonary veins is received by the left atrium. Blood traverses the mitral valve to the left ventricle. The left ventricle is a football-shaped structure, with myocardium about 10 mm thick. Contraction occurs with a complex wringing motion to expel blood through the aortic valve into the aorta at a systolic pressure of about 120 mm Hg.

The aorta distributes blood via a branching network of arteries to the organs. Within an organ the arteries branch to form arterioles, which branch further at the cellular level to form capillaries where the nutrients and oxygen are exchanged for waste products and carbon dioxide. From the aorta to the capillary, the blood vessels branch more than 20 times. As blood exits in the capillaries it is carried by venules, which coalesce to form veins, back to the heart.

Oxygen is delivered to the myocardium by the left and right coronary arteries (Figure 12-3). The left main coronary artery divides into two main branches. The left anterior descending artery supplies oxygen and nutrition to the interventricular septum and anterior wall of the left ventricle, whereas the left circumflex artery supplies the left atrium and the posterior and lateral walls of the left ventricle. The right coronary artery supplies the inferior wall of the left ventricle, the free wall of the right ventricle, and the right atrium. Blood drains from the myocardium to the coronary veins located alongside the coronary arteries and terminate in the coronary sinus of the right atrium.

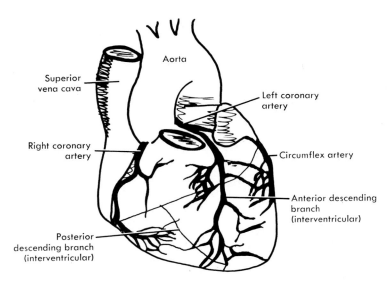

Figure 12-3 Anterior view of the heart, showing the coronary arteries.

PHYSIOLOGY

Circulation

Blood flows unidirectionally through each blood vessel under normal physiologic conditions. Deoxygenated venous blood, loaded with carbon dioxide and waste products, returns from the tissues toward the heart via the veins. Although venous pressure is low, resistance to blood flow is also low, and blood flows through the large veins at 40 cm/sec on its way to emptying into the right atrium at a pressure of less than 5 mm Hg. Blood is expelled from the right ventricle with a pressure of 25 mm Hg into the lungs. In the enormous capillary bed of the lungs the velocity of blood slows to 1 mm/sec in the capillaries of the alveoli, where carbon dioxide is eliminated and oxygen is taken up. The oxygenated blood returns to the heart via the pulmonary veins to the left atrium at a pressure of less than 5 mm Hg. The blood then flows through the mitral valve to the left ventricle, which provides sufficient kinetic energy, in the form of a systolic pressure of 120 mm Hg and a flow rate of 50 cm/sec, to permit the blood to travel to the farthest capillary bed and return to the heart. As in the pulmonary capillaries, the velocity of blood slows at the tissue capillaries to permit the exchange of nutrients for waste products.

The valves in the heart play no role in propelling or initiating flow, only in preventing backflow. The design of the mitral and tricuspid valves is different from the pulmonic and aortic valves: leaflets of the tricuspid and mitral valves are much larger and require "anchors" in the ventricle to prevent blow back during ventricular systole. To ensure that the leaflets of the valves stay in contact when the valves are closed, the leaflets are anchored by tendinous strands, the *chordae tendineae.* The chordae tendineae are attached to the papillary

muscles, which are integrated into the ventricular walls. The aortic and pulmonic valves are smaller and function without the need for special leaflet support.

Mechanical Activity of the Heart

Each cardiac cycle (one beat) consists of *systole,* the period of ventricular contraction, and *diastole,* the period of ventricular relaxation. Both sides of the heart contract in unison, but for clarity our discussion follows the left heart through a contraction cycle starting in late diastole. During this period both the left atrium and left ventricle are relaxed. Left atrial pressure is slightly higher than left ventricular pressure, the mitral valve is open, and blood passes from the left atrium through the mitral valve to the ventricle. The majority (80% to 90%) of ventricular filling takes place in this passive fashion. The aortic valve is closed during this time because aortic pressure is higher than left ventricular pressure. At the end of diastole the atrium contracts, adding 10% to 20% more volume to the left ventricle. The quantity of blood in the ventricle at the end of diastole is called the *end-diastolic volume* (about 150 ml in an average 70 kg adult).

Systole, ventricular contraction, starts as the myofibrils of the ventricular myocardium shorten and left ventricular pressure rises, causing the mitral valve to close. As the myofibrils continue to shorten, left ventricular pressure rises at a rapid rate. The interval after mitral valve closure but before the generation of sufficient pressure to open the aortic valve is called the *interval of isovolumetric* (no change in volume) *contraction.* Continued shortening of the myofibrils causes the left ventricular pressure to exceed aortic pressure; the aortic valve opens and ventricular ejection begins. During the 250- to 300-msec interval when the myofibrils shorten to their minimal length, approximately half to

Table 12-1	Cardiac output at rest and exercise	
	Fraction of cardiac output	
Organ	**Rest (5 liters/min)**	**Exercise (15 liters/min)**
Brain	15%	4%
Heart	4%	5%
Kidneys	20%	5%
Liver	10%	1%
GI tract	15%	1%
Skeletal muscle	20%	70%
Skin	6%	10%
Other	10%	4%

From McCardle WD et al: In *Exercise, physiology, energy, nutrition and human performance,* Philadelphia, 1981, Lea & Febiger.

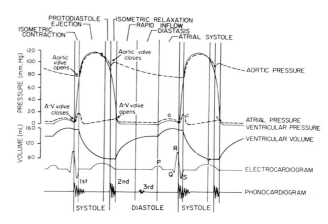

Figure 12-4 Events in the cardiac cycle, showing simultaneous relationship of the electrocardiogram and phonocardiogram to the measured pressures in the left atrium, left ventricle, and aorta and the volume of the ventricles.

two thirds of the end-diastolic volume is ejected. Blood returning to the left heart during the interval of ventricular ejection, when the mitral valve is closed, is stored in the left atrium. As a result, both the left atrial volume and pressure rise during the interval of ventricular ejection. At the conclusion of left ventricular ejection the myofibrils rapidly relax, left ventricular pressure falls, the aortic valve closes, the mitral valve opens, and the ventricle starts to fill with blood that has returned to the left atrium during the interval of ventricular ejection. Filling occurs rapidly during early diastole and slows as atrial pressure and volume decrease. This filling pattern ensures the heart's ability to function unimpaired during times of increased heart rate (as with exercise and emotional stress), when the length of diastole is shortened. In a relative sense the atrial contribution to end-diastolic volume is greater during exercise when cardiac output and heart rate are increased then at rest.

The quantity of blood ejected from the left ventricle over a 1-min interval is the *cardiac output* (usually expressed in liters/minute). A normal 70 kg adult has a cardiac output of approximately 5-6 L/min at rest. The quantity of blood ejected in a single beat is the *stroke volume* (usually expressed in milliliters). The normal adult stroke volume is approximately 80-100 ml. The cardiac output is distributed to the organs in proportion to their oxygen requirements, which change from rest to exertion as summarized in Table 12-1.

Electrical Activity of the Heart

The muscle that makes up the myocardium has an intrinsic rhythm of contraction. The sinoatrial node, a small mass of specialized cells embedded in the wall of the right atrium near the entrance of the superior vena cava, has the fastest inherent rhythm and supersedes other similar sites in the heart. As a result the sinoatrial

node usually serves as the impulse generator for the remainder of the heart.

Although the electrical signal can propagate through the muscle fibers of the ventricles causing each area to contract as it is depolarized, the left ventricular myocardium is thick, and contraction would occur in each area sequentially, rather than at the same time. To overcome this problem, the ventricular myocardium has a more efficient system to deliver the signal to all portions of the right and left ventricles in a timely fashion. A series of specialized muscle fibers, called the *conducting system*, carry the electrical message from the atrioventricular node to the far reaches of the ventricular myocardium.

The wave of electrical depolarization begins in the sinoatrial node (the fastest pacemaker) and spreads to the surrounding atrial muscle cells. There are no specialized conduction fibers within the atrium, probably because it is thin, and the wave of excitation spreads from cell to cell to cover the entire atria within 0.08 sec. As the electrical signal propagates through the atrium, it stimulates mechanical contraction. Mechanical contraction requires approximately 0.1 sec, much more time than the spread of the electrical signal.

To maximize the amount of blood in the ventricles before the onset of ventricular contraction, atrial systole must be completed before the ventricles begin to contract. This requires a delay in the transmission of the electrical signal from the atria to the ventricles. The electrical signal enters the atrioventricular node, where it is held for over 0.1 sec, before entering the specialized conducting system (named the *bundle of His*) to signal ventricular systole. As a result the electrical signal for the ventricles to contract starts at the conclusion of mechanical atrial systole. Rapid conduction along the bundle of His results in depolarization of the right and left ventricular myocardium almost simultaneously. The electrical signal is followed by the onset of mechanical systole, which requires approximately 0.3 sec.

> ### Box 12-1 Common conduction abnormalities
>
> - **Premature systoles** may originate in the atria (premature atrial contractions, PACs) or ventricles (premature ventricular contractions, PVCs) or be coupled together. If the extrasystoles occur every other beat, the rhythm is called *bigeminy*.
> - **Ventricular tachycardia** originates in a focus in the ventricle. This type of rapid rate is potentially life threatening and should be treated immediately. Ventricular tachycardia can proceed to ventricular fibrillation, which if untreated results in death.
> - **Atrial fibrillation** is defined as a totally disorganized firing at multiple sites in the atria, causing a rapid irregular ventricular rate.
> - **Left bundle branch block** is an abnormal conduction pattern associated with slower depolarization of the conducting pathway through the left ventricle than the right.
> - **Right bundle branch block** is an abnormal conduction pattern associated with slower depolarization of the conducting pathway through the right ventricle than the left.

From Zipes DP: In *Heart disease: a textbook of cardiovascular medicine*, Philadelphia, 1984, WB Saunders.

The electrocardiogram (ECG) reflects the electrical activities of the heart (Figure 12-4). It typically consists of a P wave, QRS complex, and T wave. The P wave is the electrical signal to the atria to contract, the QRS complex serves the same function in the ventricles, and the T wave identifies an electrical reset of the ventricles for the next cardiac cycle. During much of diastole the heart is electrically silent.

Irregularities or abnormalities of conduction are quite common and can have substantial effects on radionuclide studies of ventricular function. Some of the more common conduction abnormalities are listed in Box 12-1.

GENERAL IMAGING CONSIDERATIONS

Measurements

Radiopharmaceuticals determine the parameters that will be depicted in the image. There are three major categories of radiopharmaceuticals for clinical cardiac imaging:

1. Agents for evaluating myocardial perfusion (e.g., single-photon emitters such as ^{201}Tl, ^{99m}Tc-labeled perfusion agents such as ^{99m}Tc sestamibi, tetrofosmin, or teboroxime and the positron-emitting tracer ionic ^{82}Rb).
2. Agents to label the blood to measure ventricular function (e.g., ^{99m}Tc-labeled red blood cells or ^{99m}Tc albumin).
3. Agents to detect acute myocardial necrosis (e.g., ^{99m}Tc pyrophosphate or ^{111}In antimyosin).

Other agents are available to evaluate myocardial metabolism (e.g., ^{123}I fatty acids or positron-emitting radiopharmaceuticals such as ^{18}F fluorodeoxyglucose or ^{11}C-labeled fatty acids) and sympathetic innervation (^{123}I MIBG).

Planar and SPECT Data Acquisition

Data can be recorded with planar or SPECT techniques with any of the radiopharmaceuticals. However, since radionuclide imaging is relatively count poor (noisy) compared with other imaging techniques, it is best to use planar imaging when studies have a low-count rate or when data must be recorded in a short interval of time and SPECT imaging when high-count rates are available (usually with ^{99m}Tc-labeled radiopharmaceuticals). Images are recorded with either a single detector or multidetector scintillation camera with extrinsic resolution better than 5 mm full width at half maximum (FWHM). Digital image data are typically recorded in a computer, usually in a 64×64 matrix for a standard field-of-view detector or 128×128 matrix for a large-field detector (see Chapter 4).

Because most heart disease is focal, the heart should be imaged from as many perspectives as possible. Although this is best accomplished with single photon emission computed tomography (SPECT), planar images can sample the major surfaces of the left ventricle (usually in three views). SPECT imaging requires a minimum of a 180-degree sample, with data recorded from an arc spanning the 180 degrees from 30 degrees right anterior oblique (RAO) to 30 degrees left posterior oblique (LPO). Data are reconstructed into tomographic slices in transverse, sagittal, coronal, and oblique slices through the heart (see Chapters 3 and 4 for details of SPECT acquisition and processing).

SPECT images are recorded with either a single detector or multidetector rotating scintillation camera. The most common multidetector (multiheaded) cameras have either two detectors (that can assume positions ranging from 90 to 180 degrees apart) or three detectors spaced 120 degrees apart. If 180-degree sampling is desired, a dual-detector system with the detectors oriented 90 degrees to each other is preferable. If data are to be recorded with 360-degree sampling, a three-detector system is preferred. The higher sensitivity (sensitivity is a function of the total number of detectors—a two-detector system at 90 degrees can ac-

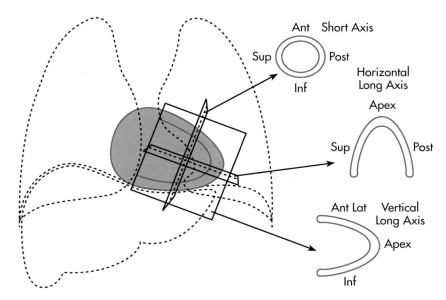

Figure 12-5 Schematic representation of the heart in the chest. SPECT data are reoriented to present the myocardium in views that are orthogonal to the major cardiac axes. The slices are called *short-axis* (cut from the apex to the base of the left ventricle), *horizontal long-axis* (cut from the septum to the posterior wall rotated with the apex pointing to the top to differentiate this view from the vertical long axis), and *vertical long-axis* views. The specific walls depicted in each view are indicated with the representative slice.

quire a cardiac SPECT in half the time of a single-detector system for the same total counts in a 180-degree acquisition, whereas a three-detector system would require one third the time to acquire data for a 360-degree acquisition). To maximize spatial resolution, the detectors should be as close as possible to the surface of the patient when recording each image. Mechanically, it is easiest to rotate the detector through a circle when recording data at steps of ≤6 degrees for 15 to 60 sec at each step. Inadequate sampling (step angles >6 degrees or gaps between the steps) can produce an artifact resembling the spokes of a wheel (star artifact). To avoid this, angular sampling of about 3 degrees or continuous data acquisition is recommended. A circular orbit maximizes the distance between the collimator and the body surface in the anterior and posterior positions, resulting in a spatial resolution of approximately 12-19 mm. Moving the detector through an ellipse as it moves around the chest keeps the detectors closer to the heart, resulting in some improvement in resolution. Setting up a noncircular acquisition is more complex, however, and the gain in resolution is small, especially for large patients.

SPECT data are acquired in a step-and-shoot or a continuous-acquisition mode. Step-and-shoot mode has greater resolution (no detector motion blurring during acquisition) but requires increased time for acquisition because an extra few seconds is required to move several thousand pounds of detector 3 to 6 degrees and bring it to a full stop before the next image is acquired. During the 20- to 30-min acquisition, the patient lies supine with the left arm above the head (a fairly uncomfortable position).

A 180-degree acquisition is typically used with single-detector and 90-degree, dual-detector gamma cameras because the detector is closest to the heart for each image, maximizing collimator resolution, and highly attenuated photons recorded from the back of the patient are not employed in the reconstruction. The 180-degree acquired studies have higher contrast than data acquired with a 360-degree acquisition. The dual-detector 90-degree gamma camera has the advantage of double the sensitivity of a single-detector machine. This increase in sensitivity can be utilized to either decrease the examination time (while maintaining the study quality), increasing study quality by doubling the count density, or slightly shortening the time to accomplish some of both. However, there are some artifacts on 180-degree studies that are eliminated when 360-degree data are employed. When a three-detector machine is used, data are typically acquired using a 360-degree acquisition. The differences in image quality between 180- and 360-degree acquisitions are reduced when a technetium-labeled radiopharmaceutical is employed.

To maximize resolution, SPECT images should be recorded with high–or ultra-high–resolution collimation.

Data can be recorded with or without synchronization to the patient's cardiac cycle (physiologic [e.g., ECG] gating). In the past, ECG gating was reserved for blood-pool studies to measure global and regional ventricular function. The increased photon flux available from ^{99m}Tc-labeled perfusion agents allows high-quality gated myocardial perfusion SPECT studies to be recorded. Data from gated perfusion scans is particularly helpful to differentiate attenuation artifacts from significant perfusion abnormalities and to assess ventricular volumes and regional wall motion.

Projection data from SPECT acquisitions are reconstructed into transverse images by filtering and back-projecting the images. The filter utilized for reconstruction should have sufficient spatial resolution to permit visualization of the myocardial borders (usually a frequency of 0.5-0.7 cycle/cm is employed). Transverse section images should provide six to eight slices through the heart (typical reconstructions are 1- to 2-pixels thick with no spaces between the slices). Before reconstruction the projection images should be reviewed as a cinematic display to detect patient motion, major changes in cardiac position during acquisition, and technical problems such as missed or duplicated angles. Single episodes of motion of ≤2 pixels can usually be tolerated. Data with multiple episodes of motion, movement >2 pixels, or loss of more than one set of projection data will have artifacts in the reconstructed tomograms that may result in an erroneous interpretation. If these situations occur, a repeat acquisition should be recorded.

Once the transverse plane data are available, the cardiac volume is realigned to present a standard orientation of the heart orthogonal to its major axes. Short-axis images depict the myocardium from the apex to the base, vertical long-axis images slice the volume from anterolateral wall to inferior wall, whereas horizontal long-axis images depict the right ventricle, septum, and posterior wall (Figure 12-5).

RADIONUCLIDE EVALUATION OF VENTRICULAR FUNCTION

The heart's ability to function as a pump can be measured by imaging a radiopharmaceutical that is retained within the blood pool throughout the time of data collection. Two approaches are generally used: data are recorded as sequential images during injection of the radiopharmaceutical, when the majority of activity is contained in the cardiac chambers, a first-pass acquisition; or data are recorded over hundreds of beats synchronized with the cardiac cycle, after the radiopharmaceutical has equilibrated in the body, multigated acquisition (MUGA) equilibrium technique. Though the recording techniques differ, the measurements made from the data are similar. These include the size and shape of the chambers, the motion of the walls during each beat, and the ejection fraction. Functional assessment of the heart should describe the ejection fraction and regional motion of both ventricles, as well as atrial size and contraction patterns. Of these measurements the single value used most often to characterize cardiac function is the left ventricular ejection fraction (LVEF), a value calculated by dividing the amount of blood ejected by the ventricle during systole by the amount of blood in the ventricle at the end of diastole.

The first-pass and equilibrium techniques place different constraints on the radiopharmaceutical. The first-pass study requires the tracer to reside in the blood pool less than a minute to traverse the chambers of interest. Optimally, the tracer is cleared rapidly from the bloodstream to allow for repeat studies in the same imaging session, if necessary. Equilibrium blood-pool images require the tracer to remain within the bloodstream for at least 30 min.

First Pass

The most common radiopharmaceutical for examinations of right and left cardiac chambers that require multiple first-pass studies in a short interval is ^{99m}Tc DTPA, because of its rapid clearance through the kidneys. Other radiopharmaceuticals that provide a high-photon flux with an acceptable radiation burden can be used to perform first-pass studies, if a single injection is all that is required. Pertechnetate is not well suited for multiple injection studies because its concentration in the gastric mucosa makes it difficult to visualize the inferior surface of the heart. Similar limitations apply to ^{99m}Tc-sulfur or albumin-colloid preparations that are trapped in the liver and spleen. Unusual agents, such as ^{99m}Tc MAA, ^{133}Xe, or ^{81m}Kr dissolved in saline, can be used if specific information about only right heart function is desired.

In the past multicrystal cameras, with maximum count rates of >500,000 counts/sec were recommended for first-pass studies. However, high-count rates were achieved at the cost of spatial resolution, which was on the order of 1 cm. Anger cameras are now used for most of these studies, since these instruments provide better spatial resolution and have maximum count rates of >100,000 counts/sec with dead-time losses of <20% (with some of the new cameras providing useful data at rates of ~250,000 counts/sec). Before recording first-pass studies routinely on an Anger camera, phantom studies should be performed to determine the count-rate characteristics of the camera/computer. Sources of increasing intensity should be placed in the field to determine that activity in each is accurately portrayed and that hot spots or lines do not appear between the known sources. A reasonable test would use ~3 cm of lucite to simulate body tissue and 3 or 4 sources with activity totaling 20 mCi in the field of view at the same time. This test should provide a count rate of ~60,000 counts/sec through an all-purpose collimator.

Data recording. Data can be recorded using either a high-sensitivity or all-purpose collimator. High-sensitivity collimation provides about twice the count rate of an all-purpose collimator, but resolution falls off rapidly as the distance between the heart and the face of the collimator increases. As a result, for patients with skin thickness >5 cm, an all-purpose collimator is preferred. The patient is positioned in either the anterior (for assessment of overall cardiac function) or the 45-degree left anterior oblique (LAO) position for optimal separation of the right and left ventricles, then data recording is started at 25 msec/frame and the tracer is injected. About 1 min of data (2400 frames) are collected.

Injection technique. Since data are recorded as the bolus of activity passes through the heart and lungs the first time, it is critical to administer the activity in a small volume, typically less than 1 ml through an indwelling line placed in the basilic (medial) vein of the forearm. The laterally located cephalic vein takes a less direct path to the subclavian vein and tends to produce a fragmented bolus, making the data difficult to analyze. Optimal results require injection via the external jugular vein, to provide the shortest, most direct path possible. To facilitate delivery of a compact bolus for left ventricular function measurement via an arm vein, the Oldendorf injection technique should be used. An 18-gauge needle or intracath is placed in the basilic vein. A three-way stopcock is placed at the end of the line; a syringe containing the activity should be connected to one port, and a syringe containing 10-20 ml of a flushing solution of either sterile saline or 5% dextrose should be connected to the other. A blood pressure cuff is placed proximal to the catheter. When palpating the radial pulse, the cuff is inflated until the pulse just disappears, then the pressure is reduced by about 10 mm Hg. Inflation is maintained for 1 min, then increased above systolic pressure; activity is slowly injected through the stopcock into the occluded vein; the computer is started; the cuff is then rapidly removed (not deflated); and the flushing dose is administered. Injection should be performed during normal respiration and care should be exercised to ensure that the patient does not alter the normal breathing pattern during the study.

Framing interval. To determine the ejection fraction, both end-systole and end-diastole must be accurately sampled. End-systole is shorter and defines the framing interval. At a heart rate of 70 beats/min, end-systole lasts less than 80 msec. To ensure that this interval is properly measured, data are recorded at 40 msec/frame or preferably 25 msec/frame.

Total data recording. Normal transit time through the heart and lungs is 15 sec, but patients with heart disease may take 45 sec for bolus transit. Since additional time is needed to start the camera/computer before injection, at least 60 sec of data should be obtained (1500-2400 frames). It may be necessary to have two people work together to record these studies: one to start the camera/computer and the other to perform the bolus injection.

Data analysis. The short interval of data collection for each frame makes it difficult to appreciate specific cardiac structures when the data are replayed. To facilitate specific chamber identification, sequential groups of 20 to 40 frames are added together and data are reviewed in intervals of 0.5 to 1 sec. Reformatted frames are displayed as an endless-loop movie to identify the superior vena cava, right and left ventricles, and lungs. Regions of interest are carefully drawn over each of these, and a time-activity curve is generated from the original short-duration frame data.

The superior vena cava curve is evaluated for the duration of the bolus. The full-width-at-half-maximum transit time of activity through this curve should be less than 2.5 sec. If the transit time is longer than this, activity enters the left ventricle before it has completely cleared the right, and the calculated left ventricular ejection fraction may be erroneous.

The right ventricle curve should appear as a sawtooth, with one or two peaks (end-diastole) and comparable minima (end-systole) (Figure 12-6). A second series of sawtooth peaks occurs as activity enters the left ventricle, since the ventricles overlap in the anterior position. Frames with activity in the left ventricle should be excluded from analysis of right ventricular function. The counts at the peak points selected from the early part of the curve, when activity is only in the right heart, should be added together, and the counts at the minimal points should be added together to give end-diastolic (ED) and end-systolic (ES) counts, respectively. The right ventricular ejection fraction (EF) is calculated as follows:

$$\text{Ejection fraction} = \frac{(\text{End-diastolic counts} - \text{End-systolic counts})}{\text{End-diastolic counts}}$$

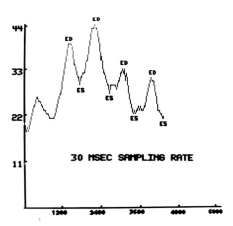

Figure 12-6 Right ventricular time-activity curve in the first-pass method.

There has been some debate about the need to subtract "background" from the data used for analysis of right ventricular function. Some investigators argue that background counts are significant relative to counts within the heart and should be subtracted for the most accurate determinations. Others argue that since the amount of activity outside the heart during this portion of the first-pass examination is minimal, a background correction plays a very small role and can usually be ignored. For most clinical applications background can be ignored. On the other hand, background must be determined and subtracted from the left ventricular data.

The lung curve (obtained from a region of interest placed adjacent to the left ventricle) should appear smooth, rising as the RV curve falls and falling before the rise of the left ventricular curve. The counts/pixel of the lung curve are determined to permit correction of the left ventricular curve for background.

The curve obtained from the left ventricular region of interest should appear as a sawtooth, starting after the peak of the lung curve. A series of small peaks can be seen in synchrony with transit of the bolus through the right ventricle due to overlap of the chambers, as just described. These peaks should be ignored when calculating the ejection fraction of the left ventricle. A minimum of three peaks occurring in conjunction with the decrease in lung activity, near the peak of the left ventricular curve, should be used to calculate the ejection fraction. The left ventricular curve must be corrected for lung activity by subtracting the lung counts/pixel (multiplied by the number of pixels in the left ventricular region of interest) from it (Figure 12-7). The counts at the peak of each cardiac cycle (end-diastole) are then added together; the corresponding end-systoles are similarly added; and the ejection fraction is computed, as described for the right ventricle.

A first-pass study can be used to provide a rough assessment of wall motion by viewing a cinematic display of the summed end-diastolic and end-systolic frames. Regional wall motion can be assessed either by subtracting the end-systolic image from the end-diastolic image, to produce a stroke volume image, or by outlining the blood pool at end-systole and end-diastole based on count thresholds. Alternatively, first-pass data can be collected in gated form and displayed cinematically, as described for equilibrium studies. Although all methods are acceptable, the low-count density at each point on the perimeter of the ventricle makes the first-pass approach relatively insensitive for the detection of modest abnormalities of wall motion.

Ultrashort half-life radionuclides. The 6-hr half-life of ^{99m}Tc technetium-labeled agents is too long for multiple first-pass studies. Several short-lived isotopes are being evaluated experimentally for the first-pass determination of cardiac function. These agents are expensive or have low energies, making it unlikely that any will see widespread clinical use. However, the agents have some unique characteristics, demonstrating some of the unique systems that can be developed for use in nuclear medicine.

Four generator-produced radionuclides have been suggested for evaluation of right and left heart function: (1) ^{195}Hg/^{195m}Au ($t_{1/2}$ 30 sec). ^{195m}Au behaves as a blood-pool agent, which traverses both the right and left ventricles; (2) ^{81}Rb/^{81m}Kr ($t_{1/2}$ 13 sec). ^{81m}Kr is a gas. It can be dissolved in saline to provide images of the right heart. As the bolus traverses the lungs, the agent enters the alveoli. Less than 15% of the administered dose remains in the blood pool to enter the left heart; (3) ^{191}Os/^{191m}Ir ($t_{1/2}$ 4.7 sec). ^{191m}Ir is a blood-pool agent, which traverses the lungs. It is difficult to use ^{191m}Ir in patients with heart failure because the agent decays before a significant fraction enters the left ventricle. The short half-life of the agent, however, and its consequent low radiation burden, make it of interest in the evaluation of infants. The final generator system that has been suggested for this purpose is the ^{178}W/^{178}Ta system. ^{178}Ta binds to plasma proteins. With its 10-min half-life, the agent is well suited to record multiple views with high-count density using equilibrium techniques.

The short half-life agents require that the generator be eluted directly into the patient, which limits the quality control procedures that can be performed on the eluate before administration. The severity of the problem is increased when the half-life of the parent radionuclide is long compared with that of the daughter. In the ^{81}Rb/81mKr generator the $t_{1/2}$ of the parent ^{81}Rb is only 4.7 hr. Breakthrough of ^{81}Rb into the eluate containing the 13-sec $t_{1/2}$ daughter ^{81m}Kr results in a relatively modest radiation burden to the patient. In contrast, breakthrough of parent ^{195}Hg ($t_{1/2}$ 10 hr) into the ^{195m}Au eluate ($t_{1/2}$ 30 sec) results in a much greater radiation burden per microcurie of parent in the eluate. Of the short-lived generator systems evalu-

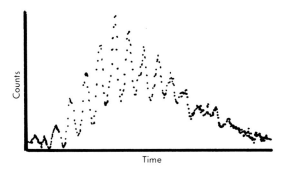

Figure 12-7 Corrected left ventricular time-activity curve in the first-pass method.

ated so far, the ^{195}Hg/^{195m}Au system is the most useful in the evaluation of all four cardiac chambers. ^{191m}Ir also can be used, but any condition that prolongs the usual 8-sec (nearly two half-lives) transit time through the lungs reduces the photon flux, making left heart interpretation difficult.

Gated Blood-Pool Studies

Equilibrium imaging records data after the radiopharmaceutical has been distributed in the vascular space. Data recording is synchronized (gated) by the patient's cardiac cycle. The patient's heart rate is computed, and the result is expressed as msec/cycle. The cardiac cycle is then divided into some number of frames ranging from a minimum of 16 to a maximum of 64. This number of frames is derived from the fact that end-systole lasts 80 msec in an adult with a resting heart rate of 80 beats/min. To sample an 80-msec interval, the computer should be collecting data at about 40 msec/frame. At 80 beats/min the cardiac cycle lasts 750 msec. Dividing this interval into 16 frames requires 46 msec/frame—about right for really sampling end-systole.

The computer is instructed to record data from the first portion of the cardiac cycle into the first frame, the second portion of the cycle into the second frame, and so on, until the last frame is reached or the next R wave is sensed, resetting the recording to the first frame to repeat the process (Figure 12-8). Data from about 500-1000 such cycles typically are added together to form an "average" cardiac cycle.

Equilibrium-gated blood-pool imaging differs from first-pass studies in several respects as follows:

1. The time required to acquire the data is much greater, typically 8 to 10 min for each view.
2. The chambers overlap, making it difficult to distinguish portions of the right ventricle from the left ventricle in the anterior view (this can be partially overcome using SPECT, but complex cardiac motion often moves chambers in and out of the slice during the cycle).
3. The count density of the images is much greater, permitting minimal abnormalities of wall motion to be readily detected.
4. Images can be recorded over several hours without the requirement for reinjecting the patient, permitting assessment of multiple short-acting drug interventions.
5. Images are usually recorded in multiple views. Typically the anterior view (to examine right atrial size and motion, tricuspid valve motion, right ventricular and pulmonary artery size and motion), 45-degree LAO (optimized to separate the right and left ventricles and to determine

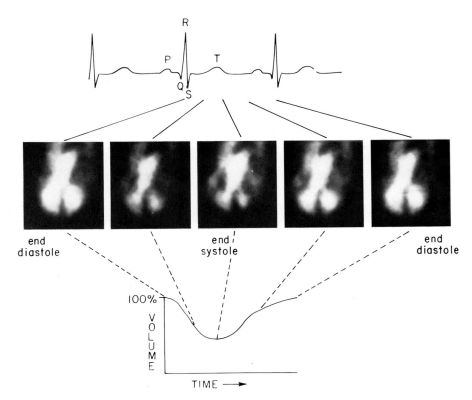

Figure 12-8 Sequential scintiphotos of the heart during a cardiac cycle shown in relation to the ECG waveform and left ventricular volume.

the timing and motion of the anterior wall of the right ventricle, posterior wall of the left ventricle, and overall motion and thickening of the septum), and either the left lateral or left posterior oblique view (to view the inferior and posterior surfaces of the left ventricle as well as the size and motion of the left atrium) are obtained. If SPECT is done, a 360-degree data collection should be performed.

Equilibrium Radiopharmaceuticals

Equilibrium blood-pool radiopharmaceuticals should have an unchanging volume of distribution over the time of observation. This can be accomplished by coupling technetium to a large molecule or cell that remains in the blood. Both red blood cells and albumin have been employed for this purpose.

Red blood cells. There are several methods available for the binding of ^{99m}Tc to the red blood cell. Each of these methods requires that ^{99m}Tc enter the red cell and bind to the beta chain of hemoglobin. Although the conditions necessary for optimal red-cell labeling are relatively well described, details of the mechanism are poorly understood. Three red-cell labeling techniques have evolved.

1. **In vivo labeled red blood cells.** Stannous ion (usually in the form of stannous pyrophosphate) is administered intravenously. Several stannous preparations including stannous glucoheptonate, stannous citrate, stannous diphosphonate, and stannous pyrophosphate all provide excellent results. More important than the type of stannous preparation is the amount of stannous ion used. In vivo labeling is obtained with doses of approximately 10 mg of stannous ion/kg of body weight (an amount approximated or exceeded by that in a typical stannous pyrophosphate kit). About 15 to 30 min after stannous administration, ^{99m}Tc pertechnetate is administered via a second intravenous access site. This second site is required to prevent adherence of reduced ^{99m}Tc to the catheter previously used for stannous ion administration or to the tissues surrounding that catheter. Although this approach is convenient, labeling efficiency is quite variable from patient to patient and is lower than that obtained with the other techniques. Typical labeling efficiencies range from 60% to 90%. ^{99m}Tc that is not bound to red cells diffuses into tissue, reducing the contrast between cardiac blood pool and adjacent tissues. The average heart-to-background contrast with this approach is 2:1 compared with 3:1 for in vitro labeling approaches. Non–red-cell bound activity is excreted through the kidneys

into the urinary bladder, making this labeling technique undesirable when patients are examined for GI bleeding. A dose of 20 mCi of ^{99m}Tc pertechnetate for in vivo red-cell labeling results in an estimated absorbed radiation dose of 2.2 rad to the bladder wall.

2. **In vitro labeled red blood cells.** At the other end of the spectrum of red-cell labeling is a procedure that completes the labeling process completely outside of the patient's body. About 12 ml of the patient's blood is drawn into a syringe containing either heparin or acid citrate-dextrose anticoagulant and a small amount of stannous ion. The mixture is incubated at room temperature for 10 to 20 min, and the blood is then transferred to a sterile test tube, which is then centrifuged. The supernatant plasma is removed, and ^{99m}Tc pertechnetate is then added. The test tube is placed in a shielded container and allowed to incubate for an additional 10 min. This time is required because the binding of technetium to hemoglobin requires several minutes. After this incubation the labeled red cells are again centrifuged, and the residual plasma is removed. Material that is injected has >95% of the activity bound to the red cells.

    A kit for in vitro red blood cell labeling (*Ultratag*, Mallinckrodt) simplifies the process and results in >95% of the readministered activity bound to the red cells.

3. **Modified in vivo labeled red blood cells.** An alternative approach combines the convenience of in vivo labeling with the improved labeling efficiencies of in vitro techniques. Stannous ions (usually in the form of stannous pyrophosphate) is administered intravenously. About 15 to 30 min later 1-5 ml of the patient's blood is withdrawn into a heparinized syringe containing ^{99m}Tc pertechnetate. The mixture is permitted to incubate for 10 min at room temperature, with occasional rotation or inversion of the syringe for mixing. The whole blood is then reinjected into the patient. Labeling efficiencies of 90% to 95% are typically obtained by this method.

    Optimal modified in vivo red blood cell labeling is affected by the length of stannous ion incubation—a minimum of 20 min appears necessary to get high-efficiency labeling. Several other factors can reduce the efficiency of red blood cell labeling. Patients with hematocrits less than 30%, chilling the syringe containing the patient's blood, and very sick patients generally have reduced labeling efficiency. In very sick patients it is not clear whether the labeling efficiency is reduced by the medication the patients are taking or some other change in the patient's plasma as a result of the severe illness. Some patients have circulating non–red blood cell antibodies that also can decrease red-cell labeling.

Albumin. ^{99m}Tc albumin is prepared from a commercial kit containing stannous-treated albumin. The kit is reconstituted and labeled with ^{99m}TcO$_4$. The advantages of ^{99m}Tc albumin are its immediate availability and minimal handling of or exposure to the patient's blood, and the fact that the kit can be used to dose multiple patients. The major problems with ^{99m}Tc albumin is its diffusion out of the vasculature, decreasing target-to-background ratios and increasing activity in the liver. In patients treated with multiple drugs that may diminish red-cell labeling, albumin is the preferred radiopharmaceutical.

Patient preparation. ECG electrodes should be placed on the chest and a baseline recording should be evaluated. Good electrode contact with the skin is ensured when the skin is lightly abraded by rubbing with alcohol or very fine sand paper before the electrodes are applied. Usually, four electrodes are placed to record one of the standard limb leads of the electrocardiogram. The ECG waveform should be reviewed to determine that the initial portion of the QRS complex is positive (Figure 12-9). Although gating will occur with either negative or positive waveforms, some triggers seek the positive deflection, creating a slight temporal offset in the data when the initial waveform is negative. As a result, it is best to standardize on one polarity. If the initial waveform is negative, the electrodes should be moved or the leads reversed to provide a positive complex. The waveform also should be reviewed to make certain that only a single, well-defined, QRS complex is observed with each cardiac cycle. Two complexes are often seen in patients with permanent pacemakers. Under the circumstances of more than one complex/cycle, the electrodes should be moved until the waveform of one complex is maximized and the other minimized to ensure that only a single triggering signal is obtained for each cardiac cycle.

If the patient has a markedly irregular heart rate (greater than 10% variation in R-R interval in more than 10% of the beats), as occurs in atrial fibrillation or with multiple premature contractions, the rates of filling and emptying of the heart change substantially from beat to beat. As a result, it is not physiologically correct to add these data together to calculate rates of filling or emptying. However, it is possible to calculate the ejection fraction from these data, since diastolic function is generally affected more by such phenomena than is systolic function.

Data recording. Data recording can begin within 2 to 3 min of administration of the radiopharmaceutical. However, if absolute ventricular volumes are measured by either a count-based method or by comparison to a blood sample, the tracer must be allowed to equilibrate for at least 15 min before data acquisition. The 5 to 10 min required to record high-quality, equilibrium blood-pool images in each projection necessitates that the data be recorded with the patient lying on a stretcher and the heart centered in the field of view. In contrast to first-pass studies, the anterior view is usually recorded in preference to the RAO, since the collimator can be positioned closer to the patient's chest, thus maximizing resolution. Although the anterior view does not allow the left ventricle to be viewed in its long axis, the left ventricle is not totally obscured by the right ventricle. The camera is then rotated to the LAO position, and using the persistence mode on the computer, the LAO view is optimized to separate the left ventricle from the right while maintaining the collimator as close to the chest as possible. Some cranial angulation of the camera (the body of the camera tilted cranially, with the crystal pointing caudally) may be necessary to accomplish this. At the conclusion of the LAO view, the patient is rotated into a steep LAO position, the left lateral position, or a left posterior oblique position, and the last view is recorded.

Data analysis. Data from equilibrium images are evaluated visually and quantitatively. Initially, the images are reviewed as a cinematic display for adequacy of count density over the cardiac blood pool and for appropriateness of positioning. The total counts in each frame are determined to ensure that the last useful frame of the sequence has less than 15% drop-off in counts compared with the beginning of the study. This can occur when there is change in rhythm or heart rate during acquisition. If there is no apparent motion of the cardiac chambers or there is more than a 15% decrease in counts, the electrodes and ECG-triggering appara-

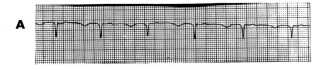

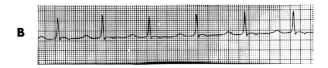

Figure 12-9 **(A),** Negative QRS complex. **(B),** Positive QRS complex.

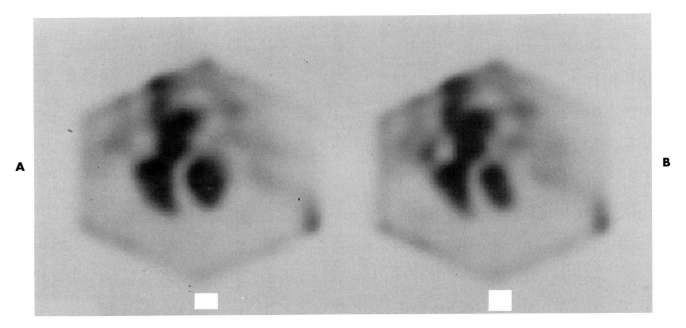

Figure 12-10   End-diastolic **(A)** and end-systolic **(B)** ventricular images demonstrating optimal ventricular separation.

tus should be rechecked and if necessary the images should be repeated.

The LAO or best septal view is analyzed to calculate the ejection fraction from the total counts in the left ventricle at end-systole and end-diastole (Figure 12-10) (after background correction). Regions of interest can be drawn over the LV automatically (using either a second derivative or threshold algorithm) or manually. Identification of the ventricular border is often facilitated by smoothing the data spatially and temporally or applying a resolution recovery (Wiener) filter before analysis. Temporal smoothing should only be used when the heart rate is regular. If the R-R interval has significant variation, temporal smoothing will cause errors. The latter frames of the acquisition, containing fewer counts, will be averaged with the initial frames, thereby lowering the counts in the early frames. If this data is used to calculate the ejection fraction, the end-diastolic counts in the left ventricle are lower than they should be, resulting in a calculated ejection fraction that is too low.

A background region, located at about 3 to 6 o'clock from the left ventricle and free of branches of the pulmonary artery, left atrium, and spleen is selected (Figure 12-11), and the counts/pixel in the lung is determined. A typical value for lung background is between 40% and 60% of left ventricular end-diastolic counts (depending on the radiopharmaceutical, window setting, and collimator). This value is then subtracted from each pixel in the left ventricular region of interest. The background subtraction step is crucial to the subsequent calculation of the ejection fraction. Subtraction of too much background will result in a falsely

elevated ejection fraction, and subtraction of too little will cause it to be falsely depressed.

The total background-corrected counts in the left ventricle on each frame are then normalized to the counts in the end-diastolic frame, and the time-activity curve from the left ventricular region of interest is displayed. The ejection fraction is calculated from the time-activity curve. Normal left ventricular ejection fraction ranges from 50% to 75%. In addition to the ejection fraction, the time of filling and emptying and the ejection and filling rates of the ventricles can be readily computed from these curves.

An alternative approach to calculating ejection fraction uses a single region of interest, based on the end-diastolic frame, to measure the time-activity curve. Left ventricular ejection fraction calculated by this approach is usually about 5% lower than that obtained with the variable region of interest method. This method has the advantage of producing a smoother curve, which is useful for calculating the filling and emptying rates. A hybrid approach is to use this fixed region of interest method to select the end-diastolic and end-systolic frames from the time-activity curve and then draw individual regions of interest on these frames to calculate the ejection fraction.

Regional motion of the left and right ventricles can be readily appreciated from visual assessment of the cinematic display. An alternative approach to depicting regional function is the stroke-volume image, obtained by subtracting the end-systolic image from the end-diastolic image. Similarly, a "dyskinesis" image can be recorded by subtracting the end-diastolic image from the end-systolic image. The stroke-volume image dem-

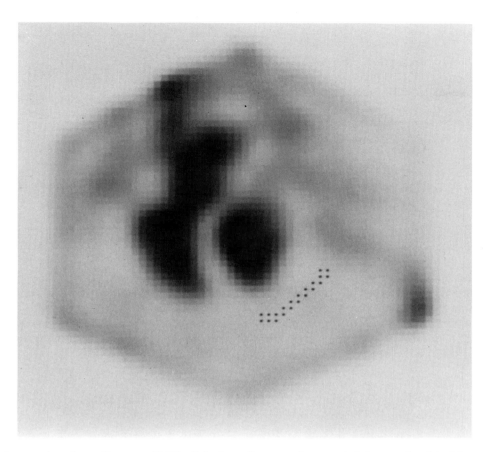

Figure 12-11   Background region of interest (ROI) *(light dots adjacent to the posteroinferior margin of the left ventricle)* selection from end-diastolic image of equilibrium-gated study.

onstrates ventricular motion and does not demonstrate the atria. The dyskinesis image shows atrial function but will not demonstrate any activity in the region of a normally contracting ventricle.

The high-count density of the equilibrium images permits another approach to the evaluation of regional wall motion, *phase* and *amplitude* images. Phase analysis assumes that the heart contracts in a specific pattern that resembles the waveform of a cosine function. Each pixel in the image can be evaluated for the timing (phase) of these changes in activity and for its amount of change (amplitude) between the maximum and minimum count value in the pixel. This information can be calculated and presented as a functional image, where specific colors or brightness represent information about amplitude or phase. An advantage of this approach is that the data are analyzed without operator interaction.

Stress Studies

Measurement of cardiac function at rest is valuable in evaluating cardiac function in patients with a history of myocardial infarction, valvular disease, shortness of breath, and suspected heart failure. Frequently, how-

ever, it is helpful to measure the reserve capacity of the heart by recording information about cardiac function while the subject is undergoing an exercise stress test. This information is particularly useful to evaluate patients for possible coronary artery disease. Exercise studies can be recorded either with the first-pass or equilibrium technique.

The basics of exercise stress testing are outlined here, with further details provided as they apply to myocardial perfusion imaging.

As the heart does more work (pumping more blood/min, pumping the same amount of blood at a higher pressure, or both) the amount of oxygen delivered to the heart must increase. In some organs the amount of oxygen extracted from the blood can be increased to deliver more oxygen without an increase in blood flow to the organ. In the heart, however, oxygen extraction is very efficient, and the only way to deliver the additional oxygen is to increase perfusion to the myocardium.

If a coronary artery supplying a region of myocardium is narrowed by more than 50%, however, blood flow cannot increase sufficiently to meet maximum increased demand for oxygen. If the blood flow to the myocardium does not increase in proportion to the increased work required to pump the blood, myocardial ischemia results. The inadequately perfused zone of myocardium stops contracting within a few seconds (if the mismatch is severe or has reduced contraction if the mismatch is less severe), causing a regional wall motion abnormality on images recorded during ischemia. If the area supplied by the stenosed coronary artery is extensive, overall function of the ventricle may be impaired, reducing the ejection fraction. A typical exercise test increases the workload the patient performs every 3 min; data is recorded during the last 2 min of each stage. Data is not recorded during the first minute of each stage because the heart rate is changing as the patient adjusts to the increased work. In 2 min only about 70-100,000 counts will be recorded from the left ventricle (about 4-6,000 counts/frame). The limited count density makes edge detection difficult, limiting the resolution for detection of small reductions in wall motion but still providing adequate data for analysis of overall (global) function (ejection fraction). Hence, lesions will only be detected when they impact overall ventricular function and result in a reduced ejection fraction.

In preparation for the exercise procedure, patients should have no food to eat for a minimum of 4 hr. A cardiac history should be obtained to plan the exercise procedure and anticipate the likely outcome. Older patients with a history of coronary disease, for example, are likely to exercise for a short time, compared with younger patients with no definite history, and are more likely to develop symptoms. A 12-lead ECG is recorded by placing electrodes in the supraclavicular and lower abdominal regions (adjacent to the pelvic crest) bilaterally, in the second intercostal space to the immediate right of the sternum (V_1), in the second intercostal space to the immediate left of the sternum (V_2), in the left midclavicular line in the fifth intercostal space (V_4), halfway between V_2 and V_4 (V_3), in the left midaxillary line in the fifth intercostal space (V_6), and midway between V_4 and V_6 (V_5) (Figure 12-12). To ensure good contact between the electrodes and skin, the skin should be shaved, if necessary; rubbed with alcohol to remove surface oils; and lightly abraded before electrodes are placed at the appropriate sites. Meticulous attention to skin preparation can reduce the resistance between the electrodes and the skin from 50,000-5,000 ohms.

Baseline ECG and sphygmomanometer blood pressure reading recordings should be obtained. If the first-pass technique is employed, an intravenous line (angiocath or intracath) is inserted at a location that will not interfere with the exercise procedure but will permit free access to the venous system for administration of the radiopharmaceutical. The subject is placed either supine or seated on the bicycle ergometer, the pedals are adjusted, and the resting radionuclide examination is recorded as previously described, using the first-pass

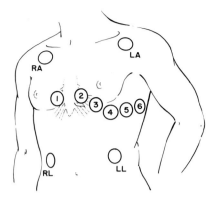

Figure 12-12 Sites of electrode placement for cardiac stress testing.

or equilibrium technique. Exercise is begun at a constant number of rpm of the pedals with adjustment of the workload (usually in 25-watt increments every 3 min). ECG and blood pressure are monitored throughout the procedure. Stress tests can cause severe ischemia, arrhythmias, hypotension, infarction, and death. As a result, these examinations should be performed only by personnel familiar with the procedure and with cardiopulmonary resuscitation. A crash cart should be kept in the immediate vicinity of the stress laboratory.

For the first-pass technique the radiopharmaceutical is administered at peak exercise, and data are recorded over the next 60 sec as described in the rest procedure. The dose of tracer utilized for the exercise study can be increased over that of a prior resting study to overcome any background from the previously administered radiopharmaceutical. Typically, a dose of 5-10 mCi is employed for the rest study and 10-20 mCi for the exercise examination. The first-pass approach is well suited for exercise, since patients can maintain their maximal effort for only a short interval.

To maximize the count rate, a high-sensitivity collimator may be employed, but an all-purpose collimator often provides better data because of its improved spatial resolution. When data are recorded with the equilibrium technique, a rest study is usually recorded in multiple views with the patient supine. Thereafter, an LAO view is recorded in the same position that the patient will use for exercise. Typically, the patient is exercised upright on a bicycle or semiupright on a modified table. At the conclusion of the exercise procedure, data are analyzed as described for equilibrium studies. Normal subjects should have at least a 5% increase in the ejection fraction from rest to the maximal level of exercise achieved. However, if a patient has an ejection fraction at rest of 65% or greater, the ejection fraction might not increase with exercise.

Nuclear medicine technologists work with the exercise team of physicians and nurses to perform the stress procedure. In addition to certification in advanced life

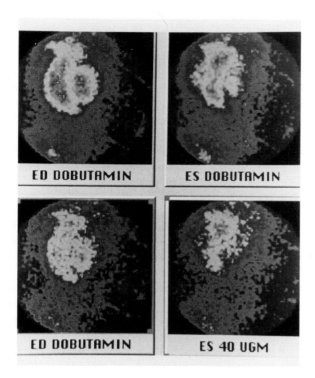

Figure 12-13 Planar-gated blood-pool scans in the 45-degree LAO position recorded at rest *(top panels)* and during dobutamine infusion *(bottom panels)* at end-diastole *(left)* and end-systole *(right)*. The right and left ventricles and great vessels are seen. Note the marked reduction in right and left ventricular size and volume from diastole to systole. During dobutamine stress, the end-systolic size of the ventricle is smaller than that at rest, suggesting an increase in ejection fraction.

support (to assist in case of catastrophe, an event that will take place about once for every 300 stress tests), technologists should be aware of the indications to terminate the tests. The following are circumstances that, if the test is continued, are likely to result in serious harm to the patient and are specific indicators to stop the test:

1. Marked arrhythmia induced by exercise (e.g., ventricular tachycardia, PVCs in pairs or triplets, and atrial fibrillation)
2. Decrease in blood pressure or heart rate as exercise progresses
3. Extreme elevation in blood pressure (systolic pressure >200 or diastolic pressure >120 mm Hg)
4. Severe chest pain
5. Achievement of greater than 85% (preferably 100%) of predicted heart rate for age (computed as 220 − age in years)
6. Severe ST depression (>3 mm)
7. Onset of advanced atrioventricular block
8. Onset of bundle branch block
9. Failure of monitoring system
10. Severe fatigue, leg pain, or breathlessness

In patients who cannot exercise, pharmacologic stress can be employed. To increase myocardial oxygen, consumption agents such as dobutamine are typically infused, and data are recorded at each phase of the infusion. Figure 12-13 demonstrates the changes in ventricular function that occur in a normal patient undergoing a pharmacologic stress test.

MYOCARDIAL PERFUSION IMAGING

Perfusion imaging is usually employed to detect the presence of myocardial ischemia and determine its location and extent. In contrast to blood-pool images performed at exercise, which detect ischemia as a result of its impact on ventricular function, perfusion imaging with injection of a radiotracer during stress can detect a relative decrease in blood flow to the myocardium directly. Myocardial perfusion images can be recorded with a number of single-photon agents. ^{201}Tl, an agent that has been used for over 20 years, is still preferred by many laboratories. Several new ^{99m}Tc-based agents are gaining favor for such studies. Each of these agents has some features that require specific tailoring of the examination. As a result, a laboratory should gain experience with one or two of these agents and become proficient in its use. The exercise tests are usually performed using a treadmill (in the United States) or bicycle (in Europe), with continuous monitoring of the patient's heart rate, ECG, blood pressure, and symptoms, as described for blood-pool imaging. The exercise test is performed to the same endpoints. The perfusion tracer is administered at the *peak of exercise,* and the patient is urged to continue exercising for at least 1 to 2 additional min to permit the tracer to deposit in the tissues.

Perfusion measurements are usually made at rest and at stress. A uniform pattern of myocardial perfusion at rest and stress makes it very unlikely that a patient has a significant risk of sudden death or myocardial infarction within the next 2 years. An abnormal scan with injection at stress and a normal scan with injection at rest suggests myocardial ischemia. Depending on the site and extent of the abnormality, the risk of an event in that patient varies from 1% to 2% up to about 15% in the next 2 years. An abnormality that is present on the rest and stress injected examinations suggests myocardial scar.

Radiopharmaceuticals for Perfusion Imaging

^{201}Tl, a monovalent cationic radiopharmaceutical, has been used for myocardial perfusion imaging for more than 20 years. This cyclotron-produced agent with a physical half-life of 74 hours, decays by electron capture with the production of mercury x rays of about 80 keV. Thallium is minimally excreted through the bowel and kidneys (only 10% is lost from the body over 10 days), resulting in a long biologic half-life. Following intravenous injection about 3.5% of the injected dose localizes in the myocardium. In myocardium that is ischemic, the relative amount of thallium in the zone of diminished perfusion is lower than that of the normally perfused zone (in direct proportion to that difference in tissue blood flow to the two regions). If serial images are recorded over several hours, the relative loss of thallium from the normally perfused zone is greater than that of the ischemic zone. At about 3 to 4 hr the relative concentration of thallium in the two areas may appear similar. This phenomenon is called *redistribution* and has made thallium very useful for identifying ischemic myocardium.

In contrast to its behavior in the myocardium, about 10% of each dose of thallium localizes in each kidney. Once in the kidney, the tracer is retained for days, resulting in a radiation burden of about 1.2 rads/mCi to the kidney. The combination of a long, effective half-life, which limits the dose that can be injected to about 4 mCi, and the low energy, which makes attenuation artifacts particularly prominent, resulted in a search for a technetium-labeled heart agent.

Three technetium-labeled perfusion tracers have been approved by the FDA: Teboroxime, sestamibi, and tetrofosmin (Table 12-3).

The short, effective half-life of these agents permits administration of up to 30 mCi of each of these agents. The kinetics of these agents differ from that of thallium. These agents do not redistribute in the same fashion as thallium. After injection the lion's share of the dose concentrates in the liver, and over the next hour the hepatic dose clears into the bowel. In contrast to thallium, there is little myocardial redistribution with the technetium-labeled agents. A lack of redistribution means that separate injections are required to define perfusion at rest and stress.

Several protocols have been developed to perform the rest and stress studies in patients with the technetium-labeled tracers. One protocol performs the rest and stress examinations on separate days, each with a dose of 20-30 mCi. To complete the study in 1 day, patients can have either the rest or stress study performed first, typically with a dose of 10 mCi, followed about 4 to 6 hr later (to permit both physical decay and biologic loss of radiopharmaceutical from the myocardium) by a dose of 20-30 mCi to complete the rest or stress examination. In summary, patients can be injected first at rest then at stress, or vice versa, using a larger dose of tracer for the second study than for the first.

An alternative approach utilizes thallium for the rest injected tracer and one of the technetium agents for the stress injected agent. Advantages of this approach are that delayed images can be recorded with thallium to detect viable myocardium and the stress test can be performed at the conclusion of rest imaging, with only minimal residual activity in the technetium window (due to the 12% incidence of gamma photons from ^{201}Tl).

Teboroxime with its biologic half-life of about 5 min in the myocardium requires completion of myocardial images within 10 min of tracer administration. To effectively use this agent patients must be injected in the immediate vicinity of the imaging device, and then images must be obtained with only a few minutes for each view. These factors limit the utility of this agent for routine imaging, and very few centers use it. In contrast, sestamibi and tetrofosmin have half-lives of >5 hr in the myocardium, allowing images to be recorded up to 90 min after injection. When possible, earlier images are preferred, and most laboratories image these agents 15 to 30 min after injection.

For the detection of ischemia, both thallium and technetium agents perform equally well. When there is a question of severe myocardial ischemia and the issue is myocardial viability, thallium is preferred. If it is important to review both myocardial function and perfusion at the same time, a gated myocardial SPECT study can be recorded. Gated SPECT studies can be recorded

Table 12-3			
Agent	**Myocardial concentration**	**Myocardial $t_{1/2}$**	**Comments**
Teboroxime	3.6%	5 min	Imaging must be completed within 10 min of injection
Sestamibi	2.4%	6 hr	Slight redistribution (not nearly as much as thallium, but images should be recorded within 90 min of injection to maximize detection of ischemic lesions); myocardial images can be recorded with gating, allowing an estimate of left ventricular ejection fraction and regional myocardial thickening
Tetrofosmin	2.0%	8 hr	Does not redistribute; myocardial images can be recorded with gating to estimate ventricular function and regional thickening

with thallium, but the higher-photon flux of the technetium-labeled agents provides data of better quality. In the following section, thallium is discussed in detail because it is still widely used as the preferred perfusion agent in many institutions.

Perfusion Imaging

^{201}Tl decays via electron capture to stable ^{201}Hg with the production of the 69-80 keV mercury x rays (100% abundant), and gamma photons of 135 and 167 keV (2% and 8% abundance, respectively). Imaging usually employs the x ray, though some institutions also utilize a dual-window approach to also record the gamma photons. The sensitivity of planar ^{201}Tl imaging for coronary artery disease is greater than 85%, despite the requirement for at least 25% difference in the distribution of perfusion between adjacent areas to be visible as a lesion on the scan. Specificity of this test also is high, typically in the 80% to 90% range.

Once deposited in the myocardium, thallium clears at different rates from normal and ischemic tissue, with faster clearance from normal tissue. Maximum contrast between normal and ischemic tissue occurs immediately after injection and persists for about 20 min. Thereafter, contrast gradually decreases, with the normal and ischemic tissues achieving similar concentrations over intervals ranging from 4 to 24 hr. The differential clearance of thallium from these zones of myocardium defines a need for immediate imaging of stress injected thallium perfusion studies to optimize the detection of altered perfusion. If imaging is delayed >20 min after injection, subtle lesions may be missed in patients with ischemia. When the tracer is injected at rest, however, the changes in myocardial uptake are less of a problem; imaging can be postponed for some time to maximize the likelihood that redistribution has occurred and that all viable myocardium is visualized.

Planar imaging. It is a good idea to record at least one or two planar views in all subjects. These images are helpful to identify attenuation artifacts and detect rapidly changing conditions, such as lung uptake or left ventricular dilation, which may normalize with 10 to 15 min after injection.

In contrast to ventricular function measurements, where imaging is performed during exercise, myocardial perfusion studies are recorded after exercise is concluded. After exercise, the patient is placed supine on an imaging table while ECG and blood pressure monitoring continue until the heart rate has decreased to within about 20% of baseline, transient ECG changes have resolved, and blood pressure is near normal. Then the patient is positioned for imaging. The scintillation camera is set to record data at the mercury x ray (centered at 80 keV and if the camera is equipped with multiple windows, the gamma photons are also imaged). A low-energy, all-purpose or high-resolution collimator is used. The anterior image is usually recorded first, since it is easiest to position, followed by the 35- to 45-degree LAO view, and finally the 70-degree LAO or left lateral view. In many (obese) patients the diaphragm obscures the inferior or posterolateral wall of the myocardium, leading some laboratories to perform the 70-degree LAO view in a decubitus position. The decubitus view is recorded with the patient lying on the right side, with the detector above the patient. The left ventricular myocardium should be located in the center of the field for all images. Images should be obtained for a preset time of 8 to 10 min/view to record a sufficient count density over the myocardium.

Data are recorded digitally in a 64 × 64 or 128 × 128 matrix (depending on the field of view of the detector) to permit review of the images with contrast enhancement and quantification of the regional distribution of ^{201}Tl. The patient is then released from the department to return for the delayed images 3 to 4 hr later. The patient should be instructed not to eat any food containing carbohydrates, since ingestion of glucose accelerates the rate of ^{201}Tl clearance from both normal and ischemic myocardium, minimizing the differential clearance necessary to detect ischemia. When the patient returns, an additional 1 mCi dose of thallium is administered at rest and another set of images is recorded for the same time as the initial series. The additional rest injected dose enhances the sensitivity for detecting ischemia in patients with moderately severe coronary stenoses.

Data recording. To maximize the likelihood of detecting coronary artery disease with perfusion imaging, the radiopharmaceutical should be administered at the peak of exercise and the exercise should continue for an additional 1 to 2 min to permit the tracer to localize in the myocardium in proportion to perfusion at the peak of exercise. Premature termination of exercise, particularly in patients with small zones of ischemia (which may rapidly normalize), will result in part of the dose delivered at a time when the tissue has decreased flow and part of the dose delivered when perfusion is normal. This phenomena will decrease contrast between the normal and ischemic tissue, making detection of the lesion difficult.

In similar fashion to performing a first-pass radionuclide angiocardiogram, an intravenous line is placed to facilitate injection at the peak of stress. Since glucose alters the clearance rate of ^{201}Tl from the myocardium, the IV line should be kept open with saline. Radiopharmaceutical injection should be followed by a flush of 10 ml of saline to minimize the time that the radiopharmaceutical is in contact with the veins of the arm. Exercise should continue for at least 1 min with thallium and preferably 2 min with the technetium-labeled tracers (because they have slightly slower blood clearance

Box 12-2

Homogeneity of tracer distribution in the left ventricular (LV) myocardium. Adjacent areas of normally perfused tissue should vary by <15% (with the exception of an occasional papillary muscle that may have markedly increased activity). Focal zones of decreased or absent tracer concentration are the hallmark of diminished perfusion.

Visualization of the right ventricular (RV) myocardium. The intensity of RV myocardial activity should be ~50% that of the LV. Failure to see the RV myocardial activity may indicate RV ischemia/infarction. Excess RV activity may indicate hypertrophy.

Size and shape of the LV and RV cavities. The LV cavity should have the shape of a football in the anterior and left lateral views. A round shape suggests disease of the myocardium. The RV cavity should have the shape of a crescent moon in the LAO view. If the borders appear rounded, dilation of the RV cavity should be considered.

Thallium used for an exercise stress test. Activity in the left lung adjacent to the heart should be <60% of the peak LV myocardial activity (assuming the peak heart rate is >120 beats/min). If the lung concentration is elevated, pulmonary congestion associated with exercise should be considered. This finding is usually associated with severe coronary disease, causing left ventricular dysfunction with exercise.

than thallium) after injection, if the patient's condition permits. Imaging should commence within 10 min with thallium and within 15 min for sestamibi and tetrofosmin.

Data analysis. Myocardial perfusion data are evaluated by viewing the images to detect zones of diminished tracer localization and by quantification of the relative regional distribution of the agent. Qualitative interpretation reviews the images for the factors listed in Box 12-2 (see Figures 12-14 to 12-17).

Data is quantified by region-of-interest analysis to express the regional concentration of thallium in the myocardium graphically (Figure 12-14). Although planar and SPECT images can be quantified, planar quantification is rarely used. SPECT images are usually quantified by stacking the reconstructed/reoriented short-axis slices onto a bull's-eye display, where the apex is at the center and the basal slice is at the periphery.

SPECT Imaging

Data recording. SPECT imaging results in a marked improvement in image contrast compared with planar imaging. However, this improvement comes with a significant price—artifacts in the data may be difficult to appreciate. Two types of artifacts occur fairly frequently: attenuation (due to breast or stomach) and motion (due to slight patient movement during the lengthy acquisition). Both of these artifacts tend to cause areas of decreased counts in the reconstructed data that can be mistaken for zones of decreased perfusion. These artifacts can be readily appreciated if the projection data are reviewed in a cinematic display. When attenuation is seen, its impact on the data can be anticipated, and the images can be interpreted correctly. Motion, on the other hand, is difficult to correct. If multiple motion episodes are seen, or if a discrete movement changes the data by more than 2 pixels, it is likely that the reconstructed data (which presumes that the data are consistent) will have focal artifacts. If this is seen, another acquisition should be recorded, rather than attempting to eliminate the motion by shifting the data in the computer.

At the conclusion of the stress test, short-duration (5 min) planar images can be recorded in the anterior and left anterior oblique positions. Thereafter, the technologist rotates the camera through a trial rotation designed to bring the camera head as close to the patient as possible without touching at the angle with the greatest body diameter. Some devices can collect data in an eliptical orbit, allowing the detector to remain closer to the patient (enhancing resolution) during rotation.

If data are to be collected in a 360-degree orbit, the patient should have both arms elevated and supported to alleviate fatigue and minimize movement. If a 180-degree orbit is chosen, then only the left arm needs to be out of the field of view, and the right arm can be at the side and held in place with an elastic chest binder. Data acquisition for the 180-degree orbit typically begins at 45 degrees RAO and ends at 45 degrees LPO.

Image acquisition time varies from 20 to 30 min, depending on several factors: (1) single detector or multidetector camera, (2) 180-degree versus 360-degree acquisition, (3) radiopharmaceutical dose, (4) step angle (3 versus 6 degree); and (4) number of counts collected at each increment. A typical SPECT protocol requires either 32 (or 64) stops for 180 degrees or 64 (or 128) stops for 360 degrees. A technologist should be present in the room throughout a SPECT data collection to prevent possible injury from a malfunction of the moving detector. It is recommended that SPECT

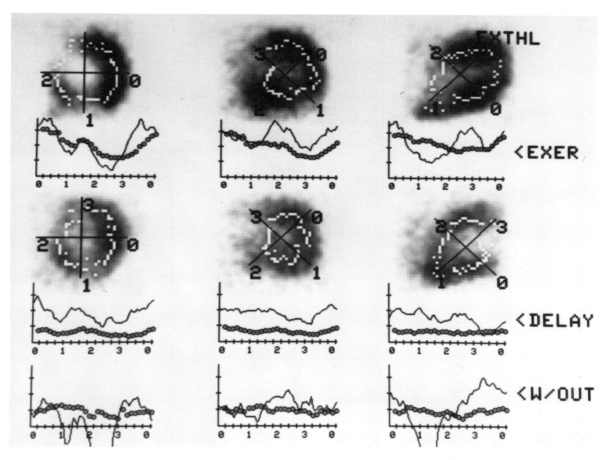

Figure 12-14 Quantitative circumferential profile analysis of planar thallium scintigrams. Upper row shows immediate postexercise images, (35 degrees LAO; anterior; 70 degrees LAO), which have been smoothed and corrected for background by interpolative background-subtraction technique. White pixels displayed in each image represent maximum pixel values located by computer along each line of radial searching from center of left ventricular cavity (determined by operator-positioned superimposed crosshairs; on each image position 1 corresponds to apex). Beneath each exercise image the corresponding plot of circumferential profile values is expressed as percentage of maximum pixel in that image (*solid line*). Lower limit of normal for circumferential profile values is shown by small boxes. In this patient both the images and circumferential profiles demonstrate subnormal activity in inferoapical region, interventricular septum (35-degree LAO view), and anteroseptal wall (70-degree LAO view). There is borderline abnormal activity in anterolateral wall (anterior view). Background-subtracted, delayed images with their circumferential profiles are displayed below each stress image. Displayed profile values are normalized maximum pixel value in corresponding immediate postexercise image. Bottom row shows wash-out profile curves expressed as percent wash-out in each radius between exercise and delay. In this patient, subnormal values, indicative of redistribution and therefore of ischemia, are apparent in inferoapical and septal regions on 35-degree LAO view, in anterolateral wall on the anterior view, and in apical and anteroseptal walls on 70-degree LAO view.

imaging begin about 10 min after strenuous exercise to avoid the phenomenon of myocardial motion due to a change in the degree of diaphragmatic excursion as the patient's respiration returns to normal. This phenomenon has been referred to as *myocardial creep* or *upward creep* and is seen mostly in patients who achieve high levels of exercise. It typically results in an artifactual lesion in the inferior or inferoseptal regions of the left ventricle.

At the conclusion of data collection the patient can be discharged to return in 3 to 4 hr for delayed images (when thallium is used) or for a second study when the technetium-labeled agents are employed. Often, even

when thallium is employed for the stress test, the patient can receive a second injection before repeat SPECT imaging or undergo a second SPECT collection without administration of additional radiopharmaceutical. The "reinjection" of thallium was found to detect a higher incidence of ischemia than redistribution imaging alone. In redistribution imaging the thallium has mixed with the body "pool" of potassium and is equilibrating in tissues. In the case of reinjection the tracer is measuring the regional distribution of perfusion at rest—a circumstance markedly different from that at stress (and similar to the conditions employed for the technetium-labeled tracers). The potential problems

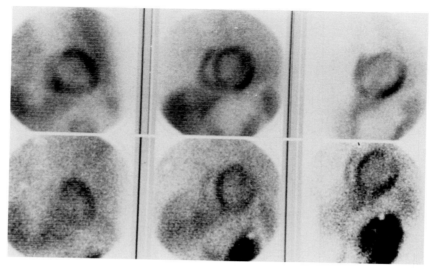

Figure 12-15 Planar thallium myocardial perfusion images recorded immediately after injection at stress *(top panels)* and at 24 hr *(bottom panels)* in the anterior view *(left)* 45-degree LAO view *(middle)* and left lateral view *(right)*. The left ventricle is markedly dilated. On the LAO view there is decreased thallium concentration in the septum, which improves on the 24-hr images, indicating an area of myocardial ischemia.

with a rest injection is that under some circumstances of severe coronary disease, the perfusion to the tissue is markedly reduced even at rest, yet the tissue is alive. The "viability" of this tissue can often be detected by redistribution imaging.

Data analysis. Analysis of SPECT data, in similar fashion to planar images, can be accomplished either subjectively or with the aid of quantification. In either case the basis of interpretation is the same as with planar imaging: perfusion abnormalities that appear less severe on rest or delayed images than they do on the stress studies indicate areas of stress-induced myocardial ischemia (Figures 12-15 and 12-16), whereas those that remain fixed on delayed imaging most likely reflect sites of myocardial scar (Figure 12-17). Interpretation is facilitated by presenting the images in a standard format, realigned along the major cardiac axes. Realignment is performed by reconstructing the projection data by filtered back-projection into transverse slices. The long and short axes of the heart are determined, and the data are reoriented and reconstructed into short- and long-axis images of the myocardium. Quantitative analysis of these slices is most sensitive for the identification of alterations in regional perfusion. Long-axis slices through the left ventricle, in both vertical and horizontal planes, also are generated for visual analysis, useful for confirmation of findings noted on the short-axis images and for assessment of the apex. Artifacts can occur due to attenuation from adjacent tissues (breast or stomach) or intense areas of adjacent activity (liver or loops of bowel). As a result, quantitative approaches should be employed as guides rather than as a primary means of interpreting SPECT data.

Tomographic images also can be analyzed using the bull's-eye type of display. For this display, the short-axis SPECT images are arranged concentrically from the apex of the ventricle (center) to the base (periphery), and the three-dimensional myocardium is thus flattened into a single-plane map of the left ventricle. Bull's-eye maps of both the stress and rest studies also can be used to quantify the tomographic data.

Pharmacologic stress. Some patients cannot exercise due to peripheral vascular disease, neurologic problems, or musculoskeletal abnormalities. Myocardial blood flow can be increased in these patients using drugs to cause vasodilation of the coronary bed or to increase myocardial oxygen demand in place of the exercise test. The vasodilator method is used most often. Two drugs are available for this purpose: dipyridamole and adenosine. Both agents cause relaxation of precapillary sphincters in the arterioles, resulting in a marked decrease in peripheral resistance and an increase in regional blood flow to the myocardium. These agents cause a generalized vasodilation, and neither is specific for the heart. The drugs work by increasing the local tissue level of adenosine, a potent dilator of the precapillary sphincter.

Dipyridamole acts by decreasing the metabolism of adenosine that is produced endogenously; the drug inhibits an enzyme called adenosine deaminase. Infusion of adenosine, on the other hand, causes a direct effect by occupying the adenosine receptors. Dipyridamole lasts for several hours after administration, whereas adenosine has a very short half-life (about 10 sec).

When the drugs are infused, coronary arteries free of atherosclerosis increase blood flow uniformly to all

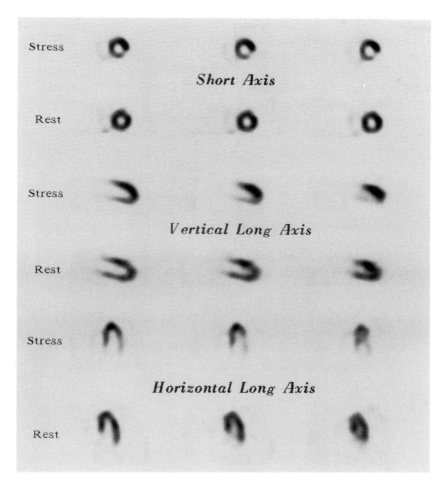

Figure 12-16 Images represent selected short-axis, vertical long-axis, and horizontal long-axis slices from SPECT ²⁰¹Tl study of patient with exercise-induced ischemia of inferolateral and inferior walls. Images obtained immediately after ²⁰¹Tl injection at peak exercise (stress) reveal a focal, marked decrease in ²⁰¹Tl activity within inferolateral myocardial segment (seen best on the short-axis and horizontal long-axis views), with a milder decrease in activity within inferior wall (seen best on the short-axis and vertical long-axis views). Repeat images obtained after a 4-hr delay (rest) demonstrate complete redistribution, with normal ²⁰¹Tl activity in these regions.

areas of the myocardium. If the perfusion tracer is administered at the time of the maximal effect of the drug, a normal scan is recorded. If a vessel is markedly narrowed, flow distal to the narrowing does not increase to the same degree as that in myocardial territories supplied by normal coronary arteries (Figure 12-18). Although this phenomenon does not usually cause ischemia, as in exercise tests, the underlying basis for detection of abnormalities (the stenosis of a coronary artery) remains the same.

The effects of dipyridamole and adenosine can be reversed by administration of aminophylline. Because the vasodilator properties of adenosine and dipyridamole result in decreased blood pressure, patients should be studied while lying supine on a stretcher, with continuous blood pressure and ECG monitoring. Typically hypotension is mild, causing a 10-15 mm Hg reduction in blood pressure. In some patients, however, the reduction in blood pressure can be profound, lead-

ing to death if not treated. In the unlikely event that patients develop serious complications during the test, a syringe of aminophylline should be available. As with exercise tests, serious side effects, such as arrhythmias, severe hypotension, cerebral ischemia, stroke, and death have been reported with this procedure. As a result the examination should be performed only in facilities equipped to handle medical emergencies.

Before performing the test, patients should be asked if they have asthma (a contraindication for using either dipyridamole or adenosine). Patients should be prepared for the test by fasting for at least 4 hr, abstaining from foods containing caffeine (coffee, tea, and many soft drinks) for at least 24 hr, and discontinuing all xanthine-containing medications 36 hr before the study. Caffeine and xanthine-containing medications will reduce the effectiveness of the vasodilator and therefore may produce a negative test in patients with coronary stenoses.

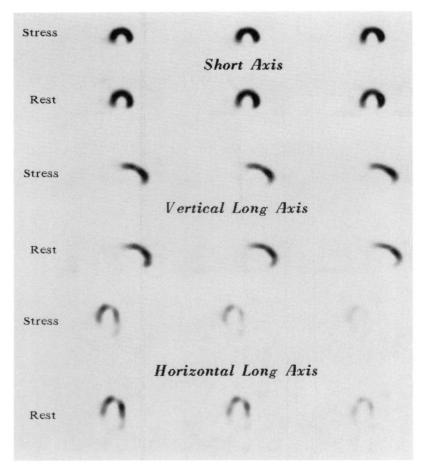

Figure 12-17 Images represent selected slices from a ^{201}Tl SPECT study of a patient with a previous inferior wall myocardial infarction. Images obtained immediately after injection of ^{201}Tl at peak exercise (stress) demonstrate a large inferior region of markedly decreased myocardial uptake of ^{201}Tl. Repeat imaging after a 4-hr delay (rest) shows no significant redistribution of activity into this region.

Blood pressure and ECG must be monitored throughout the procedure. The drugs are injected intravenously using an infusion pump. The test is performed after administration of 0.56 mg/kg dipyridamole over 4 min or 140 ugm/kg/min of adenosine for 6 min while recording serial blood pressures and ECG. The perfusion tracer is administered approximately 3 to 4 min after the conclusion of the dipyridamole infusion or during the third minute of adenosine infusion. Imaging commences about 10 min later.

Adenosine and dipyridamole administration is often accompanied by a pounding headache, a sensation of heaviness in the chest, nausea, and a feeling of breathlessness. These symptoms can be minimized with low-level exercise, either by walking on the treadmill at about 1 mile/hr or using arm weights of 2 to 5 lbs during the infusion.

An alternative to vasodilation utilizes dobutamine, a sympathomimetic drug that increases heart rate and blood pressure. This agent increases myocardial work and hence the need for increased flow in the coronary arteries. In contrast to other drugs in this category, dobutamine has a low incidence of cardiac arrhythmia. The drug has a half-life of about 1-2 min, limiting the duration of effect. As with the vasodilator agents, patients should have their heart rate, ECG, and blood pressure monitored continuously during administration of the drug. Since the drug causes increased oxygen consumption, it can cause ischemia, in similar fashion to exercise.

Dobutamine is infused at a graduated rate commencing at 5-10 µg/min and increasing every 3 min to a maximum of 50 µg/min. If the heart rate has not achieved 85% of maximum and the blood pressure is still in an acceptable range, atropine is administered in divided doses up to a total of 1 mg to produce a tachycardia. The perfusion agent is administered, and the dobutamine infusion is continued for an additional 2 min.

Although pharmacologic testing is useful in patients who cannot exercise, the vasodilator agents cause a marked increase in blood flow to the liver, which can

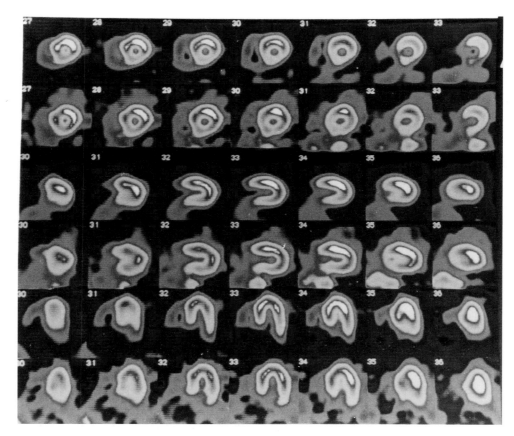

Figure 12-18 SPECT myocardial perfusion scan reconstructed in the short-axis *(top two rows)*, vertical long-axis *(middle two rows)* and horizontal long-axis views (bottom two rows), after administration of adenosine *(upper row of each pair)* and at rest *(bottom row of each pair)*. Perfusion to the inferior portion of the left ventricle is reduced following adenosine stress (best seen on the short-axis images). The distribution of perfusion improves at rest, suggesting an ischemic lesion in myocardium, usually supplied by the right coronary artery.

make it difficult to see lesions of the inferior wall. Neither the vasodilators nor dobutamine provide the breadth of information about cardiac performance that is available with an exercise study. Exercise testing offers information about the overall status of the patient's cardiovascular fitness, the duration and severity of exercise that causes symptoms, and the timing of symptoms versus objective indicators of ischemia (ST segment changes or perfusion scan abnormalities). This information frequently plays a key role in planning therapy.

Myocardial Perfusion Imaging with Technetium-Labeled Agents

The technetium-labeled agents can be substituted for thallium in the rest or stress or both portions of the examination. These agents have significant differences in selected aspects of their behavior compared with ^{201}Tl. First, the most popular agents, sestamibi and tetrofosmin, have lower myocardial extraction (about 60% for MIBI and 50% for tetrofosmin, versus 85% for thallium), so a smaller fraction of the injected dose/

mCi of injected activity localizes in the myocardium. Second, the agents have slightly slower blood clearance than thallium, making it particularly important to continue exercise for about 2 min after injection, instead of the 1 min usually employed for thallium. Third, the agents have more favorable dosimetry, thereby permitting administration of doses up to 30 mCi. The higher administered dose results in a much greater photon flux from the myocardium and allows recording of first-pass data at the time of injection. Although gated SPECT studies can be recorded with thallium, they pale in comparison with the high-quality gated SPECT of the technetium-labeled tracers. This constellation of observations makes the technetium-labeled agents very attractive, and though they are more expensive, they are gaining popularity as myocardial perfusion agents.

A disadvantage of sestamibi and tetrofosmin is their failure to have significant redistribution. These agents are lost very slowly from the myocardium, with comparable clearances from normal and ischemic tissue. Separate injections are required for the rest and stress portions of the study. There has been great debate about whether the rest or stress study should be performed first. An optimal approach performs the rest and stress examinations on separate days, thereby eliminating the problem of any residual background activity. Often, however, patients prefer to have their studies completed on a single day. Same-day studies usually use 10-15 mCi for the first examination and 25-30 mCi for the second. There appears to be little difference in the sensitivity or specificity of perfusion imaging regardless of whether a 1- or 2-day protocol is used.

Technetium-labeled agents are somewhat less sensitive for the detection of viable ischemic myocardium than thallium. The reason for this problem is unclear but may relate to the lack of redistribution. When there is a high likelihood of severe stenosis and limited collateral blood flow to a region of potentially viable myocardium, a combination of a rest injected thallium scan and a stress injected technetium-labeled tracer study may be useful. In this circumstance the dose of thallium is administered first, and images of the rest distribution of perfusion are recorded. Thereafter, the patient is stressed, the technetium-labeled tracer is administered, and stress technetium images are recorded. As

for single-radiopharmaceutical studies, the data should be carefully reviewed for technical adequacy before the SPECT data are reconstructed. When doses of 3.5-4.5 mCi are employed for the thallium study (and patient's weight is less than 180 lbs) useful data can be reconstructed using a Butterworth filter with a frequency of 0.65 cycles/cm. The technetium data should be reconstructed with a filter of about 0.75 cycles/cm to take advantage of the higher photon flux. These combined tracer data are interpreted in similar fashion to that recorded when a single radiopharmaceutical is used. If the rest and stress data appear similarly abnormal, the patient can return for imaging at 24 hr without administering any additional radiopharmaceutical. These delayed rest injected images are particularly helpful for the detection of viable myocardium, especially in patients with diminished ejection fraction.

Gated Perfusion Imaging

Gated perfusion SPECT is typically recorded using 8 instead of 16 frames/cardiac cycle because of the enor-

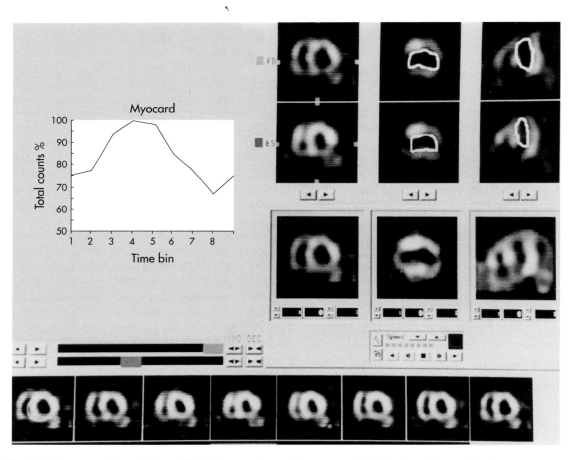

Figure 12-19 Gated myocardial perfusion SPECT in a patient with myocardial infarction. Images in the top row are midventricular slices at end-diastole (ED) in the short axis *(left)*, vertical long axis *(middle)*, and horizontal long axis *(right)*. The next row shows the same slices at end-systole (ES). Cine displays in the third row allow the viewer to see the thickening of each slice (when viewed on the computer display). The bottom row illustrates eight gated images of the midventricular short-axis slice. The graph depicts regional changes in counts in the short-axis slice, demonstrating regional wall thickening. Endocardial outlines are drawn on the long-axis images to permit calculation of left ventricular volumes and ejection fraction.

mity of the data set. When 64 angles are recorded with 8 frames/cycle at each location, a total of 512 images are obtained. Although end-systole is not correctly identified under this circumstance, the apparent loss of ejection fraction is typically on the order of 5% and is most apparent in patients with high ejection fractions at rest. This type of study has sufficient precision to differentiate patients with normal EFs from those with depressed ejection fractions.

Following reconstruction of the data, the gated slices are usually displayed as multiple cine loops on the screen for visual assessment. Thereafter, the endocardial borders of the midventricular horizontal and vertical long-axis slices are defined, and the ejection fraction and ventricular volumes are calculated. These data can be appended to the evaluation of myocardial perfusion and are particularly useful when determining the appearance of regional function in areas of diminished perfusion (Figure 12-19). Since the gated study is performed at rest, after the ischemic episode is over, zones of ischemia should have normal function (appear as areas of decreased intensity with normal thickening). Areas of scar, on the other hand, should have decreased perfusion and diminished function.

IMAGING MYOCARDIAL NECROSIS

Acute Infarct Imaging

Two agents have been proposed to image acute myocyte necrosis: [99m]Tc pyrophosphate and ^{111}In antimyosin. Myocardial infarction (irreversible damage) occurs when a zone of heart muscle is deprived of an adequate supply of oxygen for an interval longer than 15 min. Infarction usually occurs when an artery becomes occluded by a clot. The clot usually forms at the site of an atheromatous lesion that ruptures, releasing thrombogenic material into the blood. The sudden cessation of perfusion is usually associated with typical symptoms and ECG changes. In the process of irreversible damage, the cell membrane of the myocardial cell (myocyte) loses its integrity, becomes permeable to macromolecules or charged substances that are ordinarily confined to the interior of the cell, and finally develops microscopic holes. The loss of integrity of the cellular envelope leads to loss of the intracellular contents into the surrounding extracellular fluid, which are detectable as elevations of serum enzymes such as creatine phosphokinase (CPK), lactic dehydrogenase (LDH), and a number of other substances such as troponin and myoglobin. Elevations of these markers are usually used as indicators of the presence of acute necrosis in the emergency room because these assays can be done quickly, often at the bedside. Cell necrosis produces local inflammation (due to the irritation produced by the leakage of these unusual substances into the extracellular environment); followed by infiltration

of the area with white blood cells that ingest the debris; and finally by the presence of fibroblasts, which produce the fibrous tissue (scar) that replaces the dead myocytes.

Increased permeability of the cell membrane not only allows substances usually confined to the cell to escape but also allows substances that are ordinarily excluded from the cell to enter. In the case of pyrophosphate the cell loses its ability to regulate the amount of calcium. Extracellular calcium enters the cell, establishing a condition similar to that found when bone is formed. If ^{99m}Tc-labeled pyrophosphate is administered at that time, it will localize in the zone of necrosis. Conditions that lead to localization of pyrophosphate start to occur within hours of the onset of occlusion and persist for about 8 to 10 days. Thereafter, there is little localization of pyrophosphate.

An alternative, elegant approach to detecting acute necrosis uses an antibody raised against the heavy chain of cardiac myosin. One of the least soluble elements in the myocyte is the heavy chain of cardiac myosin, a key protein of the heart's contractile apparatus. When the cell membrane is intact, antimyosin antibody cannot come in contact with its antigen and no localization occurs in the heart. Loss of cell membrane integrity in irreversibly damaged cells permits antimyosin to enter the damaged cell and combine with the antigen, resulting in localization in areas of acute necrosis.

To enhance the rapidity of blood clearance (thereby enhancing image contrast), antimyosin antibody is administered as an Fab fragment. The Fab fragment has a blood clearance half-time of 10 to 12 hr, compared with about 18 to 20 hr for the intact antibody. The antibody fragment is labeled with ^{111}In using a bifunctional chelate. Localization of antimyosin can be seen within hours of occlusion and will occur in the majority of patients with acute infarction if the antibody is administered within 10 to 14 days of the event. Thereafter, the incidence of localization decreases, such that after 9 months, patients with acute infarction rarely localize antimyosin at the site of necrosis.

Although imaging with these agents provides definitive information about the site and extent of acute necrosis, these procedures are rarely used for clinical purposes because other, less expensive approaches, such as serial electrocardiograms and serum enzymes, provide similar information.

99mTc Pyrophosphate

Data recording. No special patient preparation is required. [99m]Tc pyrophosphate is administered intravenously in a dose of 20 mCi between 12 hr and 10 days after the suspected acute event. Images are recorded 4 to 6 hr after injection to minimize the possibility of residual radiopharmaceutical in the blood pool. Planar and SPECT images are recorded; planar images are recorded for at least 500,000 counts with a high-resolution or all-purpose parallel-hole collimator in at least four positions: anterior, 30-degree RAO, 45-degree LAO, and left lateral (Figure 12-20). The ribs and sternum provide anatomic landmarks but also can be sources of difficulty for detection of small sites of necrosis. SPECT imaging is particularly helpful to visualize small or faint focal areas of myocardial ^{99m}Tc-pyrophosphate uptake despite the normal thoracic cage activity.

Data analysis. The images are usually interpreted subjectively by comparing the intensity of the lesion with rib and sternal intensity. Zones of increased activity in the region of the myocardium that are seen on at least two views are considered significant.

Studies have shown that some patients have a persistently positive scan long after myocardial infarction. Occasionally such uptake reflects the formation of a ventricular aneurysm or continued ischemia of the surviving tissue. In other cases the cause of this phenomenon is unknown, but it usually signifies a poor prognosis. The intensity of uptake in these patients is typically low, and the radiopharmaceutical uptake can diffusely involve the myocardium or be concentrated in the area of previous damage.

^{111}In Antimyosin

Data collection. Planar (anterior, 45-degree LAO, and left lateral) and SPECT images are usually obtained. After intravenous administration of 1.8 mCi ^{111}In antimyosin Fab, images are recorded at 24 to 72 hr, using 20% symmetrical windows around both the 174 and 246 keV photopeaks on a camera equipped with a medium-energy collimator. Large areas of necrosis may become apparent as early as 6 hr after injection, but most small infarctions are not well visualized until 48 hr and may require an additional 24 hr for further blood clearance. If the patient is available only for a single imaging session, the most definitive images are usually obtained between 24 and 72 hr.

Data analysis. Antimyosin has been used to image acute myocardial infarction as early as 5 hr and up to 14 days after the acute insult; however, the best results are typically obtained 2 to 4 days after acute myocardial infarction. A focal area of increased activity is consistent with transmural myocardial infarction, and diffuse uptake of lower intensity usually corresponds to patchy subendocardial necrosis. Animal studies have shown a good correlation between the size of the area of infarction as defined by pyrophosphate and by antimyosin, but pyrophosphate generally overestimates the size of the infarction by a factor of 1.7. The sensitivity of antimyosin for detecting acute myocardial infarction is very similar to that of pyrophosphate (90%).

Heart Transplant Rejection and Acute Myocarditis

Antimyosin antibody also can assess myocardial necrosis associated with heart transplant rejection and acute myocarditis. Definitive diagnosis of these two entities can be obtained only by biopsy at the present time. Un-

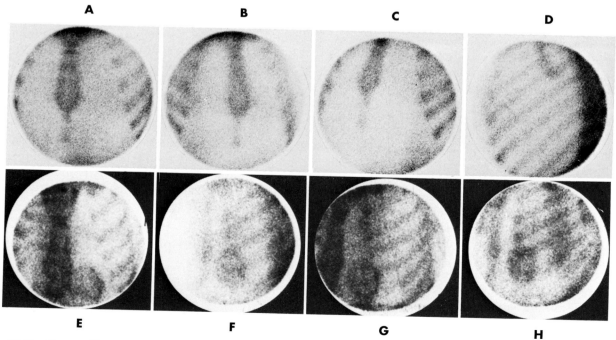

Figure 12-20 Normal ^{99m}Tc pyrophosphate myocardial images. **A,** Anterior; **B,** RAO; **C,** LAO; **D,** left lateral. Abnormal concentration of radiopharmaceutical in anterior (**E**); left lateral (**F**); 40-degree LAO (**G**); and 70-degree LAO (**H**).

fortunately, biopsy allows evaluation of only a small portion of the myocardium and is invasive. Antimyosin imaging theoretically allows evaluation of the entire myocardium noninvasively. Typically imaging is performed as described for acute myocardial necrosis. Some investigators quantify the data, using a ratio of activity in the heart to that in the adjacent lung. Values >1.5 are abnormal. Although all patients have necrosis at the time of transplantation, grafts that are not afflicted with severe episodes of rejection have minimal ongoing necrosis. Within the first year the heart/lung ratio should decrease to <1.5. Patients with values >1.5 have ongoing rejection and may require alteration in their antirejection therapy. Similarly, myocarditis may be difficult to diagnose clinically and may require endocardial biopsy. Antimyosin imaging is frequently positive in these patients and may eliminate the requirement for a diagnostic endocardial biopsy.

POSITRON EMISSION TOMOGRAPHY

Principles

Imaging the annihilation radiation resulting from positron decay can be accomplished in three ways: using a positron camera, employing high-energy collimators on a single-photon gamma camera, or with a dual-detector gamma camera modified for coincidence detection. There are substantial trade-offs with each approach. The positron camera cannot be used for single-photon imaging, but it provides images of high resolution. The collimated single-photon instrument has the lowest count rate and the lowest spatial resolution but can be employed for imaging both annihilation radiation and single photons. A hybrid dual-detector camera can be used to record both single-photon and annihilation radiation. It has slightly lower spatial resolution than a conventional single-photon instrument (because it typically uses a thicker crystal) but eliminates collimators when recording annihilation radiation (thereby enhancing sensitivity).

Positron-emitting radionuclides are important for cardiac imaging because they can be used to make radiopharmaceuticals to measure the metabolism of glucose (useful in the detection of ischemic, but viable, myocardium), fatty acids, acetate (useful for the determination of regional oxygen utilization), and catecholamines (useful to define regional myocardial innervation). PET radiopharmaceuticals can also be made for gated blood-pool studies and measurements of myocardial perfusion, but these agents generally provide similar information to that available from single-photon studies. Information on myocardial glucose metabolism is unique to the PET agent fluorodeoxyglu-

cose and can provide information that is very valuable in selected instances for patient care.

A technical advantage of annihilation radiation imaging is a straightforward means of correcting for photon attenuation, thereby eliminating a major cause of false-positive studies with single-photon instruments. As a result, absolute (rather than relative) quantitative imaging is possible with PET, and spatial resolution with PET is much better than that with SPECT.

Since positron-emitting radionuclides release beta radiation in the course of their decay, they deliver a larger amount of energy to the tissue than comparable gamma-emitting radionuclides. To minimize the radiation burden to the subject, positron-emitting radionuclides with short half-lives are usually employed. The difference in radiation burden between positron-emitting and single-photon–emitting nuclides is readily apparent when considering the radiation burden to bone from two bone-seeking radiopharmaceuticals: ^{18}F ion (physical half-life of 1.8 hr) and ^{99m}Tc pyrophosphate (physical half-life of 6 hr); 0.14 and 0.046 rad/mCi, respectively. The radiation burden from ^{18}F is threefold greater than that of ^{99m}Tc, despite the threefold longer half-life of ^{99m}Tc.

Myocardial Perfusion

Perfusion tracers. Positron-emitting radionuclides used for the assessment of regional perfusion can be classified into those tracers that are only partially extracted by the myocardium (^{82}Rb chloride and ^{13}N ammonia) and those that are freely diffusible (^{15}O water).

^{82}Rb chloride is an FDA-approved radiopharmaceutical, available from an ^{82}Sr generator, and has a physical half-life of 75 sec. It behaves physiologically in a similar fashion to ^{201}Tl and is initially concentrated in the myocardium in proportion to regional myocardial perfusion. The retention of ^{82}Rb chloride is at least partially dependent on Na$^+$/K$^+$−ATPase transport. The myocardial accumulation of ^{82}Rb chloride is partially dependent on the metabolic state of the myocardium.

^{13}N ammonia, produced by deuteron bombardment of ^{12}C in a cyclotron, localizes in the myocardium in approximate proportion to regional myocardial perfusion with the same practical limitations as ^{82}Rb chloride. Because of its 9.9 min physical half-life and favorable myocardial kinetics, image quality with ^{13}N ammonia is generally superior to shorter half-lived ^{82}Rb chloride.

^{15}O is a cyclotron-produced radionuclide with a physical half-life of 122 sec that can be used to label water (H$_2$^{15}O). Since water is virtually freely diffusible into myocytes, the extraction of this tracer by myocardial tissue is nearly 100% and is not dependent on the flow rate. In addition, this tracer is metabolically inert; thus its accumulation within the myocardium is not dependent on the metabolic state of the tissue. However, because ^{15}O water resides in both the tissue and the

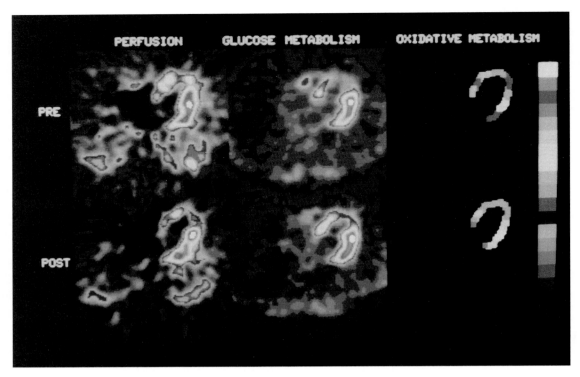

Figure 12-21 Midventricular PET images of myocardial perfusion and metabolism of patient with anterior myocardial infarction that contained nonviable myocardium, before and after coronary artery bypass surgery. Images of relative perfusion are at left, and those depicting relative glucose metabolism are shown in the middle. Images on right reflect regional differences in myocardial oxidative metabolism, measured with the ^{11}C-acetate clearance technique. White represents peak activity and black represents lowest activity. Orientation in images is septum to the left and anterior structures on top. Before surgery *(top row)* myocardial perfusion and glucose metabolism were concordantly reduced within anterior wall compared with values in functionally normal posterolateral wall. Moreover, myocardial oxidative metabolism within anterior wall was severely depressed to approximately 30% to 40% of that in normal posterolateral wall. After coronary artery bypass grafting *(bottom row)*, regional myocardial perfusion, glucose, and oxidative metabolism within anterior wall remain diminished compared with normal myocardium. (From Gropler RJ et al: *J Am Coll Cardiol* 19:989, 1992.)

blood pool, a second tracer (usually [15]O carbon monoxide, which is inhaled by the patient and subsequently binds avidly to erythrocytes) must be administered to permit the correction for ^{15}O-water activity emanating from the intravascular compartment.

To detect ischemia with PET radiopharmaceuticals, two injections are required: one set of images is recorded at rest, and a second set is recorded after stress, usually produced by pharmacologically induced vasodilation with dipyridamole or adenosine. All of these tracers yield accurate estimates of regional myocardial perfusion in relative terms. Although quantification of myocardial perfusion in absolute terms can be most accurately performed with [15]O water, [82]Rb chloride and ^{13}N ammonia can also be used.

Detection of coronary artery disease. Most of the studies designed to assess the accuracy of myocardial perfusion imaging with PET in the detection of coronary artery disease have employed either [82]Rb chloride or ^{13}N ammonia. PET and SPECT have sensitivities ranging between 80% and 95%, depending on the patient

population studied. However, because of the higher energy of annihilation radiation and improved correction for attenuation with PET, specificity tends to be about 10% to 15% higher than SPECT. The accuracy of PET has not been compared directly with that of the technetium-based perfusion agents, which have yielded results comparable to those of [201]Tl.

Myocardial Metabolism

A fundamental characteristic of the myocardium is its continuous requirement for oxygen and metabolic substrates to meet its energy needs. The heart meets its energy demands largely by oxidizing fatty acids and glucose. Under normal conditions, fatty acids are the preferred energy source for overall oxidative metabolism. When blood flow is reduced to the heart muscle and ischemia ensues, fatty acids can no longer be oxidized and glucose becomes the preferred energy source. This metabolic phenomenon is useful for the identification of myocardium that is underperfused but still viable. Such tissue is often hypokinetic or akinetic but will re-

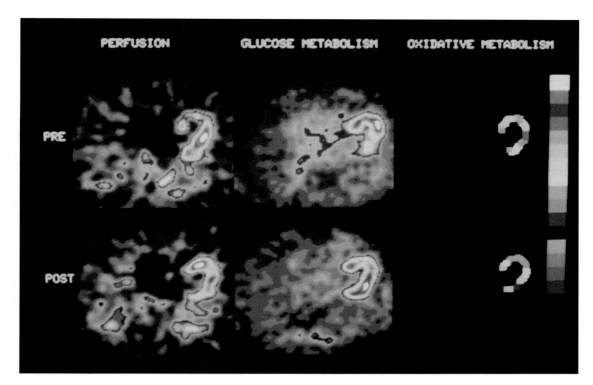

Figure 12-22 Midventricular PET images of myocardial perfusion and metabolism in patient with anterior myocardial infarction that contained viable myocardium, before and after coronary artery bypass surgery. Before revascularization, glucose metabolism in anterior wall was increased relative to that in normal posterolateral wall. In presence of anterior wall hypoperfusion, this finding indicates augmented glucose metabolism relative to flow (metabolism-flow mismatch). Although myocardial oxygen consumption in anterior wall is decreased relative to that in normal posterolateral wall, magnitude of reduction is less than that in Figure 12-21. After coronary artery bypass grafting, the regional myocardial perfusion, glucose metabolism, and oxidative metabolism in anterior wall were comparable with values in normal myocardium. (From Gropler RJ et al: *J Am Coll Cardiol* 19:989, 1992.)

turn to normal or near-normal function if blood flow is restored. Consequently, in patients with severely impaired ventricular function, combined measurements of myocardial perfusion and glucose metabolism have been advocated.

Metabolic tracers. [18]F fluorodeoxyglucose, ^{11}C palmitate, and ^{11}C acetate are typical examples of PET radiopharmaceuticals used for metabolic cardiac studies. Deoxyglucose is an analog of glucose that can be labeled with ^{18}F, a cyclotron-produced radionuclide, to form ^{18}F fluorodeoxyglucose (FDG). Its myocardial uptake reflects overall myocardial utilization of glucose. Palmitate is a naturally occurring fatty acid that can be chemically synthesized and labeled with ^{11}C, a cyclotron-produced radionuclide with a physical half-life of approximately 20.4 min. Its myocardial uptake and clearance reflect the myocardial utilization of fatty acids. The utilization of fatty acids and glucose by the heart is exquisitely sensitive to the level of glucose, fatty acids, and insulin in the blood, as well as the level of blood flow to the myocardium. Consequently, the substrate environment must be standardized when using these two tracers to study myocardial metabolism. Ac-

etate labeled with ^{11}C has recently emerged as a promising tracer of overall oxidative metabolism. The myocardial uptake and clearance of ^{11}C acetate is directly related to regional myocardial oxidative metabolism under diverse loading conditions and levels of blood flow. Unlike ^{11}C palmitate and FDG, the myocardial kinetics of ^{11}C acetate are relatively insensitive to changes in the substrate environment (Figure 12-21).

Detection of viable myocardium. Under conditions of glucose loading, a relative excess of myocardial FDG, compared with perfusion, is indicative of viable, ischemic, myocardium (Figure 12-22). Persistence of metabolic activity (demonstrated by PET with FDG) occurs in up to 50% of ^{201}Tl myocardial perfusion defects, defined as fixed on 1- and 4-hr imaging. However, the percentage of fixed myocardial perfusion lesions on 1- and 4-hr ^{201}Tl imaging, which demonstrate accumulation of FDG, is similar to the percentage of segments with fixed defects, which ultimately show improvement with ^{201}Tl reinjection. Although thallium imaging is very useful for the detection of viable myocardium, FDG imaging appears to be slightly more sensitive in patients with severely depressed ejection fractions (LVEF <30%).

SUGGESTED READING

Beller GA: *Clinical nuclear cardiology,* Philadelphia, 1995, WB Saunders.

Bergmann SR: Quantification of myocardial perfusion with positron emission tomography. In Bergmann SR, Sobel BE, eds: *Positron emission tomography of the heart,* Mount Kisco, NY, 1992, Futura.

Gerson MC, ed: *Cardiac nuclear medicine,* ed 2. New York, 1991, McGraw-Hill.

Goris ML, Bretille JA: *Colour atlas of nuclear cardiology,* London, 1992, Chapman and Hall.

Heart facts, Dallas, 1996, American Heart Association.

Wackers F, Soufer R, Zaret BL: Nuclear cardiology. In Braunwald EB, ed: *Heart disease,* ed 5, 1996, WB Saunders.

Zaret BL, Beller GA, eds: *Nuclear cardiology: state of the art and future directions,* St. Louis, 1993, Mosby.

Zipes DP: Specific arrhythmias: diagnosis and treatment. In Braunwald EB, ed: *Heart disease: a textbook of cardiovascular medicine,* Philadelphia, 1984, WB Saunders.

chapter *13*

Gastrointestinal System

Richard A. Vitti, Leon S. Malmud

Objectives

Diagram and describe the organs and structures of the gastrointestinal system.

Describe the physiology of the gastrointestinal system including the esophagus, stomach, liver, hepatobiliary collecting system and gall bladder, small intestine, and large intestine.

Describe the technique for parotid imaging.

Describe various techniques for evaluating esophageal transit using computerized regions of interest studies.

Discuss gastroesophageal reflux procedures and imaging techniques for esophageal reflux, pulmonary aspiration, and calculation of a gastro-esophageal reflux index.

Explain the clinical aspects of performing radionuclide gastric emptying studies.

Diagram the hepatobiliary system, for example, the common duct, cystic duct, gall bladder, and bile duct.

Describe the procedure used for liver and spleen scintigraphy using colloidal materials.

Describe imaging procedures using labeled red cells to detect hepatic hemangioma.

Discuss imaging procedures for the hepatobiliary system and identification of cholecystitis.

Explain procedures that can be used for the determination of enterogastric reflux.

Differentiate the advantages of sulfur colloid imaging from labeled red cells imaging techniques for the identification of gastrointestinal bleeding.

Describe the principles of performing breath test studies with ^{14}C-labeled compounds.

---

*T*he gastrointestinal system consists of the gastrointestinal tract, or alimentary canal, and several accessory organs. The alimentary canal is a continuous tube running through the ventral body cavity, originating at the mouth, and followed by the pharynx, esophagus, stomach, small intestine, and large intestine (Figure 13-1).

The purpose of the alimentary canal is to provide a route of intake for nourishment, to digest and absorb nutrients, and to eliminate waste products. For the purpose of this chapter, the accessory organs involved are the salivary glands, pancreas, liver, and gallbladder. Although not a part of the

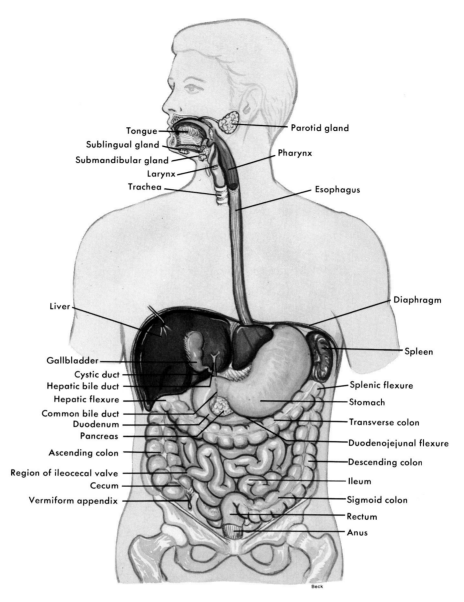

Figure 13-1   Location of gastrointestinal system organs. (From Thibodeau GA: *Anthony's textbook of anatomy and physiology,* ed 13, St. Louis, 1990, Mosby.)

gastrointestinal system, the spleen is mentioned, but only its morphology is considered.

A variety of radionuclide techniques are available for evaluation of the gastrointestinal tract, and these include techniques for imaging specific organs and those that characterize function. In this chapter methodologies are described in detail for procedures used to study the movement of luminal contents within the gastrointestinal tract. These techniques take advantage of the unique features of using radiotracers in the study of physiologic processes; that is, they permit quantitative measurement of gastrointestinal function but do not disturb the process under study. The newer methodologies include evaluation of the swallowing function and esophageal transit, the detection and quantitation of gastroesophageal reflux, the measurement of gastric

emptying, qualitative and quantitative evaluation of gallbladder function, and enterogastric reflux. Other techniques include the detection of pulmonary aspiration and ^{14}C breath testing. Techniques that have enjoyed a long clinical acceptance, such as colloid liver and spleen scanning, gastrointestinal bleeding studies, and salivary gland imaging, are also reviewed in detail.

SALIVARY GLANDS

The salivary glands consist of three paired exocrine glands that produce saliva. Saliva is a fluid that initiates the chemical breakdown of food and is continuously secreted into the mouth. The primary set of salivary glands is the parotid glands, which are located within

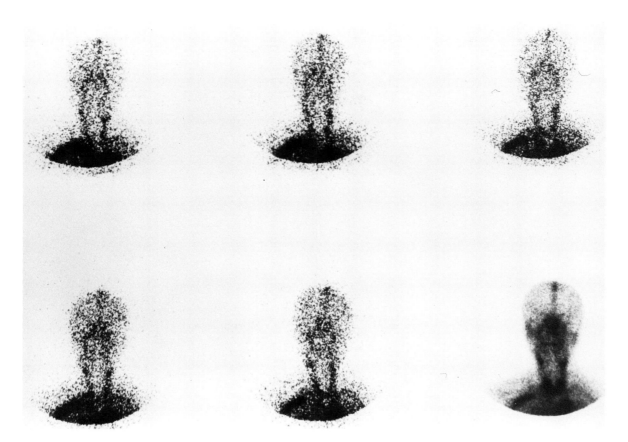

Figure 13-2 Rapid sequential images of the head and neck in the anterior projection at 2-sec intervals. There is symmetric perfusion with simultaneous and rapid localization within the salivary glands.

the cheeks, below and in front of the ears (Figure 13-1). The parotid glands empty into the oral cavity through Stensen's ducts. The second pair of salivary glands are the submandibular glands, which are located beneath the tongue in the posterior aspect of the floor of the mouth; these empty directly into the oral cavity. The third pair of sublingual glands are also located beneath the tongue and are anterior to the submandibular glands.

Salivary gland imaging, also known as nuclear sialography,[31] is used primarily in determining the size, location, and function of the salivary glands.

The salivary glands indiscriminately trap a number of ions, among them the iodides and the ^{99m}Tc-pertechnetate ion. Furthermore, these ions are actively excreted by the glands into the saliva. Hence, the production and excretion of saliva can be evaluated by using ^{99m}Tc pertechnetate.

The indications for salivary gland imaging include detection and evaluation of mass lesions involving the salivary glands as well as evaluation of the symptom of dryness of the mouth, or xerostomia. Xerostomia is a difficult clinical symptom to assess, since it may have a psychosomatic origin. However, the possibility that xerostomia is caused by a blockage of one or several of the salivary gland ducts by a benign or neoplastic mass must be considered. Xerostomia is also an important

feature and often a presenting complaint in several systemic disease complexes, notably the collagen-vascular diseases, particularly Sjögren syndrome.[31] Xerostomia can also be associated with thyroiditis and should be taken into account in the interpretation of salivary gland images. Xerostomia also occurs in sarcoidosis, following radiation therapy to the head and neck, during states of dehydration, and as a result of administration of certain drugs and pharmacologic agents.

Imaging Procedure

No patient preparation is necessary. Rinsing the mouth before the examination may decrease pertechnetate excretion into the oral cavity. The patient is seated comfortably facing the scintillation camera. The camera is peaked for ^{99m}Tc with a 20% energy window and fitted with a low-energy parallel-hole collimator. To prevent superimposition of the thyroid gland on the salivary glands, the patient's head should be tilted backward with the neck extended as far as possible, allowing the chin to make contact with the camera face.

One to 5 mCi of ^{99m}Tc pertechnetate is administered intravenously after the patient is properly positioned. Rapid sequential anterior images of the face and neck are obtained at 1- to 2-sec intervals (Figure 13-2). These should demonstrate simultaneous and symmetric up-

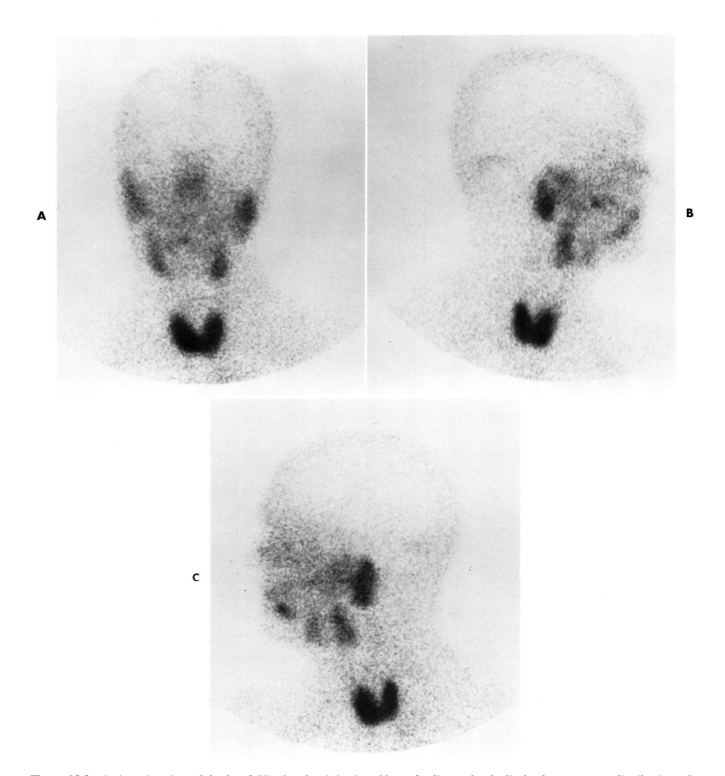

Figure 13-3 A, Anterior view of the head 15 min after injection. Normal salivary glands display homogenous distribution of ^{99m}Tc pertechnetate. Localization is symmetric within parotid, submandibular, and sublingual glands. Uptake is also seen within thyroid gland. **B,** Right lateral view of head and neck. **C,** Left lateral view of head and neck. Parotid and submandibular glands are seen particularly well in these lateral views.

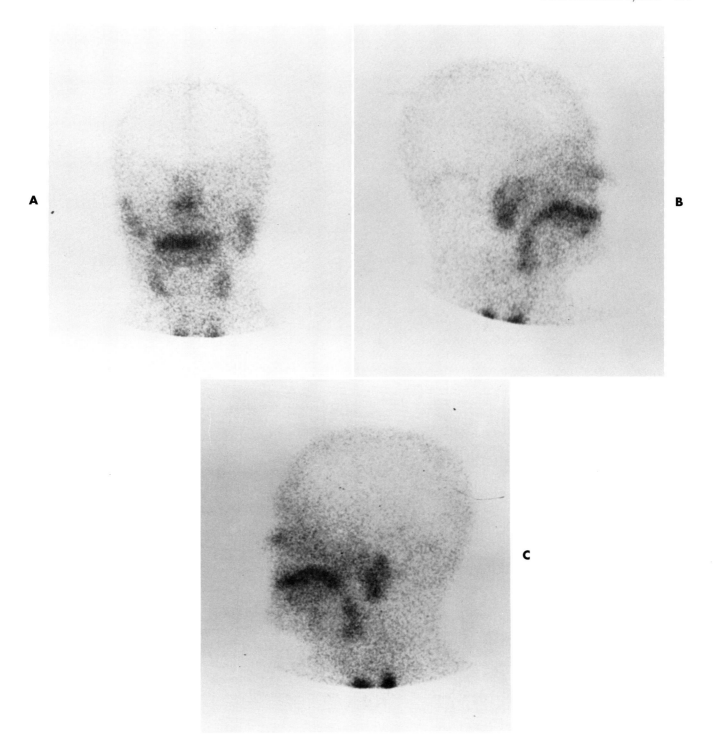

Figure 13-4   Anterior **(A)**, right lateral **(B)**, and left lateral **(C)** views of the head 20 min after oral administration of dilute lemon juice. There has been rapid, symmetric, and profound diminution of radiotracer localization within the salivary glands. Compared with Figure 13-3, most of the activity is now within the oral cavity.

take of the radiotracer within the parotid, submandibular, and sublingual glands. Thereafter, it is often useful to obtain anterior and lateral views of the head and neck (Figure 13-3) to confirm the normal presence of radiotracer within the saliva in the oral cavity.

It may be useful at this point to test the salivary gland response to gustatory stimulation.[4] A 1:1 dilution of commercial lemon juice (pH approximately 2.6) may be used; alternatively, fresh-squeezed lemon juice diluted equally with tap water may be substituted. The patient is instructed to take a mouthful of the lemon juice solution and swish the juice throughout the mouth for approximately 5 sec and expectorate fully into a disposable beaker. The patient may then be repositioned in front of the camera and imaged for an additional 20 min. In normal individuals there is usually a rapid, symmetric, and profound diminution in radiotracer localization within the salivary glands (Figure 13-4).

Prior perchlorate administration should be avoided since it will, in part, block salivary gland uptake of the radiotracer.

The estimated radiation dose to the normal parotid gland is 0.6 rad/mCi of ^{99m}Tc pertechnetate.

Clinical Aspects

Normally, there is simultaneous, rapid, and symmetric localization of the radiotracer within all three pairs of salivary glands (see Figure 13-2) with homogeneous distribution of the pertechnetate (see Figure 13-3). It was originally hoped that this examination would be capable of discerning a wide variety of mass lesions within the salivary glands, but this has not been the case. Only two types of neoplasm result in a consistent appearance on nuclear sialography: Warthin tumors, which appear as focal areas of increased uptake (Figure 13-5); and metastatic lesions, which are characteristically cold focal areas. Benign mixed tumors of the salivary glands may appear as focal areas of increased or decreased uptake. Focal cold areas are seen with other types of malignancy, cysts, some mixed tumors, enlarged lymph nodes, and inflammatory diseases. Decreased or absent uptake within a single gland or set of glands may be seen in congenital aplasia or obstructive sialolithiasis and following sialectomy, trauma, or radiotherapy. In Sjögren syndrome and other types of vascular and connective tissue diseases, there is either asymmetric arrival of the radiotracer within the salivary glands, or radiotracer uptake within the salivary glands is delayed when compared with radiotracer uptake within the thyroid. On delayed images bilaterally decreased uptake can be seen in these diseases, and there can be an absent or blunted response following the administration of a gustatory stimulant.[4] Bilaterally decreased uptake within the salivary glands can also be seen in acute suppurative parotitis, multicentric sialoangiectasis, and in some aged individuals.

Poor response to gustatory stimulation is seen in the systemic connective tissue diseases, acute parotitis (mumps), and following radiotherapy of the head and neck. If a single salivary gland, or group of salivary glands, fails to excrete, this is suggestive of stenosis or blockage of the salivary duct.

Despite lack of anatomic detail, salivary gland imaging plays a useful clinical role in the evaluation of certain morphologic and functional diseases. In some situations contrast sialography can differentiate neoplasm

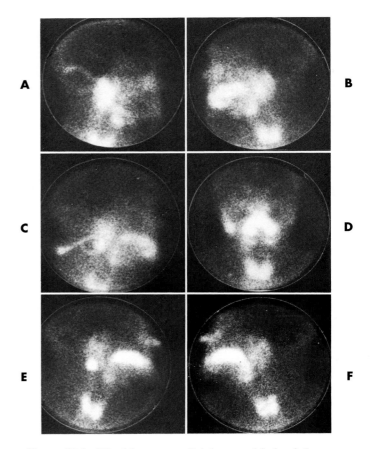

Figure 13-5 Warthin tumor of right parotid gland. Immediate right (**A**) and left lateral (**B**) views. Delayed right lateral view with radioactive string marker around palpable nodule (**C**). One hr delayed views taken in the anterior (**D**), right (**E**), and left lateral (**F**) positions.

from inflammation, benign from malignant masses, and extrinsic from intrinsic masses.

OROPHARYNX

The oropharynx lies posterior to the mouth and is a complex organ composed of numerous small muscles, cartilage, and tendons. Since the oropharynx functions in both a respiratory and digestive capacity, its components must function in a coordinated manner to accept food from the mouth and propel it from the esophagus while suspending respiration. Although radiographic studies of swallowing have been in use for some time, they are accompanied by a relatively high radiation burden and do not readily provide quantitative information of swallowing function. Because radionuclide studies are generally very sensitive and provide information that is both physiologic and quantitative in nature, the radionuclide oropharyngeal study was developed as a method for measuring clearance of liquids from the oropharynx. This technique may be combined with esophageal transit and gastroesophageal reflux studies.

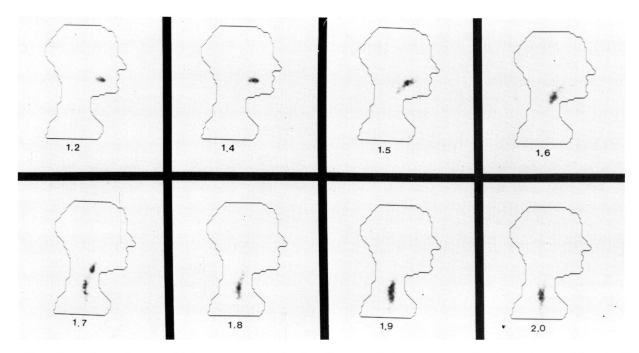

Figure 13-6 Normal oropharyngeal 0.1-sec images obtained on-line to a digital computer with the patient positioned with the right side of the face at the surface of the collimator.

Imaging Procedure

Ten ml of cold tap water is mixed with 1 mCi of ^{99m}Tc sulfur colloid by shaking for 30 sec immediately before this study. A liquid sample of approximately 10 ml is used, since this volume is easily swallowed as a bolus.

A large field of view scintillation camera fitted with a high-sensitivity collimator is used. Images should be acquired on a computer. The patient is seated erect in front of the camera in the anterior position with the neck rotated to the left. The right cheek is positioned at the surface of the collimator, as is the chest, such that a right lateral view of the mouth and oropharynx and anterior view of the chest are obtained.

The patient is instructed to sip the fluid through a straw and to hold the entire amount of the material in the mouth. On command the patient is instructed to swallow all the material at once. It may be useful to review the procedure with the patient using sips of plain water before the administration of the test dose. After swallowing the radiopharmaceutical, the patient is instructed to dry swallow every 15 sec on command. The patient should breathe quietly through the nose during the remainder of the study.

Images are acquired for 5 min in the computer for subsequent analysis. The initial 30 sec of the examination are acquired at 0.1 sec/frame, and the following 270 sec are acquired at 15 sec/frame (Figure 13-6).

Images for the first 30 sec are added by the computer to yield a composite image for anatomic definition of the oropharynx. From this summed image a manually

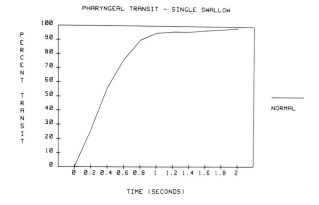

Figure 13-7 Normal time-activity curve representing oropharyngeal function. Function is biexponential with a fast- and slow-clearing component.

outlined region of interest is drawn and stored in the computer. This region of interest is then used to generate a time-activity curve from the raw data. This time-activity curve, representing the oropharyngeal count rate, is fit to a biexponential clearance model, which consists of fast- and slow-clearing components (Figure 13-7), each associated with an amplitude and half-life.

Clinical Aspects

This radionuclide imaging procedure is useful for documenting the swallowing function and pharyngeal transit time. The test may be useful to document and quantify abnormalities of the swallowing function in those patients in whom no demonstrable abnormality can be seen either by direct inspection or by other methods, such as the barium swallow. A prolonged high-amplitude slow component appears to be characteristic of an abnormal swallowing function.

ESOPHAGUS

The esophagus is a muscular tube extending from the pharynx to the stomach. Its function is to transport a swallowed food bolus from the pharynx to the stomach, which is accomplished by coordinated contractions of its muscular layers, termed *peristalsis*. The esophagus is located posterior to the trachea within the thorax and in its resting state remains collapsed (see Figure 13-1).

The esophagus is slightly narrowed, or pinched, just above the stomach, as it passes through the respiratory diaphragm. This narrowing, along with the muscular layer of the diaphragm, constitutes the physiologic lower esophageal sphincter, or gastroesophageal sphincter. Proper relaxation of the lower esophageal sphincter is necessary to allow the passage of the food bolus into the stomach. Incoordinate lower esophageal sphincter function has been implicated in a number of

disorders that affect esophageal transit, as well as in gastroesophageal reflux.

Esophageal Transit

Radionuclide esophageal transit studies[13] are useful as a noninvasive screening test for suspected disorders of esophageal motility. Usually the individual with dysphagia (any difficulty or discomfort associated with swallowing) will have a more conventional examination, such as barium swallow or endoscopy before or after a radionuclide examination. Scintigraphic studies do not provide information regarding anatomic detail, and more conventional examinations must be performed to exclude any structural lesions. Scintigraphic studies are more sensitive for detecting esophageal motor disorders and provide quantitative information.

In the act of swallowing, a bolus of solid or liquid food moves through the length of the esophagus by the forces of peristalsis and gravity. This movement is defined as esophageal transit, different from esophageal clearance, which refers to the emptying from the esophagus of refluxed material from the stomach.

Difficulty or discomfort associated with swallowing can be associated with anatomic lesions of the esophagus or an esophageal motor disorder. Severely painful

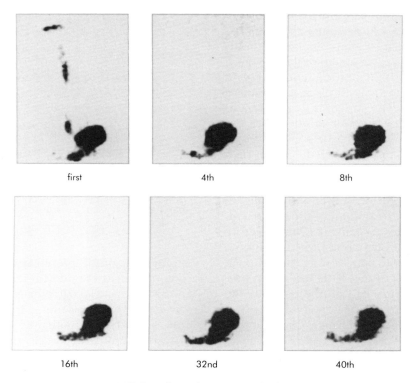

first   4th   8th

16th   32nd   40th

Multiple swallow technique—normal subject

Figure 13-8 Normal esophageal images. Images of esophagus are acquired in the anterior projection at the initial swallow and then every 15 sec with each "dry swallow" for the next 10 min. Individual images are shown for the initial swallow, first, fourth, eighth, sixteenth, thirty-second, and fortieth swallows. Images are acquired on-line, stored on a digital computer, and later retrieved for analysis. Note: Following initial swallow in the normal subject, no activity is seen within esophagus.

swallowing can be associated with mucosal destruction of the esophagus from infection, reflux esophagitis, ulcerations, or tumor. Esophageal studies are also useful for evaluating patients with suspected regurgitation or aspiration pneumonias. Motility disorders of the esophagus may be due to innate muscular or innervation disorders or can be secondary to a systemic disease, such as the connective tissue disease. There may be amotility, which is seen in achalasia and scleroderma. Hypomotility, or decreased pressure of swallowing, can be seen in aged individuals, and hypermotility can be seen in diffuse esophageal spasm.

Imaging procedure. The patient should fast for at least 2 hr before the examination.

The radiopharmaceutical is prepared by mixing 300 μCi of ^{99m}Tc sulfur colloid in 15 ml of tap water.

The patient is placed supine under the camera for an anterior view of the thorax. The camera is fitted with a high-sensitivity or low-energy all-purpose collimator and interfaced to a computer. The patient is positioned with the stomach at the bottom of the field of view. The radiopharmaceutical is administered orally through a straw, and the patient is instructed to take the entire volume into the mouth but not to swallow until instructed to do so. The computer is started and the patient is instructed to swallow the contents of the mouth as a single compact bolus. The patient is instructed to dry swallow every 15 sec for the next 10 min. Images are acquired every 0.25 sec for the first min and at 15-sec intervals for the remaining 9 min (Figure 13-8). At the conclusion of the study the data are retrieved from the computer for analysis. There are currently two methods of data analysis to measure esophageal transit. A global measure of esophageal emptying can be made by recording the counts present in the total esophagus following multiple swallows using a computer-generated rectangular region of interest over the entire esophagus (Figure 13-9). The count rate within the esophageal region of interest is used to determine the rate of esophageal transit with the following formula[13]:

$$C_t = \frac{(E_{max} - E_t)}{E_{max}} \times 100$$

where C_t represents the esophageal transit at time t; E_{max}, the maximal count rate in the esophagus, and E_t, the esophageal count rate at time t.

The second method analyzes regional esophageal transit by dividing the esophagus into proximal, middle, and distal regions of interest. Three equal-size rectangular regions of interest are drawn. A plot of counts against time is used to describe the transit of the bolus through each esophageal region (Figure 13-10).

Clinical aspects. Esophageal activity decreases rapidly, usually within 5 to 10 sec after the first swallow, and the activity is no longer visible (see Figure 13-8), although count rates of approximately 10% of peak activity may be found until the eighth swallow (2 min) (Figure 13-11). As the initial bolus passes through the esophagus, a smooth progression of sequential peaks of activity in the proximal, middle, and distal esophagus are demonstrated (see Figure 13-10). By the fortieth swallow (10 min), less than 5% of peak activity remains in the whole esophageal region of interest (see Figure 13-11). Using these methods it is possible to differentiate patients with achalasia (see Figures 13-11 and 13-12) from those with scleroderma, since in scleroderma most of the bolus activity is able to enter the stomach, whereas in achalasia there is a more marked delay in esophageal emptying. With diffuse esophageal spasm the radionuclide study shows incoordinate activ-

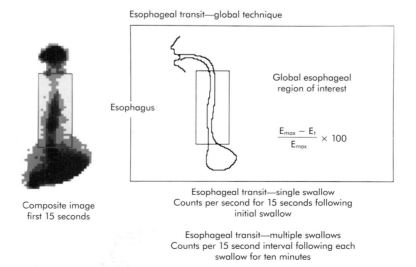

Esophageal transit—global technique

Global esophageal region of interest

Esophagus

$$\frac{E_{max} - E_t}{E_{max}} \times 100$$

Composite image first 15 seconds

Esophageal transit—single swallow
Counts per second for 15 seconds following initial swallow

Esophageal transit—multiple swallows
Counts per 15 second interval following each swallow for ten minutes

Figure 13-9 Illustration of the esophageal region of interest when esophageal transit is measured as a global function.

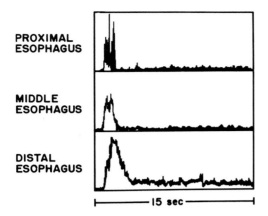

Figure 13-10 Normal esophageal transit. Three equal-sized rectangular regions of interest are used to generate time-activity curves through each of three esophageal regions.

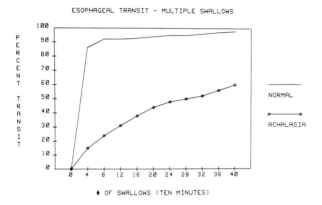

Figure 13-11 Time-activity curves of percent transit versus the number of swallows for 10 min. Both a normal individual (from Figure 13-8) and a patient with achalasia are illustrated (same patient as Figure 13-12).

ity, which is different from patients with nonspecific abnormalities.

The radionuclide method has demonstrated 100% sensitivity for detecting achalasia, diffuse esophageal spasm, and scleroderma. Radionuclide esophageal transit studies can also be useful in the evaluation of esophageal strictures, esophageal diverticula, and following radiotherapy for carcinoma of the esophagus.

A routine esophageal transit study may be combined with delayed images of the thorax in the anterior and posterior projections for the detection of aspirated radionuclide. Delayed images of the thorax can be particularly useful in the adult patient with nonspecific pulmonary symptoms in whom the diagnosis of pulmonary aspiration is often difficult to confirm. Overnight pulmonary aspiration of a radionuclide from the stomach, when demonstrable, is seen as a highly specific,

though insensitive, method for detecting this disorder (Figure 13-13). Unfortunately, a pulmonary aspiration scan can be negative, even in patients with clear symptoms.

Gastroesophageal Reflux

Gastroesophageal reflux refers to the symptom complex of heartburn, regurgitation, and chest pain. Esophageal reflux occurs when either gastric or duodenal contents enter the esophagus. Some of the anatomic abnormalities that can result in incompetence of the lower esophageal sphincter and symptomatic gastroesophageal reflux include enlargement of the diaphragmatic hiatus, disruption of the phrenoesophageal ligament, loss of the acute cardioesophageal angle of Hiss, loss of the gastric mucosal rosette, and a change in the distal paraesophageal pressure from an intraabdominal to an intrathoracic level. In short, lower esophageal sphincter incompetence must be present for acid reflux to occur.

A number of nonradionuclide studies are available for the detection of gastroesophageal reflux, including barium esophagography, barium cine-swallow, endoscopy, mucosal biopsy, manometry, acid-perfusion, clearance, and reflux testing. Of these available studies, none is as sensitive as gastroesophageal scintigraphy in the detection of reflux.[13,25] Furthermore, only gastroesophageal scintigraphy is quantitative and can be used to determine the severity of reflux as well as evaluate patient response to therapy.

The clinical significance of minimal degrees of esophageal reflux is questionable at best. It has been suggested that diminished muscle tone in the lower esophagus rather than hiatal hernia is the cause of most reflux.[29] Simple inexpensive regimens, such as the use of antacids and changes in the diet to include more protein, may resolve symptoms in most patients (only 5% of whom may eventually require surgery). Small degrees of reflux are hardly grounds for surgery, and a trial of therapy (known to be innocuous) can satisfy both patient and referring physician much more than the results of complicated diagnostic tests.[7]

Anatomically, the gastroesophageal sphincter of the distal esophagus has not been convincingly demonstrated. The concept of a physiologic sphincter is based on the fact that the proximal esophagus functions differently from the distal esophagus. The upper third of the esophagus has striated muscle and the remaining two thirds consists of smooth muscle. The body of the esophagus contracts in response to swallowing, during which time the lower esophageal sphincter relaxes. This reciprocity of esophageal function, proximally versus distally, constitutes evidence for a physiologic sphincter mechanism. Many esophageal disorders disrupt neural and muscular mechanisms that control this normal sphincter activity.

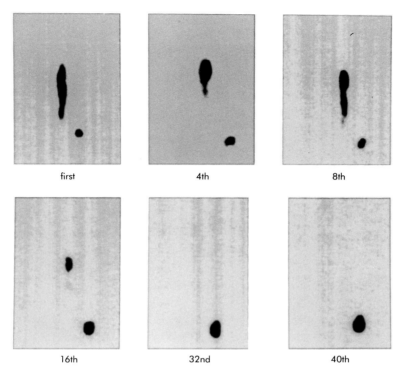

first   4th   8th

16th   32nd   40th

Multiple swallow technique in a patient with achalasia

Figure 13-12   Anterior views of the esophagus in a patient with achalasia. Note poor passage of liquid bolus within the esophagus (retention) despite repeated "dry swallows." Percent transit is illustrated in Figure 13-11.

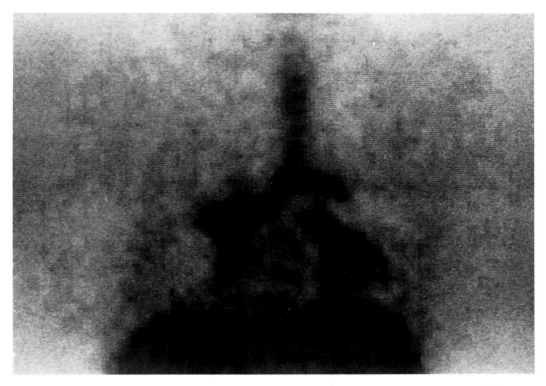

Figure 13-13   Pulmonary aspiration. Anterior view of the thorax obtained 24 hr following instillation of ^{99m}Tc sulfur colloid into the stomach via nasogastric tube. Activity is seen within trachea, bronchi, and peripheral lung fields, indicating overnight aspiration of gastric contents.

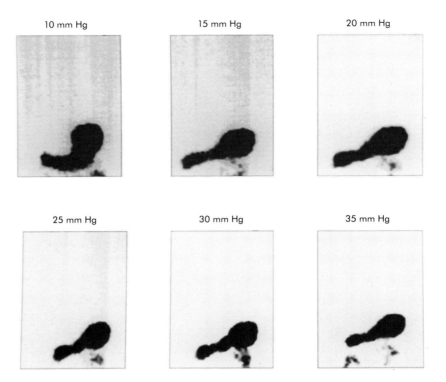

10 mm Hg   15 mm Hg   20 mm Hg

25 mm Hg   30 mm Hg   35 mm Hg

Figure 13-14 Serial scans of a gastroesophageal reflux study in a normal individual. Resting pressure across the lower esophageal sphincter is 10 mm Hg, and with each successive inflation of the abdominal binder, there is a corresponding increase of 5 mm Hg in pressure across the lower esophageal sphincter. Throughout the study, no gastroesophageal reflux is visualized.

Fat, alcohol, chocolate, and cigarette smoking are some of the factors that commonly cause depression of the lower esophageal sphincter pressure, and these have also been associated with symptomatic gastroesophageal reflux. Consequences of recurring gastroesophageal reflux are esophagitis, unrelenting heartburn, and eventual dysphagia. Often these symptoms are associated with abnormalities in esophageal clearance, and it may be beneficial to routinely perform both esophageal and gastroesophageal scintigraphic studies as a single examination.

Imaging procedure. After the patient has fasted at least 8 hr before the examination, the esophageal transit study should be performed first. This allows the technologist to visually note all the obvious abnormalities that can impair esophageal clearance. After these data for the esophagus are stored for later processing, the gastroesophageal reflux study may be performed.

The patient is given an oral solution containing 300 μCi of ^{99m}Tc sulfur colloid mixed with 150 ml of orange juice and 150 ml of 0.1 normal hydrochloric acid. The entire 300 ml of solution should be administered, since this volume of liquid in the stomach opposes induced abdominal pressure. The patient is then fitted with an abdominal binder similar to a large blood pressure cuff (Baum-Velcro Abdominal Binder). The patient is positioned supine under the camera, and the abdominal binder is readjusted so that the inflatable blad-

Patient with reflux

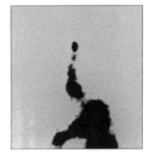

Normal subject

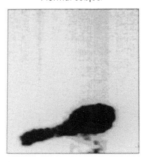

Figure 13-15 Anterior images of thorax obtained in a patient with reflux and in a normal subject, respectively. An oscilloscope with a high persistence should be used as a visual aid during the performance of this examination, since reflux can be readily visualized on the oscilloscope face.

der within it is centered over the stomach and below the costal margin. In female patients, care should be taken to not pinch the breasts. The binder should be positioned carefully so as to induce a pressure that will force the stomach superiorly. Compression of the lower ribs should be avoided because this will force the stomach inferiorly, away from the diaphragm. Four factors are required to successfully cause an induced reflux in a patient who is prone to gastroesophageal reflux: oral administration of an acidified solution; successive, increased applied pressure to the abdomen; maintenance of a supine position; and at least a 300 ml volume in the stomach to oppose the applied pressure.

No longer than 10 min after oral administration of the ^{99m}Tc-sulfur-colloid solution, center the patient under the camera so that the stomach is positioned at the bottom of the field. The entire stomach must be included on all images. As pressure is increased with the abdominal binder, the stomach image is seen to rise, but immediate repositioning is not necessary unless the esophageal region is excluded from the field of view. If activity is seen in the esophagus during positioning, either a delay in esophageal clearance or a spontaneous reflux has occurred. An additional 30 ml of tap water should clear this activity.

The use of a parallel-hole collimator on a large field of view camera is best, although a diverging collimator with a small field of view camera may be used. Images are obtained for 30 sec at the following pressure points obtained by inflating the abdominal binder: 0, 20, 40, 60, 80, and 100 mm Hg. An additional postdeflation image is also obtained. Increments of 20 mm Hg on the abdominal binder are successively applied while monitoring the sphygmomanometer attached to the binder (increments of 20 mm Hg applied externally

have been shown to increase the pressure across the lower esophageal sphincter in increments of 5 mm Hg) (Figure 13-14). Images should be acquired as quickly as possible so patient discomfort is not prolonged. It is important not to deflate the binder between successive stages of pressure. Most patients tolerate 100 mm Hg, but keep in mind that there are patients who cannot withstand this level due to debilitating surgery or to their present symptoms.

It is best that an oscilloscope with a high persistence be used as a visual aid during the performance of the examination. Reflux can be visualized during the course of the test (Figure 13-15). Computer images might warrant the need to adjust contrast in cases of subtle reflux. Subtly visualized activity within the esophagus has been shown to correspond to 3% to 4% of the 300 μCi ^{99m}Tc dose and can be used to confirm reflux. (Note: Patients who have the esophageal transit study performed before the gastroesophageal reflux study will have a greater amount of activity within the stomach at the beginning of the examination.)

Patients with known esophageal motor disorders or with a large hiatal hernia should have endogastric tube placement before performance of the reflux study. In this way the radiopharmaceutical solution can be delivered into the stomach through the tube bypassing the esophagus. The tube can then be flushed with 10 to 15 ml of tap water and removed before beginning the imaging study. This technique prevents retention of activity within the esophagus, which can be related to the motor disorder or to a hiatal hernia.

Computer analysis of this study is accomplished by recalling the separate images and then drawing regions of interest for the stomach and esophagus (Figure 13-

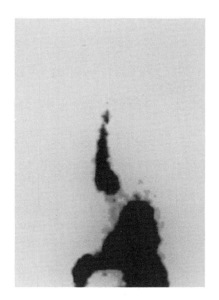
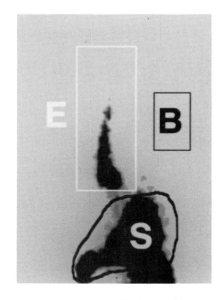

Figure 13-16 Anterior view of the thorax is recalled from the computer for analysis. Regions of interest are drawn for the esophagus *(top left)*, the stomach *(S)*, and background *(B)*. Counts within each region of interest are recorded for each pressure level and then used to calculate the gastroesophageal reflux indexes.

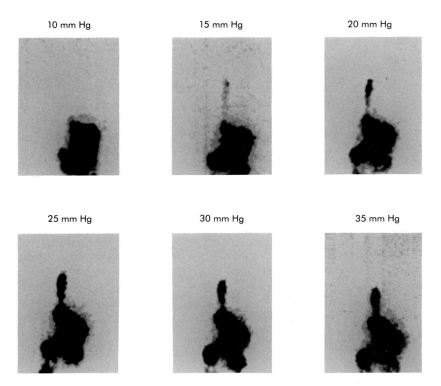

Figure 13-17 Anterior views of the thorax illustrating an abnormal examination. With progressive inflation of the abdominal binder, causing increments of 5 mm Hg of pressure across the lower esophageal sphincter, there is an increase in the amount of induced gastroesophageal reflux.

16). The counts within the stomach region of interest and within the esophageal region of interest are noted and then used to calculate a gastroesophageal reflux index for each level of abdominal pressure using the following formula:

$$\text{GERI} = \left(\frac{E_p}{G_{max}} \right) \times 100$$

where *GERI* is the gastroesophageal reflux index in percent, E_p is esophageal counts at a specific pressure point p, and G_{max} is the maximum gastric count obtained for one image in this study.

Clinical aspects. A normal gastroesophageal reflux study has a reflux index of less than 4%; this is the level at which gastroesophageal reflux cannot be visualized (see Figure 13-15). An index greater than 4% is considered to be abnormal and can usually be visualized in the images (Figure 13-17). This quantitative feature is unique to the scintigraphic study and permits the evaluation of patients before and after medical or surgical therapy for gastroesophageal reflux.

Delayed images of the thorax can be obtained up to 24 hr for the detection of reflux leading to pulmonary aspiration (see Figure 13-13). This is particularly useful in children and infants, where the radionuclide solution can be delivered through intubation or by placing the radiopharmaceutical in the bottle with the infant's formula or juice. Radionuclide studies are superior to barium studies for diagnosing reflux in children not only because of the lower radiation burden, but also because reflux occurs intermittently and fluoroscopy cannot be performed continuously due to its associated high-radiation exposure.

STOMACH

The stomach is a crescent-shaped pouchlike organ that lies just below the diaphragm (Figure 13-18). Its proximal connection is the esophagus, and its distal connection is the duodenum, the first portion of the small intestine. The stomach consists of three muscular coats, and its inner surface is lined with a membrane responsible for secreting both a protective mucous layer, as well as the hydrochloric acid used in the digestion of swallowed food particles. The stomach is divided into three anatomic regions: the fundus, the corpus (or body), and the antrum. The coordination of muscular function within the stomach is mediated by both extrinsic and intrinsic nervous pathways and is also mediated by a number of hormones (e.g., gastrin, secretin, and cholecystokinin). The proximal portion of the stomach acts as a reservoir for ingested food, and its muscular layers generate a low-level pressure gradient to propel food toward the more distal portion of the stomach. Within the antrum, intense muscular contractions act to grind

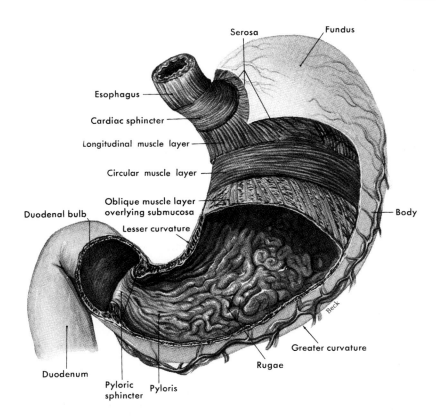

Figure 13-18   Stomach. (From Thibodeau GA: *Anthony's textbook of anatomy and physiology,* ed 13, St. Louis, 1990, Mosby.)

food particles and mix them with digestive enzymes. Furthermore, these contractions propel food out of the stomach, through the pyloric sphincter.

The control of gastric emptying of food is dependent on the volume of the meal as well as the energy density (amount of carbohydrates, fats) of the meal. Hormones such as cholecystokinin and gastrin are known to inhibit gastric emptying.

Gastric emptying studies are employed when standard radiographic or endoscopic examinations cannot adequately explain clinical signs and symptoms. These symptoms include nausea, vomiting, abdominal fullness, distention, and weight loss. Such symptoms may be due to mechanical obstruction from anatomic lesions, such as ulceration, edema, tumor, or foreign body or may be due to a gastric motility disorder. Mechanical and nonmechanical causes of gastric motility disorders are summarized in Table 13-1.

With the advent of radionuclide techniques for accurate and noninvasive assessment of gastric motility, patients with unexplained nausea and vomiting can now be shown to have an organic cause for their symptoms; furthermore, new medications have been introduced to treat disorders of gastric emptying. Emptying of both liquids and solids is significantly decreased in patients with impaired gastric emptying; rapid gastric emptying (dumping syndrome) also occurs, especially following gastric surgery. Duodenal ulcer disease, the Zollinger-Ellison syndrome, Chagas disease, and malab-

Table 13-1	Causes of gastric motility disorders
Mechanical	**Nonmechanical**
Peptic ulceration	Metabolic
Duodenal ulcer	Diabetes
Pyloric channel ulcer	Uremia
Postsurgical	Hypo- or hyperthyroidism
Pyloroplasty	Gastrinoma
Hemigastrectomy	Neurologic
Hypertrophic pyloric	Vagotomy
stenosis	Neuropathy
Cancer of the stomach	Gastroparesis
Postradiotherapy	Systemic diseases
Trauma	Scleroderma
	Amyloidosis
	Smooth muscle disorders
	Anorexia nervosa
	Drug induced
	Anticholinergics
	Opiates

sorption syndromes including pancreatic insufficiency, have been reported to increase gastric motility.

The stomach accepts a variety of both liquid and solid food, functions as a storage and mixing chamber for digestion, and then propels digested foods into the duodenum. Gastric emptying is a complex process affected by the physical and chemical composition of the ingested meal, the intrinsic and extrinsic nervous innervation of the stomach, and by circulating neuroendocrine transmitters. In terms of functional gastric emptying the stomach can be divided into the proximal region (fundus), which controls liquid emptying, and the distal region (antrum), which controls the rate of emptying for solids. Tonic contractions generated in the proximal portion of the stomach produce a pressure gradient between the stomach and duodenum, forcing liquid material into the distal stomach and through the pylorus. In the distal portion of the stomach, digestible solids are churned and liquefied before leaving the stomach. Solid particles are retained in the body of the stomach until they are smaller than 1 to 2 mm. The pylorus helps break down large solid particles not ready for digestion and restricts the rate of gastric emptying while preventing reflux of duodenal contents back into the stomach.

Numerous methods[10,11,26] have been proposed for the simultaneous radionuclide study of liquid and solid components of a meal using different radionuclide labels for both the solid and liquid portions of the test meal and dual isotope counting. Since the rate of gastric emptying varies with meal size, each laboratory must standardize meal size and composition based on the amount of carbohydrate, fat, protein, and nondigestible solids and on the caloric content. A wide variety of meals, including meat, potatoes, porridge, pancakes, cornflakes, chicken liver, eggs, French toast, and chemical resins, have been used.[8,19,27,36] [111]In and ^{99m}Tc are the radionuclides most often used, since they are well suited for imaging with the scintillation camera. Adequate images and good counting statistics can be achieved with small doses, and the radiation burden to the patient is kept to a minimum.[34]

The simplest approach to measure gastric emptying with the scintillation camera involves giving a dual solid/liquid labeled test meal and serially measuring anterior count rates from the stomach with the patient either upright or supine. Corrections for attenuation, physical decay, and downscatter from ^{111}In in the ^{99m}Tc window may be necessary to accurately measure the amount of activity remaining within the stomach during the study.[10] This is particularly true when one considers that the examination may continue over several hours. Therefore each laboratory must perform its own phantom studies to determine the appropriate correction factors.

Imaging Procedure

In preparation for the study, the patient should fast for at least 8 hr.

A number of techniques are available for preparation of a solid test meal. Among them is the in vivo labeling of chicken liver; in vitro labeled chicken liver may also be prepared. However, a simple method providing a stable in vivo solid label involves an egg sand-

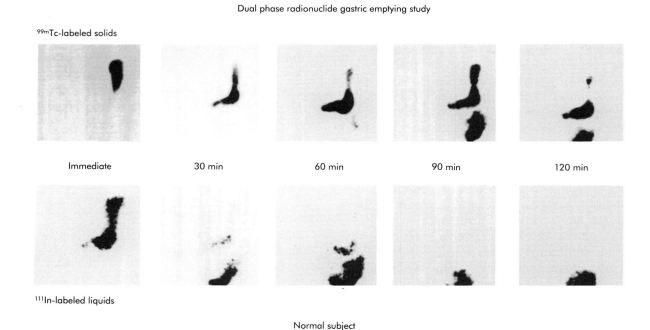

Dual phase radionuclide gastric emptying study

[99m]Tc-labeled solids

Immediate   30 min   60 min   90 min   120 min

[111]In-labeled liquids

Normal subject

Figure 13-19 Dual isotope gastric scintigraphy. Anterior images of the abdomen obtained in a normal subject following oral administration of a scrambled egg sandwich prepared with ^{99m}Tc sulfur colloid and the liquid portion consisting of ^{111}In DTPA in water. Images were obtained for 1 min at 30-min intervals at both ^{99m}Tc and ^{111}In window settings. Note the emptying of both liquids and solids from the stomach.

wich. Two raw eggs are gently broken into a disposable beaker and are injected with 500 μCi of ^{99m}Tc sulfur colloid. The eggs are allowed to incubate for 5 min behind a lead shield then scrambled well with a disposable stirrer and then fried in an electric skillet until firm and dry. The eggs are placed between two slices of toasted white bread. The liquid portion of the meal is prepared by using 125 μCi of ^{111}In DTPA[19] in 300 ml of tap water.

The patient is instructed to eat the egg sandwich within 5 min and then to drink the liquid portion of the meal. A large field of view camera is fitted with a medium-energy collimator and interfaced to a computer. The camera system is peaked for both ^{99m}Tc and ^{111}In using a pair of 20% energy windows. As soon as the patient finishes the radiolabeled meal, images of the abdomen are acquired in the anterior and posterior projections with the stomach in the center of the field of view. Images are acquired for 60 sec with the camera peaked first on the technetium setting and then on the 247 keV setting of indium. The two images are repeated every 15 min for at least the next 2 hr for both the ^{99m}Tc and the ^{111}In windows (Figure 13-19). The study may be extended beyond 2 hr if the stomach does not appear to empty.

The stored images are retrieved from the computer, a region of interest is drawn around the stomach, and the counts are generated for each image (both the ^{99m}Tc and the ^{111}In images for each 15-min interval). The total counts for each region at each time are recorded. The ^{99m}Tc counts are corrected for radioactive decay. The geometric mean of counts ($\sqrt{\text{anterior} \times \text{posterior}}$) is calculated, and the technetium and indium curves are each normalized to 100%. Other correction factors may be necessary,[10] and resultant values represent the percent of gastric retention.

The most common method for displaying gastric

emptying data is to plot the normalized percent of stomach retention for each radionuclide on linear graph paper, with the y axis representing the percent of retained activity and the x axis representing the time elapsed at each 15-min interval[26] (Figure 13-20). The most popular measure of gastric emptying is the half-emptying time ($t_{1/2}$), which is found by taking the 50% retention point from the plot and noting the time to reach this point. The $t_{1/2}$ emptying times for liquids and solids may be compared among groups of patients and between one series of examinations and another. However, the $t_{1/2}$ emptying time does not fully characterize the complex process of gastric emptying, and other methods have been described to characterize the entire pattern of gastric emptying.

Clinical Aspects

The detection of abnormally delayed or rapid emptying of liquids or solids depends on the test meal em-

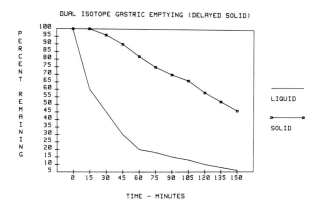

Figure 13-21 Abnormal dual isotope gastric emptying curves, generated for patient in Figure 13-23. When compared with the normal curve study, liquids empty normally, whereas solids are delayed.

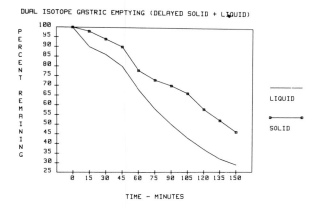

Figure 13-22 Abnormal dual isotope gastric emptying curves. Same patient as Figure 13-24. There is retention of both liquids and solids during the course of the examination. Compare with normal in Figure 13-20.

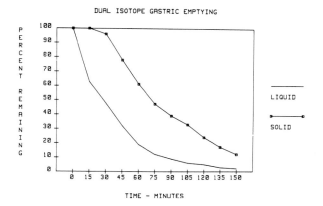

Figure 13-20 Normal dual isotope gastric emptying. Time-activity curves for both liquids and solids are graphed as percent remaining as a function of time. Note emptying of both liquids and solids. This is the same individual as Figure 13-19.

ployed. Therefore patient data are most conveniently displayed by superimposition on a normal plot for the particular test meal employed. For the test meal previously described, one may expect liquids to have a $t_{1/2}$ ranging from 10 to 45 min, and a $t_{1/2}$ for solids rang- ing from 60 to 105 min (Figure 13-20). The overall appearance of the emptying curves may be more useful in the detection of abnormalities than simple $t_{1/2}$ emptying times (Figures 13-21 and 13-22).

Abnormally delayed emptying of solids and liquids

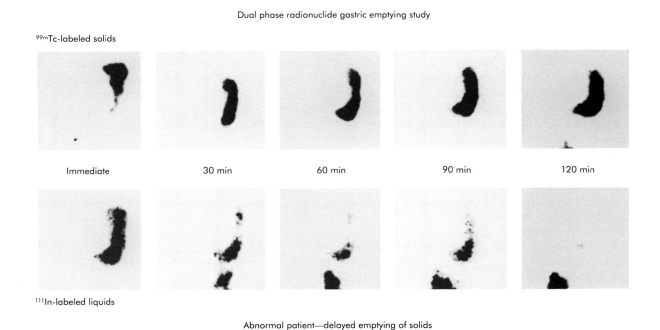

Dual phase radionuclide gastric emptying study

^{99m}Tc-labeled solids

Immediate   30 min   60 min   90 min   120 min

^{111}In-labeled liquids

Abnormal patient—delayed emptying of solids
normal emptying of liquids

Figure 13-23   Abnormal dual isotope gastric scintigraphy. Anterior images of the abdomen were obtained in this patient with delayed emptying of solids and normal emptying of liquids. Compare images with normal individual in Figure 13-19.

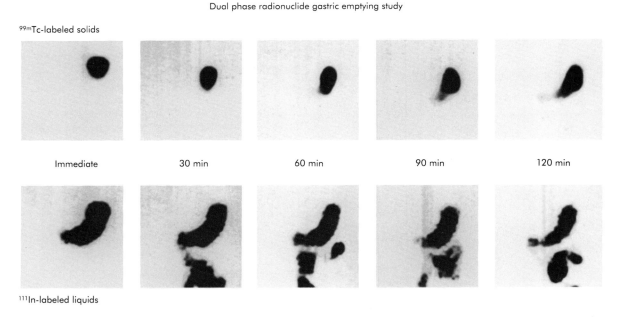

Dual phase radionuclide gastric emptying study

^{99m}Tc-labeled solids

Immediate   30 min   60 min   90 min   120 min

^{111}In-labeled liquids

Abnormal patient—delayed emptying of solids
and delayed emptying of liquids

Figure 13-24   Abnormal dual isotope gastric scintigraphy. Anterior images of abdomen obtained at 30-min intervals reveal delayed emptying of both liquids and solids. Compare with normal individual in Figure 13-19.

may be seen in peptic ulceration, diabetic gastroparesis, scleroderma, amyloidosis, smooth muscle disorders, and following radiotherapy (Figures 13-23 and 13-24). Rapid emptying of solids and liquids may be seen following gastric and duodenal surgery, in Zollinger-Ellison syndrome, duodenal ulcer disease, and in some malabsorption syndromes. A variety of medications also cause rapid gastric emptying.

PANCREAS

The pancreas is an oblong gland, 13 cm in length and 3 cm thick (see Figure 13-1), which lies behind the stomach. Its proximal portion abuts the duodenum, and its more distal portion, the tail, is nestled within the splenic hilum. The pancreas's exocrine function encompasses the excretion of potent digestive enzymes, which are carried into the duodenum through a central duct. The opening of the central duct into the duodenum is the ampulla of Vater.

The pancreas also performs endocrine functions that mediate the digestive process; for example, the pancreas secretes the hormone gastrin into the bloodstream, which inhibits gastric emptying and stimulates gastric production of acid. The pancreas also secretes both insulin and glucagon, which regulate the levels of circulating blood glucose in both the fasting and sated states.

Scintigraphy of the pancreas has been performed using selenomethionine [75]Se. However, the superior ana-

tomic resolution of ultrasound and computed tomography have replaced radionuclide imaging of the pancreas.[2]

LIVER AND SPLEEN

The liver is a solid, lobulated organ located in the right upper quadrant of the abdomen (Figure 13-25) beneath the right side of the diaphragm. In the adult male the liver weighs about 1800 g and is divided into two principal lobes, the right lobe and the left lobe, separated by the falciform ligament. The inferior quadrate and posterior caudate lobes are associated with the right lobe. The configuration of the normal liver varies widely; however, the right lobe is generally larger than the left.

The liver is composed of two major cell populations, the reticuloendothelial cells (Kupffer cells) and hepatocytes. The hepatocytes perform a variety of functions, among them the conversion of bilirubin to bile. The hepatocytes secrete bile into small canaliculi that empty into the intrahepatic ducts, which merge to become the common hepatic duct. The common hepatic duct joins the cystic duct of the gallbladder to form the common bile duct, which drains into the duodenum via the ampulla of Vater (Figure 13-26).

The liver possesses a dual blood supply: arterial oxygenated blood is received from the hepatic artery, which is a branch of the abdominal aorta; venous blood draining from the intestines is carried through the he-

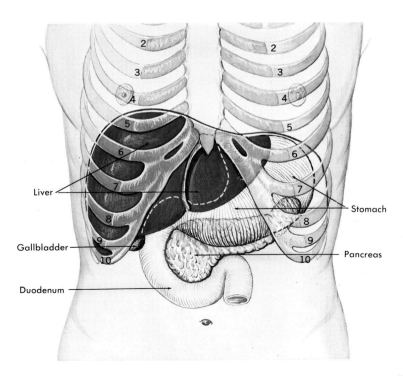

Figure 13-25 Liver in its normal position relative to rib cage, diaphragm, stomach, and pancreas. (From Thibodeau GA: *Anthony's textbook of anatomy and physiology,* ed 13, St. Louis, 1990, Mosby.)

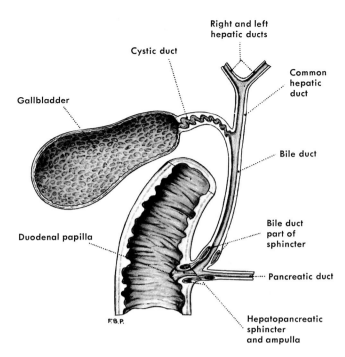

Figure 13-26 Schematic representation of extrahepatic biliary apparatus. (From Hamilton WJ: *Textbook of human anatomy*, ed 2, St. Louis, 1979, Mosby; courtesy The Macmillan Press Ltd, Houndsmill Basingstoke, Hampshire, England.)

patic portal vein into the liver. The hepatic portal system carries nutrients absorbed from the intestines into the liver for processing by hepatocytes.

The spleen is an oval mass of lymphatic tissue located in the left upper quadrant of the abdomen. It is situated between the fundus of the stomach and the left half of the diaphragm. The spleen is part of the reticuloendothelial system but not part of the gastrointestinal system.

Liver and Spleen Scintigraphy

Liver and spleen scintigraphy is the only imaging modality available for the evaluation of functional liver disease, such as cirrhosis, hepatitis, and metabolic disorders. Liver and spleen scintigraphy is also useful for the detection of hepatic lesions for biopsy and for the evaluation of hepatomegaly, jaundice, ascites, and liver enzyme abnormalities of uncertain cause.

The large field of view scintillation camera allows simultaneous imaging of the liver and spleen in most patients. A density of at least 2000 counts/cm^2 should be obtained, which corresponds to approximately 1 million counts/image.

^{99m}Tc sulfur colloid and ^{99m}Tc albumin colloid are the radiopharmaceuticals most commonly used for imaging the liver and spleen. However, this study can be combined with other imaging agents to raise the specificity of detection of certain lesions. Hepatobiliary agents, ^{99m}Tc-labeled red blood cells, and ^{67}Ga-citrate

imaging[22,23] can all be helpful in imaging certain lesions.

Rapid serial perfusion imaging[37] has been found increasingly useful and is performed routinely in some institutions. The flow images can identify the vascular nature of certain defects seen on the standard static image. All reported studies conclude that liver and spleen scintigraphy is a good screening test with a high sensitivity but a relatively poor specificity.[6] The minimum detectable lesion size is 1.5 cm, depending on camera resolution, organ size, and respiratory motion.

Imaging procedure. No patient preparation is needed; however, liver and spleen scintigraphy should be performed before the administration of any iodinated or barium-containing contrast agents. Such agents, if retained within the body, particularly barium within the colon, can result in artifactual defects within the liver or spleen.

The radiopharmaceutical is given as an intravenous bolus with the usual adult dose being 5 to 10 mCi for sulfur colloid and 1 to 8 mCi for albumin colloid.

To perform the perfusion study the patient should be positioned supine under a large field of view scintillation camera fitted with a low-energy parallel-hole collimator. The patient should be positioned with the upper abdomen included in the field of view. The camera formatter or computer should be set for 2- to 3-sec intervals. The radiopharmaceutical should be administered in the right antecubital vein and then the image

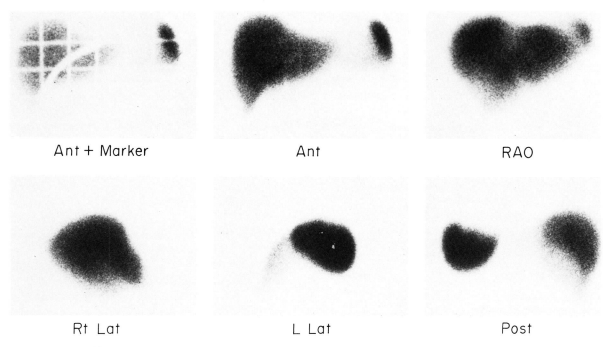

Ant + Marker   Ant   RAO

Rt Lat   L Lat   Post

Figure 13-27 Normal ^{99m}Tc-sulfur-colloid liver and spleen scan demonstrating the size and costal margin marker image as well as the anterior, RAO, right lateral, left lateral, and posterior projections. Size of the lead grid is 5 cm between bars. Note normal distribution of ^{99m}Tc sulfur colloid to the liver (85%) and spleen (10%); remaining 5% is extracted by the bone marrow and is not normally visualized.

acquisition started. Blood flow imaging should continue for at least 1 min, possibly longer, and then an immediate postinjection static image, or blood pool image, should be obtained.

After waiting approximately 15 min, planar static imaging may begin. A waiting period is necessary for the colloid particles to be completely localized within the liver and spleen. Images should be obtained for 2000 counts/cm^2 or 1 million counts total. Usually, images are obtained in the anterior, RAO, LAO, right lateral, LPO, and posterior projections (Figure 13-27). One image should be obtained using a standard size reference marker. This is usually done in the anterior view with the marker placed along the costal margin. Inspiration and expiration breath-holding views of the liver can be obtained for approximately 20 secs. These images can frequently aid in identifying defects produced by compression of the liver by the ribs.[21,28] If a defect moves with the liver, the source most likely is intrinsic disease.

Additional views can be obtained, depending on the clinical problem, or decubitus views may add valuable information.[12,38] The study may be combined with other imaging agents, such as hepatobiliary agents, ^{99m}Tc-labeled red cells, ^{67}Ga citrate,[22,23] or following the oral administration of small amounts of ^{99m}Tc sulfur colloid mixed with water to outline the stomach.

The dosimetry of ^{99m}Tc sulfur colloid and ^{99m}Tc albumin colloid for liver scintigraphy is generally low; the total body dose is 0.02 rad/mCi in each case. The dose to the gonads and liver parenchyma differ for each and are 0.2, 0.006 and 0.4, 0.3 rad/mCi, respectively, for sulfur colloid and albumin colloid.

Clinical aspects. Review of the early perfusion images usually reveals the normal dual blood supply of the liver. Absence of blood flow in these systems may be assessed in the angiographic phase, and the presence of collateral flow may be apparent. Occasionally, perfusion images help in identifying the vascular nature of a focal defect seen on the static imaging, but this has not been shown to be of value in differentiating between benign and malignant lesions. The perfusion study[37] can help identify extrahepatic disease, such as pericardial or pleural effusion. It may also reveal separation of lung and liver by a subdiaphragmatic mass.[32]

A characteristic pattern seen on the perfusion images in inferior vena caval obstruction is the concentration of the ^{99m}Tc colloid within the quadrate lobe of the liver, which is due to collateral circulation.

Planar static images are reviewed for size and shape[14] of the liver and spleen, the relative concentration and distribution of the radiopharmaceutical within these organs, and for the presence of any defects or displacements. A size marker (Figure 13-27) is useful for estimation of liver size.[9] Normally, the longitudinal axis of the right lobe of the liver is about 15 cm, measured from the dome of the right lobe. The size and shape[14] of the liver are particularly important in following the course of diseases by serial studies. The size of the spleen can also be estimated from the images. The maximum length of the spleen in one of the routine views is approximately the same size as the liver, about 14 cm, measured diagonally.

Normally the stomach lies between the spleen and the left lobe of the liver. This may be outlined by giving the patient a small oral dose of ^{99m}Tc sulfur or albumin colloid mixed in water.

Artifacts from other organs and anatomic structures are commonly seen on the liver and spleen images. In females, the breasts may cause a variety of attenuation artifacts that can mimic an intrahepatic lesion. Usually, the crescent pattern of the breast artifact is easily recognizable. Retained barium in the colon, particularly in the hepatic or splenic flexure, can produce image artifacts as well. Generally, artifacts created by overlying structures can be elucidated by obtaining supine and upright views. These demonstrate movement of the "defects." If tomographic imaging is available, the defects are seen to lie outside the liver or spleen parenchyma. Despite the advent of CT[1] and MRI scans, liver and spleen scintigraphy is still useful the in evaluation of congenital hepatic abnormalities; nutritional and metabolic diseases; infectious diseases; primary and secondary malignant neoplasms;[18] benign hepatic cell adenomas and focal nodular hyperplasia; hepatic and splenic trauma; and in the evaluation of functional asplenia, splenomegaly, and splenic variations.

Liver Hemangioma Detection Using ^{99m}Tc-Labeled Red Blood Cells

Liver hemangiomas are probably the most common benign tumor of the liver. Because of their prevalence, they are often discovered during CT or ultrasound examination of the abdomen. Yet the specific criteria for diagnosis of a hemangioma by CT or ultrasound might not always be present in an individual lesion. The radionuclide technique described herein, if performed properly, is virtually 100% accurate in the diagnosis of a hemangioma. Accurate diagnosis is essential because inadvertent biopsy of a hemangioma can lead to significant hemorrhage.

Imaging procedure. No special patient preparation is necessary, although as with any radionuclide liver imaging procedure there should be no retained radiographic contrast agents within the abdomen.

Before initiation of the imaging procedure, the position of the lesion in question within the liver should be ascertained by referring to the initial CT or ultrasound examination. If the lesion is located anteriorly within the right lobe of the liver or within the left lobe of the liver, then the patient is positioned supine for an anterior radionuclide angiogram. If the lesion is located posteriorly within the right lobe, then a posterior flow study is performed. If there are multiple lesions, then the largest lesion should be chosen as the reference. Any non–heat-treated method for labeling the patient's red blood cells can be used, and several of these techniques are outlined in the section on detection of gastrointestinal bleeding. Once the patient has been

Hemangioma detection
[99m]Tc-labeled red blood cells

CT with contrast   Planar image labeled RBCs   SPECT image labeled RBCs

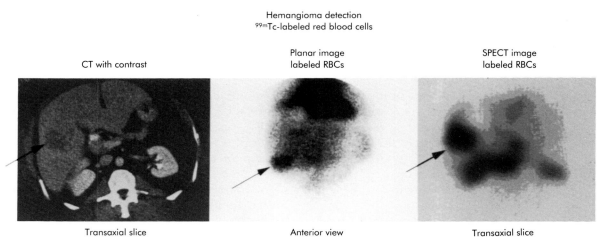

Transaxial slice   Anterior view   Transaxial slice

An ill-defined mass is seen on CT (arrow), which is seen to collect the labeled red-cells on planar and SPECT images obtained at least two hours post-dose (arrows).

Figure 13-28 Example of the use of ^{99m}Tc-labeled red blood cells to detect hepatic hemangioma. Initial image is a transaxial CT slice revealing a space-occupying lesion in the right lobe of the liver (arrow). Planar and SPECT images obtained at least 2 hr following in vivo labeling of the patient's red blood cells show accumulation of the radiolabeled cells within the lesion (arrows), indicating a hemangioma.

positioned for the radionuclide angiogram, the bolus of 15 to 25 mCi of ^{99m}Tc-labeled red blood cells can be given and rapid sequence imaging at 1 to 3 sec/frame can be done to record blood flow through the liver. Next, blood pool images should be obtained, usually in the anterior, right lateral, and posterior projections as a minimum. Steep or shallow oblique views are obtained as necessary, depending on the position of the lesion. These images should be recorded at high-count rates, usually for 500,000 to 1 million counts. At 2 hr after the dose, delayed imaging can begin. This can consist of planar images, which should be obtained in the same projections and for the same time intervals as the initial blood pool images, SPECT imaging of the liver, or a combination of both planar and SPECT imaging. Generally, single large lesions are adequately visualized using the planar technique alone; small lesions (less than 2.5 cm) and multiple lesions require SPECT imaging.[5]

Clinical aspects. The characteristic features of a hemangioma using the above method are (1) little or no blood flow to the lesion on the early angiographic images, although late angiographic images might show early uptake; (2) early accretion of the tagged cells, usually from the periphery of the lesion inward on the blood pool images; and (3) accretion of the tagged cells equal to, but usually greater than, the surrounding liver parenchyma on the delayed planar or SPECT images. Other types of lesions, such as hepatic carcinoma and metastatic disease, can exhibit increased blood flow and early accretion of the radiolabeled cells, but they do not retain the cells for long. Only hemangiomas retain red cells until the 2-hr interval. Adequate time must be allowed for the hemangioma to accumulate a sufficient quantity of the radiolabeled cells to be identified (Figure 13-28).

GALLBLADDER

The gallbladder is a hollow pear-shaped organ about 7 to 10 cm in length (see Figure 13-26). It is located against the visceral surface of the liver, where it occupies a small indentation, the gallbladder fossa. The gallbladder concentrates and stores bile, which it receives from the common hepatic duct through the cystic duct. Following the ingestion of a fatty meal, the gallbladder is stimulated to contract, and it discharges the stored bile into the duodenum. Bile is useful in digestion in the breakdown and emulsification of fats.

Hepatobiliary Imaging

Radiopharmaceutical agents that localize in the hepatobiliary system can be extremely valuable in several clinical situations.[16,17,38] The most commonly used radiopharmaceuticals are ^{99m}Tc-iminodiacetic (IDA) derivatives such as ^{99m}Tc HIDA, ^{99m}Tc DISIDA, and ^{99m}Tc mebrofenin. These agents are superior to ^{131}I rose bengal because ^{99m}Tc-IDA derivatives provide a relatively low-radiation dose to the patient,[39] have a 6-hr half-life, and provide very high-count images.

Cholescintigraphy is a valuable method for investigating patients with upper abdominal pain. Since acute cholecystitis is generally due to cystic duct obstruction, visualization of the gallbladder with the radionuclide tracers virtually excludes the diagnosis of acute cholecystitis. Conversely, lack of gallbladder visualization with these agents carries a high probability of acute cholecystitis. In this way, obstructive causes of clinical jaundice may be differentiated from the hepatocellular causes. In the neonate, suspected biliary atresia can be evaluated with these agents. ^{99m}Tc-IDA derivatives are selectively removed from the blood circulation by hepatocytes, and therefore these agents are specific for liver tissue. This high specificity allows cold defects demonstrated on colloidal liver and spleen scans to be identified as anatomic variants of the biliary anatomy. However, if the defect is not adequately explained by hepatobiliary imaging, other causes, such as benign or malignant mass lesions, must be considered.

The clinical indications for biliary tract imaging are summarized in Box 13-1.

Imaging procedure. To perform the examination, it is preferable to have the patient fast for at least 2 hr before the study; prolonged fast is to be avoided (i.e., greater than 24 hr). Failure to adhere to this guideline may cause nonvisualization of the gallbladder. Pain medications that contain opium or morphine derivatives or their synthetic counterparts should be discontinued from 2 to 6 hr before the study, since these medications can prevent transit of the radiotracer through the biliary system.

Box 13-1	Hepatobiliary imaging: clinical indications

Acute (or chronic) cholecystitis
Calculation of gallbladder ejection fraction
Evaluation of enterogastric reflux (bile reflux)
Evaluation of the biliary system following surgery
Jaundice: Obstructive versus nonobstructive
Pediatrics: biliary atresia versus neonatal hepatitis; presence of choledochal cyst
Evaluation of cold defects seen on radiocolloid liver images

The usual adult dose is 1 to 5 mCi of the ^{99m}Tc IDA given intravenously. Imaging may begin immediately with the patient supine under a large field of view scintillation camera with a low-energy, all-purpose parallel-hole collimator. The patient is positioned so that the liver appears in the upper left corner of the field of view. Sequential images are obtained in the anterior projection for time or total counts (1 million) for at least 1 hr (Figure 13-29). Supplemental views in the anterior oblique or right lateral projection may be useful in separating underlying structures such as the kidneys.

If the gallbladder or biliary ducts fail to visualize by 1 hr, imaging should be continued for up to 4 or more hr, since delayed visualization of the gallbladder and biliary tree can indicate chronic cholecystitis.

The count rate of the liver is constantly changing during the study due to the metabolism and excretion of the radiotracer into the bile ducts. Cameras with good resolution can delineate the path of the biliary ducts and the gallbladder. Supplemental pinhole views may be useful for further evaluation.

Clinical aspects. In the normal individual the radiopharmaceutical begins to concentrate within the liver during the first few min after injection. By 15 to 30 min after injection, most of the radiopharmaceutical has been removed from the bloodstream and is concentrated within the liver. This is followed by concentration of the tracer within the biliary ducts and gallblad-

der (Figure 13-29). The gallbladder is typically well visualized by 45 to 60 min, and radioactivity is identified within the gastrointestinal tract (duodenum and proximal jejunal loops) by 30 min after injection (Figure 13-30).

In acute cholecystitis the liver, common bile duct, and gastrointestinal tract are visualized within 60 min after injection. However, the gallbladder is not visualized at 60 min and if further imaging is obtained, it will still fail to visualize up to 4 hr after injection (Figure 13-31). The lack of visualization of the gallbladder is due to functional or anatomic obstruction of the cystic duct of the gallbladder, which is the basis for acute cholecystitis. In chronic cholecystitis the liver, common bile duct, and gastrointestinal tract may visualize by 60 min; there will usually be delayed visualization of the gallbladder after 60 min, usually between 2 and 4 hr after injection.

The use of pharmacokinetic agents such as cholecystokinin (CCK) analogs[15] and morphine sulfate has been advocated by some practitioners to separate those patients with acute cholecystitis from those with chronic cholecystitis without necessitating imaging to 4 hr. In general, if the administration of either of these agents during a study in which the gallbladder does not visualize by 60 min causes gallbladder visualization to occur, cystic duct obstruction is not present.

Occasionally the liver, common bile duct, and gallbladder visualize within 60 min after injection, but no

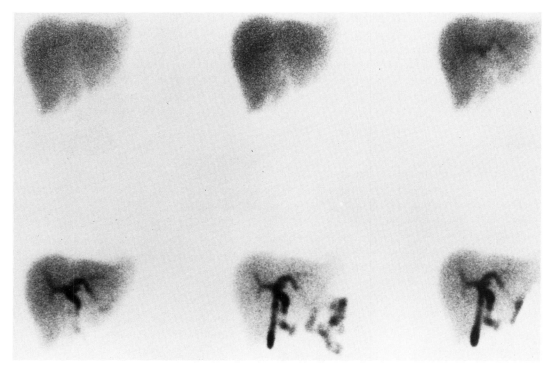

Figure 13-29 Normal hepatobiliary scan. Anterior images of the abdomen obtained at approximately 10-min intervals following intravenous administration of 5 mCi ^{99m}Tc IDA. There is rapid uptake of the radiotracer by the liver, with excretion into the biliary ducts, gallbladder, and small bowel.

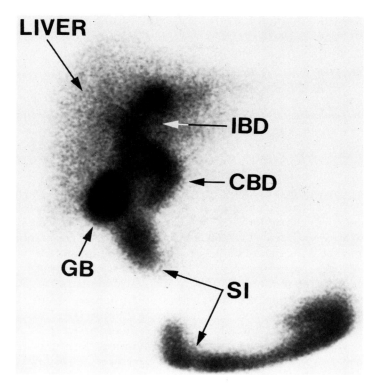

Figure 13-30 Normal hepatobiliary scan. This is a single anterior image of the abdomen obtained at 60 min following intravenous administration of a ^{99m}Tc-IDA compound. There is normal visualization of the gallbladder *(GB)*, intrahepatic biliary duct *(IBD)*, common bile duct *(CBD)*, and small intestine *(SI)*.

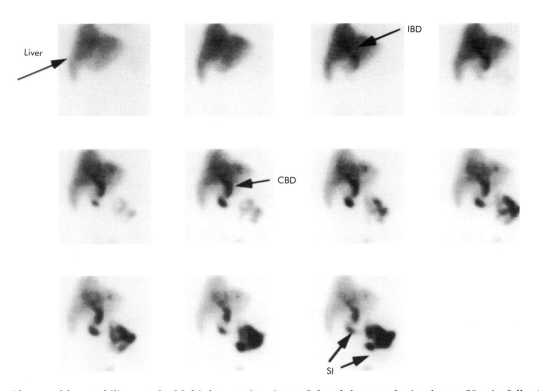

Figure 13-31 Abnormal hepatobiliary study. Multiple anterior views of the abdomen obtained over 60 min following intravenous administration of a ^{99m}Tc-IDA compound. There is normal excretion of the radiotracer through the intrahepatic biliary ducts *(IBD)*, common bile duct *(CBD)*, and small intestine *(SI)*. However, there is no radiotracer localization in the expected area of the gallbladder. Compare with Figure 13-29.

radiotracer is seen within the gastrointestinal tract. In these instances it might be necessary to obtain delayed views of the abdomen up to 24 hr after injection. Absence of excretion of the radiotracer into the gastrointestinal tract is evidence of common bile duct obstruction, either functional or anatomic.

In the evaluation of cold defects seen on ^{99m}Tc-sulfur-colloid liver and spleen scan, the use of a biliary agent can answer the question of whether the cold defect seen on the sulfur colloid liver image is due to normal anatomic structures of the biliary system. This is particularly useful when the defect is in the region of the porta hepatis or to determine whether an apparent lesion is due to an intrahepatic gallbladder.

In pediatric and congenital abnormalities ^{99m}Tc-IDA agents are extremely helpful in the detection of choledochal cysts, biliary atresia, and other congenital abnormalities. The radiation dose to the child is minimal, the study can be performed without sedation or restraints, and there is no danger of morbidity.

A common problem in performing this examination is the presence of profound jaundice in the patient. When serum bilirubin approaches 15 to 20 mg/dl, extraction of the ^{99m}Tc-IDA compounds by the hepatocytes becomes severely reduced. There may be spurious excretion of the radiotracer through the urinary system causing circulating background-level activity to be high. In these instances, delayed images may be useful up to 24 hr.

Hepatobiliary imaging is not a useful method for the detection of gallstones, either within the gallbladder or within the common bile duct. Oral cholecystography, ultrasonic examination, and computed tomography are the methods of choice for the detection of gallstones, although the presence of gallstones alone is not a true indicator of either acute or chronic cholecystitis.

Enterogastric Reflux (Bile Reflux) Imaging

Functional scintigraphy can be employed to detect and quantitate enterogastric reflux with the use of hepatobiliary (^{99m}Tc IDA) agents.[35] Enterogastric scintigraphy will confirm the presence of bile refluxing into the stomach in patients with symptoms of bile reflux gastritis.

Both alkaline gastritis and bile reflux gastritis have been used to describe patients with symptoms of nausea, bile vomiting, abdominal fullness, heartburn, gastric pain, weight loss, and anemia. In severe cases the patient may vomit bile-stained fluid that does not contain food. These patients also have high concentrations of bile acid in fasting gastric aspirates, gastritis or esophagitis, and no peptic ulcerations.

The enterogastric reflux study is particularly useful in individuals who have undergone gastric surgery, where the pyloric sphincter mechanism has been rendered incompetent, removed, or bypassed. Although gastric endoscopy may confirm the presence of bile

within the stomach in these individuals, the scintigraphic study has the advantage of being noninvasive and can also quantitate the amount of refluxed bile.

Imaging procedure. Patients fast overnight, and any medication that might affect gastrointestinal motility is stopped. Although patients can be imaged standing, sitting, or supine, supine imaging is preferred because there is less chance of patient movement, repositioning is easier, and there is minimal overlap of the stomach and small bowel.

To identify the stomach, a dual radiopharmaceutical imaging technique with a radiolabeled test meal is helpful. A 2- to 5-mCi dose of ^{99m}Tc IDA is prepared for intravenous injection, and a fatty meal is prepared by mixing 100 to 250 μCi ^{111}In DTPA with a commercial fatty meal preparation of 250 cc. Any fatty meal preparation may be used, although it is most convenient to use one of the several bottled or canned preparations available on the market, such as Meritene.

Following the intravenous injection of the ^{99m}Tc IDA, patients are immediately positioned under a large field of view camera with a low-energy, all-purpose collimator. Patients are positioned so that the liver appears in the left upper quadrant of the image. Images are recorded for 45 min until there is peak filling of the gallbladder seen on the persistence scope. At this point the patient is then instructed to drink the fatty meal labeled with the ^{111}In DTPA. At this time the liver and biliary tree are identified by imaging the technetium window, and the stomach is identified by imaging the indium window (Figure 13-32). Images are obtained at 15-min intervals for 2 hr at both the technetium and the indium window settings for 1 min each. Between imaging intervals the patient is permitted to assume the upright position, to sit, or stand. At each imaging interval the liver, gallbladder, and biliary tree are identified by the pattern of ^{99m}Tc activity seen before giving the meal (Figure 13-33).

At the conclusion of the study the images are recalled from the computer, and regions of interest are created for the stomach and for the hepatobiliary area. The hepatobiliary area includes the liver, bile ducts, and gallbladder (Figure 13-34). The counts for both the ^{111}In and the ^{99m}Tc are recorded within both regions of interest for time zero (ingestion of the fatty meal) and for each subsequent 15-min interval (Figure 13-35). Corrections must be made for the ^{111}In downscatter into the ^{99m}Tc window, and the technetium counts must be decay corrected.

Enterogastric reflux is defined as the increase in ^{99m}Tc activity in the stomach area of interest divided by the decrease in ^{99m}Tc activity in the hepatobiliary tree, using the following formula:

$$EGRI_t = \frac{(S_t - S_o)}{(HB_o - HB_t)} \times 100$$

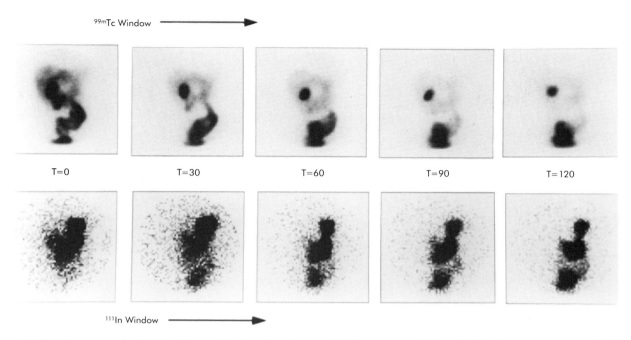

Figure 13-32   Enterogastric (bile) reflux study. Anterior images of abdomen are obtained following intravenous administration of one of the ^{99m}Tc-IDA compounds and following the oral ingestion of a fatty meal containing ^{111}In DTPA. Images are shown for ^{99m}Tc window and ^{111}In window. Presence of ^{99m}Tc tracer in the stomach is evidence for enterogastric reflux.

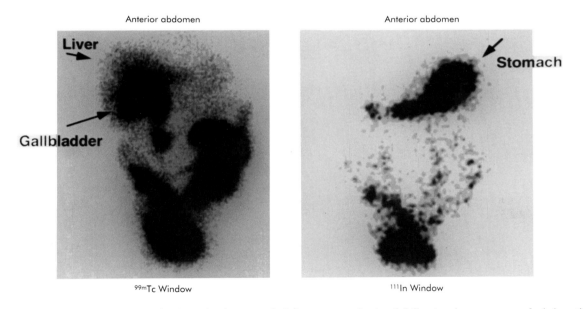

Figure 13-33   Enterogastric reflux study. Anterior images of abdomen are obtained following intravenous administration of one of the ^{99m}Tc-IDA compounds and oral ingestion of a fatty meal labeled with ^{111}In DTPA. Liver, gallbladder, and stomach are seen.

where $EGRI_t$ is the enterogastric reflux index at time t, S_o represents the ^{99m}Tc activity in the stomach at time zero (immediately after ingesting the fatty meal), HB_o represents the activity in the hepatobiliary area of interest immediately following the fatty meal, and S_t and HB_t indicate the activity within the stomach and hepatobiliary area at subsequent time intervals.

Clinical aspects. In the normal individual without previous gastric surgery, one may expect to find very little, if any, of the ^{99m}Tc counts within the stomach, usually less than 15% at 15 to 30 min. In those patients who have undergone previous peptic ulcer surgery, in which a portion of the stomach has been removed and the pyloric sphincter mechanism has either been removed, rendered incompetent, or bypassed, enterogastric re-

Anterior abdomen

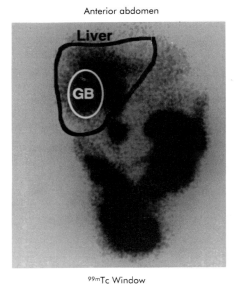

⁹⁹ᵐTc Window

Anterior abdomen

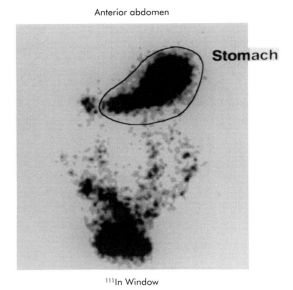

¹¹¹In Window

Figure 13-34 Calculation of enterogastric reflux index. Anterior images of abdomen are recalled from the computer, and regions of interest are created for the stomach, liver, and gallbladder (*GB*). Hepatobiliary area includes liver, bile ducts, and gallbladder. Counts for both the ¹¹¹In and the ⁹⁹ᵐTc are recorded within both regions of interest at each 15-min interval.

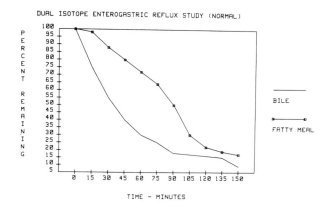

Figure 13-35 Normal dual isotope enterogastric reflux study. Percent normalized remaining ¹¹¹In counts and ⁹⁹ᵐTc counts are graphed as a function of time. There is smooth emptying of the fatty meal from the stomach area with a nearly parallel decrease in the labeled bile.

flux is usually observed, even in asymptomatic patients. In studies with asymptomatic postsurgical patients, one may expect an enterogastric reflux index of approximately 25% at 15 to 30 min. In postsurgical patients with symptoms of nausea, bile vomiting, and abdominal burning, the enterogastric reflux index can be greater than 80% at 15 to 30 min. This study is useful in the postsurgical patient in whom the degree of enterogastric reflux can be used to determine the response to therapy. A trial of medical therapy can be instituted and followed by repeat examination to determine if the degree of enterogastric reflux has decreased.

Several variations in the performance of this particu-

lar examination have been proposed, in particular, the use of cholecystokinin analogs to replace the fatty meal. Furthermore, there are several sources of error inherent in the scintigraphic determination of enterogastric reflux. Each laboratory must establish methods for background-level correction, tissue attenuation, scatter correction, and correction for interference from liver and small bowel overlap. Normal values must be established for each laboratory. Simple visual interpretation of the images can be used to determine if reflux is present (see Figure 13-32).

INTESTINAL TRACT

The small intestine is a lengthy hollow tube extending from the pyloric sphincter of the stomach to the ileocecal valve at the large intestine. The small intestine is divided into the duodenum, the jejunum, and the ileum (see Figure 13-1). It is responsible for digestion and absorption of all nutrients in the body. The inner lining of the small intestine contains glands that secrete intestinal digestive enzymes. The lining is also especially adapted for absorption of all needed nutrients; microvilli cover the entire 20-ft length of the small intestine. These microvilli are also known as the brush border.

The large intestine extends from the ileocecal valve to the anus. The large intestine is divided into the cecum, ascending colon, transverse colon, descending colon, sigmoid colon, and rectum (see Figure 13-1). Very little absorption of nutrients occurs in the large intestine, with the notable exception of some vitamins. The major function of the large intestine is reabsorption of water, which results in the formation of fecal material that is expelled through the anus.

Gastrointestinal Bleeding

Evaluation of gastrointestinal bleeding using radionuclide methods is now a routine procedure in most clinical nuclear medicine facilities.[24] Initial studies using ^{51}Cr-labeled red blood cells demonstrated the feasibility of detecting and localizing sites of gastrointestinal hemorrhage using radiolabeled markers. ^{99m}Tc-labeled agents are now widely used for the detection of gastrointestinal bleeding; however, controversy over the selection of the labeled agent exists. Two groups of agents have been proposed, based on whether they are extracted rapidly or slowly from the intravascular space. Of the rapidly extracted agents, ^{99m}Tc sulfur colloid and ^{99m}Tc-labeled heat-treated red blood cells are commonly used, with the former being preferred because it can be rapidly and simply prepared. Slowly extracted agents include ^{99m}Tc-labeled albumin and non–heat-treated ^{99m}Tc-labeled red blood cells. Non–heat-treated ^{99m}Tc-labeled red blood cells can be labeled using either in vivo or in vitro techniques.

[99m]Tc sulfur colloid has the advantage of minimizing background-level activity and promoting the highest contrast ratios. However, its rapid clearance requires that the patient be actively bleeding at the time of injection (or within minutes following injection). Non–heat-treated ^{99m}Tc-labeled red blood cells, with their prolonged retention in the intravascular pool, are preferred by those investigators who maintain that gastrointestinal bleeding is most often intermittent and slow.

Furthermore, non–heat-treated ^{99m}Tc-labeled blood cells allow repetitive imaging for up to 36 hr after injection with a far lower radiation dose to the liver and spleen and have the ability to better detect gastrointestinal bleeding in the upper abdominal region. The theoretical disadvantage of higher background-level activity with the labeled red blood cells in the heavily vascularized abdominal organs does not appear to be a significant factor in several clinical comparisons.

The methods using the rapidly extracted ^{99m}Tc sulfur colloid and the slowly extracted non–heat-treated ^{99m}Tc-labeled red blood cells follow.

Imaging procedure

[99m]Tc sulfur colloid technique. The patient is placed supine under a large field of view scintillation camera equipped with a low-energy parallel-hole collimator to include the inferior margin of the liver to the symphysis pubis. Seven to 10 mCi of freshly made ^{99m}Tc sulfur colloid are injected as an intravenous bolus, and an anterior flow study of the abdomen is obtained at 1 to 2 sec/frame for 2 to 3 min. Thereafter, 500,000- to 750,000-count anterior images of the abdomen are obtained every 1 to 2 min for 20 to 30 min at intensity settings such that the bone marrow can be visualized.

If an area of bleeding is identified, more detailed views of that area can be obtained with oblique, lateral, or posterior views. If no bleeding site is identified at the end of 30 min, a 1-million-count image of the upper abdomen is obtained with oblique views to better delineate the hepatic and splenic flexures. If these views are negative, repeat lower abdominal views can be obtained in 15 to 20 min to check for activity that may have been obscured in the areas of the hepatic and splenic flexures by liver and spleen activity. Any bowel movements by the patient during the course of the study should be scanned in the bedpan to ensure that a very low rectal source of bleeding has not been obscured by genital activity. If the scan is negative, repeat injections of the tracer may be necessary if there is clinical evidence for renewed active bleeding.

The flow study clearly delineates the aorta and other vascular structures including the liver, spleen, kidneys, and small and large bowel. As the ^{99m}Tc sulfur colloid clears the intravascular space, it accumulates in the liver and spleen and bone marrow and fades from the vascular structures. The genital areas have a significant accumulation of the ^{99m}Tc sulfur colloid, and a lateral view may be helpful to avoid confusion with a possible lower rectal bleeding source. If a fresh preparation of ^{99m}Tc sulfur colloid is used, renal and bladder activity will be minimized, since the amount of free ^{99m}Tc will be less than 2%.

Care should be taken in positioning the patient so that only small margins of the liver and spleen are seen in the images. This brings out any activity within the abdominal cavity.

Non–heat-treated ^{99m}Tc-labeled red blood cell method. ^{99m}Tc-labeled red blood cells provide a long-lived blood pool tracer that can identify areas of upper and lower gastrointestinal bleeding. This method may be able to image bleeding rates of from 0.2 to 0.4 ml/min.

Although there are several methods available for labeling red blood cells with ^{99m}Tc, either the in vitro technique (Brookhaven kit) or a modified in vivo method offers a high degree of labeling efficiency. This minimizes the amount of free ^{99m}Tc that can accumulate in the stomach and ultimately collect in the colon. A modified in vivo method is described below.

Initially, the patient is injected intravenously with 6 to 12 mg of cold stannous pyrophosphate. After a 10 to 20-min wait, the patient is placed supine under a large field of view camera fitted with a low-energy, parallel-hole collimator. The patient is positioned in such a way that xiphisternum is at the top of the field of view and the symphysis pubis is at the bottom. The patient is then given 15 to 25 mCi of ^{99m}Tc pertechnetate as an intravenous bolus (pediatric dose is 240 μCi/kg with a minimum dose of 2 mCi). An immediate flow study of the abdomen is acquired at 1 to 3 sec/frame for the next 2 to 3 min. This is primarily used to identify normal abdominal structures. Following this,

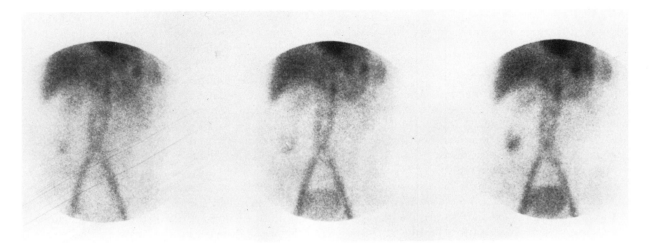

Figure 13-36   99mTc-labeled red blood cell study. Anterior views of abdomen were obtained to visualize an intermittent bleeding site. Images were obtained at approximately 5-min intervals. There is progressive accumulation of the tagged red cells within the right lower quadrant of the abdomen with apparent tracking of these cells within the ascending colon toward the hepatic flexure. Note the normally visualized structures using this method: liver, spleen, abdominal vessels, kidneys, bladder, and stomach.

1-million-count anterior abdominal views are obtained at 1 to 5 min intervals for the next 60 min to include the inferior aspect of the heart to the symphysis pubis. Oblique, lateral, and posterior views can be obtained as necessary. The images can be stored on a computer and displayed in the cine mode to help visualize both normal and abnormal movement of the tracer. If active bleeding is not identified during the first hour, delayed views at 2-, 4-, and 6-hr intervals can be obtained as clinically suggested by changes in vital signs or evidence of recurrent bright red blood per rectum. Delayed views for up to 36 hr after injection can be obtained with good results.

Normally, using this method the vascular structures of the abdomen are well visualized, including the great vessels and the highly vascular kidneys, spleen, bowel, and genital organs (Figure 13-36). It may be necessary to obtain supplemental views with lead shielding placed over certain vascular structures, since the degree of background-level activity can obscure small foci of gastrointestinal bleeding.

Clinical aspects. Using 99mTc sulfur colloid, areas of active bleeding may be seen on the flow study, but they are more commonly identified after the first 5 min. They usually appear as focal areas of increased activity that can become more intense with time as background-level activity decreases. Since blood is both a stimulant and an irritant in the bowel, the activity can pass more quickly through the colon. Retrograde motion that can occur may make localization of the site of bleeding difficult. Both arterial and venous bleeding can be identified from both small and large bowel sources. False-positive studies can occur when there is asymmetric bone marrow accumulation of the tracer, as can be seen with replacement of marrow by tumor, after radiation therapy, or due to other pathologic processes such as Paget disease. Hence the area of involvement has decreased uptake and the more normal-appearing area on the other side of the abdomen can be misinterpreted as an area of bleeding. False-positive studies can also occur in renal transplants, which will accumulate 99mTc sulfur colloid during rejection.

Using the non–heat-treated 99mTc-labeled red blood cell method, the flow study outlines the great vessels of the abdomen as well as the general position of the kidneys, spleen, small and large bowel, and genital organs (particularly in women, where the uterus may be well vascularized). Occasionally, if marked bleeding is occurring, it can be seen on the flow study. Additionally, vascular tumors can be seen as abnormal tracer collections on the arterial phase, which disappear during the venous phase. An abnormal scan demonstrates a focus of tracer activity, which usually becomes more intense with time and is not related to normal abdominal structures (Figure 13-36). Generally speaking, the tagged red cell method can identify colonic bleeding more easily than small bowel bleeding sites. It is important to get frequent images for accurate localization of the bleeding site. If early views are negative and only delayed views show activity within the cecum, it may be difficult to accurately pinpoint the site of bleeding, since bleeding may have occurred in the upper small bowel, right side of the colon, or transverse colon and has merely collected in the cecum. This is especially true if suboptimal red cell labeling has occurred and gastric activity is noted on the initial views. False-positive studies may occur when there are anatomic variants of vascular structures within the abdomen.

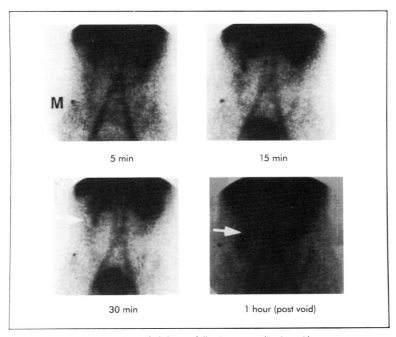

Anterior views of abdomen following premedication with
H-2 blocker and pentagastrin, and 25 mCi ^{99m}Tc pertechnetate I.V.

Figure 13-37 Meckel diverticulum in right side of abdomen. Patient received H$_2$ blockers for 2 days before the study, and 20 min before the examination pentagastrin was given. There is progressive accumulation of the radiotracer within the diverticulum *(arrow)*. M, Marker at right iliac crest.

Meckel Diverticulum

Meckel diverticulum is a common cause of gastrointestinal tract bleeding in children. The acute remnant is a small invagination of the intestine that can contain gastric mucosa. Bleeding is the presenting symptom in almost three fourths of patients, but patients may also present with symptoms of inflammation, obstruction, intussusception, or perforation of the bowel. Most Meckel diverticula are located in the ileum, usually within 1 m from the ileocecal valve. Most patients who present with gastrointestinal bleeding are found to have gastric parietal cells in the Meckel diverticulum. These cells cause peptic ulceration of the bowel by acid secretion.

^{99m}Tc pertechnetate concentrates in gastric mucosa and can be used to detect and localize a symptomatic Meckel diverticulum (Figure 13-37). Details of this procedure may be found in Chapter 18; Meckel diverticulum imaging is most frequently done in children.

Barrett Esophagus

The presence of ectopic gastric mucosa within the distal esophagus is termed *Barrett esophagus*. The scintigraphic detection of this ectopic gastric mucosa within the distal esophagus was proposed because the parietal cells contained in gastric mucosa are known to concentrate ^{99m}Tc pertechnetate. However, scintigraphy can only support the diagnosis of Barrett esophagus; mucosal biopsy is still necessary to confirm it. With the widespread use of fiberoptic endoscopy, the use of this examination has declined. However, it may still be used as an aid in locating a more specific region for biopsy.

Imaging procedure. The patient should fast for 2 hr before the examination. ^{99m}Tc pertechnetate, 5 mCi, is given intravenously. Dental sponges are placed within the oral cavity to prevent the patient from swallowing pertechnetate excreted in the saliva and to avoid confusing the origin of esophageal activity. The patient is then placed in a sitting position with the anterior chest against a large field of view camera with a parallel-hole collimator. Images are then acquired for 5-min intervals for the next 30 min.

Prior administration of atropine or atropine-like compounds, or the administration of potassium perchlorate is to be avoided. These agents are known to decrease uptake of pertechnetate ions by gastric mucosa.

Clinical aspects. Normally, activity is visualized only within the stomach and salivary glands. The presence of pertechnetate activity above the level of the diaphragm suggests the presence of ectopic gastric mucosa in the distal esophagus. The presence of Barrett esophagus is associated with dyspepsia, esophagitis, and upper gastrointestinal bleeding.

Gastric mucosal imaging has also been used for preoperative diagnosis of pulmonary and mediastinal enterogenous cysts containing gastric mucosa.

BREATH TESTING WITH ^{14}C-LABELED COMPOUNDS

Breath testing is used to diagnose bacterial overgrowth and carbohydrate malabsorption. Breath testing also shows potential in evaluating sucrose-isomaltose malabsorption, fat malabsorption, and liver function.

Gas, produced in the bowel lumen by various acid-base or metabolic reactions, diffuses to some degree into the body circulation and is excreted by respiration into the breath. Of the five principal colonic gases (carbon dioxide, hydrogen, methane, nitrogen, and oxygen), carbon dioxide and hydrogen are the two most important for breath analysis.

The isotopic carbon dioxide breath tests[33] use ^{14}C-labeled substrates, which are given orally. Labeled carbon dioxide is then excreted in the breath as a result of carbon dioxide production from absorption and breakdown of ^{14}C-labeled material.

^{14}C carbon dioxide can be measured directly by passing the expired breath through plastic filament detectors or by liquid scintillation counting of specimens in which ^{14}C carbon dioxide breath is trapped as labeled carbonic acid by a known amount of alkali such as hyamine hydroxide.

Liver Function Analysis

Measurement of ^{14}C-labeled carbon dioxide following either oral or intravenous administration of ^{14}C-labeled aminopyrine provides an estimate of hepatic mixed oxidase function.[3,20] The radiolabeled aminopyrine breath test has the clinically useful potential for differentiating patients with the cholestatic form of chronic active hepatitis from those with primary biliary cirrhosis. The correct categorization of such patients is not easily accomplished by other means, and simple blood tests do not measure actual liver function. Therefore the aminopyrine test has important therapeutic implications.

Xylose Breath Test

The most sensitive and specific breath test for bacterial overgrowth of the small intestine uses 1 g of ^{14}C-labeled D-xylose. This test has greater than 95% sensitivity and specificity for detecting abnormal proliferation of the small bowel microflora.

Breath excretion of labeled carbon dioxide is measured from 30 to 60 min after the patient drinks a solution containing 1 g of xylose with 5 to 10 μCi of ^{14}C-labeled D-xylose mixed in 500 ml of water. Rapid results make this test clinically practical and ensure that analysis occurs during the period when the test solution is still only in the small intestine. In the rare patient with extremely slow gastric emptying, it may be necessary to make a delayed analysis at 180 min to ensure bacterial content with the test substrate.

The ^{14}C-labeled D-xylose breath test is even more sensitive than a single jejunal culture. The breath test integrates the findings over a long segment of the small intestine, whereas a single culture can only be made from one site, which may not reflect the true state of the surrounding flora.

^{14}C-Labeled Bile Acid Test

This breath test was the first developed for detecting abnormal contact of intestinal bacteria with substrate. It relies on deconjugation of ^{14}C-labeled cholylglycine by anaerobic bacteria, which produces ^{14}C carbon dioxide from the labeled glycine.

Since conjugated bile salts are absorbed in the distal rather than the proximal small bowel, even normal subjects display substantial contact of the labeled substrate with their colonic flora. This contamination creates a background of labeled carbon dioxide, produced by colonic flora, against which small intestine bacterial-labeled carbon dioxide must be measured.

The ^{14}C-labeled bile acid test used concomitantly with another test to rule out bacterial overgrowth may be useful for detecting bile acid malabsorption. This condition, which can lead to vexing diarrhea, is often difficult to diagnose.

Fat Absorption Test

One of the earliest reported uses of the labeled carbon dioxide breath test was breath analysis following oral administration of fat labeled with isotopic carbon.[30] Despite earlier encouraging reports, simple carbon dioxide testing does not adequately distinguish those with moderate fat malabsorption from normal subjects. The steps between ingestion of labeled fat and excretion of labeled carbon dioxide are much more complicated than those encountered with other labeled carbon dioxide breath tests. Hence, the clinical use of these tests remains elusive.

REFERENCES

1. Alfidi RJ, Haaga J, Meaney TF, et al: Computed tomography of the thorax and abdomen: a preliminary report, *Radiology* 117:257, 1975.

2. Barkin J, Vining D, Miale AJ Jr, et al: Computerized tomography, diagnostic ultrasound and radionuclide scanning: comparison of efficacy in diagnosis of pancreatic carcinoma, *JAMA* 238(19):2040, 1977.

3. Bircher J, Kupfer A, Gikalov I, et al: Aminopyrine demethylation measured by breath analysis in cirrhosis, *Clin Pharmacol Therapeut* 20:484, 1976.

4. Blue PW, Jacison JH: Stimulated salivary clearance of technetium-99m pertechnetate, *J Nucl Med* 26:308, 1985.

5. Brodsky RI, Friedman AC, Maurer AH, et al: Hepatic cavernous hemangioma: diagnosis with ^{99m}Tc-labeled red cells and single-photon emission computed tomography, *Am J Roentgenol* 148:125-129, 1987.

6. Bryan PJ, Dunn WM, Grossman ZD: Correlation of computerized tomography, gray scale ultrasonography and radionuclide imaging of the liver in detecting space-occupying processes, *Radiology* 124:387, 1977.

7. Castell DO: The lower esophageal sphincter: physiologic and clinical aspects, *Ann Intern Med* 83:390, 1975.

8. Chaudhuri TK, Heading RC, Greenwald A, et al: Measurement of gastric emptying (GET) of solid meal using ^{99m}Tc DTPA, *J Nucl Med* 15:483, 1974.

9. Christian PE, Coleman RE, Harris CC: An accessory for estimating organ size from gamma camera images, *J Nucl Med Technol* 8:211, 1980.

10. Christian PE, Datz FL, Sorenson JA, et al: Technical factors in gastric emptying studies, *J Nucl Med* 24:264, 1983.

11. Cooperman AM, Cook SA: Gastric emptying-physiology and measurements, *Surg Clin North Am* 56(6):1277, 1976.

12. Crandell DC, Boyd M, Wennemark JR, et al: Liver-spleen scanning: the left lateral decubitus position is best for lateral views, *J Nucl Med* 13:720, 1972.

13. Datz FL: The role of radionuclide studies in esophageal disease, *J Nucl Med* 25:1040, 1984.

14. DeNardo GL, Stadalnik RC, DeNardo SJ, et al: Hepatic scintiangiographic patterns, *Radiology* 111:135, 1974.

15. Freeman LM, Sugarman LA, Weissman HS: Role of cholecystokinetic agents in ^{99m}Tc IDA cholescintigraphy, *Semin Nucl Med* 11:186, 1981.

16. Fonseca C, Greenberg D, Rosenthall L, et al: Assessment of the utility of gallbladder imaging with ^{99m}Tc-IDA, *Clin Nucl Med* 3:437, 1978.

17. Fonseca C, Rosenthall L, Greenberg D, et al: Differential diagnosis of jaundice by ^{99m}Tc-IDA hepatobiliary imaging, *Clin Nucl Med* 4:135, 1979.

18. Garcia AC, Yeh SDJ, Benua RS: Accumulation of bone-seeking radionuclides in liver metastasis from colon carcinoma, *Clin Nucl Med* 2:265, 1977.

19. Heading RC, Tothill P, Laidlaw AJ, et al: An evaluation of [113m]indium DTPA chelate in the measurement of gastric emptying by scintiscanning, *Gut* 12:611, 1975.

20. Hepner GW, Vesell ES: Quantitative assessment of hepatic function by breath analysis after oral administration of (^{14}C) aminopyrine, *Ann Intern Med* 83:632, 1975.

21. Kranzler JK, Vollert JM, Harper PV, et al: The diagnostic value of hepatic pliability as assessed from inspiration and expiration views on the gamma camera, *Radiology* 97:323, 1976.

22. Kumar B, Coleman RE, Alderson PO: Gallium citrate Ga-67 imaging in patients with suspected inflammatory processes, *Arch Surg* 110:1237, 1975.

23. Lomas F, Dibos PE, Wagner HN Jr: Increased specificity of liver scanning with the use of [67]gallium citrate, *N Engl J Med* 286:1323, 1972.

24. Lull RJ, Morris GL: Scintigraphic detection of gastrointestinal hemorrhage: current status, *J Nucl Med Technol* 14:79, 1986.

25. Malmud LS, Fisher RS: Quantitation of gastroesophageal reflux before and after therapy using the gastroesophageal scintiscan, *South Med J* 71(suppl 1):10, 1978.

26. Malmud LS, Fisher RS, Knight LC, et al: Scintigraphic evaluation of gastric emptying, *Semin Nucl Med* 12:116, 1982.

27. Meyer JH, MacGregor IL, Gueller R, et al: ^{99m}Tc-tagged chicken liver as a marker of solid food in the human stomach, *Am J Dig Dis* 21:296, 1976.

28. Oppenheimer BE, Hoffer PB, Gottschalk A: The use of inspiration-expiration scintiphotographs to determine the intrinsic or extrinsic nature of liver defects, *J Nucl Med* 13(7):554, 1972.

29. Pope CE II: Pathophysiology and diagnosis of reflux esophagitis, *Gastroenterology* 70:445, 1976.

30. Ruttin JM, Shingelton WW, Baylin GJ, et al: [131]I labeled fat in the study of intestinal absorption, *N Engl J Med* 225:594, 1956.

31. Schmitt G, Lehmann G, Strotges W, et al: The diagnostic value of sialography and scintigraphy in salivary gland diseases, *Br J Radiol* 49:326, 1976.

32. Selby JB: Radiological examination of subphrenic disease process, *CRC Crit Rev Diagn Imaging* 9(3):229, 1977.

33. Shreeve WW: Labeled carbon breath analysis. In Rocha AFG, Harbert JC, eds: *Textbook of nuclear medicine: basic science,* Philadelphia, 1978, Lea & Febiger.

34. Siegel JA, Wu RK, Knight LC, et al: Radiation dose estimates for oral agents used in upper gastrointestinal disease, *J Nucl Med* 24:835, 1983.

35. Tolin RD, Malmud LS, Stelzer F, et al: Entero-gastric reflux in normal subjects and patients with Bilroth II gastroenterostomy, *Gastroenterology* 77:1027, 1979.

36. van Dam APM: The gamma camera in clinical evaluation of gastric emptying, *Radiology* 110:155, 1974.

37. Waxman AD, Apaw R, Siemsen JK: Rapid sequential liver imaging, *J Nucl Med* 13:522, 1972.

38. Wistow BW, Subramanian G, Van Heertum RL, et al: An evaluation of ^{99m}Tc-labeled hepatobiliary agents, *J Nucl Med* 18:455, 1977.

39. Wu RK, Siegel JA, Rattner Z, et al: Tc-99m HIDA dosimetry in patients with various hepatic disorders, *J Nucl Med* 25:905, 1984.

SUGGESTED READINGS

Maurer AH, guest ed: Gastrointestinal nuclear imaging. I. Functional studies. Freeman LM, Blaufox MD, eds, *Sem Nucl Med* 25:4, 1995.

Maurer AH, guest ed: Gastrointestinal nuclear imaging. II. Freeman LM, Blaufox MD, eds, *Sem Nucl Med* 26:1, 1996.

Henry D. Royal

chapter *14*

Genitourinary System

Objectives

Describe the anatomy and physiology of the genitourinary system.

List the radiopharmaceuticals used for renal studies and discuss their characteristics.

Describe the excretion methods for renal radiopharmaceuticals.

List common renal nuclear medicine studies and their indications.

Describe the performance of functional renal study.

Discuss the procedure for diuretic renal scintigraphy.

Describe the procedure for performing renal scintigraphy with ACEI augmentation.

Describe the performance of scintigraphy for morphologic renal imaging.

Discuss the anatomy, physiology, and indications for testicular scintigraphy.

Define ERPF and GFR and describe methods to obtain these measurements.

ANATOMY

The top of the kidneys is usually located just underneath the lowest ribs in the back (Figure 14-1), spanning the distance from about the twelfth thoracic vertebra to the third lumbar vertebra. In the adult the kidneys measure about 11 to 12 cm (long axis) and are 5 to 7.5 cm wide and 2 to 3 cm thick.[10] Because of the displacement of the liver, the right kidney is usually slightly lower than the left kidney.

Determining the size of the kidney by planar scintigraphy is less accurate than determining the size of the kidney by ultrasound. With planar scintigraphy, the size of the kidney may appear smaller than the actual size if the long axis is not parallel with the surface of the crystal of the gamma camera. This artifact is called *foreshortening* (Figure 14-2).

Normally the kidneys are at about equal depths from the skin of the back, but in some patients the depth of each kidney may be unequal. When the kidneys are at unequal depths, measurements of the relative activity in each of the kidneys will be inaccurate due to the fact that there is greater attenuation of the radiation coming from the deeper kidney. As a result the relative function of the deeper kidney is underestimated. When a kidney study is obtained in the intensive care unit, imaging must be performed by placing the patient in a lateral decubitus or prone position. Either of these positions may exaggerate the asymmetric depth of the kidneys, since one kidney may fall forward more than the other. It is sometimes tempting to perform a mobile study in the anterior view. Anterior images of normally positioned kidneys are rarely satisfactory.

Sometimes the bottoms of the two kidneys are joined. This congenital abnormality of the kidneys is called a *horseshoe kidney* (Figure 14-3).

Because the spine attenuates the activity coming from the thin band of tissue connecting the lower poles of the kidneys, this congenital abnormality may be missed if only posterior views are obtained. An anterior view will often clearly show the band of functioning tissue that connects the lower poles of the kidneys. Another clue to the presence of a horseshoe kidney is the orientation of the kidneys. The lower end of horseshoe kidneys are closer together than normal kidneys. Another disease that can grossly distort the anatomy of the kidney is polycystic kidney disease. Patients with this inherited disease have multiple large cysts in their kidneys and liver (Figure 14-4). These cysts increase in size as the patient ages, often resulting in renal failure.

Occasionally a kidney may be in an unusual location. Sometimes a kidney will be located in the pelvis, particularly if the patient is sitting or standing. When the patient is imaged in the supine position, the kidney may return to a more normal position. When a mobile kidney is in an abnormal position, it is termed *ptotic*. Transplanted kidneys are most often placed in the anterior pelvis. Before beginning a kidney study, the technologist should inquire whether it is likely that the patient's kidneys are in an unusual location to make certain that the camera is optimally positioned.

The urine produced by the kidneys is excreted into the renal pelvis and then transported to the bladder through the ureters (Figure 14-5). When the renal pelvis and ureters are dilated, it is called *hydronephrosis*, which can occur when there is an obstruction of the collecting system or can simply be due to a dilated but nonobstructed collecting system. The bladder is a distensible bag that stores urine until it is eliminated through the urethra. Sometimes a patient's bladder is

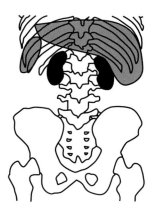

Figure 14-1 Location of kidneys on the posterior view. The right kidney is normally slightly lower than the left kidney because it is displaced by the liver. The background activity for the right kidney is usually higher than the left because of activity that accumulates in the liver. Blood flow to the spleen can be misinterpreted as blood flow to the left kidney, especially when the blood flow to the left kidney is reduced.

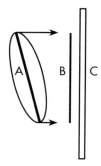

Figure 14-2 Foreshortening. The true length of the long axis of the kidney, *A*, will be underestimated, *B*, when the long axis of the kidney is not parallel to the plane of the NaI crystal, *C*.

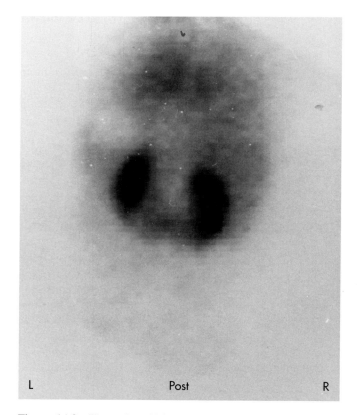

Figure 14-3 Horseshoe kidney. Posterior image of the kidneys of a 10-mo-old baby girl acquired 0 to 2 min after the injection of ^{99m}Tc MAG3. The child had bilateral hydronephrosis by ultrasound. Hydronephrosis is frequently seen with horseshoe kidneys because the connecting band of tissue compresses the ureters. The decreased activity noted superior and lateral to the left kidney is caused by a full stomach. This decrease in activity is often seen in infants after feeding.

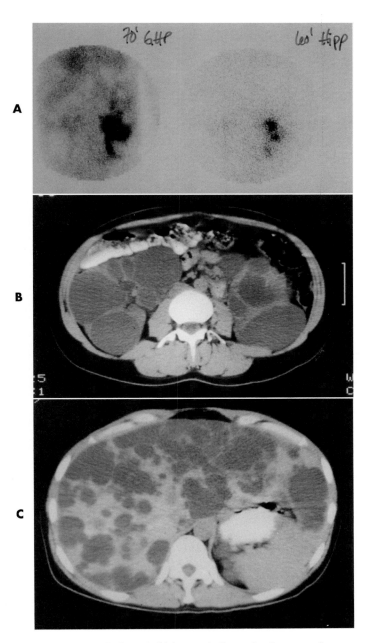

Figure 14-4 Polycystic kidneys. **A.** Posterior images of the kidneys obtained 70 min after the injection of ^{99m}Tc glucoheptonate *(left)* and 60 min after the injection of ^{131}I hippuran *(right)*. Both images are very abnormal in this patient with polycystic kidney disease and renal failure. The function of the left kidney is considerably worse than the right kidney. The areas of decreased activity seen on the glucoheptonate images are due to the renal cysts. Despite the poor renal function, most of the hippuran is in the collecting system at 60 min. The glucoheptonate is cleared from the rest of the body more slowly than hippuran and is retained in the renal parenchyma. **B.** CT scan of the kidneys showing nearly complete replacement of the renal tissue by cysts. **C.** CT scan of the liver showing extensive cystic disease of the liver. Patients with polycystic kidney disease often have cysts in their liver.

removed to treat bladder cancer. A new "bladder" called an *ileal loop* can be made from a portion of the small bowel (ilium) (Figure 14-6). Barium in the rectum can cause an artifact that overlies the bladder (Figure 14-7). The scrotum is a skin pouch that is suspended from the lower pelvis and contains the testes, epididymis and vas deferens. The testes produce spermatozoa and the hormone testosterone. The epididymis is a tortuous tubular structure where spermatozoa mature, are stored, and then transported. The vas deferens is contiguous to the epididymis and is the excretory duct of the testes.

The blood flow to and from the kidney usually is through a single artery and vein that subsequently divides into interlobar arteries. These arteries subdivide until they form the afferent arteriole to a web of capillaries called a glomeruli. The blood leaves the glomerulus through the efferent arteriole, which then courses deep into the medulla, forming the peritubular capillaries and the vasa recta.

PHYSIOLOGY

The kidney has several major functions including the excretion of waste products, reabsorption of important body constituents, maintenance of acid-base balance, and maintenance of fluid balance. To accomplish these functions, the kidney requires a large blood flow. Approximately 20% to 25% of the cardiac output goes to normally functioning kidneys. Since the resting cardiac output is 5 L/min, total renal blood flow is about 1.2 L/min (Table 14-1). Since plasma constitutes about 50% of the total blood volume, the effective renal plasma flow (ERPF) is about 600 ml/min. When the plasma and red cells pass by the glomerulus, approximately 20% of the plasma passes through the glomerulus into the renal tubules, resulting in a glomerular filtration rate (GFR) of 120 ml/min. Most of the filtrate is reabsorbed. The proportion of plasma that reaches the kidney and filtered by the glomerulus is called the *filtration fraction*. Normally, the filtration fraction is equal to about 20% (GFR/ERPF).

Only 1000 to 1500 ml of urine are produced each day. Over 170 liters of urine per day would be produced

Table 14-1	
Cardiac output	5 L/min
Renal blood flow	1.2 L/min
Effective renal plasma flow	600 mL/min
Glomerular filtration rate	125 mL/min
Filtration fraction	25%

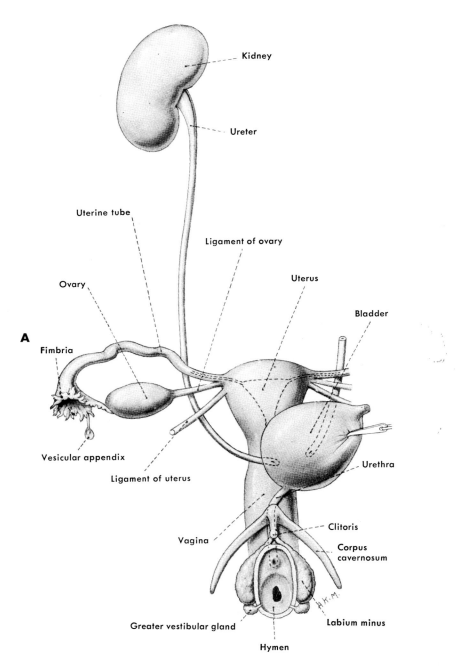

Kidney

Ureter

Uterine tube

Ligament of ovary

Ovary

Uterus

Bladder

A

Fimbria

Vesicular appendix

Ligament of uterus

Urethra

Vagina

Clitoris

Corpus cavernosum

Greater vestibular gland

Labium minus

Hymen

Figure 14-5   Schematic representation of urogenital organs in the female (**A**) and male (**B**).

if none of the plasma that was filtered through the glomerulus was reabsorbed by the tubular cells. On average, the body only contains about 42 liters of water, therefore tubular cell dysfunction that prevents reabsorption of the filtrate would rapidly cause death from dehydration. Fortunately when tubular dysfunction occurs, a number of reflex mechanisms cause a dramatic decrease in renal blood flow and glomerular filtration. Although these compensatory mechanisms have significant long-term adverse effects, rapid death from acute dehydration is prevented.

The basic functional unit of the kidney is called a *nephron* (Figure 14-8). There are millions of nephrons in a normally functioning kidney. The nephron consists of an afferent arteriole that delivers blood to a web of capillaries (vascular tuft) in the glomerulus. The blood leaves the glomerulus through the efferent arteriole. Between the afferent and efferent arterioles is an important hormone-producing mass of cells called the *juxtaglomerular apparatus.*

The porous surface of the glomerulus permits filtration of water and solutes into Bowman's capsule (Figure

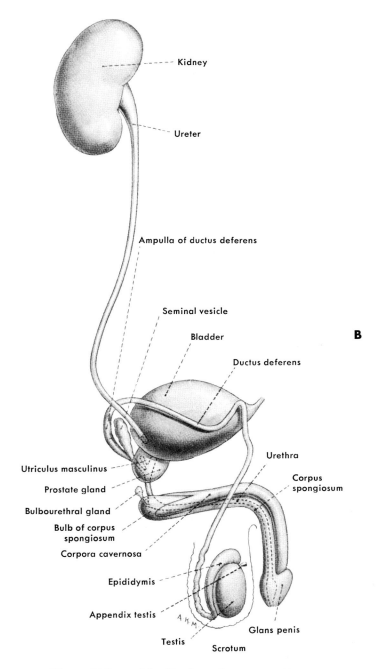

Kidney

Ureter

Ampulla of ductus deferens

Seminal vesicle

Bladder

Ductus deferens

B

Utriculus masculinus

Prostate gland

Bulbourethral gland

Bulb of corpus spongiosum

Corpora cavernosa

Epididymis

Appendix testis

Urethra

Corpus spongiosum

Glans penis

Testis

Scrotum

Figure 14-5, cont'd.   For legend, see opposite page.

14-9). The major factor that determines whether a substance will be filtered is its molecular size. Substances with a molecular size of less than 150,000 daltons are freely filterable if they are not protein bound. The filtration is a passive process whose rate is primarily determined by the perfusion pressure. The large volume of filtrate (125 mL/min) is transported to the proximal and distal renal tubules. Over 99% of the filtrate is selectively reabsorbed by the tubular cells. The nephron is oriented with the glomerulus in the cortex of the kidney, whereas the tubules are primarily in the medulla.

The kidney produces a number of important hormones. The physiology of the renin-angiotensin system is important for understanding renovascular hypertension. When renal artery stenosis is present, the perfusion pressure decreases (Figure 14-10). This decrease in perfusion pressure results in a decrease in pressure in the afferent renal arteriole and thus a decrease in filtration pressure and in glomerular filtration rate. For-

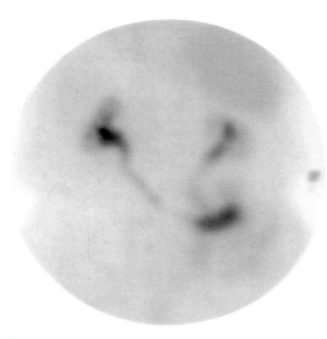

Figure 14-6   Ileal bladder. This patient's bladder has been removed. Excreted activity collects in an artificial bladder that has been created using a section of ilium. The ileal bladder usually drains into a collecting bag.

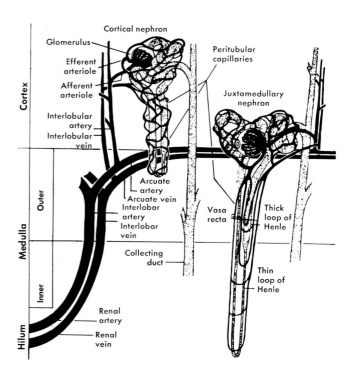

Figure 14-8   Schematic representation of nephron, circulation, and respective location in the kidney.

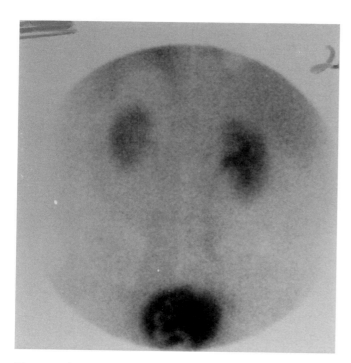

Figure 14-7   Barium in the rectum. The serpiginous area of apparent decreased activity overlying the bladder is due to barium in the rectum.

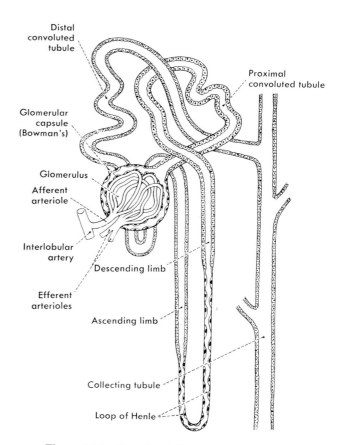

Figure 14-9   Simplified diagram of nephron.

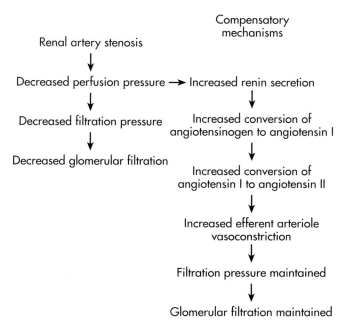

Figure 14-10 Renovascular hypertension.

Box 14-1	Characteristics of ERPF/GFR agents

1. ERPF Completely removed from plasma during its passage through the kidney (high first-pass extraction)
   GFR Freely filterable by the glomerulus
2. Not protein bound
3. Not metabolized
4. No significant excretion by other organs

tunately, the kidney has an important reflex mechanism to maintain the glomerular filtration pressure even in the presence of renal artery stenosis. The decrease in perfusion pressure in the afferent renal arteriole is a potent stimulus to the release of renin from the juxtaglomerular apparatus. Renin converts angiotensinogen to angiotensin I, which is subsequently converted to angiotensin II by the angiotensin converting enzyme (ACE). Angiotensin II causes vasoconstriction of the efferent glomerular arteriole, thus helping to preserve filtration pressure and GFR. In addition, angiotensin II causes increased aldosterone secretion, which in turn causes increased sodium reabsorption by the tubular cells. The increased salt retention increases systemic blood pressure. The increased blood pressure helps to preserve the perfusion/filtration pressure of the kidney.

When a patient with renal artery stenosis is given an ACE inhibitor, the conversion of angiotensin I to angiotensin II is blocked and the compensatory mechanisms are lost. The loss of the efferent glomerular arteriolar vasoconstriction results in a decreased filtration pressure and a subsequent decrease in GFR. ACE inhibitor decreases the vascular resistance of the abnormal kidney, therefore the blood flow to the kidney is maintained or may increase despite the decrease in GFR. For this reason when an ACE inhibitor is given, the initial uptake of a blood flow agent such as ^{99m}Tc MAG3 may be preserved even though the initial uptake of a GFR agent such as ^{99m}Tc DTPA may be markedly decreased. For both agents there is prolonged retention of the radiopharmaceutical due to the decrease in GFR.

RADIOPHARMACEUTICALS

Conceptually, it is best to divide renal radiopharmaceuticals into two categories: functional and morphologic agents (Table 14-2).[7,28] Functional radiopharmaceuticals are rapidly taken up and excreted by the kidneys by a single, simple physiologic mechanism such as ERPF or GFR. Morphologic tracers are also rapidly taken up by the kidney but by more complicated mechanisms that usually involve a complex interaction of ERPF, GFR, tubular secretion, and tubular resorption. The hallmark of a morphologic tracer is that some of the tracer is retained in the renal parenchyma for a prolonged period. Prolonged retention of the tracer in the kidney makes relatively high-resolution imaging of the renal parenchyma possible, even several hours after the injection of the tracer.

Functional agents (Table 14-2) include ^{131}I hippuran, ^{99m}Tc MAG3,[28] and ^{99m}Tc DTPA. ^{131}I hippuran is used infrequently because a high-energy collimator is required and the amount of ^{131}I hippuran administered is limited to 100 μCi due to the high radiation dose to the patient. The small amount of administered activity and use of a high-resolution collimator compromise the quality of the images that can be obtained. ^{123}I hippuran has better imaging characteristics but is not readily available due to the short (13 hour) half-life of ^{123}I. Currently, ^{123}I hippuran is not available in the United States.

Hippuran is the classic agent that has been used to measure effective renal plasma flow. The ideal characteristics of an agent to measure ERPF or GFR are listed in Box 14-1. Hippuran fulfills these requirements because there is a high first-pass extraction of this agent as it passes through the kidney. A high first-pass extraction means that almost all of the agent that is delivered to the kidney remains in the kidney. For hippuran the ratio of activity in the renal vein to the activity in the renal artery is about 0.15 because about 85% of the activity is retained in the kidney. The most accurate blood flow agent is microspheres because they have the highest first-pass extraction (~100%). The high first-pass

Table 14-2

Functional radiopharmaceuticals	Comments
[131]I hippuran	Effective renal plasma flow agent; paraaminohippuric acid analog
	High first-pass extraction
	Freely filtered; near total tubular secretion; no tubular reabsorption
	High target to background even with poor renal function
	[131]I has poor imaging characteristics and gives a relatively high radiation dose to the patient
	^{123}I-labeled hippuran has much better imaging characteristics and gives a relatively low radiation dose to the patient; however, it is expensive and not readily available due to its short (13 hr) half-life
[99m]Tc DTPA (diethylenetriamine pentaacetic acid)	Glomerular filtration agent; inulin analog
	Freely filtered; no tubular secretion; no tubular reabsorption
	Readily available
	Very good imaging characteristics; low radiation dose to the patient
[99m]Tc MAG3 (mercaptoacetyl-triglycerine)	"Effective renal plasma flow agent"; biokinetics are different from hippuran
	High first-pass extraction
	Freely filtered; near total tubular secretion; no tubular reabsorption
	High target to background even with poor renal function
	Very good imaging characteristics; low radiation dose to the patient
	Recently introduced; likely to replace all other renal radiopharmaceuticals for most applications

Morphologic radiopharmaceuticals	Comments
[99m]Tc DMSA (dimercaptosuccinic acid)	Hepatobiliary excretion with poor renal function can interfere with delayed imaging of the renal parenchyma
	Physiologic mechanisms for uptake; excretion and retention are complex
	66% of the dose is excreted; 34% is retained by the renal cortex at 6 hr after injection
[99m]Tc glucoheptonate	Physiologic mechanisms for uptake; excretion and retention are complex
	>90% of the dose is excreted; 6% to 10% is retained by the renal cortex

extraction of hippuran is due to the fact that hippuran is efficiently secreted by the renal tubule cells and is not reabsorbed from the tubular lumen.

[99m]Tc MAG3 has largely replaced hippuran as a functional agent.[28] Like hippuran, MAG3 has a high first-pass extraction fraction. Unlike hippuran, MAG3 is taken up by red blood cells, so its plasma clearance is even more rapid than is the plasma clearance of hippuran. [99m]Tc MAG3 is preferred over hippuran because of its superior imaging characteristics.

[99m]Tc DTPA is cleared from the plasma almost exclusively by glomerular filtration by the kidney. Several other radiopharmaceuticals (e.g., ^{125}I iothalamate) possess the characteristics needed to measure GFR,[16] but optimal imaging is only possible with ^{99m}Tc DTPA.

[99m]Tc DMSA and ^{99m}Tc glucoheptonate are considered morphologic imaging agents (see Table 14-2) because accumulation within the kidney is the result of a complex interaction of blood flow, GFR, tubular secretion, and tubular reabsorption. Approximately

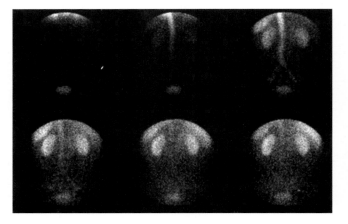

Figure 14-11 Radionuclide flow study of the kidneys. A flow study of the kidneys is obtained as the tracer is being injected. These images have been added on the computer so that each image contains 10 sec of data. Activity is initially seen in the descending aorta, then in the kidneys and in the spleen. Notice that the activity in the liver does not appear until well after the activity in the spleen. This is because most of the hepatic blood flow is from the portal circulation.

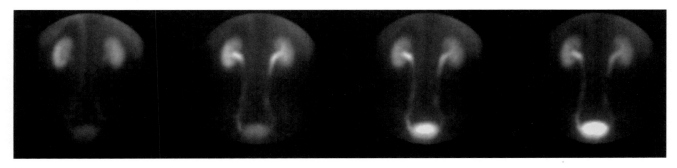

Figure 14-12 Evaluation of renal parenchyma with ^{99m}Tc MAG3. Relatively high-quality images of the renal parenchyma can be obtained using MAG3. Images from the dynamic study have been added so that each image contains 5 min of data. The evaluation of the renal parenchyma is not compromised by collecting-system activity on the earliest images.

30% of DMSA is retained in the renal parenchyma compared with 5% to 10% of glucoheptonate.

Although the choice of radiopharmaceuticals for renal imaging is quite arbitrary, there are a few major factors that guide selection. A technetium labeled agent is required to obtain a flow study (Figure 14-11). To evaluate the renal collecting system for obstruction, an agent that is rapidly excreted into the collecting system is best. To optimally visualize the renal parenchyma, an agent that is retained in the renal parenchyma is preferred.

Before the introduction of ^{99m}Tc MAG3 in 1989, different radiopharmaceuticals and different combinations thereof were chosen for different indications. Since the introduction of MAG3, our institution has used this radiopharmaceutical for most indications. With this functional radiopharmaceutical, it is even possible to evaluate the morphology of the renal parenchyma because very good images of the kidney (Figure 14-12) can be obtained within the first few minutes after the injection of the tracer.

RADIONUCLIDE PROCEDURES

Practical Considerations

To maximize the clinically relevant information obtained from radionuclide renal imaging, the reasons for doing the study must be ascertained before the study is started. Major indications for radionuclide imaging are listed in Box 14-2. Pertinent clinical information includes the number and size of the kidneys, the results of other imaging tests, the patient's creatinine level, the patient's current medication, and any specific instructions regarding the physiologic conditions under which the test is to be performed.

Common physiologic variables include the state of hydration and the position of the patient. Normally patients are hydrated by giving them 2 to 3 8-oz glasses of water by mouth. Renal imaging is usually performed in the supine position, except for diuretic renal imaging, which is performed in the upright position. Less com-

Box 14-2	Indications for radionuclide renal scintigraphy

Relative renal function
Renal transplant evaluation
Acute renal failure
Obstructive uropathy
Renovascular hypertension
Infection and inflammation
Vesicoureteral reflux

mon but potentially important physiologic variables include whether various draining tubes (e.g., Foley catheters, nephrostomy tubes, and wound drains) should be clamped.

In general, no patient preparation is necessary. A number of drugs can significantly affect the function of the kidney or directly interfere with the uptake of the radiopharmaceuticals.[17] If a renal arteriogram is performed a few days before the radionuclide renal study, an inaccurate impression of renal function (absolute and relative) may be obtained due to transient contrast-induced acute tubular necrosis (ATN). Drugs that block tubular secretion (probenecid) may interfere with the uptake of certain tracers despite normal renal function.

Technologists should reassure patients about the safety of the examination. Reactions to iodinated hippuran are extremely rare even in patients with a history of iodine contrast hypersensitivity. These agents are extremely safe because such small quantities are injected. The amount of iodine in labeled hippuran is about one billionth of the iodine injected with iodinated contrast. Patients often express concern about having a radioactive material injected into their bodies. The radiation dose is similar to the radiation dose from contrast intravenous urography.[25] The overall risk of the radionuclide examination is much less than the risk from urography due to the extreme rarity of hypersensitivity reactions with radionuclides.

Common Procedures

Functional renal imaging. Functional renal imaging using ^{99m}Tc MAG3 or ^{99m}Tc DTPA is the most common radionuclide renal imaging study performed at most medical centers. Common indications for performing this study include (1) measurement of relative renal function, (2) renal transplant evaluation, and (3) the evaluation of acute renal failure.[27]

A typical protocol for acquiring functional renal imaging consists of a rapid sequence of blood flow images (e.g., one 64 × 64 image/2 to 3 sec for 1 min) followed by a sequence of functional images obtained at a slower rate (e.g., one 128 × 128 image/20 to 30 secs for 19 min). Functional renal imaging can be used to determine both absolute and relative renal function. Most medical centers do not measure absolute renal function (ERPF or GFR) because the most accurate methods are time consuming and cumbersome, requiring several timed blood samples.[20] Measurements of absolute renal function based on imaging alone are done infrequently because, in most clinical settings, serum creatinine is a satisfactory indicator of absolute renal function. Much more useful is the ability of radionuclide renal imaging to provide an index of relative individual kidney function. A major factor in the decision to treat or remove a diseased kidney is how much the diseased kidney contributes to total renal function.

Little effort is usually expended to repair a kidney that contributes less than 10% of total renal function.

Relative renal function is calculated using an early (1 to 3 min or 2 to 3 min postinjection) image of the kidneys. The relative renal function is calculated by dividing the background corrected kidney counts by the sum of the background corrected counts from both kidneys. An early image is used because the radiopharmaceutical is primarily in the parenchyma (functioning tissue) of the kidney at this time. In later images the radiopharmaceutical may be retained in the collecting system. The collecting system activity does not correspond to relative renal function. To measure relative renal function, whole kidney regions of interest are drawn. Partial kidney regions of interests (in an attempt to avoid collecting system activity) would be unsatisfactory.

The time-activity curve (renogram) (Figure 14-13, *A*) from a normal hippuran or MAG3 study shows prompt uptake of the tracer with the activity in the kidney peaking at 3 to 5 min after the injection and decreasing to less than 50% of its peak value by 20 min. Abnormal curves can either be obtained due to abnormal renal function, retention of activity in the collecting system, or patient movement. The cause for an abnormal curve can usually be easily determined from visual inspection of the images with careful attention to the fate of activity seen in the peripheral parenchyma of the kidney. A carefully drawn crescent-shaped region of interest that excludes the collecting system may be helpful.

There are several caveats regarding the determina-

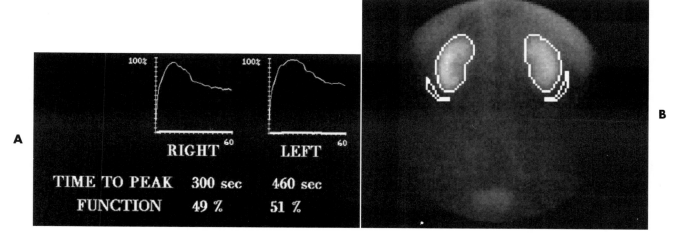

Figure 14-13 A, Renogram. The background corrected activity versus time curve from the kidney regions of interests is called the renogram. The renograms from the right and left kidneys are shown. The renogram only represents the function of the kidney when there is no significant retained activity in the collecting system. Retained activity in a dilated collecting system can give the false impression of decreased renal function. To avoid this error, the images as well as the curves need to be examined. **B,** Relative renal function. The percent of renal function that is contributed by each kidney is calculated by drawing a region of interest around each kidney. In addition, a background region of interest is drawn for each kidney. The contribution of each kidney to total renal function is calculated by dividing the background corrected counts for each kidney at 1 to 3 (or 2 to 3) min postinjection by the background corrected counts at 1 to 3 (or 2 to 3) min from both kidneys. The results are usually expressed as a percentage.

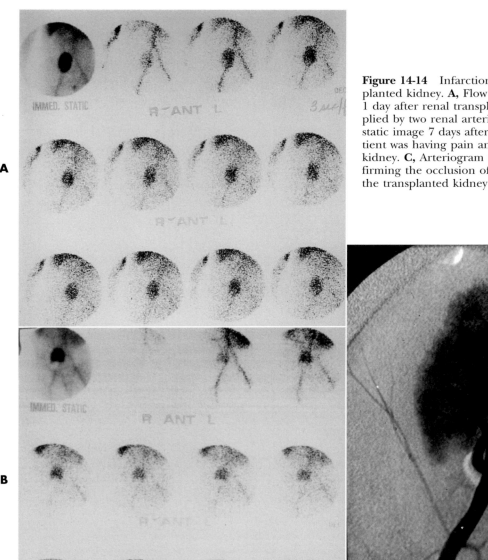

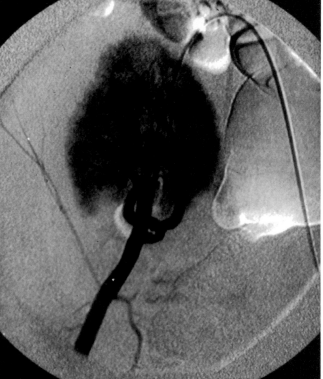

Figure 14-14 Infarction of the lower pole of a transplanted kidney. **A,** Flow study and immediate static image 1 day after renal transplant. The donor kidney was supplied by two renal arteries. **B,** Flow study and immediate static image 7 days after renal transplant when the patient was having pain and swelling of the transplanted kidney. **C,** Arteriogram of the transplanted kidney confirming the occlusion of the artery to the lower pole of the transplanted kidney.

tion of relative renal function. First, the calculation of relative renal function requires estimates of the number of counts in each kidney as well as the number of counts in a background region of interest (Figure 14-13, *B*).[12] Normally, this calculation is quite robust; however, as renal function deteriorates, the number of counts in the background region of interest increases and becomes much more important in the calculation. Under these circumstances (high background), choice of the background region of interest can significantly change the measured contribution of the diseased kidney, therefore a subjective estimate of the relative function may be just as accurate. Unfortunately, no universally accepted standards have been adopted for defining re-

gions of interests. A second source of error for the measurement of relative renal function is attenuation. Some of the radiation coming from the kidneys is absorbed by the soft tissue between the kidney and the gamma camera. If there is a significant difference in the depths of each kidney, the contribution of the deeper kidney will be underestimated. Finally, under some conditions (e.g., acute urinary obstruction, especially in young children) the loss of renal function may be reversible.

The role of functional renal imaging in the routine postoperative management of renal transplant patients is controversial. Routine postoperative radionuclide imaging is not performed at most medical centers because unexpected surgical complications from renal trans-

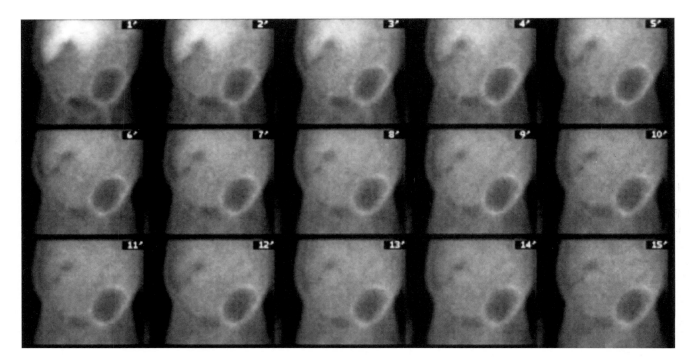

Figure 14-15 Infarction of a transplanted kidney; 20-min dynamic study (1 min per image) following the injection of ^{99m}Tc MAG3 reveals decreased activity and no function of the renal transplant.

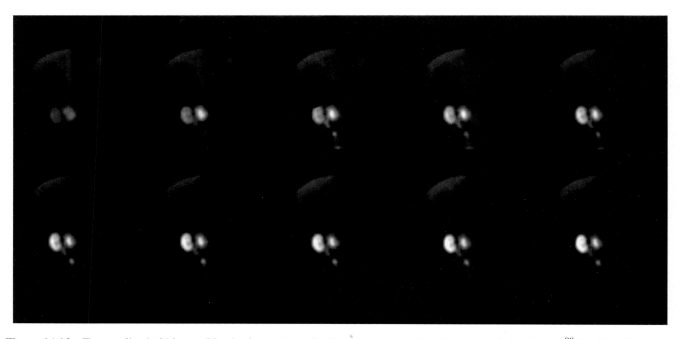

Figure 14-16 Two pediatric kidneys; 20-min dynamic study (2 min per image) following the injection of ^{99m}Tc MAG3 in an adult patient who received both kidneys from a child donor. The kidney at the iliac bifurcation is functioning normally; the other kidney has prolonged retention of activity consistent with ATN, probably due to a longer ischemic time.

plantation are rare. In selected patients, radionuclide imaging can be useful to identify urine leaks, obstruction of the urinary collecting system, and renal infarctions (Figures 14-14, 14-15, and 14-16). Differentiation of acute tubular necrosis, rejection, and cyclosporine toxicity with radionuclide imaging is imperfect.[6]

Treatable causes of acute renal failure include hypo-volemia, infection, urinary collecting-system obstruction and acute vascular obstruction. Radionuclide renal imaging is most helpful in excluding acute vascular obstruction as the etiology of acute renal failure. Acute vascular obstruction is a rare cause of acute renal failure.

Another potential use for radionuclide renal imaging in patients with acute renal failure is prognosis. Patients

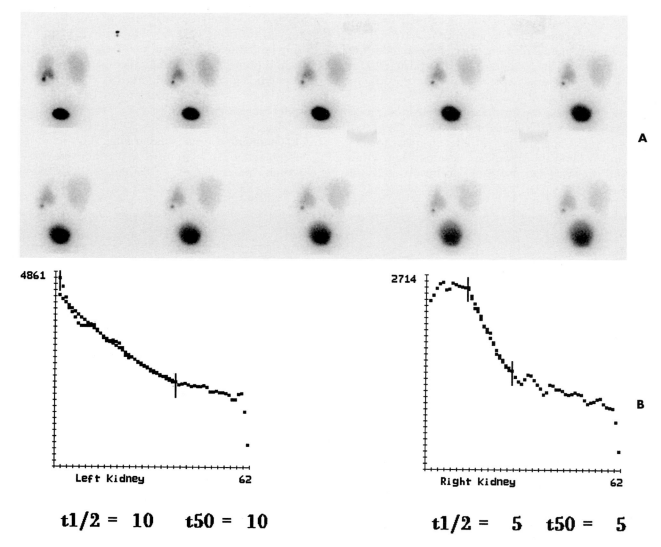

$$t1/2 = 10 \quad t50 = 10 \qquad t1/2 = 5 \quad t50 = 5$$

Figure 14-17 Diuretic renal study. **A,** 20-min dynamic study (2 min per image) following the injection of Lasix reveals normal washout of the radiopharmaceutical from the dilated but unobstructed left renal collecting system. **B,** Renogram reveals that both kidneys have a normal ($t_{1/2} \leq 10$ min) response to Lasix.

with little or no detectable renal activity on radionuclide renal imaging with hippuran (and presumably with ^{99m}Tc MAG3) are unlikely to recover significant renal function.[24] Determining the likelihood of recovery of renal function is helpful in deciding whether an arteriovenous shunt should be placed for future hemodialysis.

Diuretic renal imaging. The standard method used to differentiate a dilated renal collecting system from an obstructed renal collecting system is called the Whitaker test.[30] This invasive test requires the placement of an infusion catheter percutaneously into the collecting system proximal to the suspected point of obstruction. Saline is then infused at high, nonphysiologic flow rates ($\sim$25 mL/min) while the pressure in the proximal collecting system is monitored. If there is no significant increase in pressure, there is no urodynamically significant obstruction. Because it is invasive, the

Whitaker test cannot be used to routinely follow patients for urinary tract obstruction. In addition, some question the significance of increased pressure at high, nonphysiologic flow rates.

Diuretic renal imaging is particularly useful to differentiate a dilated renal collecting system from an obstructed renal collecting system (Figure 14-17, *A*).[2,3] Many dilated but unobstructed collecting systems will empty spontaneously during routine radionuclide renal imaging. If collecting-system activity persists on a sitting postvoid image of the kidneys obtained 20 min after the injection of the radiopharmaceutical, the intravenous injection of furosemide (Lasix) (e.g., 0.5 mg/kg) is very useful. Following the injection of furosemide, an additional 20 to 30 min of functional images are obtained. If a urodynamically significant outflow obstruction is present, the affected kidney is unable to significantly increase its urine flow rate in response to the furosemide injection. Because urine flow rate does not increase, the washout of the activity from the collecting system is prolonged (clearance half-time greater than 20 min). A dilated but unobstructed kidney is able to increase its urine flow rate in response to furosemide, therefore the washout of activity from the collecting system is in the normal range (clearance half-time less than 10 min) (Figure 14-17, *B*).

Diuretic renal imaging has a high sensitivity for detecting urodynamically significant lesions when compared with the Whitaker test. False-positive results and equivocal interpretation may arise when (1) a diseased kidney is not responsive to furosemide injection (such as very immature function in neonates, severe dehydration, and poor baseline renal function); (2) the collecting system is grossly dilated; and (3) vesicoureteral reflux or fully distended bladder (such as neurogenic bladder) is present.

ACEI augmented renal scintigraphy. The relationship between renal artery stenosis (RAS) and renovascular hypertension is complex.[4,22] Patients with hypertension

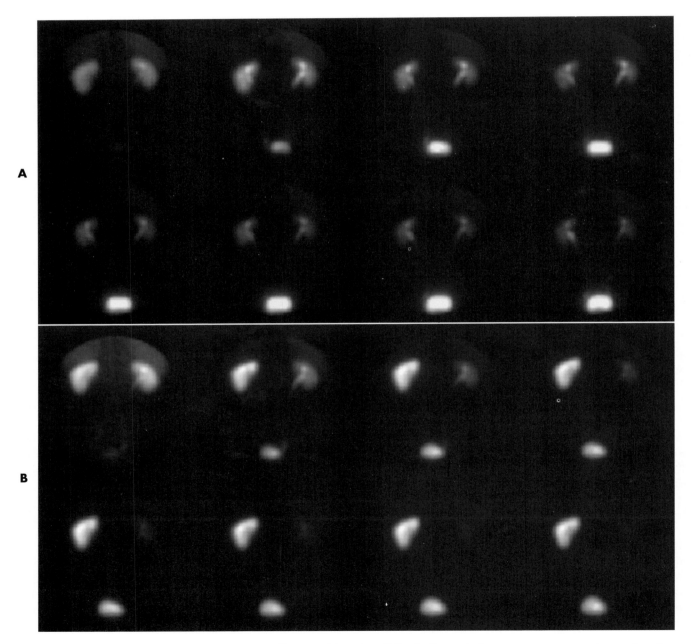

Figure 14-18 Renovascular hypertension. **A,** Baseline renal imaging (2.5 min/image) shows prompt symmetric uptake of ^{99m}Tc MAG3. There is a small amount of retained activity in the renal collecting system bilaterally. There is little retained activity in the renal parenchyma. **B,** Renal imaging (2.5 min/image) following the administration of an ACE inhibitor shows prompt uptake of activity in both kidneys. There is marked prolonged retention of activity in the left kidney. The patient had left renal artery stenosis.

may be classified into three groups: (1) those with hypertension and no significant RAS, (2) those with hypertension with RAS as a major contributor of the hypertension, and (3) those with hypertension with RAS as an insignificant contributor of the hypertension. Renal imaging with and without ACE inhibitor is intended to identify patients with renovascular hypertension.[1]

The physiology of renovascular hypertension has been reviewed. If an ACE inhibitor is given, less efferent arteriolar constriction occurs, the glomerular filtration pressure decreases, and the GFR declines. The ACE dependent change in renal function can be detected using radionuclide imaging with and without an ACE inhibitor (Figure 14-18).

A number of different parameters can be used to document the change in renal function. These parameters include a decrease in renal uptake, prolongation of renal parenchymal transit, a decrease in the relative function of the affected kidney, and an increase in the time to peak activity.[21] Different investigators have used different parameters and combinations of parameters to detect renovascular disease. Recent studies have documented the accuracy of this test in predicting normalization of blood pressure after revascularization.[5,9,11,15,18,29]

Morphologic renal imaging. Morphologic renal imaging following the injection of ^{99m}Tc glucoheptonate or ^{99m}Tc DMSA can be used to document global and regional changes in function in patients with pyelonephritis. In patients with acute pyelonephritis, areas of decreased function may improve with appropriate treatment. In children with vesicoureteral reflux and a history of urinary tract infections, the decision to repair the ureters may be influenced by the presence or absence of persistent renal cortical defects by radionuclide imaging.[14,19,23,24]

This study may also be used to detect the presence or absence of small renal infarctions. These infarctions may occur in patients at increased risk for systemic emboli, such as patients with atrial fibrillation or a left ventricular aneurysm. Infarctions that can occur as the result of a complicated renal procedure such as percuta-

neous angioplasty of a stenotic renal artery can also be detected with renal imaging.

Vesicoureteral reflux study. A conventional contrast-voiding cystourethrogram is the initial investigation of choice in selected children with urinary tract infections. The anatomic information provided by this study is far superior to the functional information provided by the radionuclide vesicoureteral reflux (VUR) study. Because of its lower radiation dose, radionuclide VUR studies are preferred for follow-up when the primary concern is the severity and presence or absence of reflux rather than anatomy.[8,26] Radionuclide cystography can be performed by catheterizing the patient and directly instilling the radionuclide into the bladder (Figure 14-19) or by injecting the patient with the tracer and allowing the bladder to fill with the tracer as it is excreted from the kidneys. Direct catheterization has a higher sensitivity and specificity than the indirect method and is the preferred method for radionuclide cystography. The clinical importance of reflux in children is its association with chronic pyelonephritic scarring and subsequent increased risk of hypertension in later years.

TESTICULAR IMAGING

Anatomy and Physiology

The testicles develop within the abdomen and they descend to their normal position in the scrotum at about the time of birth. During their descent, the testicles are draped with a fold of parietal peritoneum called the *tunica vaginalis* (Figure 14-20). Normally the tunica

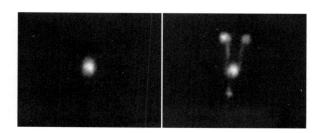

Figure 14-19 VUR. Two images from the first 2 min of a VUR are shown. Activity is initially seen only in the bladder *(left)*. There is prompt, severe reflux of activity to the level of both renal collecting systems.

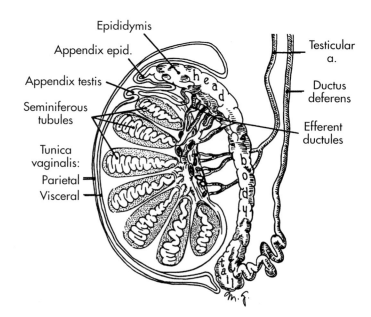

Figure 14-20 Testicular anatomy. (From Henkin RE, Boles MA, Dillehay GL et al: *Nuclear medicine*, St. Louis, 1996, Mosby.)

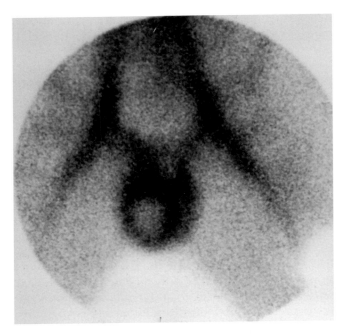

Figure 14-21 Delayed torsion. Testicular scintigraphy revealing a central area of decreased activity with a surrounding area of increased activity. The increased activity is due to inflammation that occurs after the testicle becomes nonviable.

vaginalis covers only the anterolateral surface of the testicle. The blood supply enters the posterior aspect of the testicle and prevents the testicle from rotating in the scrotum. A common variant of this normal anatomy is for the tunica vaginalis to more fully envelop the testicle. The blood supply that would normally enter posteriorly now enters superiorly and no longer tethers the testicle, keeping it from rotating. This common variant is called the *"bell clapper" deformity*, and this variant is always present in cases of acute testicular torsion. Since the "bell clapper" deformity is usually bilateral, corrective surgery on the unaffected testicle is indicated when testicular torsion has been diagnosed.

Torsion is most common in children ranging from 10 to 19 years of age. Usually there is the sudden onset of testicular pain. Since the torsed testicle will only remain viable for several hours, it is imperative to suspect the diagnosis and to operate on the patient quickly. Some testicles will no longer be salvageable after 4 hr of torsion. None will be salvageable after 12 to 24 hr of torsion. When testicular torsion lasts for more than 24 hr (delayed torsion), the testicle becomes necrotic and an inflammatory reaction occurs (Figure 14-21). Occasionally, testicular torsion can be intermittent and the patient can have recurrent episodes of pain. Because acute testicular torsion is a surgical emergency, surgery should not be delayed. Patients who are suspected of having acute torsion should be sent directly to the OR. Testicular scintigraphy should be reserved for patients who are unlikely to have acute testicular torsion.

Other diseases that can cause testicular pain include epididymo-orchitis, tumor, torsion of the appendix testis, trauma, and abscess. Usually these causes of testicular pain can be differentiated from acute torsion by the patient's history and physical exam.

Testicular Scintigraphy

Testicular scintigraphy consists of a flow study and immediate static images.[13] ^{99m}Tc pertechnetate is the most commonly used radiopharmaceutical. The penis of the supine patient should be taped over the pubis. A tape sling should be used to support the testicles between the thighs. Cephalic angulation of the camera can help separate the activity from the thighs and pelvis from the activity from the testicles. Lead shielding can be used on the immediate static images but may make interpretation of the flow study more confusing. When lead shielding is used on the immediate static images, it must be carefully placed to shield both testicles symmetrically.

The blood flow study is primarily used to detect asymmetric blood flow. It is usually impossible to distinguish low testicular blood flow from normal testicular blood flow. The main purpose of the flow study is to detect areas of increased blood flow that would be seen with diseases such as epididymo-orchitis, delayed torsion, tumor, trauma and abscess. Acute torsion will likely have normal-appearing blood flow images. In acute torsion, the immediate static images will reveal a central area of decreased activity with normal surrounding activity. A central area of decreased activity can also be seen with a hydrocele (fluid in the space formed by the tunica vaginalis). Hydroceles are usually painless and can be identified by transillumination on physical examination. Abscesses, necrotic tumors, hematomas, and delayed torsion usually have a central decreased activity surrounded by an area of increased activity due to the surrounding inflammatory reaction.

MEASUREMENT OF EFFECTIVE RENAL PLASMA FLOW AND GLOMERULAR FILTRATION RATE

How well the kidneys clear a substance from the plasma can be measured using two fundamentally different approaches. The first approach is called the UV/P (UV divided by P) method (Table 14-3). This method requires (1) measurement of the plasma concentration of the substance (P in mg/mL), (2) the rate of urine production (V in mL/min), and (3) the concentration of the substance in the urine (U in mg/mL). The units of clearance are mL/min. Conceptually, clearance is how much plasma is completely cleared of the substance (mL) per unit time (min).

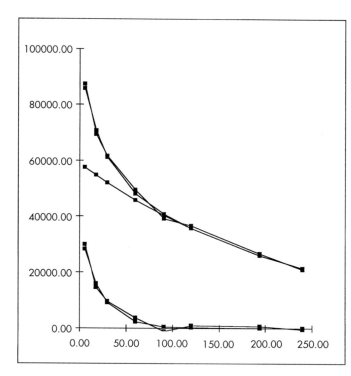

Figure 14-22 GFR plasma clearance curve. Plasma clearance curve following the intravenous injection of ^{99m}Tc DTPA. The x axis is in min and the y axis is counts/ml. The GFR is calculated by fitting a monoexponential to the slow (the last 4 points) component of the plasma clearance curve. The fitted curve is then subtracted from the original data. A monoexponential curve is then fitted to the first four points of the resulting curve (the curve on the bottom of the graph). The GFR can then be calculated based on the results of the two fitted monoexponential equations.

Table 14-3	UV/P method

U (urine concentration) = 4000 cpm/mL
V (timed urine collection) = 60 ml urine produced/20 min
P (plasma concentration) = 100 cpm/mL

$$GFR = \frac{UV}{P} = \frac{60 \text{ mL} * 4000 \text{ cpm} * 1 \text{ mL}}{20 \text{ min} * 1 \text{ mL} * 100 \text{ cpm}}$$

$$= \frac{240,000 \text{ mL}}{2000 \text{ min}} = 120 \text{ mL/min}$$

The UV/P method suffers from two major limitations. First, the method works best if there is a steady plasma concentration of the substance of interest. In practice this requires that the patient be given a constant infusion of the substance over a period of a few hours. Second, although the plasma and urine concentrations of the substance are readily measured, accurate measurement of urine production requires timed, complete urine collections. Hydration (to increase urine

production) and bladder catheterization are needed to increase the reliability of the method.

A second way to determine how well the kidneys clear a substance from the plasma is to measure the plasma disappearance curve. This method only produces reliable results when the kidneys are the only significant pathway for excretion. This important requirement is only adequately met by a few radiopharmaceuticals. Typically the plasma clearance curve is modeled as two compartments (Figure 14-22). The first compartment is the intravascular compartment (plasma), and the second compartment is the extravascular compartment. Initially, the concentration of the tracer in the plasma is very high. The initial rapid clearance (often called the fast component) of the tracer from the plasma is primarily due to diffusion into the extravascular compartment. During this time a small amount of tracer is also cleared from the intravascular space by kidney excretion. Once the tracer reaches equilibrium in the two compartments, any decrease in activity in the intravascular compartment is due to kidney excretion alone. Mathematically, the clearance curve that results from this model consists of the sum of two monoexponential equations. The plasma clearance curve method does not require the urine collections that are needed for the UV/P method. The method is still laborious because at least eight blood samples collected over a 4-hr period are needed to accurately estimate the biexponential clearance of the tracer. Methods using only one to two blood samples have been described.[20]

REFERENCES

1. Black HR: Captopril renal scintigraphy—a way to distinguish functional from anatomic renal artery stenosis, *J Nucl Med* 33:2045-2046, 1992.
2. Conway JC: The principles and technical aspects of diuresis renography, *J Nucl Med Tech* 4:208-214, 1989.
3. Conway JJ, Maizels M: The "well tempered" diuretic renogram: a standard method to examine the asymptomatic neonate with hydronephrosis or hydroureteronephrosis. A report from combined meetings of the Society for Fetal Urology and members of the Pediatric Nuclear Medicine Council—the Society of Nuclear Medicine, *J Nucl Med* 33(11):2047-2051, 1992.
4. Davidson RA, Wilcox CS: New tests for diagnosis of renovascular disease, *JAMA* 268:3353-3358, 1992.
5. Dondi M, Fanti S, et al: Prognostic value of captopril renal scintigraphy in renovascular hypertension, *J Nucl Med* 33:2040-2044, 1992.
6. Dubovsky EV, Russell CD: Radionuclide evaluation of renal transplants, *Semin Nucl Med* 3:181-198, 1988.

7. Eshima D, Fritzberg AR: Radiopharmaceuticals for renal imaging. Henkin RE, Boles MA, Dillehay GL, et al: *Nuclear medicine,* St. Louis, 1996, Mosby.

8. Fettich JJ, Kenda RB: Cyclic direct radionuclide voiding cystography: increasing reliability in detecting vesicoureteral reflux in children, *Pediatr Radiol* 22:337-338, 1992.

9. Fommei E, Volterrani D: Renal nuclear medicine, *Semin Nucl Med* 25(2):183-94, 1995.

10. Gates GF: Glomerular filtration. In Henkin RE, Boles MA, Dillehay GL, et al: *Nuclear medicine,* St. Louis, 1996, Mosby.

11. Geyskes GG, Oei H, et al: Renovascular hypertension identified by captopril-induced changes in the renogram, *Hypertension* 1:36-42, 1987.

12. Harris CC, Ford KK, et al: Effect of region assignment on relative renal blood flow estimates using radionuclides, *Radiology* 151:791-792, 1984.

13. Holder LE, Martire JR, et al: Testicular radionuclide angiography and static imaging: anatomy, scintigraphic interpretation, and clinical indications, *Radiology* 125:739-752, 1977.

14. Majd M, Rushton HG: Renal cortical scintigraphy in the diagnosis of acute pyelonephritis, *Semin Nucl Med* 22:298-311, 1992.

15. Marks LS, Maxwell MH: Renal vein renin: value and limitation in the prediction of operative results. *Urol Clin N Am* 2:311-317, 1975.

16. Perrone RD, Steinman TI, et al: Utility of radioisotopic filtration markers in chronic renal insufficiency: simultaneous comparison of 125-I-iothalamate, 169-Yb-DTPA, 99m-Tc-DTPA, and inulin, *Am J Kid Dis* 16(3):224-235, 1990.

17. Prescott MC, Johnson WG: Influence of drugs on the renogram. In O'Reilly PH, Shields RA, Testa HJ: *Nuclear medicine in urology and nephrology,* Boston, 1989, Butterworth.

18. Roubidoux MA, Dunnick NR, et al: Renal vein renins: inability to predict response to revascularization in patients with hypertension, *Radiology* 178:819-822, 1991.

19. Rushton HG, Majd M, et al: Renal scarring following reflux and nonreflux pyelonephritis in children: evaluation with [99m]technetium-dimercaptosuccinic acid scintigraphy, *J Urol* 147:1327-1332, 1992.

20. Russell CD, Dubovsky EV: Measurement of renal function with radionuclides, *J Nucl Med* 30:2053-2057, 1989.

21. Setaro JF, Saddler MC, et al: Simplified captopril renography in diagnosis and treatment of renal artery stenosis, *Hypertension* 18:289-298, 1991.

22. Sfakianakis GN, Bourgoignie JJ, et al: Single-dose captopril scintigraphy in the diagnosis of renovascular hypertension, *J Nucl Med* 28:1383-1392, 1987.

23. Shapiro E, Slovis TL, et al: Optimal use of [99m]technetium-glucoheptonate scintigraphy in the the detection of pyelonephritic scarring in children: a preliminary report, *J Urol* 40:1175-1177, 1988.

24. Sherman RA, Sherman B: Clinical significance of nonvisualization with I-131 hippuran renal scan. In Hollenberg NK, Lange S: *Radionuclides in nephrology,* Stuttgart, Germany, 1980, Thieme.

25. Snyder WS, Ford MR, et al: *Absorbed dose per unit cumulated activity for selected radionuclides and organs, MIRD pamphlet No. 11,* New York, 1975, Society of Nuclear Medicine.

26. Stork JE: Urinary tract infection in children, *Adv Pediatr Infect Dis* 2:115-134, 1987.

27. Taylor A Jr, Nally JV: Clinical applications of renal scintigraphy, *Am J Roentgenol* 164(1):31-41, 1995.

28. Taylor A, Siffer JA, et al: Clinical comparison of I-131 orthoiodohippurate and the kit formulation of Tc-99m mercaptoacetyl-triglycine, *Radiology* 170:721-725, 1989.

29. Van Bockel JH, van Schilfgaarde R, et al: Renovascular hypertension: collective review, *Surg Gynecol Obstet* 169:471-478, 1989.

30. Whitaker RH: Methods of assessing obstruction in dilated ureters, *Brit J Urol* 45:15-22, 1973.

Paul E. Christian, R. Edward Coleman

Skeletal System

Objectives

Explain the composition of bone, and list general types of bones.

Name the major bones and joints of the skeleton.

Explain the accumulation mechanism of bone-imaging agents.

Discuss advantages of whole-body imaging techniques versus spot imaging.

Describe adequate acquisition parameters for static bone imaging using spot-film and whole-body imaging devices.

Explain the advantages of performing SPECT bone scans.

Describe imaging techniques and acquisition parameters for obtaining flow studies and blood-pool imaging.

Explain the advantages of performing delayed imaging in the diagnosis of osteomyelitis.

Discuss the use of gallium and white-cell imaging techniques in correlation with bone scans.

Describe the principles of bone therapy, and discuss the characteristics of radioactive strontium.

Identify the appropriate radiopharmaceutical dose and administration technique for strontium bone therapy.

*T*he skeleton performs several functions for the body, including support, protection, movement, and blood formation. Bone, like other connective tissues, consists of living cells and a predominant amount of nonliving intercellular substance that is calcified. It is a metabolically active tissue with large amounts of nutrients being exchanged in the blood supplying the bone. Thus, the skeleton and body fluids are in equilibrium. Tracer techniques have been used for many years to study the exchange between bone and blood.[5] Radionuclides have played an important role in understanding normal bone metabolism, in addition to the metabolic effects of pathologic involvement of bone.

Radionuclide imaging of the skeleton is being used with increasing frequency in the evaluation of abnormalities involving bones and joints.[7] Several studies have demonstrated that different information can be obtained by radionuclide bone imaging compared with radiography and blood-chemistry analysis.[18,22,28,36,42] Radionuclide joint imaging has been utilized for a shorter period than has bone imaging and is still being evaluated in many diseases involving the joints.[15,31,37,38,50,51]

The anatomy and physiology of bones and joints must be well known for full understanding of the technical and clinical aspects of radionuclide imaging of the skeletal system. The first part of this chapter reviews skeletal anatomy and physiology. The remainder of the chapter discusses radionuclide imaging of the bones and joints, with an emphasis on the technical aspects and applications of the imaging procedure.

COMPOSITION OF BONE

Bone is no different from other tissues in the body in that it is maintained by living cells in addition to having amorphous ground substance and fibers like other connective tissue. The main difference between bone and other connective tissue is that it is calcified; thus it is harder. Bone matrix, the other major constituent of bone, consists of collagen, amorphous ground substance, and mineral.

The composition by weight of normal adult cortical bone is approximately 5% to 10% water, 25% to 30% organic matter (collagen, ground substance, and cellular elements), and 65% to 70% inorganic matter (bone mineral). Collagen is the main protein constituent and accounts for 90% to 95% of the organic matter of bone. Collagen is present in the form of fibrils bunched together into bundles of fibers. The ground substance is the interfibrillar cement substance in which the fibrils are embedded.

The bone salt mineral (inorganic matter) has the crystalline form of an apatite, and chemical analysis reveals the following ions: calcium, phosphate, hydroxyl, carbonate, and citrate with lesser amounts of sodium, magnesium, potassium, chloride, and fluoride. Approximately 27% of the weight of cortical bone is calcium. The main anion constituent of bone is phosphorus (as phosphate), contributing approximately 12% of the weight of cortical bone. The bone mineral consists of individual crystals so small that the electron microscope is needed for visualization of the crystals. The crystalline structure is hydroxyapatite, $Ca_{10}(PO_4)_6(OH)_2$. This formula represents the ratio of the constituent elements and is not necessarily the molecular formula.

GROSS STRUCTURE OF BONE

Bones have obvious differences in size and shape but also have certain features in common. They have a cortex (compact bone) surrounding various amounts of cancellous (spongy or trabecular) bone, which contains blood-forming (myeloid) elements or fatty marrow (Figures 15-1 and 15-2). In the adult most of the myeloid marrow is in the bones of the trunk, with some in the calvarium and upper ends of the humeri and femora. Bones are also similar in that they are covered by periosteum, except in areas of articulation or where tendons and ligaments connect them. The gross structure of bones is discussed in respect to their general architecture in the following groups: tubular, short, flat, and irregular.

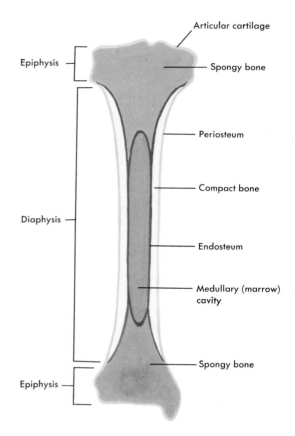

Figure 15-1 Structure of long bone in longitudinal section. (From Anthony CP, Thibodeau GA: *Textbook of anatomy and physiology,* ed 10, St. Louis, 1979, Mosby.)

Tubular Bones

The long tubular bones include the humerus, radius, ulna, femur, tibia, and fibula. The short tubular bones include the metacarpals, metatarsals, and phalanges. Often the tubular bones are all classified as long bones. The tubular bones have a shaft (diaphysis) consisting of a cortex of compact bone surrounding the medullary cavity, which contains bone marrow (see Figure 15-1). In the adult this is mainly yellow, or fatty, marrow, except for the proximal humerus and femur, where it is red (blood-forming) marrow (see Figure 15-2). The cortex is thickest at the midshaft and tapers toward the ends of the shaft. The end of a bone that previously had an epiphysis is known as an epiphyseal bone end. The juncture of the cancellous bone of the epiphyseal bone end and the spongy bone of the diaphysis is called the metaphysis.

Short Bones

The short bones include the wrist (carpals), ankle (tarsals), sesamoids (small bones forming in a tendon or joint capsule), and other anomalous or extra bones. These bones are generally cubic and have spongy osseous tissue covered by a shell of compact bone.

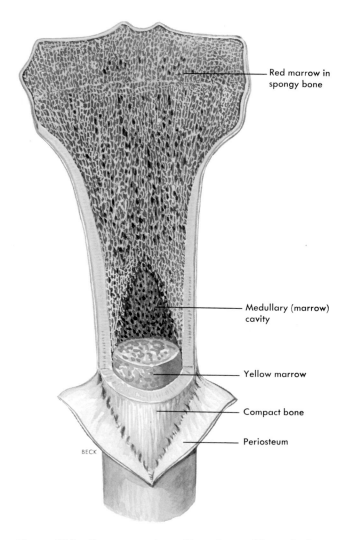

Red marrow in spongy bone

Medullary (marrow) cavity

Yellow marrow

Compact bone

Periosteum

BECK

Figure 15-2 Cutaway section of long bone. (From Anthony CP, Thibodeau GA: *Textbook of anatomy and physiology,* ed 10, St. Louis, 1979, Mosby.)

Table 15-1	Skeletal system	
Skeletal parts		**Number of bones**
Axial skeleton		
Skull and hyoid	29	
Vertebrae	26	
Ribs and sternum	25	
		80
Appendicular skeleton		
Upper limbs	64	
Lower limbs	62	
		126
TOTAL		206

bone may have no spongy tissue and be composed of two layers of compact bone.

THE SKELETON

The skeletal system (Figures 15-3 and 15-4) usually contains 206 bones and provides a supporting framework for the body, as well as forming protective chambers such as the skull and thorax. The skeleton is divided into two main parts: the axial and appendicular parts (Table 15-1). The axial skeleton is composed of the bones of the skull, thorax, and vertebral column, which form the axis of the body. The appendicular skeleton is composed of the bones of the shoulder, upper extremities, hips, and lower extremities. A detailed structure of the vertebrae is shown in Figure 15-5.

JOINTS

Joints (articulations) are spaces where bones come into contact and are bridged in some manner. The articulations have variable amounts of movement and have been classified into two main types according to the amount of movement: rigid (synarthroses) or freely movable (diarthroses).

With a synarthrosis there is absence of a joint space, with little or no movement allowed. In the formation of a synarthrosis the tissue connecting the bones is replaced by the ends of the bone growing together. The sutures of the skull are examples of synarthroses with only a thin fibrous membrane separating the ends of the bones (Figure 15-6, *A*). In some synarthroses, cartilage grows between the articular surfaces of the bones and may allow some motion. Examples of the cartilaginous synarthroses are the symphysis pubis and the joints between the vertebral bodies (Figure 15-6, *B* and *C*).

Flat Bones

The flat bones include the ribs, sternum, scapulae, and several of the skull bones. These bones are thin and have little spongy bone between two layers of compact bone. The flat bones of the skull consist of an inner and outer table (layers of cortical bone) separated by a thin layer of spongy bone (diploë). The spongy layer of the ribs and sternum contains considerable red marrow.

Irregular Bones

The irregular bones include the bones of the spine, pelvis, and some of the skull. A part of an irregular bone may fit into one of the other categories, but the entire bone does not fit into any of the previous categories. The largest part of these bones often consists of large amounts of spongy osseous tissue with a very thin surrounding cortex, whereas another part of the same

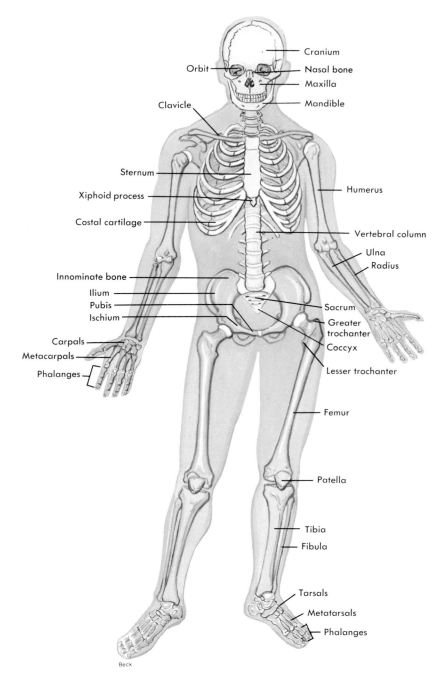

Figure 15-3 Skeleton, anterior view. (From Thibodeau GA: *Anthony's textbook of anatomy and physiology,* ed 13, St. Louis, 1990, Mosby.)

A diarthrosis permits freedom of movement and is the most common type of joint in the body. There is a well-defined articular cavity containing fluid (synovia) and lined by a synovial membrane (Figure 15-6, *D* and *E*). Intraarticular structures such as ligaments and menisci may be present. There is a thin layer of hyaline cartilage, known as articular cartilage, that cushions the ends of each bone in the joint. The synovial joint develops from undifferentiated mesenchyme between the bone rudiments. Part of the undifferentiated mesenchyme differentiates into synovial mesenchyme and subsequently into synovial membranes, menisci, and ligaments. The outer portion of the undifferentiated mesenchyme condenses and forms the joint capsule, which attaches to the bone ends of the joints beyond their articular cartilages.

RADIONUCLIDE IMAGING

Of the many different imaging procedures performed in clinical nuclear medicine, radionuclide bone and

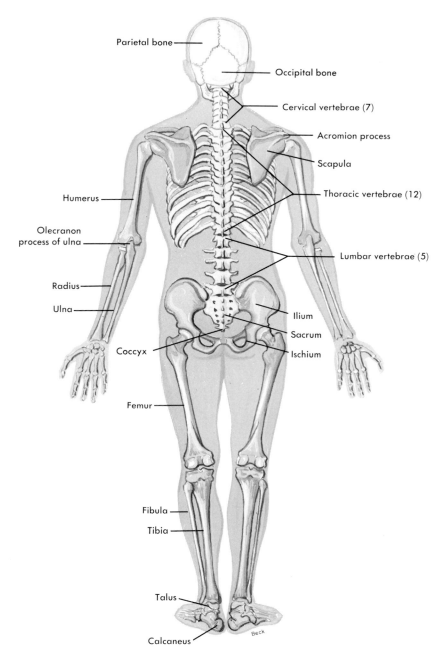

Figure 15-4   Skeleton, posterior view. (From Thibodeau GA: *Anthony's textbook of anatomy and physiology,* ed 13, St. Louis, 1990, Mosby.)

joint studies require the technologist to be thoroughly knowledgeable of anatomy and imaging techniques so that excellent images of the radiopharmaceutical distribution can be obtained. Since early disease involvement of bone may initially be subtle, improper positioning of the patient for imaging or improper exposure of the film may lead to an inaccurate interpretation. Furthermore, since these studies are frequently used to follow therapy, the technique used must be reproducible to allow careful comparison with a previous study. Several different types of radionuclide studies can be performed in the evaluation of bone and joint disor-

ders. The most commonly performed procedure is radionuclide bone imaging with a ^{99m}Tc-phosphate compound. Joint imaging is being used in the evaluation of suspected inflammatory processes involving bones and joints.

Past and Present Radiopharmaceuticals

The earliest applications of radionuclides to the study of bone were performed with phosphorus-32 and calcium-45 for observation of bone structure and function.[2,39] These radionuclides are pure beta particle

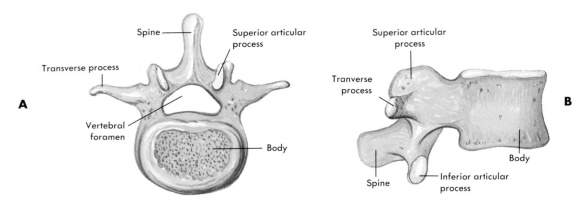

Figure 15-5 Third lumbar vertebra from **A,** above, and **B,** side. (From Thibodeau GA: *Anthony's textbook of anatomy and physiology,* ed 13, St. Louis, 1990, Mosby.)

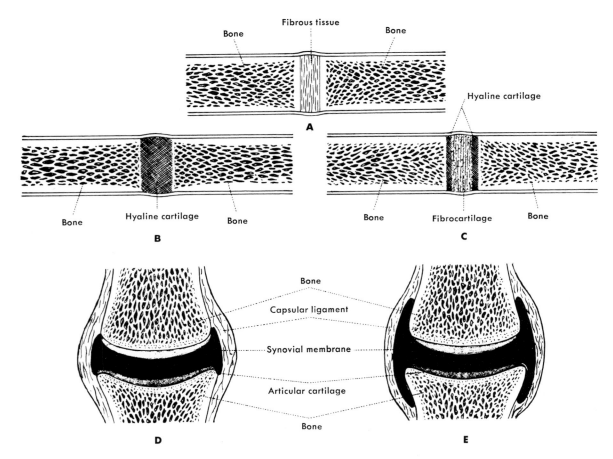

Figure 15-6 Classification of joints. **A,** Fibrous synarthrosis. **B** and **C,** Cartilaginous synarthroses. **D** and **E,** Synovial diarthrosis. (From Hamilton WJ: *Textbook of human anatomy,* ed 2, St. Louis, 1976, Mosby; courtesy The Macmillan Press Ltd, Houndsmill Basingstoke, Hampshire, England.)

emitters and accumulate in regions of increased bone mineral deposition, but their lack of gamma radiation limits external measurement. Clinical application was not made possible until the use of strontium-85, a calcium analog, whose gamma rays could be detected externally.[4,12,13] The introduction of the rectilinear scanner and [85]Sr in the early 1960s made bone scanning possible, but because of the high radiation dose its use was limited to patients with documented malignancy. [85]Sr has a half-life of 65 days and emits a gamma ray at 513 keV. The long effective half-life of this radionuclide limits the amount of activity injected to 100 μCi. With this small amount of activity, scanning time was extensive and the information density of the image was ex-

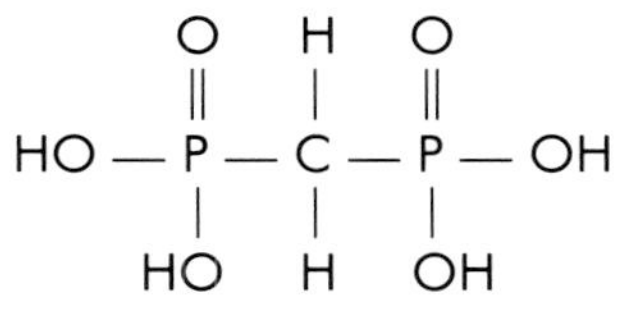

Methylene diphosphonate

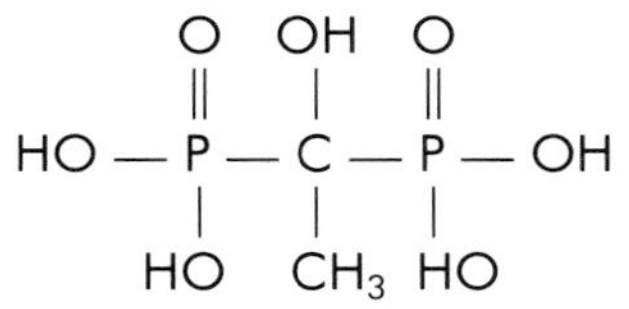

Ethylenehydroxydiphosphonate

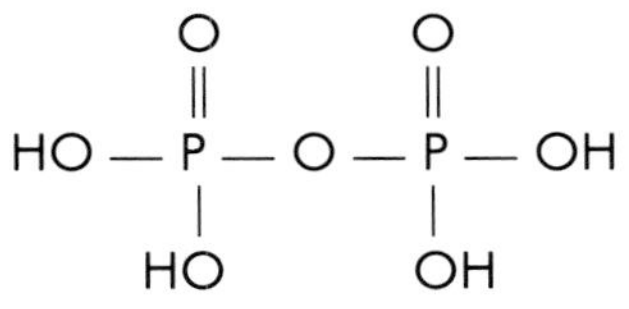

Pyrophosphate

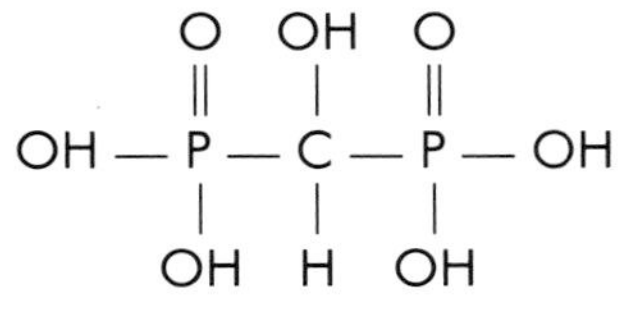

Hydroxymethylene diphosphonate

Figure 15-7 Structural formulas of various phosphate pharmaceuticals in acid form.

tremely low. Although the accumulation of strontium in bone is rapid, the blood and gastrointestinal clearances are slow; therefore a 2- to 7-day interval between the times of injection and scan was needed.

Another isotope of strontium used for bone scanning is ^{87m}Sr, which has a 2.9-hr half-life and a gamma ray energy of 388 keV.[48] The short half-life allows the administered dose to be increased to a range of 1-4 mCi, and scans can be performed 2 to 3 hr after injection. ^{87m}Sr is a generator-produced isotope from a parent product of yttrium-87, which has an 80-hr half-life. This generator-produced radionuclide was rather expensive.

Fluorine-18 was the first bone-seeking radiopharmaceutical that gave an acceptable radiation dose to the patient and provided a higher quality scan than did the isotopes of strontium, permitting a wider application of bone imaging in the late 1960s and early 1970s.[10] The rapid blood clearance of ^{18}F is advantageous for the performance of bone scans because the blood and tissue activity levels are low compared with that of bone at the time of imaging and therefore give a high ratio of bone to soft tissue. The disadvantage of using ^{18}F is its half-life of 1.87 hr, which makes it very expensive to manufacture and deliver to a large number of hospitals at any great distance from the production facility. The annihilation radiation (511 keV) from its positron emission is suitable for imaging with a rectilinear scanner but not a scintillation camera because of the high-energy photons.

The development of ^{99m}Tc-labeled phosphate complexes for bone imaging was introduced by Subramanian in 1971.[49,50] ^{99m}Tc in the form of pertechnetate does not localize to any useful extent in bone. ^{99m}Tc has excellent physical properties for nuclear medicine imaging because of its ideal characteristics for use with the Anger scintillation camera. The short half-life of ^{99m}Tc allows several millicuries of activity to be injected; images with high information density can be obtained.

Since ^{99m}Tc is the present radionuclide of choice, the phosphate compound that produces the best image needs to be determined. Figure 15-7 shows the structure of four phosphate compounds that have been utilized in routine clinical bone imaging. To evaluate these various phosphate compounds, their distribution in the body relative to the rate and amount of accumulation in various organ systems and bone must be determined.

Polyphosphate was the first commercially available ^{99m}Tc-labeled compound for bone imaging. The structural formula of polyphosphate includes a group of phosphates with a chain length of approximately 40 to 55. Phosphate chains that are extremely long can result in the formation of a radiocolloid in the bloodstream, causing hepatic localization of the pharmaceutical. Further development of this agent moved from longer phosphate chains toward shorter, more stable phosphate complexes. Among these were pyrophosphate and ethylenehydroxydiphosphonate (EHDP). Pyrophosphate is a naturally occurring compound in the body, and its P — O — P bond is subject to breakdown by phosphatase enzymes. The carbon-carbon bond of EHDP is believed to offer greater stability than pyrophosphate. Both pyrophosphate and EHDP have a faster blood and tissue clearance than does polyphosphate.

Methylene diphosphonate (MDP) and hydroxymethylene diphosphonate (HMDP) are similar to pyrophosphate and EHDP but have faster blood clearance.[33] The blood clearance of MDP and HMDP in the initial 3 to 4 hr after administration is very similar to fluorine. MDP and HMDP labeled with ^{99m}Tc provide a better image of the bones, since the lower blood and tissue concentration gives a higher ratio of bone to tissue. MDP and HMDP give comparable quality bone images.

Mechanism of Accumulation

The accumulation of radionuclides in bone is related to both vascularity and rate of bone production.[19,49] Increased blood supply to an area of bone results in a blood-pool image (obtained immediately after radiopharmaceutical administration) with increased activity.

The localization of various bone-imaging agents is related to exchange with ions in the bone. The process of exchange of an ion native to bone for a labeled, bone-seeking ion is termed *heterionic exchange*.[11,27] Calcium phosphate is the main inorganic constituent of bone; however, calcium is also found in the form of carbonate and fluoride. Calcium is located in microcrystals of hydroxyapatite.[40] Analog elements of calcium, such as strontium, are believed to exchange with the calcium. ^{18}F exchanges with the hydroxyl (OH) ion in the hydroxyapatite. The accumulation of labeled phosphate compounds is probably related to the exchange of the phosphorus groups onto the calcium of hydroxyapatite. Although these mechanisms are not completely understood, the principal of bone imaging is fairly basic. Calcium analogs or phosphate compounds have a low concentration in blood and tissue.

Radiopharmaceuticals used for bone imaging can localize in soft-tissue areas, demonstrating not only calcification but also infarction, inflammation, trauma, and tumor. The portion of any radiopharmaceutical that does not accumulate in bone and tissue or stays in the circulation is eliminated from the body by various routes, depending on the radiopharmaceutical. ^{85}Sr has some concentration in the gastrointestinal tract for several days. ^{18}F and phosphate scans labeled with ^{99m}Tc demonstrate activity in the kidneys and bladder, since these agents are excreted through the urinary tract.

Technical Considerations

The physical characteristics of the radionuclides that have been used for bone imaging present several important factors in radiopharmaceutical selection. These factors relate primarily to the amount of activity that may be administered to the patient, the gamma-ray energy, and the amount of accumulation of radiopharmaceutical in the bone.

Before the introduction of ^{18}F and ^{99m}Tc-phosphate compounds, bone imaging was a time-consuming procedure associated with a high radiation dose to the patient and poor information content in the images. The subsequent development of better radiopharmaceuticals and improved instrumentation produced images of higher quality with better information concerning bone physiology. In conjunction with the improved information in the images, the need for carefully controlling the technical aspects of the procedure became apparent.

Choosing the best radionuclide for bone imaging is currently a simple choice based on the physical characteristics. The strontium and fluorine isotopes have high-energy gamma rays and require the use of coarse-resolution collimators with thick lead septa. The high-energy gamma rays have a low attenuation coefficient resulting in a poor detection efficiency in the thin, sodium-iodide crystal of the Anger scintillation camera. Also, these radionuclides must be administered in amounts of activity smaller than those of ^{99m}Tc, yielding lower information-density images. ^{18}F is an excellent agent for bone imaging, but its short half-life and high cost limit its general availability. ^{99m}Tc-labeled compounds allow larger quantities of activity to be administered with a resultant lower radiation dose than do the other radionuclides. The monoenergetic gamma-ray emission of 140 keV and the absence of particulate radiation make ^{99m}Tc well suited for use with the scintillation camera. ^{99m}Tc is also readily available to all laboratories at a very low cost, unlike other radionuclides for bone imaging.

Patient Preparation

The preparation of the patient for bone imaging is minimal when any of the ^{99m}Tc-labeled agents are used, but several factors must be taken into consideration. The patient needs to have a complete understanding of the procedure, especially the reason for the delay between radiopharmaceutical administration and imaging. A delay of approximately 3 hr is generally an adequate time for good bone accumulation and a low soft-tissue level of the radiopharmaceutical. Radiopharmaceuticals with fast blood and tissue clearance, such as MDP and HMDP, allow imaging as early as 2 hr after administration. Unless contraindicated, patients should be hydrated to aid in clearance of the radiopharmaceutical from the body. The administration of four to six glasses of liquid during the delay period is adequate, and the patient should be encouraged to void frequently to decrease the radiation dose. Patients must also void immediately before imaging begins so that the image of the pelvis is not obscured by a large amount of radioactivity in the bladder. Because of the high concentration of radioactivity in the urine, care must be taken to avoid contamination of the patient, the patient's clothing, or the bed sheets, which can lead to a false-positive study.

INSTRUMENTATION

Several types of instruments have been used for bone imaging. Wider application of this procedure has been responsible for the design of new instruments and accessories.

The Anger scintillation camera is currently the most versatile and most commonly utilized imaging device for use with ^{99m}Tc-labeled compounds. Since the skeleton is one of the most extensive organ systems in the body, the application of the mobile camera with an approximately 10-in standard field of view requires 25 to 30 separate views for complete imaging. Performing bone imaging by this technique requires a large amount of the technologist's time and effort in positioning the patient for all these views. High-resolution or medium-resolution (140 keV) collimators are well suited for bone imaging with a standard-field camera (high-sensitivity collimators should not be used). However, a 140 keV diverging collimator can maintain good resolution and allow reduction of the total number of images because of the larger effective field of view. The currently used diverging collimators result in slight spatial distortion and loss of resolution at the image edges. The use of a large-crystal (15 in) scintillation camera with a parallel-hole collimator allows inclusion of a

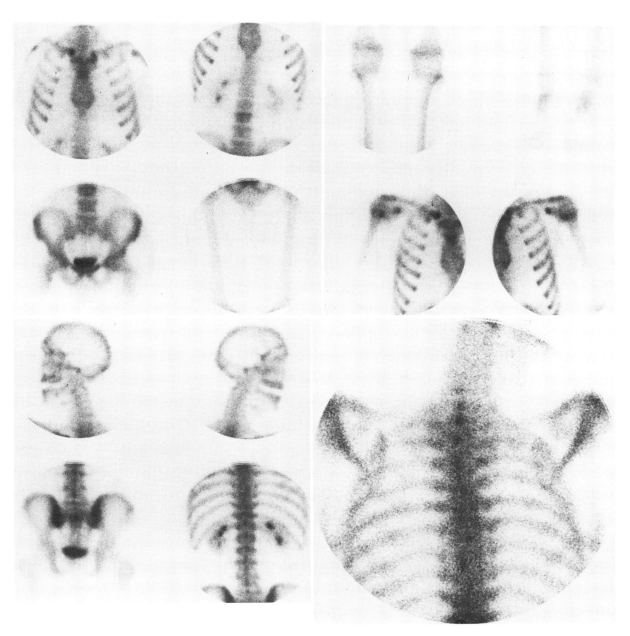

Figure 15-8   Thirteen images necessary to cover whole body with large-crystal camera. Forearms and hands are still omitted with these images.

larger area of the body in each view, reducing the total number of images to approximately 13 to 16 views (Figure 15-8). Newer cameras with extra large crystals, either square, rectangular (Figure 15-9), or circular, can image larger areas of the body and fewer images are needed for whole-body imaging.

The bone area and activity in the field of the camera can be highly variable for different portions of the body, and some images may require a long imaging time to achieve high-information density (ID). Commonly, multiple individual images are taken for an equal amount of time. This equal-time technique allows the film density in one image to be compared with the density in another image, since the exposure is made for an equal amount of time. This method is effective as long as adequate statistics are achieved. First, one area of the body (such as the anterior or posterior view of the chest) is imaged for a preset number of counts.

Between 400,000 and 600,000 counts are accumulated for a standard-field camera and between 500,000 and 1 million for a large-crystal camera. After this first exposure, all subsequent images are taken for the same interval of time. An alternative method of performing equal-time imaging is to use the ID feature available on some scintillation cameras. An area of normal bone as found in the sternum or spine is selected with the ID marker, and an exposure is made until the ID in this region reaches a range of 2500-4000 counts. The time for this exposure is then used to obtain the other images.

Individual images of certain areas can be obtained with the scintillation camera after the initial image of the total skeleton on another type of instrument is performed. The spot films provide detailed images of areas that were not well visualized on the whole-body imaging instruments or provide additional views aiding in

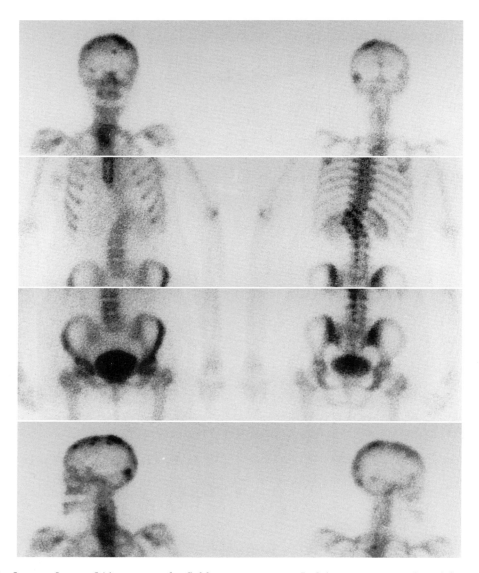

Figure 15-9 Images from a 24-in rectangular-field gamma camera. Left images are anterior; right are posterior.

the determination for presence (or absence) of abnormality. A detailed view of the pelvis can be degraded by whole-body imaging devices because of activity accumulated in the bladder before the imaging device reaches the pelvis. Images of the pelvis should be obtained immediately after the patient has voided, which can be before or after the whole-body image.

WHOLE-BODY IMAGING

The production of an image of the total body area (Figure 15-10) onto one film is accomplished by an accessory that moves either the camera detector or the patient through the camera field of view. As the body moves past the detector, the area seen by the camera is minified and advances across the film at a speed proportional to that of the patient. Some large-crystal cameras can cover the body in two passes or, when equipped with a special diverging collimator, in one pass. When multiple passes are required to produce the image, faint longitudinal lines appear on the image. This "zipper" is created because of the slight separation of each pass over the body.

When a scintillation camera is used with a whole-body imaging accessory, a portion of the crystal may be masked either electronically or by collimation into a rectangular field of view. It is essential that this region of the detector be proportional in its speed over the patient compared with the motion of the minified image area that moves across the cathode ray tube (CRT).

One determines the technique for establishing imaging parameters by monitoring the count rate, ID, or by selecting the total time for the whole-body scan. A region for measuring the count rate is usually selected anteriorly over the chest or posteriorly over the spine. The same scan speed should be used for both the anterior and the posterior images. The scan speed is determined by one of several techniques. Most camera manufacturers supply a table, chart, or nomogram for determining the proper scan speed, based on the desired ID in the image and the count rate from the patient. Some systems may have a microcomputer for automatically calculating the scan speed, determined from monitoring the count rate from the patient. All these methods are basically the same, but some additional variations from the manufacturer's method may give improved image quality. Digital cameras record the whole-body scan in a high-resolution matrix for photographing after data acquisition.

It is recommended that the whole-body image include greater than 2.5 million counts. The best positioning of the patient is to have the detector under the table and have the patient lie prone and supine to produce the anterior and posterior images, respectively. By using this technique, the detector can be nearer the patient during imaging.

Whole-body imaging with the scintillation camera provides a good esthetic relationship of overall radio-pharmaceutical distribution with only a small loss in resolution generated from the motion synchronization of the table and the CRT recording. Patients are manipulated less, and little effort is required of the technologist during the imaging procedure.

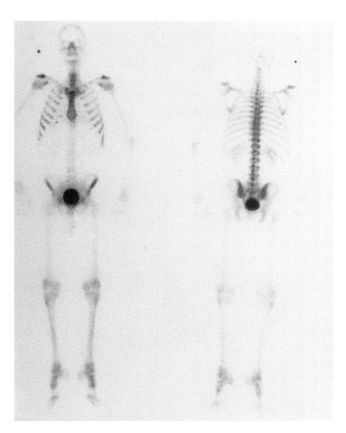

Figure 15-10 Normal whole-body bone scan with extra-large–crystal camera. Anterior *(left)* and posterior *(right)* are obtained simultaneously in the scan using two detectors.

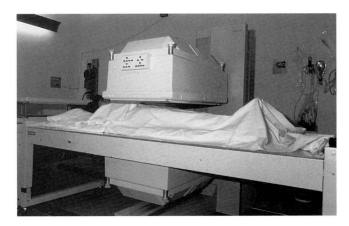

Figure 15-11 Dual-detector extra large field of view (24-in wide) for whole-body image.

Figure 15-11 shows a dual-detector large-field camera for performing whole-body imaging. Both anterior and posterior scans are obtained simultaneously using detectors that cover the full body width.

SPECT IMAGING

The potential use of single photon emission computed tomography (SPECT) in bone imaging is in examining areas in which there is substantial superimposition of bony structures. Bone studies using SPECT have mainly involved patients with suspected disease of the hips, lumbar spine, temporomandibular joints, and facial bones. Bone SPECT has been demonstrated to be the most sensitive noninvasive test for evaluating the extent of arthritis in patients with chronic knee pain examined by conventional radiography, bone scanning, and subsequent arthroscopy. SPECT offers advantages over planar imaging in evaluating patients with suspected avascular necrosis of the hip. A photopenic area is frequently seen on SPECT imaging that is not seen on planar imaging. SPECT has also been shown to be more sensitive than planar imaging in evaluating patients with evidence of spondylolysis or spondylolisthesis. SPECT is better than planar imaging in identifying the site of abnormality in symptomatic patients with defects in the pars interarticularis. SPECT is also superior to planar imaging in evaluating patients with temporomandibular joint dysfunction who undergo preoperative evaluation.

Bone SPECT imaging of the axial skeleton should be performed with high-resolution collimators. As with usual SPECT imaging, the detector-to-patient distance should be minimized. High-quality images can be obtained only with an adequate imaging time—30 to 45 min. Imaging of the lumbar spine should be done with the patient's legs slightly elevated to make the spine straight. Imaging with a single-head camera is most commonly performed using a 64×64 image matrix; some newer cameras have high enough resolution to warrant the use of a 128×128 matrix. Studies should be acquired using a large number of views (120 to 128) in 360 degrees to obtain good angular sampling. SPECT studies acquired with these parameters have very high counts and very high resolution and should

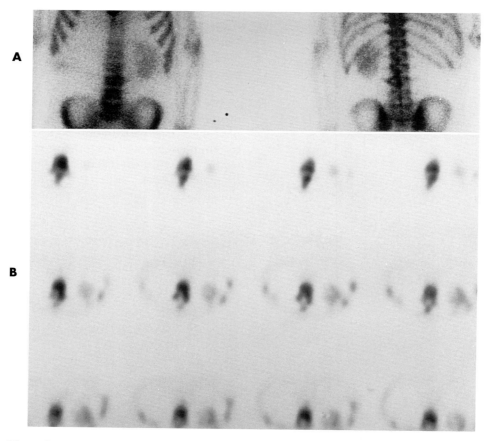

Figure 15-12 **A,** Planar images of lumbar spine with abnormal radiopharmaceutical accumulation in the L2-3 region. **B,** Reconstructed superior-to-inferior transverse slices show increased uptake in the transverse and spinous process of these vertebrae. **C,** Sagittal slices. **D,** Coronal slices.

therefore be reconstructed with high-resolution prefiltering and reconstruction filters. Reconstructed images should be reviewed by the technologist for proper orientation and should be free from artifacts. Reconstructed transverse, coronal, and sagittal slices should be oriented to the patient's anatomy for interpretation and comparison with planar images.

The importance of quality control in SPECT is stressed in Chapter 3. SPECT studies of poor quality or those performed improperly will be inferior to quality planar images. The improved image contrast for lesions makes SPECT of interest for bone imaging. The utility of SPECT in bone imaging is now being determined.

Furthermore, the removal of superimposition of bony structures results in better localization of abnormal accumulation. The widespread use of SPECT for bone imaging will determine its appropriate role in radionuclide bone imaging.

Figure 15-12 shows a SPECT study of the lumbar spine compared with planar images. SPECT applications to bone scintigraphy can add clinically useful information in nearly all parts of the skeleton, particularly the spine, skull, knees, and hips. The primary advantage is to add three-dimensional information about the extent of disease. SPECT also occasionally shows lesions not seen on planar images.

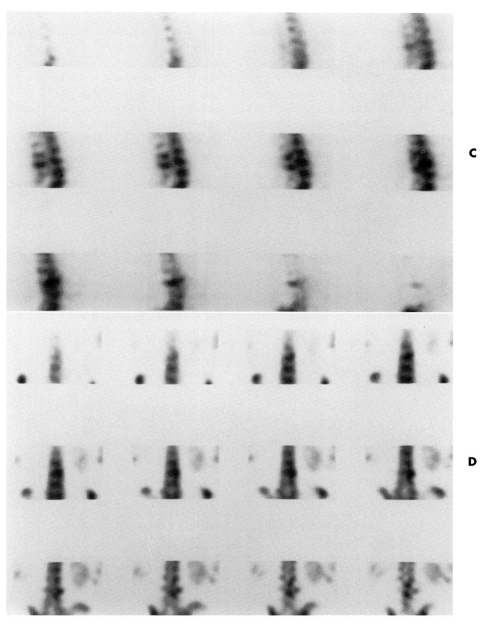

Figure 5-12, cont'd   For legend see opposite page.

CLINICAL ASPECTS

The skeleton is a complex organ system subjected to many different types of adversities. Bone disease can be generally classified into two broad categories: congenital and acquired. Of the congenital bone diseases, radionuclide imaging has essentially no role, since most of the diseases have characteristic radiographic appearances. Radionuclide bone imaging, however, is important in the evaluation of several acquired bone diseases. These can be classified as traumatic, neoplastic, inflammatory, metabolic, degenerative, vascular, and other bone diseases not fitting into these listed categories.

The localization of the bone-seeking radiopharmaceuticals is mainly dependent on two factors: bone blood flow and bone production. The relative importance of each of these parameters is not well defined, but frequently both are increased. Increased radiopharmaceutical deposition accompanying increased bone production is well exemplified by the epiphyseal growth plate in bone imaging in children (Figure 15-13). Occasionally an abnormality is detected as a focal area of decreased pharmaceutical accumulation (Figure 15-14). This decreased accumulation can be related to impaired blood flow or to complete destruction or replacement of bone by tumor, inflammatory mass, or radiation.

The indications for bone imaging are as follows:
1. Staging of malignant disease
   A. Screening of high-risk patient
   B. Localization of biopsy sites
2. Evaluation of primary bone neoplasms
3. Diagnosis of early skeletal inflammatory disease
4. Evaluation of skeletal pain of undetermined etiology
5. Evaluation of elevated alkaline phosphatase of undetermined etiology
6. Determination of bone viability
7. Evaluation of painful total joint prostheses

The most frequent reason for ordering a bone scan is staging of malignant disease by determining if spread to bone has occurred. The other indications are used less frequently, but they are important reasons for bone imaging.

Anterior and posterior images of the whole body are generally obtained (see Figure 15-10). The anterior skull, facial bones, mandible, clavicle, sternum, anterior ribs, anterior iliac spine, and pubic rami are best visualized on the anterior images. The posterior skull, spine, posterior ribs, scapulae, sacroiliac joints, and is-

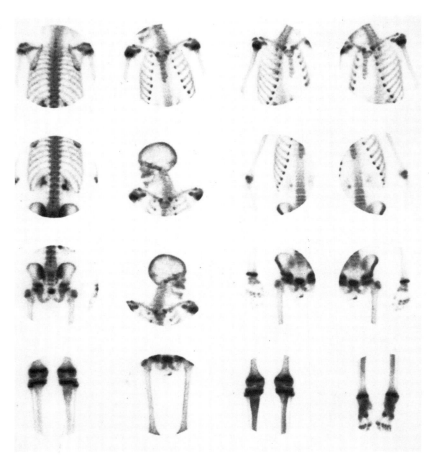

Figure 15-13   Multiple gamma camera images from a large-crystal camera of a 15-year-old boy with an aneurysmal bone cyst of the right tibia. The epiphyseal activity in multiple areas is apparent.

chia are best visualized on the posterior images. Shoulders, hips, and extremities are commonly seen well on both views, primarily dependent on patient positioning.[12] The activity within the skeleton is usually symmetric from side to side. However, some asymmetry may

be seen in the skull, shoulders, sternoclavicular joints, and anterior ends of the ribs without a pathologic condition present.[52] The activity within the kidneys is variable. With ^{99m}Tc MDP or ^{99m}Tc HMDP, the kidney activity is usually less than the surrounding bone activity. Kidney disease may be associated with pronounced asymmetry of renal activity, a focal area of absent activity (cyst or tumor), or ureteric visualization, suggesting ureteric obstruction.[9,34] Accumulation of the bone-imaging radiopharmaceutical can occur in the normal female breast as well as in various diseases of the breast[3] (Figure 15-15).

In most institutions radionuclide bone imaging has replaced the radiographic skeletal survey for the evaluation of skeletal metastatic disease. Metastases to bone are common in several primary malignancies, including lung, breast, and prostate carcinomas. Metastases to the spine are difficult to detect radiographically, since loss of approximately 50% of the mineral content of the bone must occur before lytic lesions are detected.[16] Whereas 10% to 40% of the adult patients with metastatic bone disease and an abnormal bone scan may have normal radiographs, less than 5% of bone scans are negative when the radiograph demon-

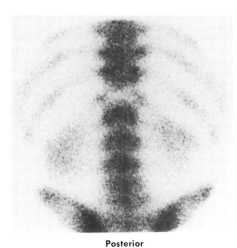

Posterior

Figure 15-14 Absent accumulation of radiopharmaceutical in vertebral body.

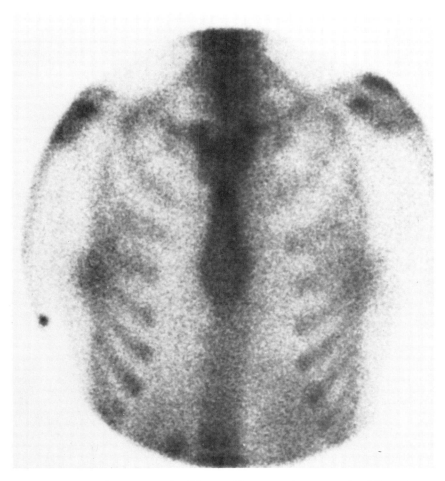

Figure 15-15 Anterior chest image in a bone scan of a 37-year-old woman demonstrating bilateral accumulation of the radiopharmaceutical in normal breasts.

strates metastatic disease.[29,47] In the pediatric population one study has demonstrated 68% of metastases identified by radionuclide imaging alone.[23] False-negative scans have been related to several factors. If the skeleton is diffusely involved with metastatic disease, the focal nature of the lesions might not be apparent.[17] The diffusely abnormal scan may be difficult to differentiate from the normal scan, but with quality images from the scintillation camera, irregularities of radiopharmaceutical deposition can generally be noted (Figure 15-16). Metastatic lesions may have no associated osteoblastic activity and thus may not be detected by bone scan or may be detected as a photon-deficient area.[24] An example of a disease in which the lesions might not produce an abnormality on the bone scan is multiple myeloma, which has a high false-negative rate. After the bone images are performed, radiographs of the abnormal areas are often recommended for a more definitive diagnosis and to exclude other etiologies of an abnormal scan in the patient with suspected metastatic disease.

The usual pattern of skeletal metastatic disease is multiple focal lesions throughout the skeleton, with the greatest involvement generally in the axial skeleton[26,28] (Figure 15-17). The area of abnormal radiopharmaceu-

tical deposition represents the edge of the metastatic deposit where osteoblastic repair is attempted. Some primary cancers that metastasize to tissue other than bone accumulate bone-seeking radiopharmaceuticals (Figure 15-18). These tumors generally tend to be calcified on radiographs, but the bone scan is abnormal before the radiographs. A few bone-producing metastatic lesions do occur, such as those attributable to osteogenic sarcoma (Figure 15-19). Accumulation of the agent in soft-tissue metastases may prove helpful in detecting extraskeletal involvement.[44]

The malignancies in which bone imaging has demonstrated importance for the staging of the disease are breast, lung, and prostatic carcinomas.[28,36,43] These are common malignancies with a high incidence of bony metastatic disease. Other malignancies are now evaluated with bone imaging, and there is a higher incidence of bony metastases than previously suspected. Therefore most patients with malignancies now have a bone scan as part of their evaluation.

Bone scanning is also used for the evaluation of primary bone neoplasms. Usually the patient has already had radiographs of the primary tumor, and the bone scan offers no additional information of that area. The extent of the abnormality on the bone scan is gener-

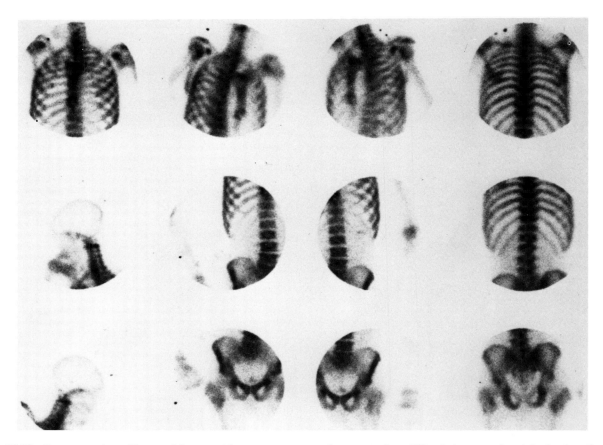

Figure 15-16 Bone scan in a 61-year-old man with prostate cancer demonstrating diffusely increased activity in the ribs, spine, and pelvis. Irregular distribution of activity is noted in the ribs and minimal activity in the soft tissue and kidneys. This is a "superscan" from widespread metastatic disease.

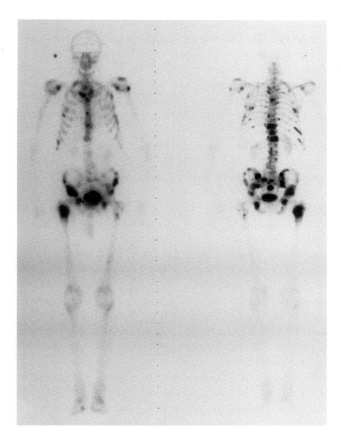

Figure 15-17 Multiple focal lesions in bone of patient with prostate carcinoma.

ally not much different from the radiographically apparent lesion. The value of bone scanning in patients with primary bone malignancy lies in the detection of the disease elsewhere.[23] As many as 30% of the patients with Ewing sarcoma may have lesions in other bones, a finding that significantly alters the therapy of the disease.[8,23,53] Metastatic deposits in soft tissue from osteogenic sarcoma can be detected by scan before the appearance of radiographic abnormalities.[44]

In addition to being used in the evaluation of malignant disease involving the skeleton, radionuclide bone imaging is used in the evaluation of several other nonmalignant processes. Bone imaging has been demonstrated to be useful in the evaluation of patients with suspected osteomyelitis and diskitis.[20,30,45,54] The bone scan may be positive within 24 hr after the onset of symptoms, whereas the radiographic changes are not apparent for 10 to 14 days.

Early images are important in evaluating inflammatory processes; therefore a three- or four-phase bone scan should be performed. A three-phase bone scan is performed by acquiring a rapid flow sequence of images over the area of interest during radiopharmaceutical injection. Flow images are taken every 2 to 4 sec for 40 to 60 sec. Static images are then immediately ob-

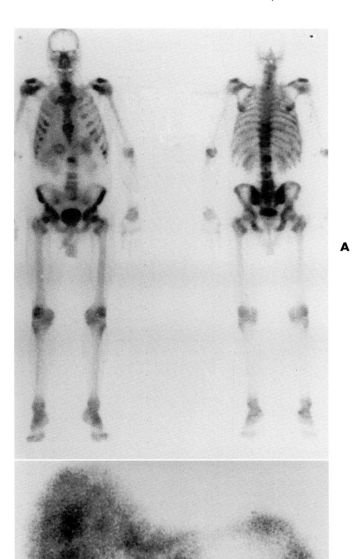

Figure 15-18 Metastatic colon cancer. **A,** Anterior whole-body scan reveals a doughnut-shaped area of abnormal accumulation in the right upper quadrant. **B,** ^{99m}Tc–sulfur-colloid liver-spleen scan reveals areas of diminished colloid localization. This abnormality is a metastatic lesion from a primary colon cancer.

tained for 300,000 to 500,000 counts without moving the patient, and additional projection images are taken as necessary. Both osteomyelitis and cellulitis cause early increased activity due to an increased vascular response to the affected area. The second phase is routine scanning at 2 to 3 hr after injection. The third

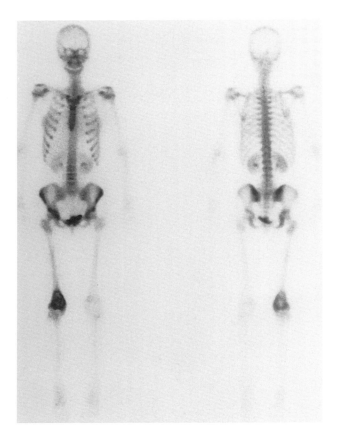

Figure 15-19 Osteogenic sarcoma of distal femur in a 16-year-old girl shows tumor restricted to femur without evidence of metastatic disease.

phase is to evaluate persistent increased activity at 5 hr. A fourth phase can be added by taking images after a 24-hr delay. The third- and fourth-phase images should be taken for 100,000 to 250,000 counts to allow comparison of these delayed images with respect to changes in activity in the affected area (Figure 15-20).

With cellulitis, there may be increased blood-pool activity diffusely throughout the area of involvement, as well as some diffusely increased activity on the regular bone images obtained 2 to 3 hr after injection. Osteomyelitis, however, demonstrates focally increased activity in the involved bone on both the blood-pool and routine images (Figure 15-20). Since the use of bone imaging for detecting osteomyelitis, it has been found that several patients do not subsequently develop the typical radiographic changes because the early treatment prevents the development of radiographic abnormalities.

Diskitis, an inflammatory process of the disk space, is usually secondary to a bacterial infection. The bone scan reveals increased activity in the vertebral bodies on each side of the disk space (Figure 15-21).

In some instances trauma is being evaluated with bone scanning.[42] Immediately after a fracture, for the first day or two, there may be decreased activity visualized at the site. After day 3, there is generally diffusely increased activity in the area of fracture, which becomes focally increased by day 10. Depending on angulation of the fracture and stress, for example, the activity decreases with time but may remain abnormal for years if the fracture is complicated and bone remodeling continues. The bone scan has been used to evaluate patients with normal radiographs suspected of having fractures (Figure 15-22). Some of these patients have normal radiographs at the time the bone images are abnormal.

Radionuclide bone imaging is also used in several other conditions. Paget disease is associated with greatly abnormal radiopharmaceutical accumulation typically involving the greater part of a bone[1,46] (Figure 15-23). The bone scan has been used to evaluate therapy for this disease.[1] The determination of the cause of pain after a total joint replacement is frequently difficult. Radionuclide imaging has been demonstrated to be a sensitive method of detecting a complication, such as loosening or infection of the prosthetic implant[21] (Figures 15-24 and 15-25). Radionuclide imaging is also very sensitive for the detection of osteoid osteomas, a cause of skeletal pain that may be undetected for years.[32]

Avascular necrosis of the hip is difficult to diagnose by clinical examination and radiographs of the hips, and radionuclide imaging is frequently used in the evaluation of these patients. Early in the course of the disease, decreased blood flow and blood pool, in addition to decreased accumulation of the bone-scanning radiopharmaceutical on the delayed images, can be seen. Magnetic resonance imaging (MRI) may also detect abnormalities before radiographic changes (Figure 15-26).

Joint Imaging

Radionuclide imaging of the joints has been used in several institutions for the evaluation of inflammatory joint disease.[6,15,31,35-38,50,51] This imaging has been performed with either ^{99m}Tc-pertechnetate or ^{99m}Tc-phosphate compounds. The ^{99m}Tc-pertechnetate images are obtained immediately after injection of the radiopharmaceutical, and abnormal accumulation is noted in areas of increased blood flow as found in synovitis. The ^{99m}Tc-phosphate compounds localize in areas of joint inflammation, since there is an increased turnover rate and vascularity of the adjacent bone as well as increased synovial vascularity (Figure 15-27). Either of these radiopharmaceuticals can be used to detect early joint inflammation, often before radiographic abnormalities occur. When compared with physical examination, radiographs, and arthrography, joint imaging with the ^{99m}Tc-phosphate complex is the most sen-

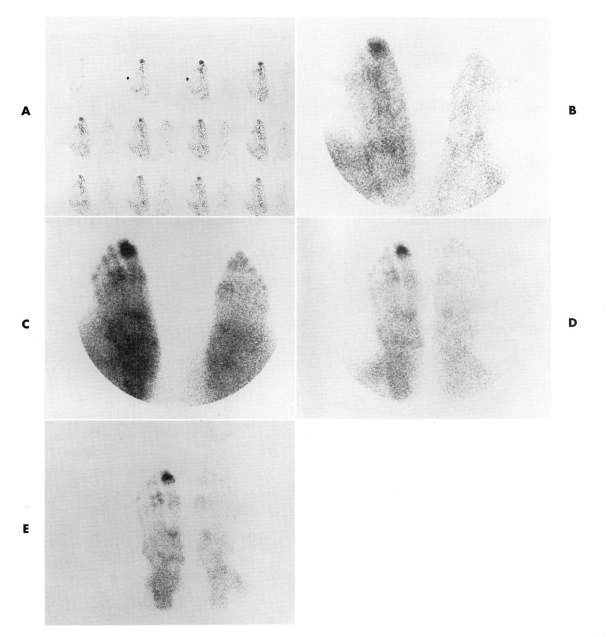

Figure 15-20   A, Plantar view flow images at 4 sec/frame show increased perfusion to the first right distal phalanx. **B,** Blood-pool images also demonstrate abnormal accumulation. Images at 2 hr **(C),** 5 hr **(D),** and 24 hr **(E),** have persistent radiopharmaceutical collection consistent with osteomyelitis.

sitive indicator of early degenerative disease of the knee.[51]

Several recent studies have demonstrated the utility of ^{99m}Tc-phosphate imaging in the early detection of sacroiliac inflammatory disease[15] (Figure 15-28). Detection of the inflammatory process before radiographic changes has been demonstrated. The technique utilizes a computer to quantify areas of bone activity and compares the activity in the sacroiliac joint region with an area of·equal size in the midsacrum.

Bone Pain Therapy

Skeletal metastases occur in more than half of patients with prostate, breast, or lung cancer. Pain from these metastases is caused by tumor infiltration and expansion of periosteal membranes or by encroachment on nerve roots. Localized areas of bone pain are frequently treated by single-field radiotherapy to relieve pain.

For more than 40 years, bone-seeking, beta-emitting radiopharmaceuticals have been used to provide pain

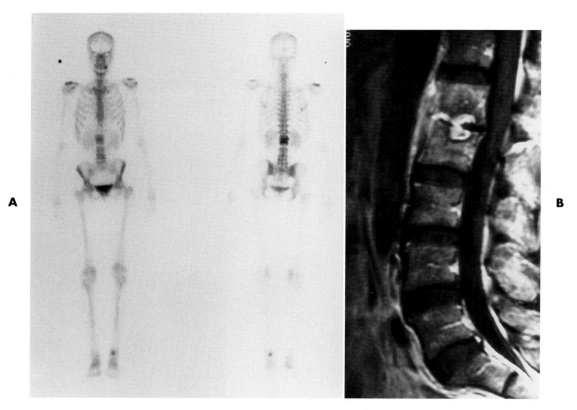

Figure 15-21 **A,** Whole-body bone scan reveals diffusely increased radiopharmaceutical accumulated in T10 and L2 vertebral bodies. **B,** T2 weighted MRI image reveals abnormal signal intensity in disk space between L1 and L2 with the abnormal signal extending into the vertebral bodies in this patient with diskitis.

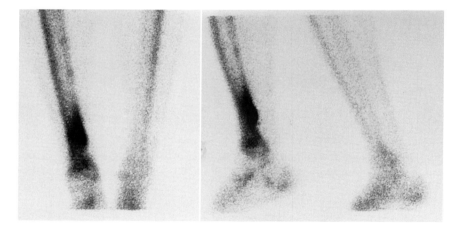

Figure 15-22 Delayed static images of the lower extremities of a 20-year-old male athlete with pain in the tibia and normal plain radiographs. The bone scan shows marked abnormal accumulation in the distal tibia (anterior and lateral) with the abnormality extending through the cortex, characteristic of a stress fracture.

relief in patients with metastatic carcinoma to the bone. For most of this time, ^{32}P orthophosphate has been used in certain patients to relieve bone pain. A series of ^{32}P orthophosphate injections were given in a total dose not to exceed 21 mCi. However, phosphorus-32 orthophosphate causes hematologic toxicity. Pancytopenia is dose dependent and occurs in the fourth or fifth week postinjection. Acute leukemia has also been reported to occur but rarely before 2 years after administration. The life expectancy of patients with painful

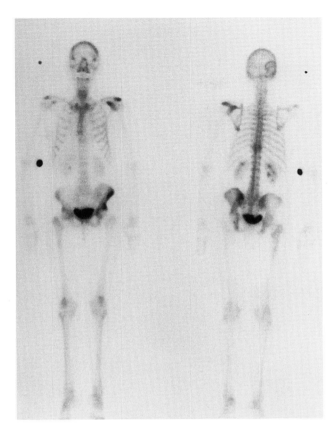

Figure 15-23   Paget disease. Whole-body images demonstrate abnormal uptake in the left ilium, left scapula, thoracic spine, right proximal femur, and skull.

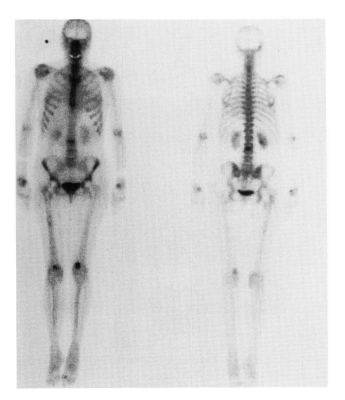

Figure 15-24   Loosened total hip prosthesis. Patient with bilateral hip protheses has focal abnormal accumulation in the right femoral lesser and greater trochanters and tip of prosthesis, typical of loosening.

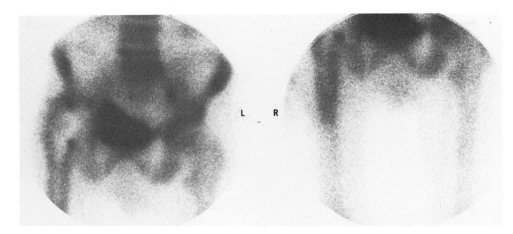

Figure 15-25 Infected total hip prosthesis. Diffusely abnormal accumulation around entire prosthesis in right hip is characteristic of infected implant.

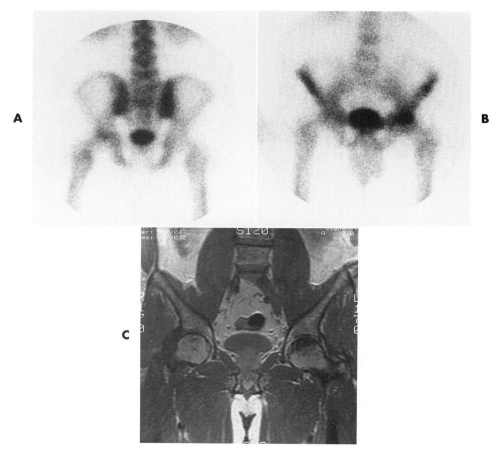

Figure 15-26 Patient with left hip pain from aseptic necrosis. **A** and **B**, Anterior and posterior bone scan demonstrates increased uptake in left femoral head with slightly increased uptake in right femoral head. **C,** Coronal magnetic MRI demonstrates decreased signal in 30% to 40% of left femoral head and 10% to 15% of right femoral head.

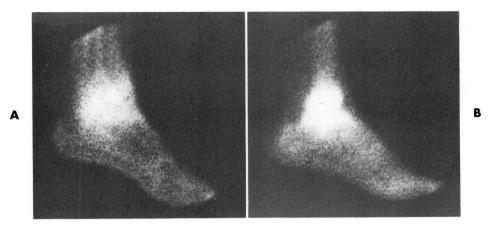

Figure 15-27 Septic arthritis of tibiotalar joint. **A,** Blood-pool image obtained after administration of ^{99m}Tc methylenediphosphonate (^{99m}Tc MDP) demonstrates abnormal accumulation in ankle joint area. **B,** Routine image obtained 2 ½ hr later demonstrates focal accumulation in distal tibia and talus. Joint fluid was aspirated, and aspirate grew pathogenic organisms. Radiographs revealed no joint abnormality.

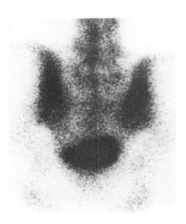

Figure 15-28 Sacroileitis. Posterior pelvis image in patient with low back pain. Quantification revealed ratio of activity in sacroiliac area to midsacrum to be greater than 2, with normal being less than 1.5.

bone metastases is rarely greater than 1 year. An improved radiopharmaceutical, ^{89}Sr, is now commercially available.

^{89}Sr is a pure beta emitter with a 50.6-day half-life that is capable of delivering a high radiation dose to cortical and trabecular bone. Patients may be considered candidates for ^{89}Sr-chloride therapy on confirmation that metastatic disease is the cause of their bone pain. ^{89}Sr may be administered in conjunction with external beam radiotherapy and/or chemotherapy. Patients should have platelet counts above 60,000 and white cell counts greater than 2400. Any patient with impending pathologic fractures or spinal cord compression should not be considered candidates for this therapy. As part of the screening process, bone scans should be performed with ^{99m}Tc MDP to document that there is abnormal bone turnover identified at the site of pain.

The dose of ^{89}Sr is 40-60 μCi/kg or 4 mCi.[41] The therapeutic radiopharmaceutical should be handled using good radiation safety practices including gloves, plastic syringe shields, and an absorbent pad under the injection area. The dose should be injected into an indwelling catheter using a three-way stopcock and at least a 10-ml saline flush to ensure the complete delivery of radiopharmaceutial intravenously. The syringe, three-way stopcock, and catheter should be disposed of appropriately, and the area where the dose was administered should be monitored with a Geiger counter. Patients should be routinely monitored for 30 min after therapy administration due to rare adverse reactions of nausea or tachycardia. The radiation dose to metastatic sites may be in the range of 300-2500 rads/mCi.

Patient follow-up should be carried out to monitor the hematologic status of patients and the effectiveness of pain relief. Radiostrontium relieves pain in approximately 80% of patients. Some reports indicate that an increase in bone pain during the first week after injection is a positive prognostic indicator for later pain relief. Depending on the hematologic status of patients, repeat therapeutic injections may be administered at 3-month intervals. Although the cost of a single radiostrontium treatment may exceed $3000, this is a cost-effective treatment in bone pain patients compared with the cost of radiotherapy, chemotherapy, and analgesic palliative strategies.

^{67}Ga and ^{111}In White Blood Cell Imaging in Bone and Joint Disease

Several studies have recently demonstrated the value of ^{67}Ga-citrate scanning in patients with inflammatory bone and joint disease.[25,30,31,32] Some patients with osteomyelitis or septic arthritis may have normal ^{99m}Tc-phosphate complex images but abnormal ^{67}Ga images.

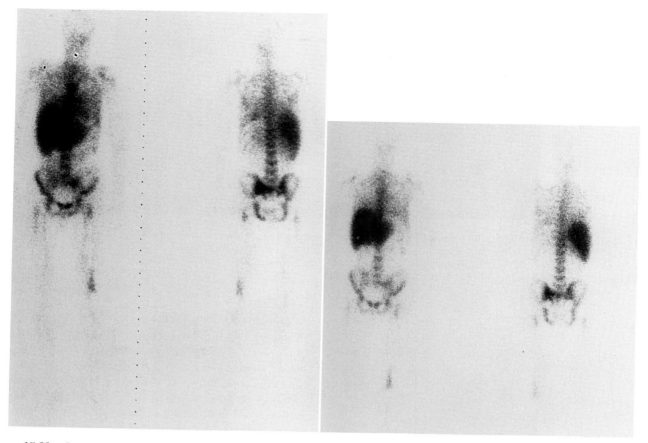

Figure 15-29 Osteomyelitis. Whole-body images obtained 4 *(left)* and 18 *(right)* hr after administration of ^{111}In leukocytes in a patient after splenectomy. Abnormal accumulation in left sacroiliac joint, left ischium, left proximal femur, and left distal femur in this patient with multifocal osteomyelitis.

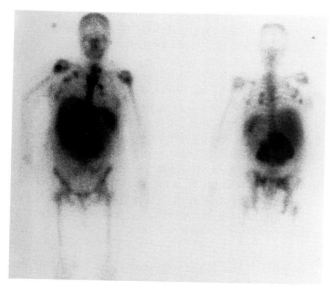

Figure 15-30 Whole-body ^{67}Ga-citrate imaging demonstrates markedly abnormal accumulation in abdominal lymphadenopathy and in multiple ribs in this patient with Hodgkin lymphoma.

^{111}In-labeled white blood cells (see Chapter 17) have also been used for evaluating patients with suspected bone and joint infections.[14] The results of using ^{111}In white cells have varied, which is most likely related to the patient populations studied. One study had only a 50% sensitivity (Figure 15-29) in detecting skeletal infection, but the patient population included many patients with chronic infection. Another study reported a 98% sensitivity in patients with suspected bone and joint infection. Although ^{111}In white cells can be comparable with ^{67}Ga-citrate imaging in detecting inflammatory bone and joint disease, ^{67}Ga-citrate imaging does not require the handling of blood products and is the preferred procedure at some institutions. Recent reports of patients with diabetes mellitus and skin ulcers of the feet have demonstrated a high frequency of osteomyelitis and a high accuracy of ^{111}In white cells in this patient population.

^{67}Ga-citrate imaging is used for staging certain malignancies such as Hodgkin lymphoma and malignant melanoma. The study is typically used to detect the soft-tissue involvement of these malignancies, but skeletal involvement can be detected (Figure 15-30).

REFERENCES

1. Altman RD, Johnston CC, Khairi MRA, et al: Influence of disodium etedronate on clinical and laboratory manifestations of Paget's disease of bone (osteitis deformans), *N Engl J Med* 28:1379, 1973.

2. Anderson J, Emergy EW, McAlister JM, et al: The metabolism of a therapeutic dose of calcium-45 in a case of multiple myeloma, *Clin Sci Mol Med* 15:567, 1956.

3. Bassett LW, Gold RH, Webber MM: Radionuclide bone imaging, *Radiol Clin North Am* 19:675, 1981.

4. Bayer GCH, Wendeberg B: External counting of Ca-47 and Sr-85 in studies of localized skeletal lesions in man, *J Bone Joint Surg* 41B:558, 1959.

5. Belchier J: An account of the bones of the animals being changed to a red color by aliment only. In Bauer GCH, ed: Tracer techniques for the study of bone metabolism in man, *Adv Biol Med Phys* 10:228, 1965.

6. Bekerman C, Genant HK, Hoffer PB, et al: Radionuclide imaging of the bones and joints of the hand, *Radiology* 118:653, 1975.

7. Bernier DR, Coleman RE: Impact of computed cranial tomography on radionuclide imaging and cisternography, *J Nucl Med Technol* 4:180, 1976.

8. Bhansali SK, Desai PB: Ewing's sarcoma: observations in 107 cases, *J Bone Joint Surg* 45A:541, 1963.

9. Biello D, Coleman RE, Stanley RJ: Correlation of renal images on bone scan and intravenous pyelogram, *Am J Roentgenol Radium Ther Nucl Med* 127:633, 1976.

10. Blau M, Nagler W, Bender MA: Fluorine 18: a new isotope for bone scanning, *J Nucl Med* 3:332, 1962.

11. Charkes ND, Philips CM: A new model of ^{18}F-fluoride kinetics in humans. In *Medical radionuclide imaging*, vol 2, Vienna, 1977, International Atomic Energy Agency.

12. Charkes ND, Sklaroff DM: Early diagnosis of metastatic bone cancer by photoscanning with strontium-85, *J Nucl Med* 5:168, 1964.

13. Charkes ND, Valentine G, Cravitz B: Interpretation of the normal ^{99m}Tc polyphosphate rectilinear bone scan, *Radiology* 107:563, 1973.

14. Coleman RE, Welch DM, Baker WJ, et al: Clinical experience using indium-111-labeled leukocytes. In Thakur ML, Gottschalk A, eds: *Indium-111 labeled neutrophils, platelets, and lymphocytes*, New York, 1980, Trivirium.

15. Davis P, Thomson ABR, Lentle BC: Quantitative sacroiliac scintigraphy in patients with Crohn's disease, *Arthritis Rheum* 21:234, 1978.

16. Edelstyn GA, Gillespie PJ, Grebbel FS: The radiological demonstration of osseous metastases: experimental observations, *Clin Radiol* 18:158, 1967.

17. Frankel RS, Johnson KW, Mabry JJ, et al: "Normal" bone radionuclide image with diffuse skeletal lymphoma, *Radiology* 111:365, 1974.

18. Galasko CSB: The detection of skeletal metastases for mammary cancer by gamma camera scintigraphy, *Br J Surg* 56:757, 1969.

19. Galasko CSB: The mechanisms of uptake of bone-seeking isotopes by skeletal metastases. In *Medical radionuclide imaging*, vol 2, Vienna, 1977, International Atomic Energy Agency.

20. Gelfand MJ, Silberstein EB: Radionuclide imaging: use in diagnosis of osteomyelitis in children, *JAMA* 237:245, 1977.

21. Gelman MI, Coleman RE, Stevens PM, et al: Radiography, radionuclide imaging, and arthrography in the evaluation of total hip and knee replacement, *Radiology* 128:467, 1978.

22. Gerber FH, Goodreau JJ, Kirchner PT, et al: Efficacy of preoperative and postoperative bone scanning in the management of breast carcinoma, *N Engl J Med* 297:300, 1977.

23. Gilday DL, Ash JM, Reilly BJ: Radionuclide skeletal survey for pediatric neoplasms, *Radiology* 123:399, 1977.

24. Goergen TG, Alazraki NP, Halpern SE, et al: "Cold" bone lesions: a newly recognized phenomenon of bone imaging, *J Nucl Med* 12:1120, 1974.

25. Handmaker H, Giammona ST: The "hot joint"—increased diagnostic accuracy using combined ^{99m}Tc phosphate and ^{67}Ca citrate imaging in pediatrics, *J Nucl Med* 17:554, 1976.

26. Hart G, Hoerr SO, Hughes CP: Detection of bone metastases from breast cancer: an accurate, four film roentgenographic survey, *Cleve Clin Q* 38:1, 1971.

27. Jones AG, Francis MD, Davis MA: Bone scanning: radionuclide reaction mechanisms, *Semin Nucl Med* 6:1, 1976.

28. Krishnamurthy GT, Tubis M, Hiss J, et al: Distribution pattern of metastatic bone disease—a need for total body skeletal image, *JAMA* 237:2054, 1977.

29. Legge DA, Tauxe WN, Pugh DG, et al: Radioisotope scanning of metastatic lesions of bone, *Mayo Clin Proc* 45:755, 1970.

30. Lisbona R, Rosenthall L: Observations on the sequential use of ^{99m}Tc-phosphate complex and ^{67}Ga imaging in osteomyelitis, cellulitis and septic arthritis, *Radiology* 123:123, 1977.

31. Lisbona R, Rosenthall L: Radionuclide imaging of septic joints and their differentiation from periarticular osteomyelitis and cellulitis in pediatrics, *Clin Nucl Med* 2:337, 1977.

32. Lisbona R, Rosenthall L: Role of radionuclide imaging in osteoid osteoma, *Am J Roentgenol Radium Ther Nucl Med* 132:77, 1979.

33. Littlefield JL, Rudd TG: Tc-99m hydroxymethylene diphosphonate and Tc-99m methylene diphosphonate: biologic and clinical comparison: concise communication, *J Nucl Med* 24:463, 1983.

34. Maher FT: Evaluation of renal urinary tract abnormalities noted on scintiscans, *Mayo Clin Proc* 50:370, 1975.

35. Merkel KD, Brown ML, Fitzgerald RH, et al: Prospective In-111 WBC scan vs Tc-99m-MDP-Ga67 scan for low-grade osteomyelitis, *J Nucl Med* p 72, 1983.

36. Merrick MV: Review article—bone scanning, *Br J Radiol* 48:327, 1975.

37. Namey TC, Rosenthall L: Periarticular uptake of ^{99m}technetium disphosphonate in psoriatics, *Arthritis Rheum* 19:607, 1976.

38. Park HM, Terman SA, Ridolfo AS, et al: A quantitative evaluation of rheumatoid arthritic activity with Tc-99m HEDP, *J Nucl Med* 18:973, 1977.

39. Pecher C: Biological investigations with radioactive calcium and strontium, *Proc Soc Exp Biol Med* 46:86, 1941.

40. Rasmussen H: Parathyroid hormone, calcitonin and calciferols. In Williams RH, ed: *Textbook of endocrinology*, ed 5, Philadelphia, 1974, WB Saunders.

41. Robinson RG, Preston DF, Schiefelbein M, et al: Strontium 89 therapy for the palliation of pain due to osseous metastases, *JAMA* 274:420-424, 1995.

42. Rosenthall L, Hill RO, Chuang S: Observation on the use of ^{99m}Tc-phosphate imaging in peripheral bone trauma, *Radiology* 119:637, 1976.

43. Schaffer DL, Pendergrass HP: Comparison of enzyme, clinical, radiographic and radionuclide methods of detecting bone metastases from carcinoma of the prostate, *Radiology* 121:431, 1976.

44. Schall GL, Zeiger L, Primack A, et al: Uptake of ^{85}Sr by an osteosarcoma metastatic to lung, *J Nucl Med* 12:131, 1971.

45. Shirazi PH, Rayudu GVS, Fordham EW: ^{18}F bone scanning: review of indications and results in 1500 cases, *Radiology* 112:361, 1974.

46. Shirazi PH, Rayudu GVS, Ryan WG, et al: Paget's disease of bone: bone scanning experience with 80 cases, *J Nucl Med* 14:450, 1973.

47. Sklaroff DM, Charkes DN: Diagnosis of bone metastasis by photoscanning with strontium 85, *JAMA* 188:1, 1964.

48. Spencer R, Herbert R, Rish MW, et al: Bone scanning with ^{85}Sr and ^{18}F: physical and radiopharmaceutical considerations and clinical experience in 50 cases, *Br J Radiol* 40:641, 1976.

49. Subramanian G, McAfee JG, Blair RJ, et al: Radiopharmaceuticals for bone and bone-marrow imaging. In *Medical radionuclide imaging*, vol 2, Vienna, 1977, International Atomic Energy Agency.

50. Sy WM, Bay R, Camera A: Hand images: normal and abnormal, *J Nucl Med* 18:419, 1977.

51. Thomas RJ, Resnick D, Alazraki NP, et al: Compartmental evaluation of osteoarthritis of the knee—comparative study of available diagnostic modalities, *Radiology* 116:585, 1975.

52. Thrall JH, Ghaed N, Geslien GE, et al: Pitfalls in Tc^{99m} polyphosphate skeletal imaging, *Am J Roentgenol Radium Ther Nucl Med* 121:739, 1974.

53. Wang CC, Schulz MD: Ewing's sarcoma—a study of 50 cases treated at the Massachusetts General Hospital, 1930-1952 inclusive, *N Engl J Med* 284:571, 1953.

54. Waxman AD, Bryan D, Siemsen JK: Bone scanning in the drug abuse patient: early detection of hematogenous osteomyelitis, *J Nucl Med* 14:647, 1973.

SUGGESTED READINGS

Probst-Proctor SL, Dillingham MF, McDougall IR, et al: The white blood cell scan in orthopedics, *Clin Ortho Rel Res* 168:157, 1982.

Subramanian G, McAfee JF: A New complex of ^{99m}Tc for skeletal imaging, *Radiology* 99:192, 1971.

Helen H. Drew, Ursula Scheffel, Patricia A. McIntyre

chapter 16

Hematopoietic System

Objectives

List the normal components of blood in the plasma compartment and cellular compartments.

Define a hematocrit value, how it is performed, and how to interpret it.

Describe the function, life span, and survival problems of a red blood cell.

Describe how to label platelets with ^{111}In oxine.

State the isotope dilution principle.

Explain the ascorbic acid technique for labeling red blood cells with ^{51}Cr.

Describe the correct procedure and calculation for performing a total red cell volume measurement, including sample collection, processing, and counting.

Describe the correct procedure and calculation for performing a total plasma volume measurement, including sample collection, processing, and counting.

Describe the limitations imposed when attempting to compare measured red cell and plasma volumes to normal volumes.

Describe the technique used to perform a red cell survival, and calculate the results.

Describe the technique used to perform a splenic sequestration.

Describe the technique of performing an in vivo cross match.

Describe the calculations and interpretation of an in vivo cross match.

Describe the performance and calculate the results of a stage 1, 2, and 3 Schilling test, including patient preparation, test administration, sample collection, sample processing, and counting.

List the sources of errors in performing a Schilling test, and explain the role of the "flushing" doses.

BLOOD COMPONENTS

Circulating blood is an extraordinarily complex mixture. Some of the representative components are listed in Table 16-1. When blood is collected with an anticoagulant (a substance that prevents normal clotting), the whole blood divides into a plasma compartment and a cellular compartment. If it is collected without an anticoagulant, the fluid that can be separated from the clot is known as serum. The clot contains most of the cellular elements as well as the proteins consumed in the coagulation process. It is important to recognize this fundamental difference between the terms *plasma* and *serum.* Many of the anticoagulants routinely used by hematologists are not applicable to

Table 16-1 Representative components of blood (not all-inclusive)

1. Plasma compartment
   a. Water
   b. Simple solutes, such as Na^+, K^+, Cl^-, Mg^{2+}, Ca^{2+}, HCO_3^-, and sugar
   c. Proteins
      (1) Albumin
      (2) Immunoglobulins, such as gamma globulin (IgG) and macroglobulins (IgM)
      (3) Transport proteins, such as transferrin, transcobalamin I, and transcobalamin II
      (4) Lipoproteins (and other lipids)
      (5) Precursors and active components of the complex coagulation-fibrinolysis system
2. Cellular compartment
   a. Erythrocytes (red blood cells, RBC), about $5 \times 10^6/mm^3$
   b. Leukocytes (white blood cells, WBC), about $5 \times 10^3/mm^3$
      (1) Granulocytes
      (2) Lymphocytes
      (3) Monocytes
      (4) Plasma cells and fragments of, or whole, megakaryocytes—rarely present in routine preparations of peripheral blood for microscopic examination
   c. Platelets (thrombocytes), about 3.5×10^5 mm^3

nuclear hematologic studies because they prevent clotting by chelating calcium (a requirement for normal clotting) and other heavy ions such as tracer iron, which is used in some nuclear medicine studies.

The relative numbers of the basic cellular types present in circulating blood are listed in the lower portion of Table 16-1. One rarely measures the number of red blood cells in a given volume of blood to assess whether a patient has anemia unless it is included with the information routinely printed out by an automated electronic particle counter. A much simpler method is to measure the hematocrit value. This is done when one places a well-mixed sample of anticoagulated blood in a suitable tube and centrifuges it for an appropriate period to use *g* force (multiples of gravity) to separate the cellular elements from the plasma phase. When hematocrits are performed on normal blood, the red cells comprise the majority of the volume of packed cells (Figure 16-1, *A*). This is attributable to their relatively great number and size. The layer just above the red cells known as the buffy coat, which is slightly grayish, is the white cell population in that sample of blood; just above this is an even more minute layer of creamy-colored cells, representing the platelets. Because of their smaller number and, in the case of platelets, their minute size, the hematocrit value cannot be relied on

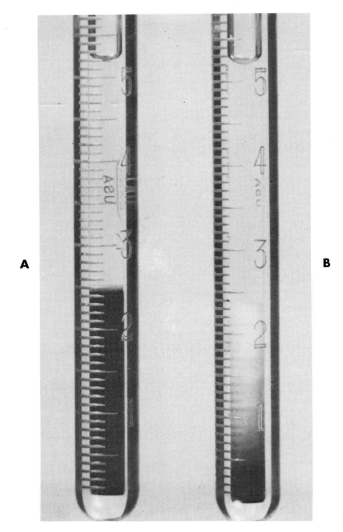

Figure 16-1 Tube **A** contains normal blood sample and **B** contains a sample of blood from a patient who has basic hematologic abnormality. Cellular elements have been separated from plasma by centrifugation.

to measure the quantity of these cells, and they must be counted separately, preferably with an electronic particle counter. In contrast, Figure 16-1, *B* shows the blood of a patient who had a basic hematologic abnormality. The overwhelming majority of packed cells are made up of platelets and white cells, with the lower portion being a poorly separated mixture of white cells and red cells. If one gave only a casual glance at this hematocrit value, especially if it were done as a routine in a microcapillary tube, one could easily make the serious error of overlooking the severe degree of anemia and greatly abnormal increase in white cells and platelets present.

There are two important things to remember about the interpretation of a hematocrit value. First, it represents merely the ratio of the cellular compartment volume to the total volume of a given sample of blood. Accordingly, alterations (for example, dehydration) in the plasma compartment can make the hematocrit value seem falsely elevated. Second, a very careful examination of the hematocrit tube is necessary to make sure that one is indeed dealing with a normal red cell population in the packed cells and not a preponderance of white cells or platelets. Should the latter condition prevail and be unrecognized, tracer-labeling studies give false and misleading results. One should use a hand-held magnifying glass or the magnifier supplied with the reading equipment when using the microhematocrit tubes.

In Table 16-2 we have summarized some of the important features of the cellular elements of the blood. Since most clinical nuclear medicine laboratories are doing cell-labeling studies of the erythrocytes, this chapter chiefly deals with those tests that deal directly, or indirectly, with the mature red blood cells and factors that may influence their production. Random platelet labels and white cell labels are also discussed.

The mature circulating red blood cells (RBC), or erythrocytes, are critical to the survival and proper function of each cell within each tissue of the body because of their oxygen transport function. RBC survive for approximately 100 days, even though with each complete transit of the circulation they are shot out of the aorta during the left ventricular contraction at speeds that come close to those of a jet airliner. At the other extreme the RBC are required to weave their way slowly through the tiny, intricate openings in the splenic sinusoids, which are much smaller than the cells themselves. In their transit through the spleen, the RBC actually are required to deform themselves, with only a tiny portion initially emerging through an opening and the rest being pulled slowly after it; after this they are still able to regain their normal biconcave shape and maintain their normal functions.

Their life of approximately 100 days has a profound implication; every day the bone marrow must replace 1% of the total circulating mass of RBC that have died of old age. When one considers that the mean hematocrit value is approximately 45% and the total blood volume in adults averages 5 L, one can see that the normal bone marrow performs a most efficient assembly line function to maintain homeostasis; the same is obviously true for the production by the marrow of all the other cellular elements of the blood. Furthermore, the normal marrow contains reserves of mature cells, which can be quickly released into the circulation when needed, and with continuing stress, the normal marrow can gradually increase its daily rate of production many fold (up to eight times normal in the case of RBC).

A complete listing of all known causes and types of anemia would require several pages of this textbook; however, the following list summarizes the basic mechanisms by which anemia may be caused:

1. Excessive rate of removal from circulation
   a. Blood loss
   b. Hemolysis

2. Deficient production
   a. Lack of proper building blocks, such as iron, vitamin B_{12}, and folic acid
   b. Suppression of marrow activity by a wide variety of acute and chronic diseases
   c. Primary disorders of the bone marrow

Obviously anemia can result either from an excess rate of removal of RBC or from deficient production. Blood loss, be it chronic or acute, remains high on the list of causes of anemia. Accelerated destruction of the RBC within the patient's body is a process known as hemolysis and has the same end result as blood loss, provided that either occurs at a rate that exceeds the ability of the normal bone marrow to compensate. Deficient production can result from the lack of proper building blocks, suppression of marrow activity by a wide variety of acute and chronic diseases, or, least common of all, a primary disorder of the bone marrow. Iron-deficiency anemia, a simple and rapidly curable condition, remains the most common worldwide hematologic disorder. Vitamin B_{12} and folic acid are listed, not because they represent the only other building blocks of importance but because nuclear medicine can provide useful information regarding the differential diagnosis in patients presenting with manifestations of their deficiency.

Acute, self-limited, or rapidly cured disorders, such as the common cold or acute pneumonia, cause temporary, essentially complete, cessation of marrow RBC production. Since normal RBC live approximately 100 days, such a short-term illness does not result in a recognizable degree of anemia. Certain patients who have a compensated hemolytic anemia (that is, a significantly shortened life span of their RBC but a very active marrow that is maintaining a normal hematocrit value by its increased rate of erythrocyte production) may very rapidly develop a severe degree of anemia because of marrow suppression from such otherwise mild illnesses. In addition, there is a wide variety of chronic diseases (for example, rheumatoid arthritis and malignant disorders) that may cause chronic suppression of marrow activity and consequent anemia.

Last are the primary disorders of the bone marrow. It is often in these complex hematologic problems that the judicious choice of nuclear medicine procedures gives unique and valuable information that could not be gathered in any other fashion.

ISOTOPIC LABELING OF CELLULAR ELEMENTS

All isotopic labels of the cellular elements of the blood are of two general types: cohort, or pulse, labels and random labels. It is important to recognize the fundamental difference between the information to be gained by the use of each of them.

Table 16-2	Circulating cellular elements: origin, function, approximate life span		
	Erythrocytes	**Granulocytes**	**Monocytes**
Tissue of origin in normal adults	Red (hematopoietically active) marrow	Same	Same; circulating through blood to become the tissue macrophages
Earliest recognizable precursor cell in the bone marrow	Proerythroblast	Myeloblast	Promonocyte
Function of mature cell	Oxygen transport to tissues	Phagocytosis	Phagocytosis; processing of antigens
Life span	90 to 110 days	50% to 60% of mature granulocytes in blood are adhering to vascular endothelium, the so-called marginal pool, and are freely exchangeable with those circulating; $t_{1/2}$ in blood is 6 to 7 hr; may survive up to 5 days after migration into tissues	Experimental data less firm but probably very similar to granulocytes in blood; once they enter and are converted to tissue, macrophages may survive months to years

Platelets	Lymphocytes	Plasma cells
Same	Same	Some if not all are derived from immunologically stimulated lymphocytes
Megakaryocyte	Certain small marrow lymphocytes are morphologically indistinguishable from pluripotential stem cells; however, other evidence suggests that lymphocytes are not derived from same stem cell as are the erythrocytes, granulocytes, and platelets	
Vital components of normal coagulation process	After release from marrow they differentiate into (1) B lymphocytes (precursors of plasma cells) with production of circulating humoral antibody and (2) T lymphocytes (participants in cellular immunity)	Produce humoral antibody specifically directed against antigen to which they are exposed
8 to 10 days	B lymphocyte—unknown T lymphocyte—long lived; continue to recirculate	Highly variable; some may persist for many months

Cohort or Pulse Labels

This type of label is only available to the marrow precursors of a given cell type for a specific and limited length of time; thus it will not label cells already circulating. Incorporation of this type of label in the marrow erythroid precursors results in the appearance in the circulation of mature labeled RBC of the same age. An ideal cohort label that met all these necessary criteria and had the appropriate gamma-emitting nuclide would permit study of the rate of production of RBC, their kinetics, longevity, manner of death, and ultimate disposal within the body. None of the currently available radioisotopes for cohort labeling of RBC satisfies all these requirements, and none is used in routine clinical studies.

Random Labels

Random labels are radiopharmaceuticals that are applied to the circulating cells of the peripheral blood in vitro. This process labels all cells in the sample, that is, from the youngest to the oldest circulating blood cells or, as classically expressed, blood cells of random age; thus these are applicable to the study of mean cell survival or other direct measurements of the circulating cells of the blood. It is important to emphasize that isotopic labeling of circulating blood cells provides reasonably precise data only if separating, labeling, and reinfusing these cells are performed in such a way as to minimize damage to them. Strict adherence to aseptic techniques is also obligatory.

PLATELET KINETICS

The only isotopic labels available for platelets are of the random type, that is, applicable to determination of the fate of platelets already circulating in the blood. ^{51}Cr chromate has been extensively used as a random platelet label and was recommended in 1977 by the International Panel on Diagnostic Application of Radioisotopes in Hematology[3] as the only available satisfactory agent for studies in humans. The major limitations of ^{51}Cr are due to the physical characteristics of the radionuclide. Only 9% of the emissions of ^{51}Cr are useful gamma photons. Furthermore, the 27.8-day half-life of ^{51}Cr is long for studies of human platelets, which have a mean survival of approximately 10 days. An additional limitation is placed on these studies because of the low platelet labeling efficiency of ^{51}Cr chromate; large amounts of blood (up to 500 ml) must be withdrawn even from normal subjects to maximize the final platelet-bound ^{51}Cr activity. Even with optimal harvesting and labeling procedures, the amount of ^{51}Cr infused labeled to platelets is limited to approximately 10-30 μCi. As a consequence of this low labeling efficiency and the 9% gamma emission of ^{51}Cr, the circulating platelet-associated measurable radioactivity is low, particularly in the latter days of the study. External quantitative organ localization or imaging studies cannot be performed with adequate statistics despite the 320 keV energy of ^{51}Cr because of the restricted number of photons available for such studies.

The discovery of ^{111}In oxine as a random cellular label has made possible precise platelet kinetic and organ distribution studies.[19]

In 1988 the International Panel on Diagnostic Application of Radioisotopes in Hematology recommended the use of ^{111}In as a random label for platelets.[11] Platelet labeling with ^{111}In is possible at lower platelet counts than with ^{51}Cr.

This ^{111}In-oxine complex easily penetrates the cell membrane due to its lipophilic nature, and the ^{111}In label has been shown to possess great stability. The viability of the cells is reportedly not affected by the ^{111}In-oxine labeling procedure if care is taken to avoid cell damage during separation and washing procedures and labeling is carried out in the presence of plasma.

Since all cellular elements of the blood (red and white cells, leukocytes, and platelets) are labeled with ^{111}In oxine, platelets must first be separated by differential centrifugation before the ^{111}In-labeling complex is introduced. After incubation of platelets with the ^{111}In oxine, the unbound ^{111}In radioactivity has to be removed. For this purpose the cells are washed with plasma, centrifuged, and resuspended in fresh plasma.[17,18,20]

^{111}In has a 2.8-day half-life. Its gamma photon energies of 173 and 247 keV and their relatively high yield (84% and 94%, respectively) make quantitative external imaging of sites of platelet distribution and deposition, as well as precise determination of platelet survival, possible.

Clinical Application

^{111}In-labeled platelets are used for the study of platelet kinetics and for in vivo quantification of sites of platelet distribution and deposition. They have also been employed extensively in the investigation of thrombotic and vascular disorders and in monitoring the therapeutic effectiveness of platelet-active drugs in these conditions.

Platelet Survival Studies

The mean platelet survival time (MPST) in a normal person is 8 to 10 days. The normal recovery of the labeled platelets, that is, the percent of ^{111}In platelets in the circulation shortly after injection, is approximately 60%; the rest of the dose (about one third) accumulates in the splenic pool. To determine the mean platelet survival, multiple venous blood samples must be drawn. If a normal or nearly normal platelet life span can be expected, blood samples are obtained at 90 min after infusion and daily thereafter for 10 days. In patients with idiopathic thrombocytopenia (ITP) in which the MPST can be as short as 1 day or even less, blood samples have to be drawn much more frequently, for example at 10, 30, and 60 min after injection, then at 2-hr intervals until whole blood indium activity is approximately 10%.

The hematocrit value and platelet count are determined in each sample. Duplicate samples of 5 ml of whole blood, lysed with saponin, and 2 ml of platelet-free plasma (PFP) diluted with 3 ml of water are prepared for measurement of the radioactivity. Standards are made by adding 20 µl of the injectate to 5 ml of water. All samples are counted with less than 3% statistical error in a scintillation-detector system. The results are expressed as a percent of the injected dose in circulating platelets as follows:

$$\% \text{ Injected dose in circulating platelets} = \left[\frac{\text{cpm (1 ml WB)} - (\text{cpm [1 ml plasma]} \times \text{Plct})}{\text{cpm (Std)} \times \text{Dilution factor}} \right] \times (BV) \times (100)$$

where *cpm* is counts per minute, *Plct* is decimal plasmacrit (1.00 − decimal hematocrit), and *WB* is whole blood.

The data are then subjected to computer analysis. Several mathematical models have been proposed for formal curve fitting. Of these models, the maximum likelihood estimate of the interger-ordered gamma function is preferred.

[111]In-oxine–labeled white blood cells (WBC) are used routinely in nuclear medicine departments for imaging inflammatory lesions. Simple sedimentation techniques are routinely used to separate the WBC from the RBC. This technique yields a variety of labeled WBC, including polymorphs, lymphocytes, and monocytes. The mixed cell types cannot be used to study the kinetics of a specific cell type but are acceptable for abscess location. Detailed labeling techniques for WBC are outlined in Chapter 17.

ERYTHROKINETICS

Measurement of Circulating RBC Mass

The determination of RBC mass and plasma volume is based on the simple radioisotope dilution technique.[4] The larger the volume into which the label is mixed, the lower the counts in the sample withdrawn; conversely, the smaller the volume, the higher the counts in the sample. This dilution technique is true only if you are working with a closed system and no radiopharmaceutical is allowed to leak out of the system you are measuring. Also, the volume of the unknown must not change significantly during the measurement. RBC volume measurements are performed in a closed system using ^{51}Cr-labeled RBC.

Whole blood is collected by use of the appropriate anticoagulant in the correct ratio to the volume of whole blood. If citric acid, trisodium citrate, and dextrose (ACD)-NIH solution A or Strumia ACD solution is used, the ratio is 1:5. Because of the wide variance in the composition of the many citric acid, sodium citrate, sodium biphosphate, and dextrose (CPD) solutions, now judged to be at least as good and in some instances preferable, it is imperative to consult the manufacturer's recommendation as to the proper ratio of whole blood to CPD. Heparin and ethylenediaminetetraacetic acid (EDTA) are unsatisfactory for use in this procedure. There are several satisfactory methods, both for preparing the ^{51}Cr-labeled RBC and for performing the necessary measurements. We describe in detail the one we routinely use, but readers interested in other methods should refer to a publication of the International Panel on Diagnostic Applications of Radioisotopes in Haematology.[1]

[51]Cr is not an entirely ideal label for RBC mass measurements. Only 9% of its emissions are gamma rays; so one must inject a substantially larger amount of radioactivity to obtain statistically significant counting rates compared with an isotope having 100% gamma emission. Furthermore, the relatively long half-life of [51]Cr (27.8 days), coupled with its relatively slow rate (1% per day) of removal from circulating RBC, means that serial RBC volume measurements require undesirable increases in the amount of ^{51}Cr injected for each subsequent study. For these reasons labeling of RBC with ^{99m}Tc and trace amounts of stannous ion is a useful alternative method for measuring RBC mass.[7,8,12] [99m]Tc has a 6-hr half-life and for practical purposes can be considered a pure gamma-ray emitter. Therefore physically it is nearly ideal for RBC mass measurements. It can be used in amounts that greatly reduce the radiation dose to patients who undergo serial RBC mass measurements. Because of the more rapid loss of the ^{99m}Tc label, however, ^{51}Cr-labeled RBC should be used when sampling times for a single study must extend beyond 60 min after injection.

[51]Cr Ascorbic Acid Method for Labeling RBC

Ten ml of venous blood is withdrawn from the patient into a 20-ml syringe containing 2 ml of Strumia ACD formula and is transferred into a sterile 20-ml vial. About 30 µCi of ^{51}Cr in the form of chromate ion is added to the vial. A resultant prompt transport of 80% to 95% of the chromate ion across the RBC membrane occurs and binds to the beta chain of the hemoglobin molecule. During labeling within the RBC the hexavalent chromate ion is reduced to a trivalent chromic ion.

After 15 min of incubation, ascorbic acid (50 mg) is added to reduce the free chromate to chromic ion, which immediately stops the tagging procedure, since the chromic ion is unable to penetrate the RBC membrane.

Exactly 5 ml of the labeled blood is drawn into a syringe, and the remainder is kept to make a standard. The 5 ml is injected intravenously, with care taken not to infiltrate any of the dose. After adequate time to ensure complete mixing of the labeled RBC within the circulation, a sample is withdrawn from a vein other than that used for the injection. In normal subjects 10 min is sufficient to ensure complete mixing. However, in disease states like splenomegaly or severe polycythemia, mixing may be greatly delayed. In this case serial samples should be taken until there is no significant difference in their counts.

In other seriously ill patients a less pronounced delay of mixing may occur. For this reason the routine in our clinic is to wait 30 min to obtain the postinjection sample (with use of a heparinized syringe).

Hematocrit (Hct) value determinations are performed on the well-mixed standard and blood samples. Four counting tubes are prepared to contain 1-ml volumes of the following:

Whole blood from the standard = Std WB
Plasma from the standard = Std Plas
Whole blood from the sample = Samp WB
Plasma from the sample = Samp Plas

The standards and samples are counted in a well counter with the spectrometer centered about the 320 keV photopeak of ^{51}Cr and counted for sufficient time to ensure a counting accuracy of 1% error or less. Usually there are so few counts in the postinjection plasma sample that a shorter counting time is acceptable for this tube.

$$\text{RBC volume (ml)} = \frac{[\text{cpm Std WB} - (\text{cpm Std Plas} \times \text{Std Plct})] \times \text{Volume injected} \times \text{Samp Hct}}{[\text{cpm Samp WB} - (\text{cpm Samp Plas} \times \text{Samp Plct})]}$$

where *Plct* is decimal plasmacrit (1.00 − decimal hematocrit) and *Samp Hct* is decimal hematocrit of sample.

Falsely high results are found if a faulty intravenous injection technique is used, and the entire dose is not injected into a vein. Damaged RBC or excessive binding of the ^{51}Cr by WBC or platelets when these are abnormally elevated also yields spuriously high values. Falsely low values are caused by a failure to obtain a preinjection blood sample in a patient who has had previous administration of radioactive tracers. Contamination of equipment with radioactivity also yields spuriously low results.

The ^{51}Cr should not be added to the ACD solution

before the patient's blood is added to the vial. Dextrose contained in the ACD solution acts as a reducing agent.

For the measurement of circulating RBC mass, 10 μCi of ^{51}Cr is an adequate amount of activity and provides enough counts so that statistically significant sample counting can be performed in a reasonable time. The specific activity of the ^{51}Cr chromate must be such that less than 2 μg of chromium ion is present per milliliter of packed RBC. This becomes particularly critical when this technique is used for RBC survival studies that require larger doses of ^{51}Cr.

Plasma Volume

Iodinated human serum albumin is the conventional agent used for estimation of plasma volume. Albumin does not remain within the intravascular space but diffuses rapidly into extravascular compartments. Since this vascular space is now an open system, using the closed system isotope dilution principle for calculations causes errors in the plasma volume measurement. An extrapolation procedure can be used to calculate the volume if the injected tracer leaves the open system at a rate that is slow compared with the rate of mixing uniformly within that system, and samples are taken only after mixing has been completed.[22]

^{125}I-labeled human serum albumin is provided by radiopharmaceutical manufacturers in a concentration of 10 μCi per 1.5 ml. Not more than 2% of the radioactivity can be in the free form. The free form is removed from the intravascular space more rapidly than the labeled albumin, causing an overestimation of plasma volume. ^{99m}Tc-labeled albumin can also be used but must be 98% bound on injection.

The patient should be at rest or supine for at least 10 to 15 min before starting the study because plasma volume decreases when standing due to increased venous pressure in the legs, causing water to move from the intravascular to extravascular space.[22] It is recommended that thyroid blockage of radioiodine be performed at least 30 min before injection of the radiotracer by the oral administration of 5 drops (150 mg) of a supersaturated solution of sodium iodide (SSKI).

The dose of 10 μCi of ^{125}I-labeled human serum albumin is injected intravenously, with care being taken that it all enters the vein. Using a site different from the injection site, collect three timed heparinized samples of blood at 10, 20, and 30 min. These samples are centrifuged, and 1-ml aliquots of plasma are counted.

The radioactivity in each of these samples is measured and plotted against time on semilogarithmic paper (Figure 16-2). The best straight line is drawn through these points, with only the earlier points being used if the later points deviate from the initial linear slope. The zero-time activity is estimated by extrapolation and used for the calculation of the plasma vol-

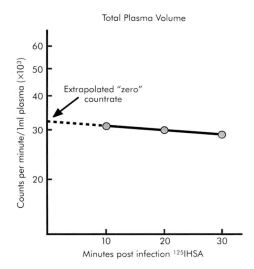

Total Plasma Volume

Figure 16-2 Extrapolation graph used to determine zero-time activity for the calculation of plasma volume.

Table 16-3	Normal blood volume compartment values (ml/kg)	
	Males	**Females**
Total blood volume	55-80	50-75
Red blood cell volume*	25-35	20-30
Plasma volume†	30-45	30-45

*95% confidence limits.
†Because of the many variables that may influence plasma volume in normal subjects, it is not possible to place confidence limits on these values.

ume. A standard is prepared and counted. All counts are performed with the spectrometer adjusted to count ^{125}I (20-50 keV) for a time long enough to ensure a 1% error or less. The plasma volume is calculated as follows:

$$\text{Plasma volume (ml)} = \frac{\text{Volume injected} \times \text{cpm in 1 ml Std} \times \text{dilution factor}}{\text{cpm of plasma sample obtained by extrapolation}}$$

Having precisely measured the RBC or plasma volume and knowing the venous hematocrit value, one can safely calculate the volume of the other compartment and thus estimate the total blood volume in normal subjects only. The reason is that in normal subjects there is a fixed relationship between the whole-body hematocrit (Hct_b) and the venous hematocrit (Hct_v); the ratio of Hct_b to Hct_v on the average is 0.90. It is believed that two factors are responsible for the difference observed between the Hct_b and Hct_v: (1) the hematocrit value of blood in small capillaries is lower than that found in larger vessels and (2) the iodinated albumin used to measure the plasma space is immediately distributed into a space larger than that of the vascular space in which the RBC are distributed.

It is important to recognize, however, that most of the patients referred to the clinical nuclear medicine service for measurement of either RBC volume or plasma volume are severely ill and the predictable normal relationship most likely will not be present in these individuals. For instance, in patients in whom there is moderate or gross splenomegaly, the ratio of Hct_b to Hct_v may be substantially and unpredictably increased to greater than 1; in patients with severe polycythemia, abnormalities may also be present in the plasma volume as well as in the RBC mass. Thus, in clinical circumstances total blood volume can be reliably esti-

mated only by doing simultaneous measurements of red cell mass and plasma volume.

A limitation in the interpretation of these studies is that normal values for blood volume in any given individual cannot be simply predicted from such parameters as height and weight despite the many elaborate formulas that have been proposed. In interpreting studies in adults, the simplest method of calculating the values in milliliters per kilogram is probably at least as reliable as using any of the various formulas or nomograms. The normal values published by the International Panel on Standardization in Haematology are shown in Table 16-3. Note the wide range in plasma volume observed in normal subjects; this immediately tells us that this is less than a precise test. The undesirable rapid diffusion of the radiolabeled albumin from the vascular space is but one factor making this procedure less than precise, even in normal subjects. Body position, recent exercise, and a number of other factors cause rapid significant changes in plasma volume. Therefore although we can precisely measure the circulating RBC mass, it is best always to report the plasma volume as estimated.

Other factors seen in patients referred for study, such as obesity, recent weight loss, and prolonged bed rest, may make it impossible to estimate the RBC and plasma volume solely from height and weight measurements in a given patient. Since RBC mass is related to lean body mass, patients who are exceptionally obese or have had recent significant weight loss should have their measured values compared with those based on ideal or recent body weight.

There are several specific circumstances in which blood volume measurements have proved to be of considerable value. The use of ^{51}Cr-labeled RBC to measure the RBC mass allows a precise determination as to whether true polycythemia is present or whether the patient has an elevated hematocrit because of a reduced plasma volume. Hematologists see several patients each year because of a persistent elevation of the hematocrit, but the RBC mass is normal when this is measured by the ^{51}Cr technique. Usually these are normal subjects whose RBC mass is near the upper limits of normal and whose plasma volume is near the lower limits of normal. The performance of this one, simple, relatively inexpensive test, proving that they have a normal red blood cell mass, saves these patients an elaborate, expensive, and prolonged series of other diagnostic procedures.

Patients with polycythemia vera and myelofibrosis may have a pronounced expansion of their plasma volume, which is apparent only if this parameter is directly measured. Because of the combined abnormality of plasma volume and red cells, serial measurements of both the RBC and plasma volume may become essential to the management of patients with polycythemia vera. In these circumstances availability of ^{99m}Tc RBC becomes invaluable.

Paradoxically, in the acutely hemorrhaging patient or patient with recent severe trauma, the hematocrit may remain normal or disproportionally high for some time. In this circumstance direct measurement with ^{51}Cr-labeled RBC will reveal the true RBC mass of the patient.

Erythrocyte Survival and Splenic Sequestration Studies

RBC are labeled by use of the same technique as in the RBC volume determination with the exception that the dose of ^{51}Cr is adjusted to 1.5 μCi/kg of body weight. After labeling, the cells are reinjected and the first sample is obtained 24 hr later (to permit removal from the circulation of any cells accidentally damaged during the labeling procedure; during this same interval, any injected plasma radioactivity is cleared from the cir-

culation). Samples are then obtained every other day for the next 3 weeks; a 6-ml sample of blood is withdrawn and placed into a tube containing an anticoagulant (preferably solid EDTA or concentrated heparin).

Five milliliters of whole blood is pipetted from the tubes as it is collected. (To ensure thorough mixing, tubes should be inverted 12 to 15 times before samples are pipetted and hematocrit values are determined.)

Hematocrit determinations are made on each sample on the day of collection. Next, a tiny amount of saponin powder is added to each tube, and they are again gently tilted several times to ensure mixing and complete lysis of the RBC. Care is taken not to allow the sample to touch the cap of the counting tube.

On the last day of the study, all the samples are counted on the gamma spectrometer with settings of 280-360 keV for ^{51}Cr.

The samples are counted to give a sample error of 1% or less (for approximately 10 min each).

To calculate the half-time of disappearance of the labeled RBC, net counts per minute of each sample are plotted on semilogarithmic paper as a function of time (Figure 16-3). The best straight line is drawn through all the points. The $t_{1/2}$ is obtained as follows: extrapolate the line to time zero. This is the y intercept. Divide the y intercept value by 2. At this value on the y axis, draw a straight line parallel to the x axis until it intersects the best straight line drawn through the observed data points. Drop a perpendicular line to the x axis. This is the labeled RBC half-time disappearance rate or survival time as measured by the ^{51}Cr technique, not corrected for elution of the isotope.

Occasionally one encounters patients whose data do not permit a satisfactory "eye fit" of a single straight line

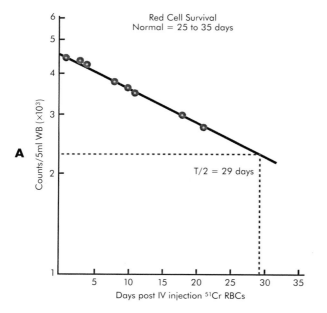

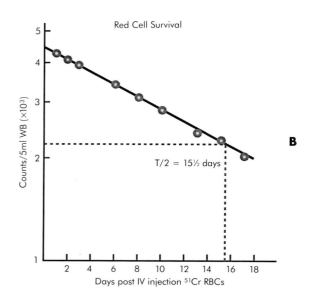

Figure 16-3 Red cell survival graph showing normal $t_{1/2}$ of 29 days (**A**) compared with an abnormal $t_{1/2}$ (**B**) indicating a hemolytic process causing shortened survival of chromium-51–labeled erythrocytes.

to the data points. The International Panel on Diagnostic Applications of Radioisotopes in Haematology's publication on RBC survival studies[2] describes alternative methods, including computer programs for handling such data. Now that most clinical nuclear medicine laboratories have one or more dedicated computers, it is suggested that the appropriate programs be added to their software for use as needed.

The mean half-life of normal ^{51}Cr-labeled RBC is 25 to 35 days. Normal RBC are removed from the circulation when they become senescent at a rate approximating 1% per day; the true mean life span of the normal RBC therefore is between 50 and 60 days. However, this approximately 1% per day removal of senescent RBC from the circulation coupled with the approximately 1% per day elution of the ^{51}Cr label from the RBC combine to give the mean half of 25 to 35 days when measured with this technique. Tables are available for correcting for this elution, but they were derived from studies in normal subjects, and their relevance in disease states where the elution rate is known to vary is uncertain. However, the more severe the hemolytic process or bleeding and thus the more rapid the rate of removal of the ^{51}Cr-labeled RBC, the less significant this ^{51}Cr elution becomes.

Determination of the mean RBC life span from a label randomly applied to cells of all ages is meaningful only in a patient who is in a steady state with regard to the rate of production and destruction of RBC. If either of these rates changes, the mean age of the circulating RBC will be changed and will affect the ^{51}Cr results, even though the actual longevity of each individual RBC has not changed. A constant hematocrit value before and during the period of study is one index of a steady state. Obviously, inaccurate results will be obtained in a patient who is being or has recently been transfused.

The study of splenic sequestration should be a routine part of any ^{51}Cr-RBC survival study. Organ counting is begun 24 hr after labeled cells are reinjected and continued approximately every other day for the next 3 weeks.

The counting probe should be equipped with a flat-field collimator designed to exclude radiation from areas other than the organs of interest but still permit sampling of a large enough organ volume to give adequate count rates. The spectrometer is adjusted to count gamma rays from 280-360 keV.

Place the patient on the examining table in the positions as follows:

Precordium: The detector is centered over the left third intercostal interspace at the sternal border, with the patient in the *supine* position.

Liver: The detector is placed over the ninth and tenth ribs on the right, in the midclavicular line with patient in the *supine* position. In elderly subjects and patients with chronic obstructive pulmonary disease, the exact location of the liver should be checked by percussion.

Spleen: The detector is placed two thirds the distance from the spinous process to the lateral edge of the body at the level of the ninth and tenth ribs, with the patient in the *prone* position.

The skin is marked with indelible ink, which in turn is covered by transparent nonallergenic tape to indicate the position of the external detector from one day to the next. Each area must be counted with the same geometry each time by having the detector touch the patient's skin. The areas are counted to give a sample error of 5% or less.

The results are expressed as the ratio of the count rate over the spleen to the count rate over the precordium. The count rate over the liver is also expressed relative to the count rate over the precordium. These ratios are graphed as a function of time on linear graph paper (Figure 16-4).

In normal subjects the spleen-to-liver ratio is less than or may approximate 1:1. In patients with active splenic sequestration of cells, this ratio often rises to 2:1 or even to 4:1. The spleen-to-precordium ratio is judged to be clearly abnormal if the ratio is greater than 2:1. An initial and persistent elevation of spleen-to-precordium ratio is attributable to increased splenic blood pool. A progressive gradual increase indicates active sequestration of the labeled cells.

Sources of Error

Sources of error include the following:

1. Inaccurate probe positioning will cause spurious results.
2. Blood loss from the gastrointestinal tract or surgical sites will cause a shortened half-life.
3. Blood transfusions during the procedure will also cause an apparent shortening of the half-life (by increasing the volume of the unlabeled cells).

Obviously, neither 2 nor 3 will affect the outcome of the splenic sequestration study and therefore do not warrant discontinuing the test, unless the hemorrhage is truly massive, leaving an insignificant amount of circulating radioactivity.

Quantitation of Blood Loss

Occult blood loss is difficult to demonstrate with sensitivity and specificity. Over the years, many methods of stool collection, homogenation, and counting have been devised by a great number of technologists to make this procedure more esthetic. Our current procedure has been demonstrated to be sensitive, specific, and acceptable to the technical staff. RBC are labeled as in the RBC survival and sequestration study and returned to the patient intravenously. The patient is instructed to collect all stools for 4 days in clean paint cans and to avoid contaminating the collection with urine. Five milliliters of concentrated phenol in water

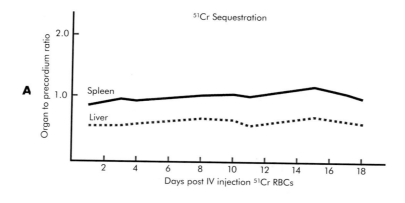

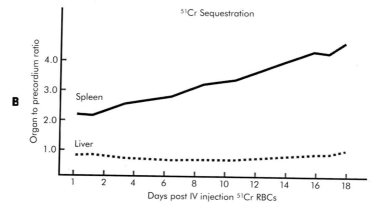

Figure 16-4 Organ localization of chromium-51–labeled erythrocytes. **A,** Normal liver-to-precordium and spleen-to-precordium ratios are depicted compared with increasing spleen-to-precordium ratios, **B,** showing active splenic sequestration.

is added to the stool collections as they arrive in the lab. The total weight of the can containing the fecal specimen and phenol is then brought to 2 kg by the addition of tap water, and the lid is tightly shut on the can. The stool is homogenized in the can by shaking the can on a commercial paint shaker for about 10 min. Blood samples are drawn on the first and third days and counted with identical geometry and compared with the counts of the homogenized stool samples for determination of blood loss.

$$\frac{\text{Total net cpm in 24-hr stool}}{\text{Net cpm in 1 ml of WB}} = \text{Blood loss (ml)}$$

Normal values are 1.2 ± 0.5 ml with a range of 0.3-2.8 ml/24 hr. Any blood in the stools in excess of this amount suggests enteric blood loss.

In Vivo Cross Matching

There are rare instances when blood banks are unable to identify a satisfactory donor for a patient requiring transfusion.[4] In these unusual circumstances, the use of chromium-labeled *donor* RBC to do an in vivo cross match may provide a life-saving service.

The general principle is to infuse the patient with no more than 1 ml of donor cells after they have been labeled with ^{51}Cr. Carefully timed serial blood samples are then taken from the recipient at 3, 10, and 60 min, and both whole blood and plasma radioactivity are measured in the samples. The technique follows.

Using a sterile technique, add 50 μCi of sodium ^{51}Cr chromate to 5 ml of the donor blood in a sterile test tube. Invert this mixture gently several times to ensure proper mixing and allow to incubate for 15 min at room temperature with occasional inverting. Centrifuge the tube and aseptically withdraw the supernatant plasma using an 18-gauge spinal needle. Fill the tube with sterile isotonic saline and centrifuge as before, after having gently inverted the tube several times. Repeat the washing procedure, and then resuspend the cells in isotonic saline to the initial volume. Draw 1 ml of the ^{51}Cr-tagged washed cells into a 3-ml syringe, and keep the remaining labeled cells to make a standard.

Technique and Sample Preparation

Determine a hematocrit value on the 3-min sample and pipette 1 ml of whole blood from each of the blood samples into the tubes, then label. Centrifuge the remaining whole blood from the 10- and 60-min samples and pipette 1 ml of the plasma into the tubes, then label. Pipette 2 ml of labeled whole blood from the dose tube into a 100-ml volumetric flask containing 50-60 ml of distilled water. The volume in the flask is then filled to the mark with water and mixed. Pipette a 1-ml sample from the flask into counting tubes, and label. All samples are then counted in a well counter with spectrometer settings for ^{51}Cr (280-360 keV) and count for a sufficient time to give a counting accuracy of 1% error or less.

Interpretation. Estimated RBC mass is obtained from tables based on the sex, body weight, and venous hematocrit value of the recipient. The predicted RBC mass is compared with the calculated value by use of the 3-min sample.

$$\text{Red blood cell mass (ml)} = \frac{\substack{\text{Volume injected} \times \text{cpm in 1-ml Std} \\ \times \text{Dilution factor} \times \text{Samp Hct}}}{\text{cpm of 1-ml blood sample at 3 min}}$$

If there has not been immediate removal of a significant portion of the donor RBC from the circulation, the estimated and the calculated RBC masses should be the same order of magnitude.

When compatible RBC have been injected, about 99% of the radioactivity in the 3-min whole-blood sample is found in the 60-min sample (range: 94% to 104%) and no radioactivity is seen in any of the plasma samples. In cases of urgency or when there is great difficulty in finding completely compatible RBC, donor cells may be transfused with minimal hazard when 70% of the radioactivity in the 3-min sample is found in the 60-min sample and the amount of radioactivity in the 10- and 60-min plasma samples is less than 5% of the radioactivity injected.

MEASUREMENT OF ABSORPTION AND SERUM LEVELS OF ESSENTIAL NUTRIENTS

Vitamin B₁₂ (Cyanocobalamin) Absorption

Nuclear medicine has furnished important tools for the diagnosis of vitamin B_{12} deficiency. The consequences of untreated vitamin B_{12} deficiency include anemia, thrombocytopenia, leukopenia, crippling spinal cord degeneration, and death.

The importance of measuring vitamin B_{12} absorption in patients with unexplained anemia deserves emphasis, since the principle that anemia is not a disease per se but only a symptom of some underlying disorder is not always reflected in practice. The onset of clinical symptoms from vitamin B_{12} deficiency is noto-

Table 16-4	Causes of vitamin B_{12} deficiency

1. Inadequate intake
2. Malabsorption
    A. Caused by gastric abnormalities
        1. Absence of the intrinsic factor
            a. Congenital
            b. Addisonian pernicious anemia
            c. Total gastrectomy
            d. Subtotal gastrectomy
        2. Excessive excretion of hydrochloric acid: Zollinger-Ellison syndrome
    B. Caused by intestinal malabsorption
        1. Destruction, removal, or functional incompetence of ileal mucosal absorptive sites
        2. Competition with host for available dietary vitamin B_{12}
            a. *Diphyllobothrium latum* (fish tapeworm)
            b. Small bowel lesions associated with stagnation and bacterial overgrowth (such as jejunal diverticula, strictures, blind loops)
        3. Drug therapy*
            a. Para-aminosalicylic acid (PAS)
            b. Neomycin
            c. Colchicine
            d. Calcium-chelating agents
    C. Caused by genetic abnormality in the transport protein transcobalamin II

*Although any of these agents may produce abnormalities in vitamin B_{12} absorption, only patients on long-term PAS therapy have been reported to develop clinical evidence of vitamin B_{12} deficiency.

riously insidious, and the initial complaints of the patients are often vague; in the early stages the classic RBC changes are not present.

Table 16-4 summarizes the causes of vitamin B_{12} deficiency. Table 16-5 summarizes factors important in vitamin B_{12} nutrition and absorption in humans. The absorption of this vitamin through the terminal ileum depends on secretion by the stomach of the intrinsic factor, which exists as a dimer and binds two molecules of B_{12}. The intrinsic factor does not in itself get absorbed at the sites in the terminal ileum but is required in an active transport mechanism. Ionic calcium and a pH of ileal contents greater than 6 are also required. Once absorption takes place, a normal transport protein transcobalamin II must be present in the bloodstream to convey the B_{12} to areas of the body for utilization or storage.

Isolated "pure" (apart from severe prolonged protein deprivation) dietary deficiency is very rare. Therefore the overwhelming number of cases of vitamin B_{12} deficiency are caused by some underlying disorder at-

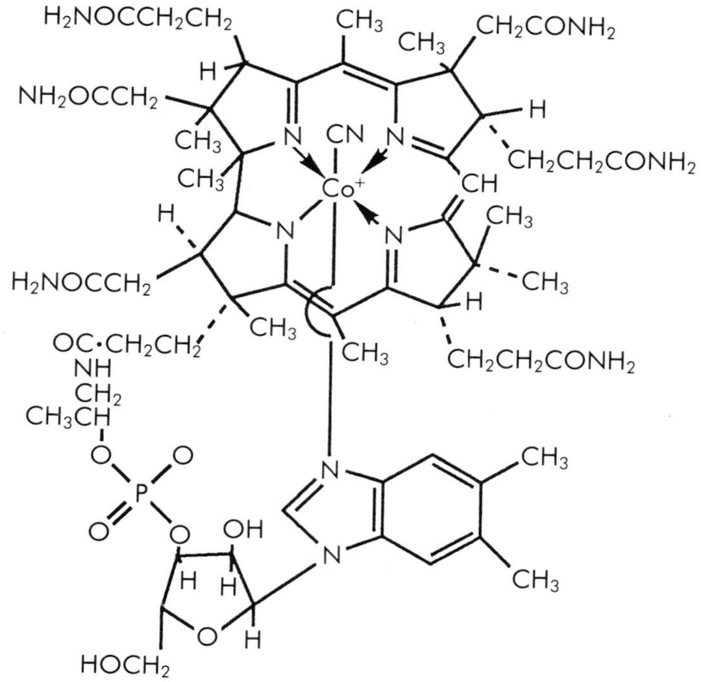

Figure 16-5 Structure of cyanocobalamin, the most widely administered form of vitamin B_{12}.

Table 16-5	Absorption of dietary vitamin B_{12} in humans*

1. Available for human nutrition only in animal food sources.
2. Vitamin B_{12} is bound to the intrinsic factor by the gastric mucosa.
3. Normal ileal mucosal absorptive sites depend on the presence of ionic Ca^{2+} and on the pH of ileal contents of more than 6.
4. Normal transport protein (transcobalamin II) conveys vitamin B_{12} from ileal absorptive sites to areas of active utilization and storage.

*The same factors apply to the absorption of tracer amounts of radioactive vitamin B_{12} used in absorption studies.

tributable to malabsorption. The most common cause of vitamin B_{12} malabsorption is a deficiency in the intrinsic factor, a protein secreted by the parietal cells of the stomach, which is an obligatory requirement for normal vitamin B_{12} absorption by the terminal ileum.

The availability of radioactive vitamin B_{12} for specific testing of a patient's ability to absorb physiologic amounts of this essential nutrient has been a great clinical value. Vitamin B_{12} is a complex corrinoid compound (Figure 16-5), the central ligand of which is cobalt; several radioactive isotopes of cobalt are available.

The earliest in use was ^{60}Co, but ^{57}Co and ^{58}Co are now preferred for routine clinical studies because of their shorter half-lives and smaller radiation doses (Table 16-6). The Schilling test of urinary excretion is generally accepted as the standard method of measuring absorption of radioactive vitamin B_{12}. This test requires (1) the oral administration and retention of a tracer dose of vitamin B_{12} (it is important that this oral dose be in the range of 0.25-2 µg, a quantity similar to one that might be present in a normal meal, because quantities above this level may be absorbed by mechanisms not dependent on the intrinsic factor) and (2) a transient saturation of normal binding sites in the plasma that is achieved by injection of a flushing dose of 1 mg of nonradioactive vitamin B_{12}.

Patients may drink water before and after the test; however, they should have nothing to eat after midnight on the day before the test and should remain fasting for 2 hr after the oral dose of ^{57}Co vitamin B_{12}. The patient's physician should be instructed not to give enemas or laxatives or schedule the patient for a barium enema or intravenous pyelogram for the duration of this study. The patient should be questioned before the dose is given regarding the medications that may interfere with the results: vitamin B_{12} injections, colchicine corticosteroids, and ACTH. Because of hepatobiliary recirculation, it is theoretically possible to block all the absorptive sites (in the terminal ileum) if large (1 mg or greater) daily doses of vitamin B_{12} are being administered. If the patient has normal renal function,

---

Table 16-6   Characteristics of selected radioisotopes of cobalt

Isotope	Physical half-life	Effective half-life in liver*	Radiation	Principal photon energies (meV)	Relative dose to liver
^{57}Co	270 days	161 days	Electron capture	0.122 (87%)	1†
^{58}Co	72 days	60 days	Electron capture, β^+, γ	0.810 (99%) 0.511 (30%)	2
^{60}Co	5.2 years	331 days	β^-, γ	1.17 (100%) 1.33 (100%)	29

Compiled from McIntyre PA. In *Textbook of nuclear medicine: clinical applications*, Philadelphia, 1979, Lea & Febiger; adapted from Rosenblum C: In Heinrich HC, ed: *Vitamin B-12 und Intrinsic Factor. 2. Europäisches Symposium über Vitamin B-12 und Intrinsic Factor*, Hamburg, 1961, Stuttgart, 1961, Ferdinand Encke Verlag, p. 306.
*Assuming a biologic half-life of 400 days after administration as radioactive cobalt-labeled vitamin B_{12}.
†Approximately 0.051 rad per 0.5 μCi of ^{57}Co-labeled vitamin when parenteral dose of 1 mg of vitamin B_{12} is given, resulting in renal excretion of approximately 30% of the absorbed dose of radioactive vitamin B_{12}.

Table 16-7   Representative results of schilling test using two 24-hr urine collections (single nuclide without intrinsic factor)

Patient	First 24-hr urine			Second 24-hr urine		
	Volume	Specific gravity	% of dose excreted	Volume	Specific gravity	% of dose excreted
A	640	1.010	3.0	1230	1.010	0.8
B	1210	1.012	3.0	1120	1.012	0.8
C	1200	1.010	3.0	1150	1.010	3.0
D (normal)	1210	1.012	14.0	1200	1.012	0.3

Patient A had an incomplete first 24-hr urine collection because of inadvertent loss of urine during cleansing enemas.
Patient B subsequently had normal excretion when the test was repeated with the addition of a potent intrinsic factor. Other studies confirmed the diagnosis of addisonian pernicious anemia.
Patient C was recognized on reexamination to have benign prostatic hypertrophy with significant bladder retention. The delayed pattern of excretion of the radioactive vitamin B_{12} was the first clinical indication of this condition.
Patient D was a cooperative, normal volunteer.

---

however, all excess vitamin B_{12} is promptly excreted in the urine and the test needs to be delayed only 24 to 48 hr after discontinuing the vitamin B_{12} injections.

If the patient has previously been given radioactive materials, a 24-hr urine collection is obtained for background. The dose of 0.5 μCi of ^{57}Co vitamin B_{12} is administered orally, and 2 hr later 1 mg of stable vitamin B_{12} is given intramuscularly. Two 24-hr urine collections are obtained, one for each 24-hr period. The patient is instructed to collect all urine during this period and avoid losing any urine during defecation.

The total volume and specific gravity of each 24-hr collection is measured. The urine samples and a standard are counted in a well counter with the spectrometer set to count gamma rays from 105-145 keV.

% of ^{57}Co vitamin B_{12} in 24-hr urine =

$$\frac{\text{cpm in urine} \times \dfrac{\text{Urine volume}}{\text{Sample volume}} \times 100}{\text{cpm in Std} \times \text{Dilution factor}}$$

Malabsorption of vitamin B_{12} can be documented by the appearance of less than 9% of the administered dose in the first 24-hr urine collection.

The major problem with this test is its dependence on a complete 24-hr urine collection. The loss of just one urine specimen may cause falsely low results. The 24-hr test also requires that urinary function be intact. Erroneously low values result from abnormal urinary retention, as in men with benign prostatic hypertrophy or in patients with renal disease. In such patients the amount excreted in the first 24 hr is reduced, but significant radioactivity continues to be excreted for the next 24 to 48 hr; total excretion will eventually be within normal limits. For this reason and because it often indicates when the first 24-hr collection was incomplete, our routine is to have the patient collect two separate 24-hr urine specimens after the single flushing dose. We measure volume, specific gravity, and the percent of the administered dose of radioactivity separately in each 24-hr specimen. Table 16-7 gives some typical patient results and illustrates the value of this minor modification of the Schilling test.

If less than 6% of the dose is excreted in 24 hr, a stage II Schilling test should be performed with 10 mg of the intrinsic factor given along with the ^{57}Co-labeled vitamin B_{12}. About 3 to 7 days must elapse before the stage II test. A normal urinary excretion value after the administration of the intrinsic factor occurs in intrinsic factor deficiency.

Several factors can contribute to a false-negative stage II Schilling test. When both the radioactive vitamin B_{12} and the intrinsic factor are given in separate capsules, there can be incomplete binding of the two in the stomach. Before administration the radioactive vitamin B_{12} and the intrinsic factor should be mixed together in water.[16] If hog intrinsic factor is used, a negative result does not completely rule out intrinsic factor–dependent malabsorption. Some patients who have previously been exposed to hog intrinsic factor (as present in many multivitamin preparations) may have antibodies against it. Vitamin B_{12} deficiency can produce small bowel megaloblastosis with atrophy, which can cause ileal malabsorption. Vitamin B_{12} therapy may be necessary to allow the ileum to heal before performing a stage II study.[10]

If it is determined that the stage II study is truly abnormal, other causes of malabsorption must be determined and treated if possible, followed by another stage I Schilling test.

Dual-isotope method for measuring vitamin B_{12} absorption. The conventional Schilling test for vitamin B_{12} absorption is done in two stages, requiring at least 1 week for a final result if stage I is abnormal. A dual-isotope method is available in which vitamin B_{12} labeled with two different isotopes of cobalt is administered. One form, ^{57}Co vitamin B_{12}, is bound to the intrinsic factor by prior incubation with normal human gastric juice, and the other contains non-protein–bound ^{58}Co vitamin B_{12}.

The two capsules are ingested orally by a fasting patient followed by the flushing injection of 1 mg of nonradioactive vitamin B_{12}. Two 24-hr urine samples are collected. Differential isotope counting is then performed to determine the percent of administered dose of each isotope that has been excreted in the urine. A patient with normal vitamin B_{12} absorption excretes equal amounts of both isotopes, whereas a patient lacking the intrinsic factor excretes greater quantities of intrinsic factor–bound ^{57}Co vitamin B_{12}. In patients with bacterial overgrowth or bowel lesions resulting in vitamin B_{12} malabsorption, both isotopes are excreted in abnormally low quantities.

The dual-isotope Schilling test has several advantages over the conventional method. The advantage of taking only 2 days compared with 1 week to obtain results leads to earlier diagnosis and treatment and saves

money. The use of ^{57}Co vitamin B_{12} bound to human gastric juice eliminates the use of hog intrinsic factor preparations, against which some patients may have developed antibodies.

Although the same conditions in the patient for comparing the absorption of free and bound vitamin B_{12} are present in this method, small bowel changes caused by vitamin B_{12} deficiency are not considered. The absorption of the ^{57}Co vitamin B_{12} bound to gastric juice will be falsely low, along with a low ^{58}Co vitamin B_{12} absorption. This leads to a false-negative result.[9]

Serum vitamin B_{12} assays. The first assay for vitamin B_{12} was introduced in the early 1950s and employed the microorganisms *Lactobacillus leichmannii* and *Euglena gracilis*. The rate of growth of these organisms in the appropriate media is directly related to the concentration of vitamin B_{12} in the sample added. An assessment of organism growth thus provides an estimate of vitamin B_{12} concentration. These methods were tedious and time consuming, and antibiotics introduced in the patient's sample interfered with the assay.

In the early 1960s the first radioisotopic dilution assay was introduced using competitive protein-binding principles. Competition between radioactive and nonradioactive vitamin B_{12} for the binding sites on the protein-purified intrinsic factor occurs, followed by separation of the protein-bound vitamin B_{12} from the free vitamin. The accuracy of these first radioassays for serum levels of vitamin B_{12} was questioned for several years. In the late 1970s Cooper and Whitehead reported that 10% to 20% of patients diagnosed with pernicious anemia had normal serum B_{12} levels using these assays.[6] At the same time studies by Kolhouse[13] showed that the intrinsic factor used in these assays contained contaminants called R-proteins, which can bind to biologically inactive vitamin B_{12} analogs, causing erroneously elevated levels in vitamin B_{12} deficient patients.

In 1980 the National Committee for Clinical Laboratory Standards (NCCLS) under direction from the FDA published standards for each manufacturer and laboratory to follow to validate their assay and ensure correct measurement of serum vitamin B_{12} levels. Today serum vitamin B_{12} radioassays using competitive protein-binding techniques are still in widespread use. A highly purified intrinsic factor is used as the binder. Recently an enzymatic nonisotopic-binding protein assay for measuring serum vitamin B_{12} levels was reported to be equal to the conventional competitive protein-binding radioassay.[21]

Serum vitamin B_{12} levels, when performed by a reliable assay, are an early indicator of vitamin B_{12} deficiency falling before macrocytosis, megaloblastic changes, or neuropathy occurs.[15]

Even though current assays are reliable, normal results obtained in any patient who otherwise has clinical evidence suggestive of vitamin B_{12} deficiency should be confirmed by a radioactive vitamin B_{12} absorption study. A single injection of vitamin B_{12} results in a normal serum value that can persist for many weeks, despite the patient's inability to absorb dietary vitamin B_{12}.

Anti-intrinsic factor–blocking antibodies. The most common cause of vitamin B_{12} malabsorption is due to pernicious anemia. Approximately 51% to 76% of affected patients have anti-intrinsic factor–blocking antibodies in their serum.[5] A diagnosis of pernicious anemia can be made if these antibodies are present.

Blocking antibodies interfere with the formation of the intrinsic factor–B_{12} complex in the stomach. A commercially available assay for measuring blocking antibodies uses a highly purified intrinsic factor covalently bound to microscopic glass particles. Blocking antibody in the patient's serum combines with the intrinsic factor to form a solid phase complex. This complex is separated from endogenous B_{12} binding proteins by centrifugation before the addition of ^{57}Co B_{12}.

The blocking antibodies prevent binding of the tracer to the intrinsic factor. A second centrifugation step separates the bound complex from the free ligand. The presence of blocking antibodies in serum is extremely suggestive of pernicious anemia. The combination of megaloblastic anemia, low serum vitamin B_{12} levels, and serum-blocking antibodies to the intrinsic factor is diagnostic of pernicious anemia.

Serum Folate Assay

Serum folate concentrations were traditionally measured microbiologically using *Lactobacillus casei*. As with vitamin B_{12} microbiologic methods, these assays were tedious, time consuming, and inhibited by antibiotics present in blood specimens. A competitive protein-binding (CPB) assay of serum folate, with use of a folate-binding protein (β-lactoglobulin) present in cow's milk, has been developed and forms the basis for commercially available kits. Commercial folate CPB assays vary in selection of folate form for use as standards, folate form for tracer, and in methods utilized in denaturing endogenous folate binders.[14]

Since serum folate deficiency can be caused by several mechanisms, including vitamin B_{12} deficiency, and serum levels respond quickly to dietary intake of folate, RBC folate levels are a much better indicator of folate stores. Folate is incorporated into RBC during their formation and remains there during their life span. Serum folate and RBC folate levels are both low in folate deficiency megaloblastic anemia; red cell folate levels are also low in vitamin B_{12} deficiency. Since serum folate levels can be either elevated or normal in vitamin B_{12} deficiency, it is necessary to measure both before diagnosing folate deficiency. RBC folate and serum vitamin

B_{12} levels reflect the status of tissue stores. The serum folate level reflects fluctuations due to intake and changes in body demand.[17]

The most important recent development in the folate radioassay was its combination with the vitamin B_{12} radioassay into a simultaneous procedure. Since both assays are routinely requested on the same patient sample, this combination reduces performance time by half, thus lowering the cost of folate and vitamin B_{12} assays. Mixtures of ^{57}Co cyanocobalamin and ^{125}I folate are used as the tracers, mixtures of folic acid and vitamin B_{12} are used as standards, and a mixture of the intrinsic factor and milk-binding protein is used as binders. The assays can be simultaneously counted in a dual-channel gamma counter with the appropriate window settings.

Serum Ferritin Assays

Ferritin is an iron-binding protein that contains virtually all of the soluble iron stores in the body. Serum ferritin concentrations in normal subjects parallel the body iron stores; levels reflect iron deficiency and iron overload states and are clinically useful in the diagnosis and management of patients with these disorders. Serum ferritin measurements are a useful screening test for early iron deficiency and can be substituted for a bone marrow biopsy.

Serum ferritin assays utilize immunoradiometric techniques employing the ^{125}I-labeled antibody and a second antibody attached to a solid support. This two-site principle involves sandwiching the ferritin (either in patient sample or standard) molecule between the two antibodies generated against different portions of the ferritin molecule. As the concentration of ferritin increases, the amount of radioactivity increases in direct proportion. This technique allows accurate laboratory measurements of body iron stores over a wide concentration range.

Serum ferritin levels must be interpreted with caution because the direct relationship between serum ferritin and iron stores is not always reliable. Disorders that cause a disproportionate elevation in ferritin levels include liver disease, anemia of chronic disease, and disorders associated with increased or abnormal erythropoiesis.

REFERENCES

1. Belcher EH, Berlin NI, Dudley RA, et al: Recommended methods for measurement of red cell and plasma volume, *J Nucl Med* 21:793-800, 1980.
2. Belcher EH, Berlin NI, Dudley RA, et al: Recommended methods for radioisotope red-cell survival studies, *Br J Haematol* 21:241-250, 1971.

3. Belcher EH, Berlin NI, Eernisse JG, et al: Recommended methods for radioisotope platelet survival studies by the panel, *Blood* 50:1137-1144, 1977.

4. Belcher EH, Berlin NI, Eernisse JG, et al: Standard techniques for the measurement of red cell and plasma volume, *Br J Haematol* 25:801-814, 1973.

5. Chanarin I: *The megaloblastic anaemias*, ed 2, Oxford, 1979, Blackwell.

6. Cooper BA, Whitehead VM: Evidence that some patients with pernicious anemia are not recognized by radiodilution assay for cobalamin in serum, *N Engl J Med* 299:816-818, 1978.

7. Ducassou D, Arnaud D, Bardy A, et al: A new stannous agent list for labeling red blood cells with ^{99m}Tc and its clinical application, *Br J Radiol* 49:344-347, 1979.

8. Eckelman W, Richards P, Hausen W, et al: Technetium-labeled red blood cells, *J Nucl Med* 12:22-24, 1971.

9. Fairbanks JF, Wahner HW: Clinical interpretation of the DICOPAC test of B_{12} absorption, *Nucl Med Communications* 5:47-51, 1984.

10. Haurani FI, Sherwood N, Goldstein F: Intestinal malabsorption of vitamin B_{12} in pernicious anemia, *Metabolism* 13:1342-1348, 1964.

11. International Committee for standardization in hematology panel on diagnostic applications of radionuclide (ICSH), *J Nucl Med* 4:564-566, 1988.

12. Jones J, Mollison PL: A simple and efficient method of labelling red cells with ^{99m}Tc for determination of red cell volume, *Br J Haematol* 38:141, 1978.

13. Kolhouse JF, Kondo H, Allen NC: Cobalamin analogues are present in human plasma and can mask cobalamin deficiency because current radioisotope dilution assays are not specific for true cobalamin, *N Engl J Med* 299:785-792, 1978.

14. Kubasik NP, Volosin MT, Sine HE: Comparison of commercial kits for radioimmunoassay: III: radioassay of serum folate, *Clin Chem* 21:1922-1926, 1975.

15. Lindenbaum J: Status of laboratory testing in the diagnosis of megaloblastic anemia, *Blood* 4:624-627, 1983.

16. McDonald JW, Barr RM, Barton WB: Spurious Schilling test results obtained with intrinsic factor enclosed in capsules, *Ann Intern Med* 83:827-829, 1975.

17. Nickoloff EL, Drew H, Hagan J: *In vitro techniques: radionuclides in haematology*, London, 1986, Churchill Livingstone.

18. Scheffel U, Tsan MF, McIntyre PA: Labeling of human platelets with (^{111}In)-8-hydroxyquinoline, *J Nucl Med* 20:524-531, 1979.

19. Scheffel U, Tsan MF, Mitchell TG, et al: Human platelets labeled with In-111-8-hydroxyquinoline: kinetics, distribution, and estimates of radiation dose, *J Nucl Med* 23:149-156, 1982.

20. Tsan MF, Hill-Zobel RL: Should platelets be radio labelled in plasma medicine? *Am J Hemat* 25:355-359, 1987.

21. Vander Weide J, Homan HC, Rheenen EC, et al: Nonisotopic binding assay for measuring vitamin B_{12} and folate in serum, *Clin Chem* 5:766-768, 1992.

22. Wright RR, Tno M, Pollycove M: Blood volume, *Semin Nucl Med* 5:63-77, 1975.

David F. Preston

Inflammatory Process and Tumor Imaging

Objectives

Discuss the pathogenesis of cancer cells.

Discuss the formation and pathogenesis of an abscess.

Describe the properties of carrier-free gallium citrate and its biodistribution.

Describe the technical considerations and instrumentation used for gallium imaging.

Explain the labeling methods for white cells using indium-111.

Describe the imaging techniques for performing indium-111 white blood cell scans.

Describe the principles of imaging using radiolabeled antibodies.

Describe PET imaging in oncology.

*C*arrier-free gallium-67 citrate is the most frequently used radiopharmaceutical for the detection and staging of cancer and for identifying inflammation and abscess. Imaging for inflammation with indium-111–labeled white blood cells (leukocytes) has proven to be an excellent alternative to ^{67}Ga citrate. Recently white cell labeling with ^{99m}Tc hexamethyl propylene amine oxime (HMPAO) has been shown to be useful in searching for inflammation.

PATHOGENESIS

Cancer

Cancer is an uncontrolled overgrowth of cells often associated with the development of tumor nodules at sites remote from the original tumor. It is these remote tumor modules, *metastases,* that usually lead to the death of the patient. In the last two decades remarkable improvement in life expectancy has occurred for victims of several types of cancer. Early stages of Hodgkin disease, choriocarcinoma, and some leukemias are now considered curable. The concept of cancer as a systemic process, involving the entire body, perhaps through altered immune mechanisms, has gained acceptance only in the last several years. The increasing success of chemotherapy, radiation therapy, and surgery is to a great extent dependent on early diagnosis. Staging and defining the extent of the disease at the time of diagnosis have permitted appropriate therapy to be instituted. The stage of the disease, type of treatment, the tumor's response to treatment are recorded in a data base.

Results of new innovations in therapy are measured against the recorded results of established therapeutic modalities.

No one is sure when a cancer begins. Biochemical changes must precede the histologic changes by years. Currently cancer is defined by cellular changes seen by the pathologist. A premaglignant lesion is a progressive cellular change whose final outcome is frank cancer. An incomplete list of organs where premalignant lesions have been identified includes the skin, breast, lung, cervix, and colon. The pathologist identifies the premalignant lesions by unusual changes in the nuclei of the cells, by changes in the cytoplasm, and by loss of the usual orientation of cells. If the atypical cells have invaded the surrounding tissue or blood vessels, a malignancy is considered to exist. The initial site is considered to be the primary cancer. The primary site can often be excised by surgery. For cancer to kill a human it must be in a critical location or must disseminate to distant parts of the body, for example, a colon cancer establishing itself in the liver or lymph nodes. This is metastatic cancer.

For cancer to continue to grow, new blood vessels must develop. When a cancer reaches a certain size, about a centimeter in diameter for breast cancer, capillaries from surrounding tissue grow toward the cancer and provide it with an adequate blood supply. Cancer implants in the anterior chamber of rabbit eyes appear to release a substance that causes local capillary proliferation. The increased blood supply permits increased nutrients, white cells, and antibodies to be exposed to the cancer. Many cancers are associated with large accumulations of serum proteins.[24]

On many occasions the center of a cancer becomes necrotic because the central blood flow is insufficient to maintain cellular life. Often these fast-growing cancers usurp the blood at the periphery that is needed centrally. The anoxic center has implications for radiation therapy. Decreased oxygenation is associated with decreased radiation responsiveness. The surface of a tumor cell contains antigens that are characteristic of the tumor. Antibodies to these antigens have been labeled with gamma-ray–emitting radionuclides.[25] Labeled antibodies are now approved by the FDA to localize colon cancer and ovarian cancer. Labeled antibodies are available but unapproved by the FDA for localization of breast cancer and melanoma.

Abscess

A pyogenic abscess is a localized collection of dead white cells and bacteria. Typically an abscess begins with a small nidus of inflammation, increased capillary permeability, capillary leakage of serum proteins, and increasing concentrations of white cells. The increased permeability of the surrounding capillaries is caused by

release of histamine and the capability of some bacteria to release toxins. Pyogenic abscesses may be found in any part of the body.

There are two major types of white cells, granulocytes and lymphocytes. The neutrophil is the granulocyte most involved in the defense against pyogenic (pus forming) bacteria. If the blood supply does not bring adequate neutrophils to the nidus of infection, the bacteria increase in number. The process of inflammation causes release of certain substances called *leukotaxines*, which cause neutrophils to migrate to the area of inflammation. Some bacteria such as staphylococci release a toxin, a coagulase, that causes deposition of fibrin, thereby walling off the bacteria from neutrophils and antibiotics. Streptococci produce hemolysins, which cause destruction of red blood cells (erythrocytes). A large cluster of vigorously growing bacteria can produce toxins that destroy neutrophils. As local blood flow brings more neutrophils to the scene, the neutrophils attempt to engulf the bacteria and digest them with packets of enzymes called *lysosomes*. The mixture of dead bacteria, dead granulocytes, and fluid is commonly known as pus. If the pus accumulates faster than the local circulation can remove it, the inflammatory volume expands and its center becomes a small volume of pus with viable bacteria. This is an abscess. At the periphery of the abscess new neutrophils arrive, fibrinogen and other serum proteins accumulate, fibrin is deposited, and the abscess becomes walled off. This wall is called the *pyogenic membrane*. The pyogenic membrane helps to isolate the abscess and limit its spread. Unrecognized abscesses are a common cause of death in seriously ill hospitalized patients.

There are five major areas of localized infection in which ^{67}Ga imaging can play a major role. Bacterial endocarditis is a serious medical emergency in which bacteria colonize a heart valve, usually the aortic or mitral valve. If not detected in time, the valve can be destroyed or scarred to the point of deformity and incompetence. Additionally, small particles of fibrin and bacteria can break off from the valve and be carried by the bloodstream to embolize any area. Embolization of the brain, eyes, and kidneys is most common. The diagnosis of bacterial endocarditis is difficult, especially in a patient with previous unsuccessful antibiotic therapy. Recent dental extractions, intravenous drug abuse, and infections from other areas of the body can precede and cause bacterial endocarditis.

Lung abscesses can result from certain types of pneumonia or from chronic lung disease or infection anywhere in the body. Lung cancer obstructing a bronchus can cause a localized pneumonia and eventually an abscess behind the obstruction.

A pelvic abscess can occur from pelvic inflammatory disease, a ruptured diverticulum of the colon, appendicitis, regional ileitis, or prior surgery. Subdiaphragmatic and intraabdominal abscesses are associated with perforated duodenal ulcers. Even in the antibiotic era, an abscess usually requires surgical drainage. Successful antibiotic treatment of a well-organized abscess might be impossible and can result in organisms resistant to antibiotics; therefore precise localization is imperative.

It is especially in the pelvic and abdominal region that gallium's poor diagnostic specificity for abscess has led to its replacement by ^{111}In-labeled leukocytes.

GALLIUM IMAGING

Historic Perspective

Gallium has 14 known isotopes ranging in mass number from 63 to 78. Because of an inappropriate half-life, type of emission, and production problems, only ^{67}Ga, ^{68}Ga, and [72]Ga seem likely to be useful in clinical nuclear medicine. Between 1949 and 1951 [72]Ga was first investigated by Dudley[14-16,50] as a diagnostic and therapeutic agent for osteogenic sarcoma and metastases to bone. [72]Ga was not especially valuable in these situations, but the bone-seeking property of gallium was demonstrated. In the early 1960s Brookhaven National Laboratories developed a germanium-68/gallium-68 generator. [68]Ge has a long half-life (280 days) and decays to ^{68}Ga, a positron emitter with a half-life of 68 min. The long-lived germanium parent and the short-lived gallium daughter looked like a promising combination for clinical use. [68]Ga as ethylenediaminetetraacetic acid (EDTA) was used with some success as a brain-imaging agent.[2,57] The citrate was investigated as a bone-imaging agent; however, neither radiopharmaceutical was widely used. By 1965 the technetium generator was commercially available, and pertechnetate quickly became the agent of choice for brain imaging. The early scintillation camera with its ½ in thick sodium iodide crystal was rather inefficient in stopping the 511 keV annihilation photon of [68]Ga. A 360-keV collimator was the standard high-energy collimator provided, and resolution was greatly impaired by septal penetration. In 1967 a prototype two-detector positron camera was available but was not mass produced. With the advent of newer positron imaging devices the [68]Ge/^{68}Ga generator may return to nuclear medicine.

In 1965 there was no technetium-labeled phosphate for bone imaging. That year the Medical Division of the Oak Ridge Institute of Nuclear Studies[1] reconfirmed earlier work[9] showing ^{67}Ga administered with carrier gallium to localize in bones within hours. Experiments with carrier-free ^{67}Ga demonstrated concentration in bones much later. Two to 3 days after injection of carrier-free ^{67}Ga, Edwards and Hayes[18] noted intense uptake in the tumor. In this initial report they found that carrier-free ^{67}Ga citrate concentrated in soft-tissue tumors, especially in those without prior radiation therapy or chemotherapy. They also found that false-negatives did occur, and they found new tumor sites not previously detected by other modalities. With this evidence of tumor detection, Oak Ridge Associated Universities (ORAU) in a cooperative study with 16 universities performed nearly 3000 scans between 1970 and 1974, firmly establishing the utility of carrier-free ^{67}Ga citrate in staging and detecting tumors.[12,27,41]

Benign tumors and inflammatory diseases such as sarcoidosis,[66] pneumonia,[13,14] pyelonephritis, active tuberculosis, dermatomyositis,[59] asbestosis, silicosis,[58] inflammation/fibrosis[47] and fevers of undetermined origin[49] can also be detected by ^{67}Ga imaging. Computers permit calculation of an index of inflammatory activity based on ^{67}Ga lung uptake. This index of ^{67}Ga lung accumulation has been demonstrated to correlate with histopathologic scores of inflammation and fibrosis in lung tissue.[6,47] Gallium has great avidity for all AIDS-related causes of inflammation, especially *Pneumocystis carinii* pneumonia.

Chemical Toxicity

Gallium toxicity[15] is characterized by vomiting, skin rash, proteinuria, anemia, and leukopenia and results from doses of 71 mg/kg or greater. Toxicity is variable in experimental animals.[8] Six millicuries of ^{67}Ga contain only 10 ng of elemental gallium, providing a substantial chemical toxicity safety factor.[61] Carrier-free gallium citrate is the radiotracer used. In early preparations excess citrate became bound to calcium and caused hypocalcemia.[53] This has not been a problem with the amounts of citrate currently used (2 mg of sodium citrate/2 mCi of ^{67}Ga). In the past, differences in citrate concentration between manufacturers were found and were thought to account for diagnostic differences reported in the literature.[64] This has not been a problem in the last 10 years.

Production

Carrier-free ^{67}Ga is cyclotron produced by several methods involving the proton bombardment of a zinc-oxide target. The reactions are as follows:

$$^{67}Zn(p,n)^{67}Ga$$
$$^{68}Zn(p,2n)^{67}Ga$$

[67]Zn and [68]Zn occur with a natural abundance of 4% and 18%, respectively.

How "free" is carrier-free? If natural zinc targets are used, as much as 4 μg of stable gallium can contaminate each milliliter of the final carrier-free gallium, depending on the amount of stable gallium in the target.[37] Ten millicuries of ^{67}Ga contain 15×10^{13} atoms of ^{67}Ga. The 40 µg of stable gallium in 10 ml contains 36×10^{16} atoms, about 2400 stable gallium atoms for each radioactive atom when the target is from natural zinc. Carrier-free gallium made from a natural zinc target is not really carrier free. Recent improvements have been made in enriching the target so that it is 99% ^{68}Zn. ^{67}Ga made from such a target contains no stable gallium in the final injectate.

Additional production methods, such as alpha particle bombardment of a zinc target, deuteron bombardment of a zinc target, and alpha particle bombardment of a copper target, are available.

Biodistribution Differences Between Carrier-Free and Carrier-Added Gallium Citrate

When nanograms of carrier-free ^{67}Ga per kilogram of body weight are injected into humans, the percent activity per organ is far different from the percent activity per organ when the same amount of ^{67}Ga is accompanied with milligram per kilogram body weight quantities of stable gallium.[1] In the carrier-free state ^{67}Ga concentrates first in the liver, soft tissues, abscesses, and

some cancers. After 2 to 3 days it concentrates slightly in bone. With carrier gallium added, ^{67}Ga initially concentrates more heavily in bone.

Distribution of Carrier-Free Gallium Citrate

After the intravenous injection of carrier-free ^{67}Ga citrate, there is binding to serum proteins (probably transferrin)[10,28] and alpha and beta globulins with little activity in albumin and gamma globulins.[19,29] Blood clearance is fairly rapid initially, with only 25% of the injected dose remaining in the blood at 3 hr. Only 7% remains at 24 hr, 5% remains at 40 hr, and only 2% remains in the intravascular space at 5 days. Once gallium has entered a tissue, it remains there. About 10% to 15% of the injected dose is excreted in the urine in the first 24 hr, whereas approximately 10% of the injected dose is excreted in the stool. Accounting for decay, 65% remains in the body.[5] About 20% of the dose is eliminated with an effective half-life of 69.5 hr[27] (Figure 17-1).

There have been attempts in the past to increase the target-to-background ratio of gallium images. They first involved the administration of stable scandium, an element with chemical properties similar to gallium. Ad-

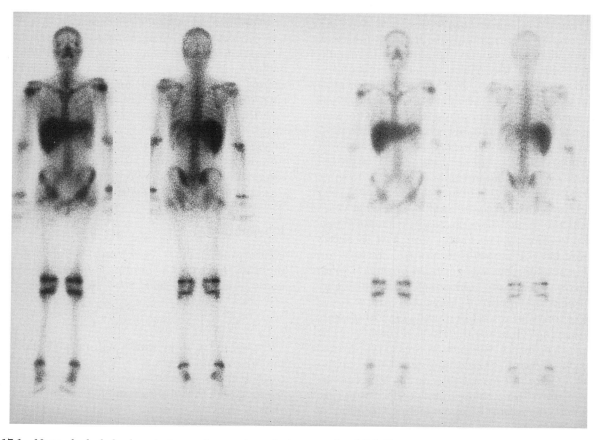

Figure 17-1 Normal whole-body anterior and posterior scintigrams of a child. Note normal uptake in liver and spleen. Normal symmetric uptake is seen in epiphyses and lacrimal glands.

ministered to animals, scandium caused a definite decrease in background gallium. When scandium administration was tried with humans, a hemolytic anemia was caused. In animals there has been success with the administration of iron-dextran complex (Imferon) to decrease the blood background and significantly enhance the target-to-background ratio.[36,52]

From autopsy studies the five organs with the greatest mean percent injected dose per kilogram are the spleen (4%), the renal cortex (3.8%), bone marrow (3.6%), liver (2.8%), and bone (1.4%).[51] From patient to patient, there was a tenfold range of activity for each organ. Brain and muscle contained one seventh to one fortieth the activity of the five most active organs. Several mechanisms of gallium localization have been suggested: (1) a role of iron-binding molecules,[46,55,65] (2) a unique tumor-specific protein,[34] and (3) gallium exchange with intracellular calcium-binding sites.[3] Data from a variety of experimental techniques[33-35,45,46] plus data in humans[20] suggest that transferrin, the iron-binding protein in serum, is involved in ^{67}Ga delivery to the tissue. At the tumor or abscess site the ^{67}Ga is transferred into the cell in a manner not totally understood. At this point calcium-binding components, ferritin, the iron storage protein, or a unique tumor-specific protein could deposit ^{67}Ga into the cell. The ^{67}Ga is eventually deposited in small structures, lysosomes present in the cell's cytoplasm.[61]

Great variations in tumor uptake are seen from one tumor to another within the same patient. In general, tumors with a significant fibrotic or necrotic content accumulate lesser amounts of gallium. Tumors with less than 5% of injected dose per kilogram are very difficult to visualize, as are those tumors under 2 cm in diameter.

Do gallium concentration by a tumor and the rate of DNA synthesis have an association? This question was examined in experimental animals with tumors. In small tumors—Harding-Passey melanomas—there was decreased gallium uptake with increased DNA synthesis, but in larger tumors there was increased gallium uptake associated with increased DNA synthesis. Chemotherapy of some experimental tumors caused a sharp reduction in DNA synthesis but no change in gallium uptake.[60] In everyday gallium imaging, loss of gallium uptake by a tumor is an indication of successful radiation therapy or chemotherapy. Continued uptake of ^{67}Ga citrate indicates continued tumor activity.[23,40,42,43]

Technical Considerations

Imaging protocols consist of establishing guidelines for dosages, optimal time after injection for imaging, photopeak settings, information density, collimation, and positioning. Certain data, such as decay mode and dosimetry, must be presented as a rationale for these guidelines. Variations of the guidelines depend on the instrumentation available.

Preparation before scanning with ^{67}Ga citrate must be twofold: physical and emotional. The physical preparation primarily concerns the elimination of gallium-containing feces from the colon. Some 9% to 15% of the gallium is excreted through the bowel, especially in the first 24 hr. At 24 hr, gallium that accumulates in the bowel is seen as areas of increased activity that may be mistaken for cancer, abscess, or inflammation. In the first 24 hr, gallium can attach itself to newly forming colon mucosal cells, which over the course of several days shed into the lumen of the colon. During the time when the gallium is in the mucosa, bowel cleansing is not successful in removing activity from the abdomen.

The more commonly used bowel preparations are a combination of bisacodyl tablets and magnesium citrate or cleansing enemas. Little research has been done on the efficacy of this type of preparation. Zeman and Ryerson[67] reported that patients given bisacodyl tablets and magnesium citrate showed no greater bowel clearance than did patients without preparation. Other reports claim bowel preparation to be necessary.[4] The patient's diet is another variable. It is likely, but as yet unproven, that patients on a normal or high-fiber diet have a greater clearance of gallium from the bowel than do patients on a low-bulk or liquid diet. If possible, a regular diet should be continued. If the patient has diarrhea, bowel preparation is unnecessary and can aggravate dehydration and electrolyte loss. Accumulation of gallium in the abdomen in patients with diarrhea is almost always indicative of a pathologic condition.

The emotional aspect of gallium scanning is important and often unappreciated. Adequate emotional preparation can yield many benefits: decreased motion, decreased imaging time, fewer repeat views, and less time spent explaining the examination after the fact. Credibility is greater when the explanation is initiated by the person performing the test. Do not expect the referring physician or nurse on the ward to adequately explain the test to the patient. Ethically and practically, a technologist should never inform a patient of anything related to the patient's specific condition or supply a patient with any records that his physician has not cleared.

Before injection the patient should be informed of the duration of the overall gallium study. Depending on the type of equipment and the dose, this ranges from 40 min to 3 hr. A longer examination than expected can be a threatening experience that can be prevented by the patient's prior knowledge of the duration of the test. The patient should also know of the need to remain still during the procedure and that various views might be required. The need to take images even 7 days later must be considered.

Using a camera with a scanning table or its equivalent, place the patient comfortably supine and image posteriorly from below the table and then anteriorly from above to include all the body from the top of the head to approximately midthigh. If a prone position is used, the head, neck, and perhaps shoulder will be rotated in an undesirable semioblique position that will require static images of the neck so that both right and left cervical areas can be compared. In addition, the prone position is usually painful if there has been recent abdominal surgery.

Doses for intravenous injection of carrier-free ^{67}Ga citrate range from 6-10 mCi for a 70-kg adult. The injection site should be chosen to avoid a potential site of clinical interest. The technologist should always record the date, time, and site of injection.

Radiation Characteristics

^{67}Ga has a 78-hr (3.25 day) half-life and decays by electron capture. It has four principal gamma-ray energies,

Table 17-1 ^{67}Ga radionuclide characteristics

| Nuclide | Production | Half-life | Principal radiations | |
			MeV	%
^{67}GA	^{67}Zn(p,n)^{67}Ga	78 hr	0.093	40
	^{68}Zn(p,2n)^{67}Ga		0.184	24
			0.296	22
			0.388	7

From Bureau of Radiological Health: *Radiocological health handbook*, Washington, DC, 1970, U.S. Department of Health, Education, and Welfare.

Table 17-2 Radiation dosimetry for ^{67}Ga citrate

Organ	^{67}GA citrate (rad/5 mCi)
Whole body	1.3
Skeleton	2.2
Liver	2.3
Bone marrow	2.9
Spleen	2.65
Kidney	2.05 (calyx)
Ovary	1.4
Testes	1.2
Stomach	1.1
Small intestine	1.8
Upper colon	4.5

From Medical Internal Radiation Dose (MIRD): Dose estimate report No. 2, *J Nucl Med* 14:755, 1973.

shown in Table 17-1. The radiation-absorbed dose from 5 mCi of ^{67}Ga citrate is recorded in Table 17-2.[48]

Imaging Time After Injection

Imaging of a patient injected with ^{67}Ga citrate can take place from 6 hr to 1 week after injection. Gallium remains in tissue once it is deposited, and the target-to-background ratio increases with the passage of time as blood clearance progresses. Considerations other than target-to-background ratios, such as the urgency of possible surgery for an abscess, the cost of hospitalization, the fact that imaging time increases with physical decay, and the necessity of delaying other studies that might interfere, may dictate earlier rather than later imaging.

Hopkins and Mende[39] have evaluated ^{67}Ga-citrate imaging for subphrenic abscess 6 hr after injection. They found no additional positive sites at 24 or 72 hr when compared with the 6-hr scans. In another study[38] it was noted that gallium citrate was not yet in the bowel at 6 hr, and in that study focal activity in the abdomen was indicative of a pathologic condition. Beihn[5] combined ^{99m}Tc-sulfur-colloid and ^{67}Ga imaging for abscess detection. He subtracted technetium counts in the liver from gallium counts and showed that increased gallium counts were associated with early detection of intrahepatic abscesses.

Our own results with imaging at 12 to 24 hr have been less than optimal. Although it is true that many abscesses have been demonstrated at this time, we have found that more than half were equivocally detected and that reimaging at 48 and 72 hr was required. Kaplan[43] has published his extensive experience with 7-day delayed gallium scans. He has found the 7-day delay to be vital to producing improved sensitivity and specificity of the gallium scan. Our experience fully supports his enthusiasm. The much reduced body background more than makes up for the reduced count rate. We have obtained clinically important diagnostic information as long as 16 days after the injection of 10 mCi of ^{67}Ga citrate.

Kaplan and others[23,40,42,43] have found a negative gallium scan to be an accurate predictor of successful therapy of lymphoma. A normal gallium scan, even in the presence of residual radiographic masses, indicates those masses are tumor free, whereas an abnormal gallium scan provides strong evidence of tumor activity in the area, even in the absence of radiographic masses.

Instrumentation and Technique Variations

A variety of equipment can be used for gallium imaging. Initially, rectilinear scanners, especially those with whole-body and minification capabilities, were used. In recent years the evolution of the scintillation camera with its increase in field size and the introduction of multiple pulse-height analyzers have supplanted the rectilinear scanner. Scintillation cameras with whole-body and SPECT imaging capabilities are necessary for modern gallium imaging.

For whole-body imaging the patient receives 6-10 mCi of ^{67}Ga citrate intravenously. After a 2- to 7-day delay, imaging is performed. Two million count whole-body images are obtained. Simultaneous anterior and posterior whole-body images require from 15 to 30 min and are usually obtained with two different analog outputs to film so the dynamic range of the data can be displayed within the limited gray scale capability of film.

The use of high-energy to medium-energy collimators (rated at a minimum of 300 keV) is necessary because of the physical characteristics of gallium photon emission. If a low-energy collimator is used and the pulse height analyzer is set at the 93-keV peak, scatter and septal penetration from the high-energy photons destroy meaningful resolution. If two photopeaks can be summed, the 93- and the 184-keV peaks are chosen. Optimally, the 93-, 184-, and 296-keV peaks are utilized. Regardless of the photopeak chosen, a high- to medium-energy collimator is needed to collimate the higher energies and reduce septal penetration even if only lower energies are selected for imaging. When three peaks can be used, the imaging time is halved with a constant information density when compared with the 93-keV peak alone. With all peaks we use a 20% window centered on each photopeak.

Technically suboptimal images are the major cause of difficulty in the confident, accurate interpretation of ^{67}Ga studies. There must be adequate counts, and the intensity of those counts must be distributed over the dynamic range of the film. Ideally the diagnosis should be made from the digital data displayed on a monitor. In whole-body scanning the sternal activity is made to correspond to a midpoint in the dynamic range of the film. Areas of increased or decreased activity usually remain within the dynamic range of the film. If equivocal areas are noted, additional static images of 300,000 counts for a standard-field camera and 500,000 counts for a large-field camera are adequate. Repeating selected views, especially of the abdomen at 48 hr, and occasionally more delayed views at 72 and 96 hr are important for accurate clinical results.

SPECT imaging with ^{67}Ga can produce exceptional clinical results. Inflammation and gallium-avid tumors, especially Hodgkin disease and squamous cell carcinoma of the lung, can be detected and the extent of disease and response to treatment can be accurately estimated.

In the past, most SPECT imaging with gallium has been performed with single-head cameras. Dual- and triple-detector cameras with large rectangular fields of view are current state-of-the-art. Satisfactory imaging can be performed 48 hr after injection. The 184- and 296-keV peaks can be summed. A 64 × 64 acquisition matrix, 64 stops at 35 sec per stop, requires almost an hour. Filtered back-projection reconstruction using a Butterworth filter, cutoff 0.4, order 6, or its equivalent is suggested. Currently, the dual- and triple-detector SPECT systems offer greater count acquisition, better statistics, and better spatial resolution.

Figure 17-2 shows an example case for gallium imaging. The patient was a 35-year-old male who was seen in an infectious disease department for recurrent fevers and night sweats. The chest x-ray was normal as were the CT, MRI, sonography, and initial hematologic studies. The patient received an intravenous injection of 10 mCi of gallium citrate. Forty-eigth hours later, a whole-body scan from head to feet was performed (only head to knees is shown in Figure 17-2). The whole-body image contains 2 million counts. The anterior image on the left reveals intense cardiac uptake best seen in the anterior view with lesser focal uptake seen in the region of the celiac axis. Colonic uptake in the transverse colon is within normal limits. The spleen was remarkable by its lack of gallium avidity. Asymmetric uptake was noted on the posterior image with increased gallium retention in the right kidney.

Because of activity within the heart, the celiac nodes and right kidney lymphoma were the primary consideration. Myocarditis could produce such cardiac uptake but the intraabdominal and right renal uptake and a normal cardiac status could not be explained by the diagnosis of myocardityis. Following biopsy of the intraabdominal lymph node, T-cell lymphoma was found with involvement of heart, right kidney, and intraabdominal lymph nodes. SPECT imaging of the abdomen provided definitive localizing information not available by standard diagnostic techniques.

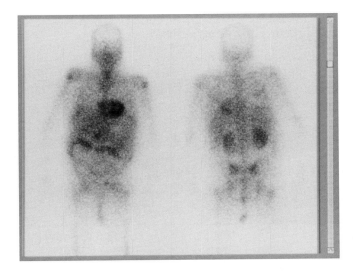

Figure 17-2 ^{67}Ga whole-body scan demonstrates uptake by lymphoma with involvement of the heart, right kidney, and intraabdominal lymph nodes.

Future Trends

At this time there is no radiopharmaceutical that is specific for cancer. The greatest clinical experience has been with carrier-free ^{67}Ga citrate. Even so, some nuclear medicine departments find it difficult to produce results that are helpful to clinicians. A nuclear medicine physician must have an optimal image based on standard technical factors. Without a stable technique, the physician's report becomes an expensive "weather report," which points in all directions and does little to aid the clinician. The nuclear medicine physician must develop confidence in the accuracy of his or her interpretation. Without confidence in the ability of gallium imaging to detect abscesses and tumors, the report will be equivocal and nondiagnostic. The typical response of the insecure physician is to "let's do CT or MRI instead."

The future of nuclear medicine lies in the development of new radiotracers that demonstrate altered biochemistry and physiology before the occurrence of an anatomic defect. To some degree nuclear medicine has this capability now with carrier-free ^{67}Ga citrate. New radiotracers, labeled antibodies, and labeled peptides can dramatically improve the specificity of tumor imaging in the future.

INDIUM-111 WHITE CELL IMAGING

In the early 1970s ^{111}In chloride was used as a tumor and abscess imaging agent. ^{111}In chloride had the advantage over ^{67}Ga of not concentrating in the gastrointestinal tract,[11] but clinical results of tumor and abscess imaging revealed ^{111}In chloride to be slightly inferior to ^{67}Ga. ^{111}In possesses unusually good imaging characteristics, and interest in its use progressed.

Radiation Characteristics

^{111}In has a physical half-life of 67.4 hr. It decays by electron capture, producing two gamma photons with a combined frequency of 1.8 photons for each disintegration. Both photons have excellent energies for external imaging. The end product of ^{111}In decay is stable cadmium-111 (Table 17-3).

Table 17-3	^{111}In radionuclide characteristics		
		Principal radiations	
Nuclide	**Half-life (hr)**	**keV**	**%**
^{111}In	67.4	171	90.0
		247	94.2

White Blood Cell as a Complex Imaging Agent

White blood cells are of two general classes, granulocytes and lymphocytes. Neutrophils, the type of granulocyte involved with defense against pyogenic bacteria, can be tagged with ^{111}In oxine or ^{99m}Tc HMPAO. The ability of the labeled neutrophils to migrate to the area of infection is maintained. This provides a specific method of localization of infectious processes. With the development of new diagnostic procedures of medical value, in the future the eosinophil, a granulocyte involved in the allergic response, and the basophil might be selectively tagged.

Lymphocytes can be separated into groups based on specific antibody production. If these selected populations of lymphocytes could be tagged and their location and degree of concentration measured, specific diagnostic information could be developed that could revolutionize medical practice. At present, most work has been performed with labeled neutrophils to detect localized infectious processes.

Most major advances in nuclear medicine are the result of radiopharmaceutical progress. The diagnostic potential of labeled white cells has been recognized for years, but to develop a nondestructive tag that would not interfere with their biologic properties appeared to be a serious problem. The lipid coating of white cells and the presence of plasma protein prevented a straightforward approach. If plasma proteins were present, the ^{111}In tagged the protein instead of the neutrophil. Removal of the plasma from the white cells causes a loss of cell viability. Labeling with ^{111}In oxine is a balance between efficiency of tagging and cell viability.

There have been many attempts to label white cells. ^{99m}Tc sulfur colloid will label granulocytes[20] and has satisfactorily demonstrated experimental abscesses in animals but has not been so successful in humans. When technetium sulfur colloid is incubated with white blood cells, the neutrophils phagocytize some of the colloid. However, the cells recognize this as a signal to activate their own bactericidal mechanisms. During this process the cell enlarges, activates its lysozymal system to digest the colloidal particle, and in the process loses its ability to migrate to an area of infection. It is soon destroyed by its own lysozymal enzymes. Of course, not all the technetium sulfur colloid is phagocytized, so a significant residual remains to be injected and be phagocytized by the Kupffer cells of the liver and spleen, thereby presenting an unwanted background in the exact regions that need to be most critically observed for intraabdominal abscess formation.

^{111}In-Oxine Complex

In 1977 Thakur[62] demonstrated a method for labeling white cells with ^{111}In oxine and showed it to be superior to ^{67}Ga citrate for localizing experimental abscesses in dogs. Since his initial report, numerous other publications have demonstrated the utility of ^{111}In-labeled white cells in the diagnosis of localized infectious processes in the clinical situation. The ability to tag white cells in a clinical setting provides nuclear medicine with a powerful new diagnostic agent.

The structural formula of ^{111}In oxine is shown in Figure 17-3. Three oxine molecules surround the ^{111}In, creating a lipophilic complex able to penetrate the lipid cell membrane. Within the cell the ^{111}In-oxine bond is broken, the ^{111}In binds to cytoplasm, and the oxine is released from the cell. The cell's ability to recognize its environment and to migrate to areas of inflammation is associated with its surface. Specialized protein molecules extend through the lipid membrane and provide communication between the external environment and the cell itself. The oxine labeling method seems to spare the surface of the cell.

Labeling Method

The usual method is to take approximately 50 ml of the patient's blood and to use the patient's own white cells. Some patients do not have an adequate number of white cells in the peripheral blood, known as *granulocytopenia*. The absence of granulocytes is called *agranulocytosis*. In this situation a donor, properly typed by the blood bank, can provide the granulocytes to be tagged.

Care must be taken to separate the white cells from the red cells and platelets. Several methods have been proposed for this separation, but it is vital that it be performed satisfactorily. The initial separation may remove the bulk of the red cells, but additional means are necessary to eliminate the remainder. Consider the problems. There are usually 5 million red cells/mm^3 and 5 thousand white cells/mm^3. If the initial gross separation method is 99.9% complete in eliminating the red

cells, the mixture will still contain 5000 red cells and 5000 white cells/mm^3.

After the initial separation by gravity, red cells may be more thoroughly separated by hypotonic hemolysis, by the addition of ammonium chloride solution, or by using methyl cellulose. With hypotonic hemolysis, water is added to the mixture of red and white cells. Since red cells are more sensitive to osmotic changes than are white cells, the red cells hemolyze and the red cell fragments are removed, leaving behind the white cells. The specific method we use is the method of Thakur and Gottschalk,[63] which appears in Table 17-4. Injection of 500 μCi of ^{111}In-labeled white cells provides an adequate count rate at 24 hr. Local commercial nuclear pharmacies offer the service of tagging an individual's white cells with ^{111}In oxine.

The viability of the cell, after undergoing the stress of labeling, can be measured by its ability to exclude trypan blue dye, which enters and stains a nonviable cell but will not stain a viable cell. Chemotaxis, the granulocyte's ability to migrate in response to an appropriate chemical stimulus, can be measured by special assays described by Boyden.[7] Observation of a portion of the labeled cells by light microscope is a simple procedure that can detect clumping of white cells. Dutcher[17] has estimated that their patients were injected with approximately 6-15 million granulocytes, labeled with 360-560 μCi of [111]In. Using this method approximately 95% of the cells were granulocytes. The entire labeling process can be completed in 2 hr or less. Labeling efficiencies of 85% to 90% can be expected.[44] Speed of labeling is important. The life of a neutrophil is about 9 hr. If it takes 6 hr to draw blood, separate cells, transport the blood, and reinject cells, the majority of labeled neutrophils will be nonviable.

Technical Considerations

A slow injection through a large needle (20 gauge or later) is required. Injection through a small needle will cause serious shearing forces at the needle tip, which will destroy all cells involved. The larger needle decreases mechanical trauma to the cells during injection. The less plastic tubing the cells must contact, the better. Polypropylene is a satisfactory plastic. Glass syringes should be avoided because blood components can react with it. Silicon lubricant, found in glass and some plastic syringes, interferes with the oxine and labeling.

There is some debate as to the optimal time to image. Several investigators[54] suggest imaging at 3 to 4 hr and again 24 hr after injection, although one study in granulocytopenic patients found excellent results at 30 min.[17] We will scan at 4 hr after injection and again at 24 hr. If scans are taken at 1 to 2 hr, there will be excessive labeled neutrophils in the lungs. This is a normal event. Labeled white cells are retained in the lungs as a normal event for the first 1 to 2 hr.

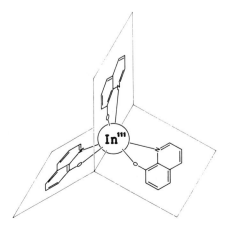

Figure 17-3 ^{111}In-oxine complex: three oxine molecules surround the ^{111}In atom.

Table 17-4 Preparation of ^{111}In-labeled white cells

Materials

^{111}In oxine (from 3.5.1. or purchased commercially)

Hank's balanced salt solution (HBSS):

2.00 g NaCl	0.025 g MgCl$_2$ .6 H$_2$o
0.010 g K CI	0.25 g glucose
0.035 g CaCl$_2$	0.065 g Hepes buffer
0.025 g MgSO$_4$.7 H$_2$O	

Add 250 ml of H$_2$O, adjust pH to 7.4 and filter into sterile, pyrogen-free vials.

Ammonium chloride solution:

2.07 g NH$_4$CI

0.25 g KHCO$_3$

0.093 g EDTA

Add 250 ml of H$_2$O adjust pH to 7.4 and filter into sterile, pyrogen-free vials.

50 ml polypropylene centrifuge tubes

Oxford Macroset pipet and sterile tips

2% (w/v) methylcellulose solution

Heparin

Method (using sterile technique and supplies)

1. Collect 50 ml of blood in 60-ml syringe containing 1-2 ml of heparin (250-1000 units) and 1.5 ml of 2% methylcellulose solution.
2. Clamp the syringe barrel to a ring stand in an upright position and tilt the syringe about 20 degrees from the perpendicular. This allows the red blood cells (RBC) to settle and produces a leukocyte-rich plasma (LRP).
3. Remove needle and replace with butterfly.
4. Express the LRP into a 50-ml sterile polypropylene centrifuge tube, taking care not to collect RBC. Remove 0.5 ml for white blood cell (WBC) count.
5. Centrifuge LRP at 450 × g for 5 min to obtain WBC button.
6. Remove leukocyte-poor plasma (LPP) supernatant and save at 37° C.
7. Resuspend WBC in 5 ml of ammonium chloride solution (to destroy RBC) and immediately centrifuge at 450 × g for 5 min.
8. Resuspend WBC in 5 ml of HBSS with gentle agitation and centrifuge at 450 × g for 5 min.
9. Resuspend WBC in 5 ml of HBSS and add about 2 mCi of ^{111}In oxine.
10. Incubate 20-30 min at 37° C. Gently agitate the mixture 3 or 4 times during the incubation to ensure adequate mixing.
11. Centrifuge LPP at 1000 × g for 15 minutes while WBCs are incubating with ^{111}In. Save the supernatant platelet-poor plasma (PPP).
12. After incubation add 5 ml of PPP obtained in step above to WBC and mix gently. The plasma aids in the removal of loosely bound ^{111}In.
13. Centrifuge mixture at 450 × g for 5 min.
14. Remove supernatant and add 5 ml of PPP and repeat step above. Count activity in supernatants and pellet and determine labeling efficiency. Include supernatant from previous spin in efficiency calculation. There should be at least 500 μCi of activity in the cells.
15. Add 5 ml of PPP to WBC, gently mix and measure activity. Now the WBC are ready for injection. Remove 0.5 ml for count differential cell smear and trypan test.

Modified from McAfee JG. In Thakur ML, Gottshalk A, eds: *In-111 labeled neutrophils, platelets and lymphocytes,* New York, 1980, Trivirum.

Collimation should be accomplished with a medium- to high-energy collimator. If dual-pulse-height analyzers are available, they can be set to 173- and 247-keV photopeaks. If only one analyzer is available, both peaks can be observed; however, the instrument must have a window capability of at least 60% width (centerline of 208 keV, window of 146-270 keV). Some discriminators have a maximum window of only 50%.

Kipper[44] suggests that the first image be taken of the liver with an information content of 700 counts/cm^2 over the liver, that time be recorded, and other views be taken for preset time. If information density is not available on the camera, preset count of 300,000 counts over the liver followed by that time for preset time for other views is suggested. Recording the images on a nuclear medicine computer is an excellent method to avoid having to repeat the view because the photographic exposure was not appropriate for the number of counts acquired. If labeling efficiency is low and the count rate is low from the patient, images with fewer counts may have to be accepted. The general rule still holds that febrile and demented patients have great difficulty in remaining motionless for more than 5 min. Therefore a maximum time of 5 min per view may be a reasonable protocol criterion if adequate counts can be obtained. Both the anterior and posterior views of the head, neck, thorax, abdomen, and pelvis should be obtained. The technologist should ask if there are any sites of suspected involvement in the extremities.

There is a normal pattern of uptake following intravenous injection (Figure 17-4). In the first minutes after injection there is rapid accumulation of labeled

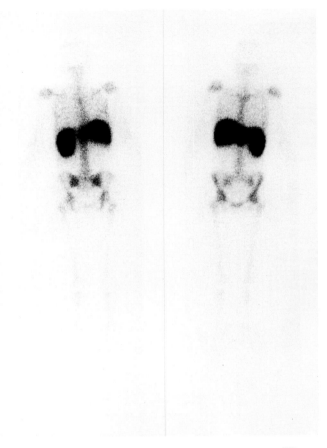

Table 17-5	Radiation dosimetry for ^{111}In-labeled white cells*

Organ	^{111}In-labeled white cells (rad/mCi)
Whole body	0.50-0.53
Liver	1-5
Spleen	18-20.4

*Dose distribution depends on amount of red cells present. From Freeman LM, Weissman HS, eds: *Nuclear medicine annual,* New York, 1982, Raven Press; and Segal AW: *Lancet* 2:1056-1058, 1976.

Figure 17-4 This is a normal posterior and anterior ^{111}In white blood cell whole-body scan performed approximately 24 hr after injection. Initial images are usually presented with the liver and spleen displayed at maximum film density. Such presentation is good for visualization of the liver and spleen. The initial method of display, scaled to the intense liver and spleen activity, causes the abdomen and pelvis, common sites of pathology, to be presented as areas of such faint activity that mild to moderate inflammation will not be seen. Images have been windowed so as to visualize some minor background in the abdomen and pelvis. This is usually necessary for adequate examination of the abdomen and pelvis.

granulocytes in the lungs, liver, and spleen. It is thought that the uptake in the lungs is not due to simple embolism of aggregates of granulocytes; rather, it is a process called *margination* in which the granulocytes reside temporarily in the lungs. Clearing of the lungs begins at around 30 min. Granulocyte accumulation in the liver and spleen persists for at least 48 hr.

The estimated radiation dose is reported in Table 17-5. Absorbed dose varies with the tagging efficiency and regional localization but in general appears to be acceptable, especially when one considers the seriousness of failing to diagnose an abscess.

There are numerous publications attesting to the clinical utility of ^{111}In white cell imaging (Figure 17-5). Several articles demonstrate a sensitivity (true-positive

rate) of greater than 90% and a specificity (true-negative rate) of greater than 90%. One investigator reporting 312 cases found a sensitivity of 95% and a specificity of 97%. When ^{111}In-labeled white cells and ^{67}Ga citrate were both compared with an assumed sensitivity of 90%, the ^{111}In–white cell specificity was 97%, whereas the ^{67}Ga-citrate specificity was 64%.[26] In one report, ^{111}In white cells were superior in detecting focal infections in the first 2 weeks of the infectious process, whereas ^{67}Ga was the superior diagnostic agent in focal infections of longer than 2 weeks' duration.[56] In a comparison of ^{111}In white cells and computed tomography (CT) body scans in the diagnosis of intraabdominal abscess, ^{111}In-labeled white cells appeared to be diagnostically superior. The labeling of white cells permits us to monitor important physiologic parameters and has the promise of making significant improvements in patient care.

New methods of labeling are under development. Neutrophils contain on their surface a specific binding site for specific peptides. The peptide is labeled with a tracer, ideally ^{99m}Tc.

Tumor Antibody Imaging

Antigens are large molecules recognized as foreign by the immune system. They are capable of causing the immune system to develop specialized proteins (immunoglobulins) called *antibodies.* Repeated or prolonged exposure to bacteria, viruses, human or animal cells, or certain chemicals can stimulate the immune system to develop antibodies. The development and magnitude of an immune response by an antigen depends on molecular weight, duration of exposure, and structure of a specific region called the *epitope.* The same epitope can exist on various tissues. The same epitope existing on multiple tissues decreases the otherwise specific nature of identifying a target tissue. If the antigen has been released from the surface of the tumor into the blood, in an imaging situation there is localization of the labeled antibody in the blood pool rather than at the site of the tumor. This produces a decreased tumor-

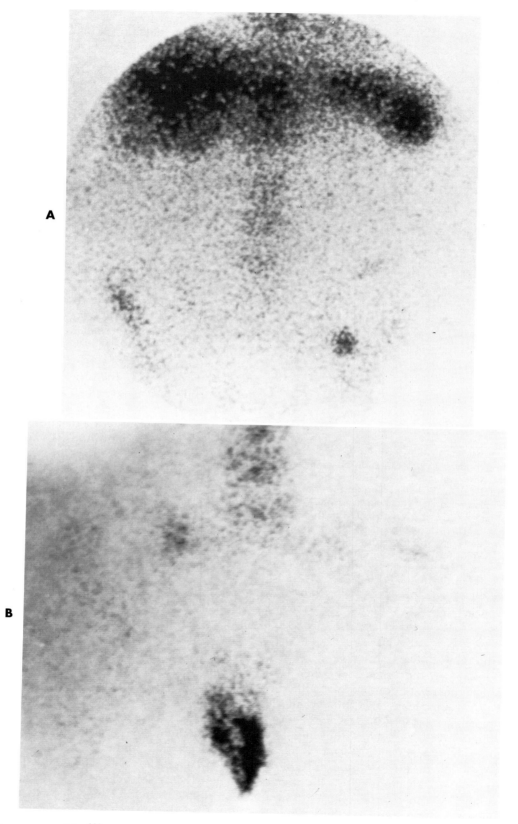

Figure 17-5 Demonstrated by ^{111}In white cells: **A,** Diverticular abscess. **B,** Perirectal abscess. Abscesses in these locations are demonstrated with a clarity that gallium cannot provide. (From Kipper MS, Williams RJ: Indium-111 white blood cell imaging, *Clin Nucl Med* 8:449-455, 1983.)

Table 17-6	Monoclonal antibody vocabulary
Antigen	Large molecule recognized by the immune system as foreign and capable of stimulating antibody formation
Antibody	Protein (immunoglobulin) synthesized by plasma cells in response to an antigen; the antibody has a specific and precise affinity for the antigen; the antibody locates on a specific site of the antigen, which is called the antigenic determinate
Hapten	Small foreign molecule that by itself is not antigenic
Haptenic determinate	The macromolecule to which a hapten binds; the combination of the hapten and the carrier macromolecule can elicit specific antibody formation
Plasma cell	Secretors of antibody molecules; derived from B lymphocytes
T lymphocytes	Mediates the cellular immune response, which aids the humoral immune response
IgA	Mass of 180-500 kd concentration (3 mg/ml) found in external secretions such as saliva, tears, mucus
IgD	Mass of 175 kd concentration 0.1 mg/ml; function not yet known
IgE	Mass of 200 kd concentration (0.001 mg/ml); function not yet known; IgE does have a harmful effect in allergic reactions
IgM	The first antibody to appear in the serum after stimulation by antigen; mass of 950 kd concentration (1 mg/ml)
IgG	Mass of 150 kd, concentration 12 mg/ml; shape of the molecule is a flexible Y, which consists of two kinds of polypeptide chains—light (L) and heavy (H); disulfide bonds connect the light chains to the heavy chains and additional disulfide bonds connect the two heavy chains
Multiple myeloma	Malignant disorder of antibody-producing plasma cells
Hybridoma	Fusing of an antibody-producing cell with a myeloma cell; large amounts of homogeneous antibody can be produced by the hybridoma

From Köhler G, Milstein C: Continuous culture of fused cells secreting antibody of predefined specificity, *Nature* 256(5517):485, 1975; and Milstein C: Monoclonal antibodies, *Sci Am*, Oct 1980, p. 66

to-background ratio and also decreases test sensitivity. Tumor surface antigens that are not shed into the blood are a preferred antigen to use to make a labeled antibody.

Molecules of less than a certain mass usually are nonantigenic. A molecule too small to cause an immune response by itself may combine with a larger molecule and become capable of producing an immune response. The small molecule is called a *hapten*.

An antigen can sensitize a B lymphocyte. At some later time, when that antigen encounters a B lymphocyte previously sensitized to that antigen, the B lymphocyte is transformed into a plasma cell. Antibodies are produced by plasma cells. A single plasma cell produces many molecules of a single antibody—a monoclonal antibody (Table 17-6). When the antibody meets the precise antigen for which it was created, the antibody adheres to the antigen. During imaging, many labeled antibody molecules finding specific antigens on the tumor cell surface demonstrate the location of the tumor.

A single bacterium, virus, or tumor has many antigenic sites. Each antigen sensitizes a different B lymphocyte. Each B lymphocyte becomes a plasma cell able to produce multiple copies of a single antibody. Multiple monoclonal antibodies result in a polyclonal antibody mixture. In an imaging situation the mixture of antibodies can aid in identifying the tumor target, since each antibody localizes to its specific antigen. Since a particular tumor may or may not express a single specific antigen on its surface, the polyclonal antibody mixture may have a better chance of visualizing the tumor.

Antibodies are immune globulins. There are several types of immune globulins: IgG, IgD, IgA, IgE, and IgM. The immune globulins can be separated from each other, but it is very difficult to separate IgG into unique purified components. Polyclonal IgG is currently used to image tumors. The IgG molecule has a mass of 150,000 (150 kd).

The shape of the molecule is that of a Y (Figure 17-6). IgG is composed of two short and two long chains of protein. One short chain and one long chain are joined by disulfide bonds. At the upper tips of the Y are the sites that react to the particular antigen. This is the variable region, which recognizes its specific target antigen. The lower part of the stem of the Y contains the Fc region, which appears to be rather constant within a species. The Fc region of human antibody is different from a mouse Fc region. The Fc region can be removed from mouse antibody before injection into a human with resultant decrease in human antibody production to the mouse antibody.

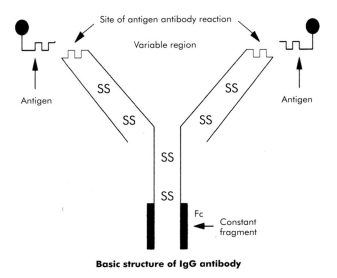

Figure 17-6 Simplified structure of IgG. The antigen-antibody reaction site is restricted to the ends of the Y.

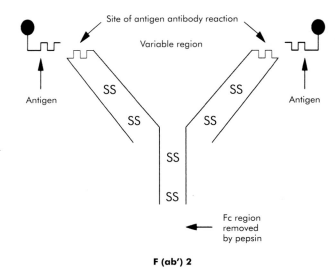

Figure 17-7 Removal of the Fc region is associated with a reduction in HAMA reaction.

The IgG molecule is large and relatively immobile in comparison with smaller molecules. It is not easy for such a large molecule to leave the intravascular space and travel to sites of tumor or infection. Plasma clearance $t_{1/2}$ of the intact IgG molecule is in the range of 40 hr. An IgG molecule can be divided into small fragments F(ab) by the enzymes pepsin and papain. Pepsin removes the Fc region and produces the F(ab)$'_2$ fragment (Figure 17-7), which has a plasma $t_{1/2}$ of approximately 20 hr. Papain also removes the Fc region but in addition divides the molecule into two identical fragments F(ab), each with only one variable site (Figure 17-8). The plasma $t_{1/2}$ of the F(ab) fragment is in the range of 1 hr.[21,22]

As of early 1996, monoclonal antibodies used in medicine are of mouse origin. The human immune system recognizes mouse antibody as a foreign antigenic substance. Human antibodies are made to mouse antibody. When a human receives a second injection of mouse antibody, the human immune system is activated with creation of variable amounts of human antimouse antibodies (HAMA), with resultant rapid removal of mouse antibody from the system. This HAMA reaction could be avoided if human antibodies were used instead of mouse antibodies. At this time technology is most advanced using the mouse immune system. Techniques must be developed that decrease the intensity of the HAMA reaction. Antibodies of human origin are being developed. Despite the known presence of HAMA reaction, it is detected in only 50% of humans following a mouse-based radiolabeled antibody tracer. By 6 months mouse antibodies are detected in only 4%.

Clinical trials have demonstrated the ability of radiolabeled antibodies to detect various cancers.[48] Malignant melanoma, small cell carcinoma of the lung, co-

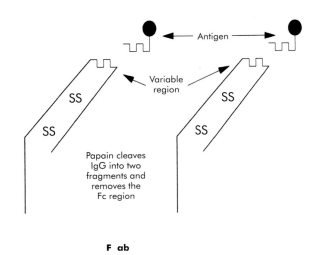

Figure 17-8 Removal of Fc region and division into two fragments results in much faster blood clearance.

lon cancer, rectal cancer, and ovarian cancer have been detected by both planar and SPECT imaging (Figure 17-9). The labeled antibody approach to colon and rectal cancer has demonstrated the ability to stage the disease in preoperative patients and to aid in postoperative follow-up and in the management of patients with elevated carcinoma embryonic antigen (CEA). In one study, immunoscintigraphy favorably changed medical management. Sensitivity and specificity are almost twice that of CT and ultrasound of the extra hepatic abdomen and pelvis.

Positron emission tomography (PET) has demonstrated unique capabilities in the detection of cancer.[31] One property of many tumors is the presence of an increased metabolic rate. This increase in glucose utiliza-

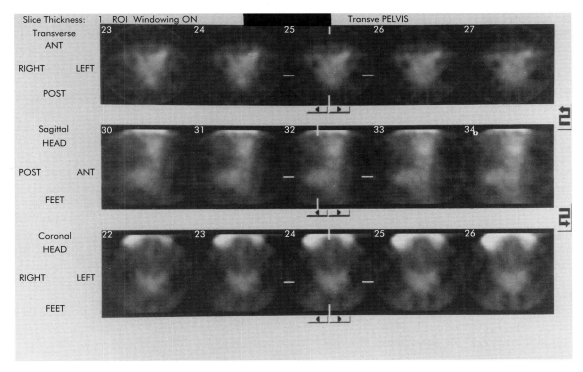

Figure 17-9 ^{111}In-oncoscint (3.5 mCi) SPECT image of pelvis after 4-day delay. Acquisition was 360 degrees, 64 × 64 matrix, 64 stops at 35 sec per stop. Reconstruction was by filtered back projection using Parzen filter. This 55-year-old woman had colon cancer resected 3 years ago. There was clinical recurrence in the pelvis. The SPECT images show a midline rectal mass approximately 4 in in diameter. The posterior extent is best seen on the sagittal views. As the tumor extends anteriorly, it extends to the left. This is best seen in the transverse images. These findings were confirmed at surgery. A low-pass filter limits noise but produces a "smooth" image with reduced spatial resolution. Given a lesion of 4 in in diameter, a minor reduction in spatial resolution is of no consequence.

tion was discovered by Warberg and resulted in his receipt of a Nobel Prize in the 1930s. Increased glucose utilization can be detected following intravenous administration of the glucose analog 2{F-18}fluoro-2-deoxy-D-glucose (FDG).

After intravenous administration the FDG molecule is phosphorylated by hexokinase, is retained in tissue, and can be imaged by PET. Increased glucose metabolism is associated with an increased degree of malignancy in many tumors. With some added effort, regional metabolic activity can be calculated. PET imaging for oncology diagnosis is quite sensitive. Metabolically active tumors can be found before their detection by CT or MRI. Failure of therapy can be identified by continued increased regional glucose uptake in the tumor bed or at distant sites. Continued tumor activity can be seen when anatomic tests, such as CT and MRI, are considered to show cure.[30,32]

The ability of nuclear medicine to examine regional metabolism or antigenic characteristics of potential cancer sites over the entire body is a unique diagnostic capability. CT measures the electron density of tissue, MRI measures the proton density, and ultrasound measures the acoustic properties of tissue. Since cancer begins as a chemical change, long before there are changes identifiable by CT, MRI, or ultrasound, the po-

tential exists for early cancer diagnosis before the development of a mass.

REFERENCES

1. Andrews GA, Knisley RM, Wagner HN: *Radioactive pharmaceuticals,* AEC Symposium Series 6, Washington, DC, 1966, U.S. Atomic Energy Commission/Division of Technical Information.

2. Anger HO, Gottschalk A: Localization of brain tumors with the positron scintillation camera, *J Nucl Med* 4:326-330, 1963.

3. Anghileri LJ, Heidreder M: On the mechanism of ^{67}Ga by tumors, *Oncology* 34(2):74-77, 1977.

4. Bakshi SJ, Parthasarathy KL: Combination of laxatives for cleansing of ^{67}Ga-citrate activity in the bowel, *J Nucl Med* 15:470, 1974.

5. Beihn RM, Damron JR, Hafner T: Subtraction technique for the detection of subphrenic abscess using ^{67}Ga and ^{99m}Tc, *J Nucl Med* 15:371-373, 1974.

6. Bisson G, Drapeau G, Lamourex G, et al: Computer-based quantitative analysis of gallium-67 uptake in normal and diseased lungs, *Chest* 84:513-517, 1983.

7. Boyden S: The chemotactic effect of mixtures of antibody and antigen on polymorphonuclear leukocyte, *J Exp Med* 115:453-466, 1962.

8. Bruner HD, Cooper BM, Rehback DJ: A study of gallium: Part IV: toxicity of gallium citrate in dogs and rats, *Radiology* 61:550-555, 1953.

9. Bruner HD, Hayes RL, Perkinson JD: Preliminary data on gallium-67, *Radiology* 61:602-612, 1953.

10. Clausen J, Edeling CJ, Fogh J: ^{67}Ga binding to human serum proteins and tumor components, *Cancer Res* 34:1931-1937, 1974.

11. Coleman RE, Black RE, Welch DM, et al: Indium-111 labeled leukocytes in the evaluation of suspected abdominal abscesses, *Am J Surg* 139:99-103, 1980.

12. DeLand FH, Sauerbrunn BJL, Boyd C, et al: ^{67}Ga-citrate imaging in untreated primary lung cancer: preliminary report of the cooperative group, *J Nucl Med* 15:408-411, 1974.

13. Dige-Peterson H, Heckscher T, Hertz M: ^{67}Gallium-scintigraphy in nonmalignant lung diseases, *Scand J Resp Dis* 53:314-319, 1972.

14. Dudley HC, Imirie GW Jr, Istock JT: Deposition of radiogallium (Ga^{72}) in proliferating tissues, *Radiology* 55:571-578, 1950.

15. Dudley HC, Levine MD: Studies of the toxic action of gallium, *Exp Ther* 95:487-493, 1949.

16. Dudley HC, Maddox GE, LaRue HC: Studies of the metabolism of gallium, *J Pharm Exp Ther* 96:135-138, 1949.

17. Dutcher JP, Schiffer CA, Johnson GS: Rapid migration of 111-indium-labeled granulocytes to sites of infection, *N Engl J Med* 304:487-589, 1981.

18. Edwards CL, Hayes RL: Tumor scanning with ^{67}Ga citrate, *J Nucl Med* 10:103-108, 1969.

19. Engelstad B, Luk SS, Hattner RS: Altered Ga-67 citrate distribution in patients with multiple red blood cell transfusions, *Am J Radiol* 139:755-759, 1982.

20. Ensslen RD, Jackson FI, Reid AM: Bone and gallium scans in mastocytosis: correlation with count rates, radiography, and microscopy, *J Nucl Med* 24:586-588, 1983.

21. Freeman LM, Blaufox MD, eds: *Seminars in nuclear medicine: monoclonal antibodies I,* Philadelphia, 1989, WB Saunders.

22. Freeman LM, Blaufox MD, eds: *Seminars in nuclear medicine: monoclonal antibodies II,* Philadelphia, 1989, WB Saunders.

23. Front D, Ben-Haim S, Isreal O, et al: Lymphoma: predictive value of Ga-67 scintigraphy after treatment, *Radiology* 192:349-363, 1992.

24. Ghose T, Nairn RC, Fothergill JE: Uptake of proteins of malignant cells, *Nature* 196:1108-1109, 1962.

25. Goldenberg DM, Preston DF, Primus FJ, et al: Photoscan localization of GW-39 tumors in hamsters using radiolabeled anticarcinoembryonic antigen immunoglobulin G, *Cancer Res* 37:1-9, 1974.

26. Goodwin DA, Doherty PW, McDougall IR: *Clinical use of Indium-111-labeled white cells: an analysis of 312 cases, neutrophils, platelets and lymphocytes,* New York, 1982, Trivirum.

27. Greenlaw RH, Weinstein MG, Brill AB, et al: ^{67}Ga-citrate imaging in untreated malignant lymphoma: preliminary report of the cooperative group, *J Nucl Med* 15:404-407, 1974.

28. Gunasekera SW, King LJ, Lavendar PH: The behavior of tracer gallium-67 towards serum protein, *Clin Chem Acta* 39:401-406, 1972.

29. Hartman RF, Hayes RL: Gallium binding by blood serum, *Fed Proc* 26:780, March 1967 (abstract).

30. Hawkins RH, Hoh CR, et al: PET-FDG imaging in cancer, *Appl Radiology* May 1992, pp 51-57.

31. Hawkins RH, Hoh CK, et al: PET cancer evaluation: with FDG, *J Nucl Med* 32:1555-1558, 1991.

32. Hawkins RH, Hoh CK, et al: Whole body PET finds promising clinical niche, *Diag Imaging* June 1992, p 88.

33. Hayes RL, Nelson B, Swartzendruber DL, et al: Gallium-67 localization in rat and mouse tumors, *Science* 167:289-390, 1970.

34. Hayes RL, Rafter JJ, Byrd BL, et al: Studies of the in-vivo entry of Ga-67 into normal and malignant tissue, *J Nucl Med* 22:325-332, 1981.

35. Hayes RL, Rafter JJ, Carlton JE, et al: Studies of the in-vivo uptake of Ga-67 by an experimental abscess: concise communication, *J Nucl Med* 23:8-14, 1982.

36. Hill JH, Merz T, Wagner HN Jr: Iron-induced enhancement of ^{67}Ga uptake in a model human leukocyte culture system, *J Nucl Med* 16:1183-1186, 1975.

37. Hirsch JI, Fratkin JM, Sharpe AR Jr: Gallium-67 citrate, drug intell, *Clin Pharm* 7:519-523, 1973.

38. Hopkins GB, Kan M, Mende CW: Early Ga-67 scintigraphy for the localization of abdominal abscesses, *J Nucl Med* 16:990-992, 1975.

39. Hopkins GB, Mende CW: Gallium-67 and subphrenic abscesses—is delayed scintigraphy necessary? *J Nucl Med* 16:609-611, 1975.

40. Israel O et al: Residual mass and negative gallium scintigraphy in treated lymphoma, *J Nucl Med* 31:365, 1990.

41. Johnston G, Benua RS, Teates CE, et al: ^{67}Ga-citrate imaging in untreated Hodgkin's disease: preliminary report of the cooperative group, *J Nucl Med* 15:399-403, 1974.

42. Kaplan WD: *J Nucl Med* 31:369, 1990 (editorial).

43. Kaplan WD et al: Gallium imaging: a predictor of residual tumor viability and clinical outcome in patients with diffuse large cell lymphoma, *J Clin Oncol* 8:1966-1970, 1990.

44. Kipper MS, Williams RJ: Indium-111 white blood cell imaging, *Clin Nucl Med* 8:449-455, 1983.

45. Larson SM, Grunbaum Z, Rarey JS: The role of transferrins in gallium uptake, *Int J Nucl Med Biol* 8:257-266, 1981.

46. Lawless O, Brown DH, Kubner KF, et al: Isolation and partial characterization of Ga-67 binding glycoprotein from Morris 5123C rat hepatoma, *Cancer Res* 38:4440-4444, 1978.

47. Line BR, Fulmer JD, Reynolds HY, et al: Gallium-67 citrate scanning in the staging of idiopathic pulmonary fibrosis: correlation with physiologic and morphologic features and bronchoalveolar lavage, *Am Rev Resp Dis* 118:355-365, 1978.

48. Medical internal radiation dose (MIRD) report number 2, *J Nucl Med* 14:755-756, 1973.

49. Misami T, Dokoh F, Yagi K, et al: Gallium-67-citrate imaging in the detection of focal lesions for anemia, proteinuria, and prolonged fever, *J Nucl Med* 31:512-515, 1990.

50. Mulry WC, Dudley HC: Studies of radiogallium as a diagnostic agent in bone tumors, *J Lab Clin Med* 37:239-252, 1951.

51. Nelson B, Hayes RL, Edwards CL, et al: The distribution of gallium in human tissues after intravenous administration, *J Nucl Med* 13:92-100, 1972.

52. Oster ZH, Larson JM, Wagner HN Jr: Possible enhancement of ^{67}Ga-citrate imaging by iron dextran, *J Nucl Med* 17:356-358, 1976.

53. Porter J, Kawana M, Krizek H, et al: [67]Ga production with a compact cyclotron, *J Nucl Med* 19:351, 1970 (abstract).

54. Segal AW, Thakur ML, Arnot RN, et al: Indium-111-labeled leukocytes for localization of abscess, *Lancet* 2:1056-1058, 1976.

55. Sephton R: Relationship between the metabolism of Ga-67 and iron, *Int J Nucl Med* 8:323-331, 1981.

56. Sfakianakis GN, Al-Shiekha W, Heal A, et al: Comparison of scintigraphy with In-111 leukocytes and Ga-67 in the diagnosis of occult sepsis, *J Nucl Med* 23:618-626, 1982.

57. Shealy CN, Aronow S, Brownell GL: Gallium-68 as a scanning agent for intracranial lesions, *J Nucl Med* 5:161-167, 1964.

58. Siemsen JK, Sargent N, Grebe SF, et al: Pulmonary concentration of Ga-67 in pneumoconiosis, *Am J Roentgenol* 120:815-820, 1974.

59. Smith WP, Robinson RG, Gobuty AH: Positive whole-body ^{67}Ga scintigraphy in dermatomyositis, *Am J Roentgenol* 133:126-127, 1979.

60. Subramanian G, Rhodes BA, Cooper JF, et al, eds: *Radiopharmaceuticals,* New York, 1975, The Society of Nuclear Medicine.

61. Swartzendruber DC, Nelson D, Hayes RL: Gallium-67 localization in lysomal-like granules of leukemic and non-leukemic murine tissues, *N Natl Cancer Inst* 46:941-952, 1971.

62. Thakur ML, Coleman RE, Welch MS: Indium-111 labeled leukocytes for the localization of abscess: preparation, analysis, tissue distribution and comparison with gallium-67 citrate in dogs, *J Lab Clin Med* 89:217-218, 1977.

63. Thakur ML, Gottschalk A, eds: *Indium-111 labeled neutrophils, platelets and lymphocytes,* New York, 1980, Trivirum.

64. Waxman AD, Kawada T, Wolf W, et al: Are all gallium citrate preparations the same? *Radiology* 117:647-648, 1975.

65. Weiner RE, Schreiber GJ, Hoffer PB: In vitro transfer of Ga-67 from transferrin to ferritin, *J Nucl Med* 24:608-614, 1983.

66. Weiner SN, Patel BP: ^{67}Ga-citrate uptake by the parotid glands in sarcoidosis, *Radiology* 130:753, 1979.

67. Zeman RK, Ryerson TW: Bowel preparation in ^{67}Ga-citrate scanning, *J Nucl Med* 18:886-889, 1977.

BIBLIOGRAPHY

Goswitz FA, Andrews GA, Viamonte M: *Clinical uses of radionuclides,* AEC Symposium Series 27, Washington, DC, December 1972, U.S. Atomic Energy Commission Office of Information Services.

Susan C. Weiss, James J. Conway

Pediatrics

Objectives

Discuss considerations of dealing with pediatric patients and parents.

List and discuss methods for immobilization of pediatric patients.

Describe techniques to interact with pediatric patients and their parents.

List materials needed for performing injections on pediatric patients, and list possible injection sites.

Discuss techniques for determining the administered dose of radiopharmaceuticals for pediatric patients.

Describe imaging considerations for bone scintigraphy in pediatrics.

Discuss renal scintigraphy, renography, crystography, and diuresis studies.

Describe imaging procedures for the pediatric patient gastrointestinal system including hepatobiliary, Meckel diverticulum, gastroesophageal reflux, and gastric emptying.

Describe imaging procedures for pediatric cardiovascular nuclear medicine.

---

*T*he disease processes of the pediatric age group and their technical requirements for imaging differ significantly from those encountered in adults. The nuclear medicine technologist should have an understanding of the differences to perform adequate pediatric nuclear medicine studies. A busy nuclear medicine department that primarily performs procedures on adults may find the occasional pediatric patient to be disruptive to the smooth flow of the day's workload. From the moment the child enters the department, the routine methods of operation must be modified to respond to the child's needs. Several factors must be considered, including the equipment and its ability to resolve small structures, patient safety and nursing care, immobilization techniques, patient and parent psychology, the injection technique, and technical factors required for specific procedures.

TECHNICAL CONSIDERATIONS

Instrumentation

A good rule of thumb is that a pediatric nuclear medicine study should be performed with a gamma camera that has the highest state-of-the-art resolution. Another good rule is only to include the area of interest in the field of view. For example, when studying the kidneys of an infant, including the entire torso only contributes unnecessary counts and reduces the information from the site of interest. Therefore the instrument should also have the capability to magnify images. Computer zooming is not effective, since it does not enhance resolution. Given the choice, for example, between the use of a large–field-of-view camera with no magnification and a standard–field-of-view camera with magnification for the performance of a neonatal bone imaging procedure, the standard–field-of-view instrument should be chosen. The use of magnifying devices such as converging and pinhole collimators is also recommended for the imaging of small parts.

Patient Safety and Care

Safety is essential when dealing with a pediatric patient. The child should never be left alone in an imaging room or on an imaging table. Immobilization devices such as sandbags, Velcro straps, or adhesive tape should be used as a "safety belt." Ideally, two individuals should perform the pediatric study: a technologist to acquire the images and another to remain close to the child. The second person serves two functions. First, and of primary importance, is safety. The individual, who may or may not be a nuclear medicine technologist, should be close enough to the patient to be able to prevent falls or other catastrophes. Second, the technologist can position the patient while the other person starts the imaging sequence, thus increasing efficiency. The second person can immobilize or entertain the child.

Nuclear medicine technologists should be certified in cardiopulmonary resuscitation (CPR) as well as trained to deal with various intravenous infusion equipment and monitoring devices such as pulse oximeters. Special emphasis on pediatric resuscitation techniques should be provided during CPR training programs. It may be necessary to request special training from resource groups such as nursing or respiratory therapy to ensure the appropriate use of pediatric infusion and monitoring devices.

To produce a high-quality pediatric nuclear medicine study, the technologist should have an attitude that the child deserves only the best that is available. One should embrace the concept that any amount of absorbed radiation dose is significant and that the study therefore must be justified. A repeat study because of technical deficiency is unjustified.

Immobilization Techniques

Immobilization is required if the patient is either unable or unwilling to remain still for the time required. Various immobilization techniques are available, including wrapping, sandbagging, and sedation.[14] In addition, some nuclear medicine technologists become adept at entertaining the child as distraction from the boredom of holding still for long intervals. It is a good practice to ask the parent to bring along a favorite toy, blanket, or object that can provide comfort and assurance to the child and may serve as an aid in holding the child's attention. When available, the use of televi-

sion with children's programing is successful. Other distractions such as tape recorders with stories or music are helpful. A supply of small toys and books in the nuclear medicine department is a good idea. Sleep deprivation or delaying the patient's normal nap time before the scheduled study might induce sleep. Many younger children are accustomed to having a story read to them just before bedtime, and simulation of that situation might induce calm or even sleep.

Mechanical. Wrapping or swaddling, sandbags, and Velcro straps or adhesive tape immobilization techniques have been advocated. Each technique has its advantages and disadvantages and should be used judiciously. Wrapping effectively immobilizes the child, but monitoring the respiratory rate, skin tone, pulse, and blood pressure is inhibited by this technique. Overheating can occur as well. If an emergent situation arises with the patient's condition, the time necessary to unwrap the child can be frustrating.

Sandbags are also used to stabilize the patient's arms or legs in an appropriate position. However, in the neonate or infant, sandbags may be too heavy or cause ischemia, particularly if used for prolonged imaging times. Sandbags also attenuate photons and can create artifacts in the image. They are primarily used as safety devices positioned alongside the body to prevent the child from rolling off the table.

Surgical adhesive tape can be used to help immobilize, but tape should never be applied directly to the skin. Many children are allergic to adhesive tape, and it can stick to the skin or hair and cause pain on removal. Adhesive tape is more practical as a safety device and should be used like a seat belt. Allergy to rubber tourniquets is also a problem. Velcro strap devices attached to the imaging table may be preferable to adhesive tape. Immobilization, particularly with infants, can also be accomplished by the technologist or the parent simply by holding the child in place with gentle pressure on the part being imaged.

Sedation. Sedation is an effective means of achieving immobilization. However, sedation should be used judiciously and with the appropriate monitoring protocol so that complications are minimized and the patient can adequately recover from the effects of the sedation before discharge. Rarely, following idiosyncratic reactions to the sedation, it may be necessary to keep the child in the hospital overnight to ensure complete recovery. Sedation is most frequently used for 1- to 4-year-old patients, especially for bone imaging, SPECT imaging, and for patients with mental retardation or behavior problems. Special consideration must be given to sedating the child with a brain injury, respiratory distress, cyanosis, or a history of an adverse reaction to sedation. The technologist must be aware of all medications the child is receiving and the time of the last dose.

The American Academy of Pediatrics has published guidelines for the sedation and recovery of children.[7] These guidelines emphasize the use of approximate doses to reach various levels of consciousness and appropriate monitoring of vital signs using modern devices such as electronic oxygen saturation monitors. All personnel monitoring sedated children must be pediatric CPR certified, and all information regarding the sedative, dose administered, monitoring, and recovery must be permanently documented as part of the patient's record. There may be state or local laws that govern sedation, such as who can administer it. The responsible physician must be readily available. Finally, the parent must be cautioned that delayed reactions can occur, and they must be given written instructions and emergency phone numbers to call if any are observed. It is highly preferable that an institutional policy and procedure for the use of sedation that follows the guidelines is in place before the use of any sedatives. The policy should include quality improvement processes and oversight.

Our current pharmaceutical of choice for sedation in the healthy child is chloral hydrate. It is the most commonly used drug for the sedation of children for diagnostic tests.[28] Chloral hydrate can be administered orally or rectally and is usually effective within 20 to 30 min. The child usually loses consciousness long enough for a bone scintigram using the multiple spot image technique. The failure rate of chloral hydrate is relatively high (approximately 13%),[45] but it is also relatively safe. Others have reported the use of midazolan as a nasal spray to achieve patient cooperation, particularly for studies of the bladder. The drug also produces an amnesialike effect, which is advocated by some because catheterization of the bladder for some patients is a traumatic event.[29] Lower doses of all sedatives are recommended for children who are debilitated or have respiratory or neurologic deficits.

The effectiveness of chloral hydrate is variable; some children may require a longer time to go to sleep. Providing a quiet, darkened environment can help. Individual imaging rooms help to segregate the patient from the noisy department. Some children never fall asleep completely but are quieted enough to enable the technologist to perform the imaging procedure, particularly when the child is reassured that no further pain is associated with the procedure. An occasional child might exhibit an adverse or opposite effect to the sedation, that is, become more combative and uncontrollable. This is particularly so if the child is allowed to become extremely agitated before sedation. For this reason we recommend to the parents that they not discuss the procedure with the child before coming to the hospital, especially if the child is easily agitated regarding such medical procedures. Frequently, a history of sedative use indicates whether a given pharmaceutical

is appropriate to use for sedation. If chloral hydrate is not indicated or if there are other medical reasons, an anesthesiologist should be consulted. Very rarely, the child may need to be admitted to the hospital and be given a general anesthetic for performance of the procedure.

The possible risks and implications of any sedation should be discussed with the parents to allay concern and to prepare for the possibility of the child being admitted to the hospital for adequate recovery. Formal arrangements should be agreed on between the nuclear medicine and anesthesiology departments for the recovery of patients sedated late in the workday or for those who have adverse reactions to the sedation.

Patient-Parent Interaction

A major consideration is the psychologic interaction between the child and the parent.[48] A pediatric study usually necessitates dealing with a family unit, that is, the parent, the child, and at times other members of the family as well. Frequently, either the parent or the child indicates apprehension about the procedure. The examination should be explained to the child as well as the parent. One explanation is given in terms that the parent will understand and another at the level of the child's understanding. The nuclear medicine technologist must assess the situation and determine which of the explanations should be given first. If the patient is under 3 years of age, it is of little value to discuss the study with the child. If the patient is an older child, the parent's explanation becomes secondary.

If the patient is of child-bearing age, the importance of inadvertent radiation exposure of the fetus must be considered. The technologist should directly address the issue of possible pregnancy. A girl's sexual activity may begin as early as 10 years of age. It is appropriate to determine the date of the patient's last menstrual cycle and to inquire if the patient is sexually active. The adolescent may deny sexual activity in the presence of the parent or others; therefore the technologist should question the patient privately.[9] That information should be noted in the patient's nuclear medicine record.

An assessment of the patient-parent relationship and interaction is important for the successful performance of a nuclear medicine examination of the pediatric patient. The parent may convey apprehension or other emotions to the child in many ways, both verbally and nonverbally. This communication has a direct effect on the child's behavior. The parenting philosophy may have a direct effect on the child's behavior as well. For example, if the parent is permissive, the child might refuse to cooperate, and the parent might not intervene or even perceive a need to intervene to correct the child's behavior. Other parents exhibit strict authoritarian parenting techniques, and the child might be passive.

It might be appropriate for the technologist or the nuclear medicine physician to privately discuss with the parent the effect of the parent's behavior on the child and the technologist's ability to perform a successful examination. Generally, it is preferable to allow the parent to accompany the child into the imaging room to observe the entire procedure.[6] It is usually more comforting to the child to have the parent in attendance. However, in those instances when the child is uncooperative and the technologist cannot gain the child's cooperation with the assistance of the parent, it may be necessary to request that the parent leave the room until the child agrees to cooperate. The technologist must be firm and authoritative in the approach to the child to maintain control of the situation. Patient cooperation should be praised, both to the child and to the parent. Allowing the child to participate in the study, for example, by letting the child control the remote stop-start switch on the gamma camera, enhances further cooperation. Cooperation is often accomplished by dealing truthfully with the child. For example, if an injection is necessary, it is preferable to tell the child that there will be some discomfort. To do otherwise ensures loss of trust and cooperation. The technologist must also listen to the child's complaints and respond to them appropriately. Never allow the child to become abusive, either physically or verbally.

Injection Technique

For the successful intravenous administration of a radiopharmaceutical to the pediatric patient, the injection should be performed by those individuals whose attributes include a delicate manual dexterity, a calmness under stressful conditions, and a capability for empathy. The nuclear medicine technologists might be the most capable for this task, since they receive formal training in phlebotomy and, unless otherwise prohibited by state regulation, are readily available to perform the majority of radiopharmaceutical administrations.

There is a common belief that an intravenous injection in an infant or child is more difficult. However, when proper technique is used, the procedure is successful in the vast majority of instances. The following technique has been used with a very high success rate at the Children's Memorial Hospital in Chicago.[14] The technique requires an appropriate explanation to the child, the ready availability of the required materials, and preferably two individuals, one to insert the needle and the other to assist in immobilizing the patient.

A tray should be prepared that includes all the necessary items for administration of the radiopharmaceutical. Included on the tray should be scalp vein infusion sets of a variety of sizes, usually 21-, 23-, and 25-gauge needles, and a three-way disposable stopcock with the radionuclide syringe attached to one port and a syringe of normal saline (minimum 10 ml) attached to the side port (Figure 18-1). Alcohol wipes, dry 2×2 sterile sponges, a pediatric size tourniquet, disposable sterile gloves, nonallergenic tape for fixation of the needle, and various sizes of support boards are also needed. The tray is lined with plastic-backed disposable paper to prevent contamination in case the radionuclide spills. The syringe containing the radiopharmaceutical should be enclosed within a lead syringe shield.

The injection should be performed using aseptic and universal precautions techniques. The selection of

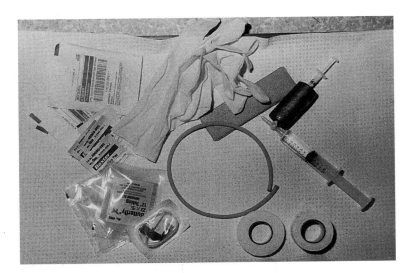

Figure 18-1 Injection tray used to transport all required materials from the preparation area to injection room. Note that some materials are duplicated in the event that more than one attempt to insert the IV is required.

an injection site is of utmost importance. One should examine all of the preferred injection sites before attempting to insert the needle. Several sites are objectionable and should be used only under unusual circumstances. The antecubital veins are often deeply situated and are not visible or palpable in young children.

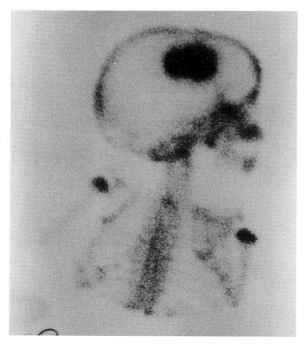

Figure 18-2 Scalp vein injection that extravasated caused an easily recognized artifact on images of the head.

They are often used for blood sampling and, as a consequence, are traumatized before the child reaches the nuclear medicine department. It is possible to infiltrate the entire radiopharmaceutical dose into the antecubital space without observing any indication of extravasation. Scalp veins are not only esthetically objectionable and more frightening to the child, but often trauma to the scalp and extravasation produce significant artifacts on subsequent images (Figure 18-2). Serious complications such as hip joint infection and femoral artery thrombosis have been reported from the attempted use of femoral veins.[33] Last, the use of the jugular veins is difficult because of the manipulations necessary to produce venous dilatation, such as extending the head and neck and forcibly restraining the child's head to the side. It is also esthetically objectionable to the parents and a very frightening experience for the child.

Preferred sites include the veins on the dorsum of the hand and the foot. The veins in these sites are usually not already traumatized, since they are rarely used for blood sampling, are usually visible because of their superficial location, and are usually oriented in a linear fashion. In addition, during a dynamic study the hands and feet are usually more accessible if the child is beneath the camera, and they are easily immobilized for the injection.[11]

Immobilization of the hand or the foot can be easily accomplished by holding the wrist or the foot between the index and middle finger and holding the patient's fingers or toes down with the thumb (Figure 18-3). Extension of the joint at the elbow and flexion at

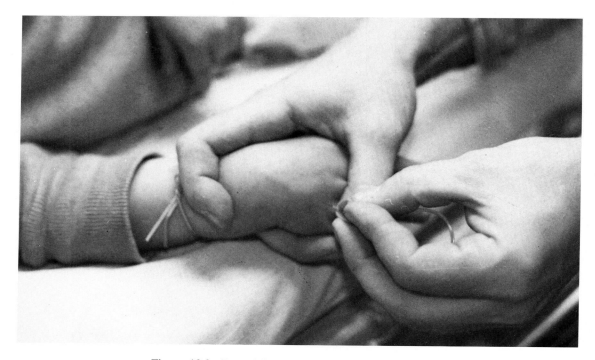

Figure 18-3 Immobilization of the hand for injection.

the wrist serves to further immobilize the hand veins and reduce the patient's capability of withdrawing the extremity. Extension of the knee and ankle joints helps to immobilize the veins on the dorsum of the foot. In older children it is helpful to have a second person gently restrain the arm or leg. If this is done, one must remember that all restraints should be loosened for a short interval before the injection of the radiopharmaceutical so as not to produce a tourniquet effect artifact[50] (Figure 18-4).

The size of the scalp vein needle should be selected to match the caliber of the vein. The needle is connected to the three-way stopcock with the valve on the stopcock positioned such that the saline syringe portal is open to the scalp vein needle. Saline is flushed through the scalp vein needle set before use. The venipuncture should be performed with the bevel of the scalp vein needle in the down position. In this manner the needle bevel enters the vein in a parallel fashion and not at an angle. It is preferable to direct the needle toward the confluence of branching vessels into a single vein. As soon as the needle has entered the vein, blood immediately refluxes into the infusion tubing at the needle hub. The application of suction by drawing back

on the saline syringe is unnecessary in children because blood in the needle hub does not appear unless the needle is intravenously located and one can safely conclude that the vein has been entered. In adults the larger caliber veins may not exhibit sufficient pressure beyond the tourniquet to reflux blood into the needle hub.

When blood is seen in the tubing, no further manipulation of the needle should be attempted, such as threading the needle into the vein, because further manipulation frequently results in perforation of the opposite venous wall or dislodgement from the vein. The tourniquet should be immediately released and a test injection of saline made to confirm the intravenous placement. Any immediate swelling about the site of the needle tip indicates an extravascular location and necessitates removal of the needle and the use of another site. If the test injection of saline confirms an appropriate placement of the needle, then the stopcock is switched to the radionuclide syringe for administration of the radiopharmaceutical. A short delay before injecting the radiopharmaceutical is suggested to eliminate the tourniquet effect artifact. During the injection, passage of the saline or radiopharmaceutical through the veins over the wrist or foot can be observed and felt beneath the technologist's index finger. Once the radiopharmaceutical syringe is empty, the residual activity within the stopcock and tubing is flushed with the remaining saline.

Radiopharmaceutical Administered Dose

Methods proposed to calculate the amount of radioactivity for a specific study are based on the child's weight, body surface area, estimation of organ volume, percentage of adult dose, and fixed dose. However, these methods tend to underestimate doses at the low end of the scale or overestimate them at the upper end of the scale. There is a minimum amount of activity required for adequate imaging, even in the smallest child. The selection of a method or individual dose should be based on the principle of as low as reasonably achievable (ALARA). Conversely, a maximum limit should be established. The method used for radiopharmaceutical dose determination at the Children's Memorial Hospital is empirically derived. That is, administered dose and dose ranges are determined by experience based on several factors, including the patient's condition, the imaging technique desired (that is, static versus dynamic imaging and limited bone imaging versus SPECT imaging), the imaging equipment to be used, the radionuclide energy, the biologic half-life of the radiopharmaceutical, and the percent localization in the organ of interest.

The empirically determined radiopharmaceutical dose is primarily based on the interval for which most patients are able to remain still. When they are being

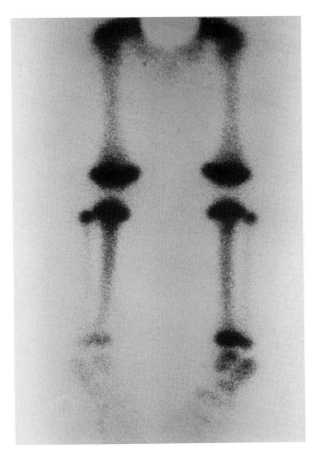

Figure 18-4 Increased localization in left lower extremity caused by tourniquet effect of restraint during injection of radionuclide in the foot.

fed, most children and even babies are able to remain still for an interval as long as 5 min. Based on that assumption the empiric method estimates the radiopharmaceutical dose required to obtain a specific type of image at the appropriate time interval after injection, which can be acquired in 5 min for a specific imaging technique, that is, the use of magnification, choice of collimation, and the sensitivity of the camera. Based on the empiric method and experience, recommended radiopharmaceutical dose ranges for common radionuclide studies used at the Children's Memorial Hospital are provided in Table 18-1.

Some radiopharmaceutical package inserts contain information regarding the recommended administered dose to be used in children. Some do not, however, since many radiopharmaceuticals have not been tested specifically for safety and efficacy in the pediatric population. This is because phase II and III clinical trials are costly and difficult to perform in the pediatric popula-

tion. The Food and Drug Administration (FDA) in cooperation with its Radiopharmaceutical Drug Advisory Committee and members of the Pediatric Nuclear Medicine Council of the Society of Nuclear Medicine have worked to provide labeling information for pediatric radiopharmaceuticals and continue to do so. Most radiopharmaceutical companies provide technical support services to give assistance in cases where the package insert information is not available. These services maintain information derived from the literature on pediatric administered doses for their products to disseminate to their customers. Other sources of information in regard to recommended pediatric administered doses are the local commercial radiopharmacies.

Positioning

It is preferable to obtain as many images as possible with the gamma camera beneath the patient. This

Table 18-1	Pediatric administered doses (the Children's Memorial Hospital, Chicago)			
Procedure	**Radiopharmaceutical**	**Administered dose***	**Minimum**	**Maximum**
Brain scintigram	^{99m}Tc DTPA	400 μCi/lb	10 mCi	20 mCi
Brain SPECT perfusion	^{99m}Tc HMPAO	285 μCi/kg	5 mCi	20 mCi
Angiogram	^{99m}Tc pertechnetate	200 μCi/lb	2.5 mCi	15 mCi
Liver scintigram	^{99m}Tc sulfur colloid	25 μCi/lb	500μCi	2 mCi
Lung scintigram	^{99m}Tc MAA	25 μCi/lb	500 μCi	2 mCi
Renal scintigram	^{99m}TC DTPA	50 μCi/lb	2.5 mCi	15 mCi
	or			
	^{99m}Tc glucoheptonate	50 μCi/lb	2.5 mCi	15 mCi
	or			
	^{99m}Tc MAG3	22 μCi/lb	1 mCi	5 mCi
Renogram	^{131}I hippuran	100 μCi	50 μCi	100 μCi
Bone scintigram	^{99m}Tc diphosphonate	300 μCi/lb	5 mCi	20 mCi
Limited bone scintigram	^{99m}Tc diphosphonate	200 μCi/lb	5 mCi	20 mCi
Cystogram	^{99m}Tc pertechnetate	1 mCi	1 mCi	1 mCi
Thyroid uptake	^{123}I sodium iodide	100 μCi	2 μCi	100 μCi
Thyroid scintigram	^{99m}Tc pertechnetate	1-2 mCi	1 mCi	2 mCi
Plasma volume	^{123}I HSA	3 μCi	1 μCi	3 μCi
Gallium scintigram	^{67}Ga citrate	3-10 mCi	3 mCi	10 mCi
Subarachnoid scintigram	^{111}In DTPA	300 μCi	100 μCi	300 μCi
Dacryoscintigraphy	^{99m}Tc pertechnetate	200 μCi/drop	400 μCi	800 μCi
Gastroesophageal reflux	^{99m}Tc sulfur colloid	150 μCi	150 μCi	150 μCi
MUGA study	^{99m}Tc pertechnetate	350 μCi/lb	10 mCi	20 mCi
Meckel's scintigram	^{99m}Tc pertechnetate	100 μCi/lb	2.5 mCi	15 mCi
Gastrointestinal bleeding	^{99m}Tc sulfur colloid	5 mCi	1 mCi	5 mCi
Hepatobiliary study	^{99m}Tc mebrofenin	100 μCi/kg	1.0 mCi	8.0 mCi
Testicular scintigram	^{99m}Tc pertechnetate	200 μCi/lb	5.0 mCi	15 mCi
MIBG scintigram	^{131}I MIBG	500 μCi	2 mCi	

*The nuclear medicine physician might double or increase the dose depending on the clinical situation, such as an uncooperative or retarded child or critical condition, to expedite the study and optimize results.
MUGA, Multiple gated acquisition; *MIBG*, metaiodobenzylguanidine; *DTPA*, diethylenetriaminepentaacetic acid; *MAG3*, mercaptoacetyltriglycine; *MAA*, microaggregated albumin; *HSA*, human serum albumin.

serves two purposes. First, it is a frightening experience for the child to have the massive detector overhead. Second, it is easier to monitor condition and vital signs without the detector obscuring the view of the child. In addition, older children are able to watch television, read a book, or be otherwise distracted. For anterior images the child can be placed prone on the imaging table. In fact, many children sleep in the prone position, and such positioning helps to calm them. A small patient can be placed directly on top of the collimator for imaging.

Of paramount importance is the appropriate positioning of the child within the field of view of the gamma camera. The determination of abnormal radionuclide localization depends on the comparison of one site with its contralateral side. This can readily be accomplished only if the patient's position is anatomic and symmetric (Figure 18-5). If it is impossible to position the patient anatomically because of the clinical condition, then both sides should be malpositioned identically and symmetrically to allow comparison. Anatomic positioning for SPECT imaging is even more important in that a slight rotation can cause the appearance of increased or decreased activity on individual tomographic slices as an artifact of positioning. Current state-of-the-art SPECT software can correct some poor positioning rotational artifacts. When using the SPECT imaging table, it might be preferable to place the patient in the prone position, since many children sleep in this manner and are therefore more comfortable. It also may be advantageous to position with the feet first rather than head first in the gantry, so that the patient can look up from that position and see something other than the back of the gantry.

Of particular concern is the safety of the patient on the narrow SPECT imaging table. We devised a patient safety restraint that wraps around the child and the imaging table using Velcro strapping, thus securing the patient to the table to prevent falling (Figure 18-6) and ensure immobilization. The device does not attenuate, as it is made of vinyl and Velcro strapping.

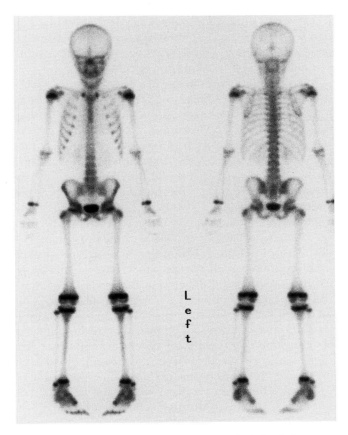

Figure 18-5   Symmetric positioning for whole-body bone scan allows comparison of one side to the other.

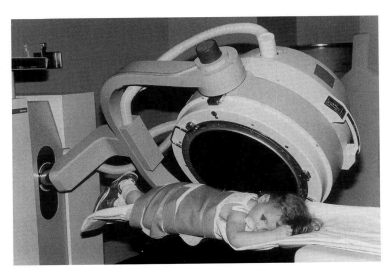

Figure 18-6   Patient restraining device used for safety belt during SPECT imaging. Note patient position with feet toward the detector and prone position, which is comforting to some patients.

CLINICAL APPLICATIONS

In this section the most commonly performed pediatric nuclear medicine procedures are reviewed with particular attention to technique. This is not meant to be a comprehensive review of all pediatric nuclear medicine procedures. For specific topics not included in this section, the reader should examine the current literature and the other chapters of this textbook related to specific imaging procedures.

Skeletal System

Bone scintigraphy in our pediatric nuclear medicine practice comprises almost 40% of the studies performed annually. It requires particular attention to technical detail. The technologist should be familiar with the appearance of normal pediatric bone localization, as well as skeletal anatomy, to perform appropriate positioning and to recognize artifacts when they occur.

The development of ^{99m}Tc-phosphate radiopharmaceuticals, as well as improved resolution and increased sensitivity instrumentation, has made bone scintigraphy a practicality in the pediatric population. Technetium-phosphate radiopharmaceuticals give acceptable radiation absorbed dosimetry, and the improved resolving power of the gamma camera over older instrumentation allows adequate bone scintigraphy, even in full-term and premature neonates.

The clinical indications for the performance of bone scintigraphy include infection, occult trauma, tumor localization, sports injuries, and orthopedic disorders such as avascular necrosis.[12] These conditions often include pain, which can inhibit the patient's ability to cooperate for a lengthy imaging procedure. Sedation or pain medication might be required to obtain adequate images. Since the technique of bone scintigraphy requires a 2 to 3 hr delay between the injection of the radiopharmaceutical and acquisition of the static images, the technologist has adequate time for assessment of the patient's ability to cooperate and to arrange for appropriate medication and monitoring. Chloral hydrate should be administered approximately 30 to 45 min before the scheduled imaging time to allow adequate time for the sedation to take effect. If SPECT imaging is to be performed, it is desirable to obtain the SPECT image as soon as the patient has fallen asleep, if possible, to ensure adequate sedation throughout the SPECT acquisition. At times this is not possible, since the site of the abnormal localization is unknown and routine static images must be acquired first to identify the location.

For specific clinical indications, bone scintigraphy is performed in one, two, or three phases. A one-phase bone scintigram consists of delayed static images acquired at 2 to 3 hr after injection. A two-phase bone imaging procedure includes an immediate extracellular (blood-pool) image of a minimum of 500,000 counts of the area of interest, which is acquired within the first few minutes after injection and the delayed static images at 2 to 3 hr. The three-phase bone scintigram includes a dynamic acquisition of the area of interest begun immediately after injection at a frame rate of 5 sec/frame for 12 frames. The dynamic acquisition is then followed by blood-pool images and the routine static images at 2 to 3 hr after injection.

Whole-body images allow the interpreter to survey the entire skeleton. This is helpful in recognizing patterns of distribution, malposition, and subtle asymmetric localizations. The distribution pattern often defines the disease process, such as in child abuse, where diaphyseal localization in the extremities is characteristic of the shaken child. A normal distribution pattern in the physes of the child is recognized. The physes at the knees have greater activity than the physes at the ankles, which in turn have greater activity than the physes of the hips. The reverse is true in the upper extremities. The physes at the shoulder have greater activity than the physes at the wrists, which have greater activity than the physes at the elbows. A knowledge of these patterns can allow one to differentiate abnormalities, increased or decreased, at any given joint.[10] The differences in the various physes are altered if the images are obtained in the anterior or posterior position because of varying distances from the camera. Single spot images of the extremities do not allow detection of subtle differences in localization because an exact positioning of the areas of interest is difficult to achieve.

Careful attention should be paid to the statistics of the images acquired. When a whole-body imaging device is used, a minimum of 1 million counts per image is required. Both anterior and posterior whole-body images with the patient positioned anatomically and symmetrically are necessary for an adequate survey (Figure 18-7). Patients under 5 years of age or older patients of short stature should have survey images done as spot films with magnification as necessary to provide sufficient detail. In addition to the whole-body survey images, spot images should be acquired for a minimum of 500,000 counts each. Subsequent spot magnification films of particular areas of interest should have a minimum of 250,000 counts/view. Limited one-phase bone scintigraphy is used only for follow-up examination such as for Legg-Calvé-Perthes disease. Such a study consists of one posterior total-body film, spot films of the pelvis (anterior anatomic projection of the hips and posterior frog-leg lateral of the hips), and pinhole anterior and frog-leg lateral views of the hips. These magnified views should exclude the bladder and include only the acetabulum and hips to the level of the lesser trochanter (Figure 18-8).

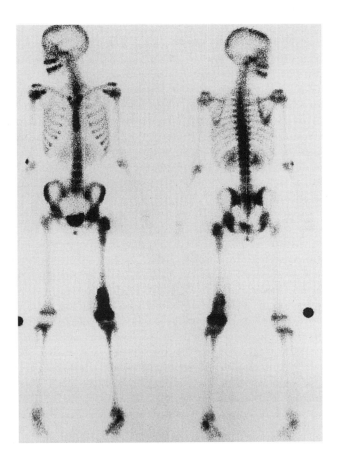

Figure 18-7 Whole-body images allowed recognition of abnormal localization of radionuclide in the scapula, which was not recognized on limited bone scan performed at another institution.

Infection. Bone scintigraphy is the most sensitive and specific imaging technique currently available for differentiating septic arthritis, cellulitis, and osteomyelitis.[27] Frequently x-ray examinations are completely normal in these disorders. Musculoskeletal infection includes pain and limitation of motion, and the patient usually but not always exhibits an elevated erythrocyte sedimentation rate and frequently fever. In the neonatal population, however, the only clinical finding may be the lack of movement of an extremity. The early identification of septic arthritis or osteomyelitis is imperative to prevent bone or joint destruction and subsequent deformity. For example, in our experience an untreated septic arthritis of the hip of greater than 5 days' duration has a 50% probability of developing avascular necrosis of the proximal femoral epiphysis.[8]

The typical scintigraphic appearance of acute osteomyelitis is a well-defined focus of increased radionuclide localization or hot lesion seen on all three phases of the bone scan. The lesion is invariably in the metaphysis of the bone. On occasion, however, it presents as a photopenic or cold lesion when the vascular supply to the bone is compromised by surrounding tissue edema (compartment syndrome) or vascular thrombosis.[3] The detection and identification of ischemic osteomyelitis resulting in a cold area on the bone scintigram warrant an emergency surgical drainage procedure to diminish the pressure in the tissues and enhance the return of blood flow.

Trauma. Because radionuclide scintigraphy has a high sensitivity for defining bone changes due to trauma, it

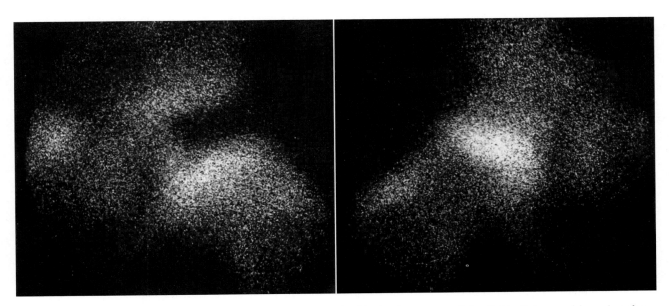

Figure 18-8 Pinhole views of hips are acquired by positioning the hip in the center of the field of view and lowering the camera until the collimator is pressing on the patient's skin. Left hip demonstrates total avascularity of the epiphysis. Right hip is normal.

is an extremely useful tool for several disorders in the pediatric population. The normal bumps and bruises of childhood play do not produce abnormalities on bone scintigraphy. Significant or repeated trauma is required to produce perfusion and metabolic changes that are evident on bone scintigraphy. Several entities are well recognized and include the occult fracture,[44] child abuse,[47] sports injuries,[36,39,40,52] and stress changes in the spine associated with spondylolysis.[23] Other entities readily obvious on bone imaging and thought to be related to trauma include reflex sympathetic dystrophy[26] and myositis ossificans.[35] It is important to note that all of these disorders have normal x-ray appearances in their early and sometimes even their late stages.

The young toddler who is limping or refusing to walk and has a normal x-ray will demonstrate increased localization of radionuclide at a site of occult trauma. The lesion might be an occult undisplaced fracture or a microtrabecular bone injury. Frequent sites include the calcaneus, the cuboid, the patella, and metatarsal bones. The identification of abnormal radionuclide localization in the bones of the foot, particularly in the small child, requires magnification images to adequately differentiate which bone is involved (Figure 18-9). Because of the prolonged imaging time required to acquire adequate magnification images of the hands or feet, lower count images (50,000) at higher intensity settings are necessary.

Correlative studies of bone scintigraphy versus x-ray survey examinations have documented that scintigraphy has a greater sensitivity (27%) for recognizing bone trauma in child abuse.[47] Although x-rays provide bet-ter evidence of healed fractures and undisplaced hairline skull fractures, bone scintigraphy better demonstrates injuries of flat bones such as the ribs, pelvis, and spine as well as soft tissue injury. X-ray and bone scintigraphy, therefore, are used in a complementary manner to document evidence of child abuse. The technical quality of bone scintigraphy in child abuse is important, since the majority of child abuse occurs in infants and young children under the age of 2. Their small bone structure requires high-resolution magnification imaging to define the appropriate information for interpretation.

Organized competitive sports for children have become more popular in recent years. Because athletic activities require repeated practice of a particular motion or series of motions, there can be chronic and repeated stress effect on the bones. This can produce focal metabolic changes that are evident on bone scintigraphy and often are related to a particular type of sport. For example, teenagers who train as runners often develop shin splits or stress fractures of the tibia. Speed skaters, because of uneven stresses on the feet due to the specific direction in which they race, may have a stress injury in one foot and not the other. Baseball pitchers demonstrate hypertrophy of their throwing arms. Frequently an athlete overlooks a specific trauma incident and is brought to the nuclear medicine department because of chronic and persistent bone pain. The information that the child participates in a particular sport frequently is either not conveyed or is not known by the referring physician. Often it is the nuclear medicine technologist who, when seeking a cause for the abnormal appearance on the bone scin-

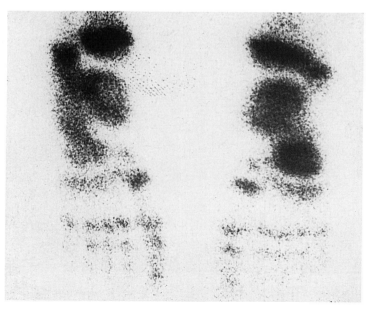

Figure 18-9 Electronically magnified image of both feet, which required 10 min of acquisition time, are required to adequately visualize abnormal localization.

tigram, finally elicits the history of a specific sports trauma, which explains the scintigraphic findings.

Stress on the pars interarticularis of the vertebrae can cause spondylolysis, which can be evident on bone scintigraphy as a focal area of increased localization. The patient develops back pain without fever. It is common in weight lifters and in football and basketball players. SPECT imaging is necessary in this disorder if the routine static images fail to demonstrate an abnormality or are equivocal.[15] SPECT imaging detects approximately one third more abnormalities than planar scintigraphic images. Radionuclide scintigraphy is much more sensitive than x-ray in recognizing all the forms of sports trauma.

Hip pain. Hip pain in the child may be due to a variety of causes, including toxic synovitis, septic arthritis, slipped capital femoral epiphysis,[43] and avascular necrosis of the femoral head.[12] Adequate imaging of the hip is achieved through the use of magnification techniques with a pinhole collimator.[37] The technologist should initially position the patient's normal hip with the pinhole collimator raised about 1 to 2 feet above it. Once the hip is visualized in the center of the field of view, the camera is lowered until the pinhole is touching and pressing lightly on the patient's skin. An anterior image is acquired for at least 100,000 counts. Subsequent images of the normal hip in the frog-leg lateral position and the painful hip in the anterior and frog-leg lateral positions are acquired for the same time as for the anterior image of the normal hip. The bladder must be emptied before imaging so that the activity from a full bladder does not degrade the images by lessening the number of counts from the area of interest. If the child is unable to void, the bladder should be excluded from the image by a lead shield.

Oncologic disorders. Children with oncologic disorders benefit from bone scintigraphy for the diagnosis, staging, and assessment of disease response to therapy. These patients can also exhibit a variety of focal abnormalities on bone scintigraphy that are unrelated to their neoplastic disease and might be confusing in their interpretation. Children with oncologic disorders may have osteoporosis from chemotherapy or poor nutrition; their bones are weaker; furthermore, they may be more susceptible to trauma or injury because of a physical handicap, such as an amputation. As a consequence, traumatic bone lesions are frequently evidenced on bone imaging performed for oncologic reasons. Amputees can display abnormal radionuclide localization at the end of the stump or in the hemipelvis because altered ambulation caused by a prosthetic device induces stress in the bone.[1] The use of crutches frequently causes increased radionuclide localization on the inner aspect of the proximal portion of the humeri. Conversely, diminished radionuclide localization, which ap-

pears as an asymmetry in the images, may be related to radiotherapy. It is important that the technologist who performs the bone scintigraphy procedure document such potential causes of abnormal localization to alert the nuclear medicine physician to allow for an appropriate interpretation of the abnormality.

SPECT technique. As mentioned previously, SPECT bone scintigraphy is extremely valuable because of its greater sensitivity in detecting subtle localization abnormalities from occult metastases, occult trauma, or localized early infection. This is especially true when examining the spine. The anatomy of the spine is complex, x-ray changes appear late in the disease, and planar scintigraphy defines relatively gross abnormalities. SPECT techniques require stringent quality control that is very time consuming. In addition to the routine daily quality control procedures for the gamma camera, pediatric SPECT scintigraphy requires the generation of flood-correction matrices and centers-of-rotation (COR) measurements for every possible combination of collimator and magnification factor that might be used. Because of the age range of patients imaged, this may necessitate a 2-week cycle of nightly quality control acquisitions.

When using a single-head SPECT instrument, data acquisition requires 45 to 60 min for statistical adequacy. Younger patients might require sedation or immobilization, sometimes even when they are cooperative.

For studies of the hips and pelvis, artifacts caused by radionuclide accumulation in the bladder can be controlled by catheterization of the bladder with continuous drainage. The upper extremities in the field of view for chest SPECT are an additional problem, which can be controlled by strapping the arms above the head for studies of the thorax.

Data processing is time consuming because on many studies the data are derived from statistically poor frames due to the limitation of the radionuclide dose or patient motion. Such poor data may require deletion of frames or other manipulation techniques. Standard protocols should not be used for data processing, since the information varies greatly from patient to patient. Computer systems that allow single-slice reconstruction with a variety of filters are helpful in determining the appropriate filter to be used for each individual patient. For SPECT images of the spine, quantification of abnormal localization of the radionuclide can be performed by placing regions of interest over the abnormal area and the contralateral normal site to derive a ratio of activity (Figure 18-10).

Genitourinary System

Radionuclide studies of the genitourinary tract comprise about 30% of all radionuclide studies performed

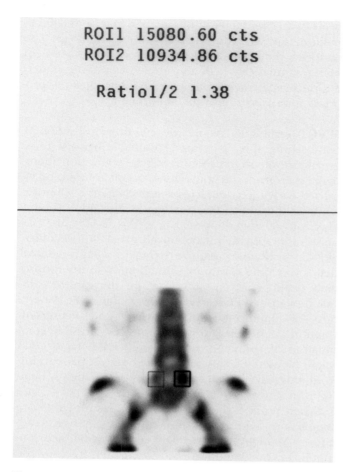

```
ROI1 15080.60 cts
ROI2 10934.86 cts

Ratio1/2 1.38
```

Figure 18-10 Quantitation of localization of radionuclide for bone SPECT imaging. Note typical hot appearance of spondylolysis.

on the pediatric population. The primary examinations include renography and renal scintigraphy, diuresis renography, direct radionuclide cystography, and scrotal scintigraphy. Radionuclide cystography and frequently renography require the placement of a urinary bladder catheter to provide adequate drainage. It is useful to develop the skill of bladder catheterization or to have an identified individual readily available to expedite the procedure and to prevent increased anxiety in the child by unnecessary delays in beginning the study. The technique of catheterization is described in the discussion on radionuclide cystography.

Renal scintigraphy, renography, and diuresis renography. Several disorders in childhood necessitate imaging and function studies of the urinary tract. These include infection, ureteropelvic or ureterovesical junction obstruction, neonatal hydronephrosis or hydroureteronephrosis, renal transplantation, renal vein thrombosis, and congenital anomalies in the neonate. Horseshoe kidneys, duplications, hypoplastic kidneys, and ectopic kidneys all can be diagnosed with radionuclide studies.[19]

A variety of radiopharmaceuticals have been developed for scintigraphic imaging and the functional evaluation of the kidneys. Most recently ^{99m}Tc mercaptoacetyltriglycine (MAG3) has become the radiopharmaceutical of choice for imaging and functional analysis in pediatric genitourinary nuclear medicine. Renal cortical scintigraphy is performed using either ^{99m}Tc glucoheptonate (GH) or ^{99m}Tc dimercaptosuccinic acid (DMSA). We prefer the use of ^{99m}Tc GH over ^{99m}Tc DMSA. The absorbed dose per millicurie is much less with ^{99m}Tc GH, and therefore higher activity angiographic images can be obtained with ^{99m}Tc GH. We have not experienced significant bowel, liver, or collecting system localization to interfere with the interpretation of the cortical regions of the kidneys using magnification and oblique projections.

Techniques such as the measurement of glomerular filtration rate (GFR) and effective renal plasma flow (ERPF) are performed occasionally; however, these techniques are time consuming when performed using multiple blood samples and are considered to be technically unreliable in the young child when using gamma-camera techniques. Only relative estimates ($\pm$ 10% to 20%) are realistically derived even with meticulous techniques.

It is well known that the state of hydration significantly affects the excretion of radiopharmaceuticals, particularly with diuretic stimulation.[16] Because of this, it is appropriate to control and monitor the patient's state of hydration for renography. Oral hydration to tolerance for at least 2 hr before the study should be encouraged. An intravenous line, using either a butterfly needle or intracath, is inserted for administration of a dilute normal saline (5% dextrose in 0.3 normal saline) at a rate of 15 ml/kg over a 30-min interval beginning at least 15 min before injection of the radiopharmaceutical. Hydration is continued through the remainder of the study as a maintenance fluid volume at a rate of 200 ml/kg/24 hr.

If the patient is unable to void on demand, the bladder should be catheterized to ensure adequate drainage during the study. Continuous bladder drainage reduces the absorbed radiation dose to the bladder and gonads and precludes patient movement due to impending urination. If the catheter does not adequately empty the bladder as observed on the persistence scope, then urine should be aspirated using syringe suction.

Twenty-two μCi/lb of ^{99m}Tc MAG3 is injected as a bolus with the patient positioned supine and the lumbar region in the field of view of the gamma camera. Magnification is used as needed to include only the area from the xiphoid to the symphysis pubis. Static images are obtained at intervals for 20 min. Digital information is acquired to derive renal function curves. A rate of 15 or 20 sec/frame is acceptable. At the conclusion of the acquisition, background-subtracted time-activity curves are generated on the computer.[16] The choice of an appropriate background region of interest (ROI) is a hotly debated topic among nuclear medicine practitioners; since each method described has its own related pitfall,[17] the best course of action is to choose one method to be used consistently. We currently prefer a circumferential ROI around the kidney for derivation of the renogram curve. Different background ROIs are preferred for the diuretic phase. ROIs must approximate as closely as possible the organ being monitored, for example, the renal pelvis during the diuretic phase of renography, to be accurate in reflecting the appropriate activity.

If there is delayed excretion of the radiopharmaceutical from the collecting system, furosemide (Lasix)[21] diuresis renography is performed. If a urinary catheter is not in place, the patient should be requested to empty the bladder. Furosemide diuresis is induced utilizing an administered dose of 1 mg/kg. Acquisition is continued utilizing the same parameters as the renogram phase of the study. The background ROI for the Lasix curve should exclude the ureter, and the ROI should closely approximate only the renal pelvis. A separate ROI for the ureter is used when there is hydroureteronephrosis.

A variety of data analyses, in addition to the generation of time-activity curves for the whole kidney, can be performed. Percent differential renal function is the total counts from the renogram curve for each kidney minus background counts during the interval between 60 sec and the initial appearance of radioactivity in the calyces. The time is best determined by viewing the computer images sequentially. The significance of percent differential renal function in the presence of bilateral disease is questionable. Parenchymal transit time has been advocated as an effective means of differentiating obstruction from other causes of hydronephrosis.[51] Cortical renal function is derived from areas of interest over the kidney cortex as opposed to the entire kidney. Clearance half-life ($t_{1/2}$) response for the diuresis phase of the renogram is a simple quantitative calculation of the disappearance half-life. Unfortunately, there are at least eight ways in which the $t_{1/2}$ can be measured.[17] All have differing $t_{1/2}$ values for the same data. It is no wonder that the correlation of diuresis renography with surgical results and clinical outcomes has been variable. Although there are computer software programs commercially available to calculate $t_{1/2}$, the validity of these automatic programs may not be documented.

Radionuclide cystography. Direct radionuclide cystography (RNC) for the detection of vesicoureteral reflux (VUR) is more advantageous than the conventional x-ray method because there is a major reduction in the absorbed radiation dose to the patient by a factor of at least 100,[18] various functional parameters relating to bladder function and reflux can be quantified, and the quantitative data have prognostic significance regarding the spontaneous cessation of reflux. The techniques of direct and indirect RNC have evolved, beginning with the use of ^{131}I-labeled x-ray contrast agents in early investigations by Winter and colleagues,[54] to an indirect method used by Dodge[20] in an attempt to eliminate catheterization. The indirect method depends on the rapid and complete clearance of the radionuclide through the kidneys after an intravenous injection of the radiopharmaceutical. Imaging is then performed during and after voiding. A sudden increase in radioactivity in the upper tracts after voiding indicates reflux. Direct radionuclide cystography enables quantification of the bladder volume at which VUR occurs,[34] measurement of the volume of VUR into the upper tracts,[53] determination of the drainage time of refluxed urine after voiding, and quantification of the residual urine volume.[46] The direct radionuclide technique is more advantageous than the indirect method because it provides continuous monitoring during the filling, voiding, and postvoiding phases of bladder function, whereas the indirect technique examines the urinary tract only during voiding. Thus the direct technique is more sensitive in detecting VUR, since a significant percentage of VUR occurs during the filling phase at low bladder pressure and low bladder volume, which is not recognized by the indirect method.

A major consideration for the use of RNC over the conventional x-ray technique is the marked reduction in absorbed radiation dose to the patient. The dose to the bladder wall from a 1-mCi dose of ^{99m}Tc pertechnetate instilled into the bladder for a 30-min imaging interval is 30 mrem.[18] The radiation dose to the gonads is much lower, in the range of 2-5 mrem to the testes. The absorbed radiation dose from conventional x-ray cystography varies from hundreds of mrem to several rem per examination, depending on how much fluoroscopy is used. When one considers the increasing use of radiation modalities for the diagnosis of urinary tract abnormalities, then modalities that provide the same or greater information with lower absorbed radiation dose should be utilized. Radionuclide cystography is strongly recommended for follow-up studies evaluating the efficacy of therapy for VUR.

Radionuclide cystography can be performed at any nuclear medicine facility that has a scintillation camera. A computer is not necessary. The procedure is simple to perform and can be accomplished in less than 45 min with a cooperative patient. The responsibilities of the technologist can be significant, especially if he or she is trained in the technique of catheterization. Catheterization can be a simple and atraumatic experience if performed properly. Both physical and psychologic trauma can occur if the procedure is poorly performed by improperly trained or inexperienced personnel. Our belief is that individuals who regularly perform catheterization become more efficient and less traumatic in their technique. Whether the technologist performs catheterization or not, the technique of direct radionuclide cystography requires careful attention to multiple details to achieve an adequate study with clinically useful information. Because VUR is a dynamic process and may appear only fleetingly and in minimal amounts, technologists must constantly monitor the persistence scope to initiate imaging at the appropriate time to document the reflux. Complete filling of the bladder is required for the adequate performance of cystography, and there usually is a serious urge to void associated with it, which can affect the patient's ability to cooperate. Be sensitive to the patient's complaints, yet in a calm, authoritative manner maintain control so that the procedure can be accomplished as quickly as possible with minimum discomfort to the patient and with any VUR adequately documented.

A Foley catheter is inserted into the bladder after aseptic preparation of the glans penis or perineum. The size of the catheter used depends on the sex and age of the child. A soft size 8 French Foley catheter is used for girls up to 1 year of age. For girls between ages 1 and 3 a size 10 French Foley catheter is recommended, and after 3 years of age a size 12 French Foley catheter can be used. Generally, a catheter one size smaller is used in boys for each age group. Nonballoon catheters are not recommended, since patients tend to void around them and eject the catheter out of the bladder. Stiff feeding tubes are not recommended because they are more hazardous, and perforation of the urethra or bladder can occur. The Foley balloon is distended carefully during observation of the child's reaction to prevent injury in case of urethral or ureteral location of the balloon.

Quantitative data. After successful catheterization the bladder is emptied of residual urine, which is collected, measured, and recorded. The expected bladder capacity can be estimated based on the patient's age according to the formula developed by Berger and colleagues.[2] Normal bladder capacity in milliliters equals (age + 2) × 30. After 9 years of age, bladder capacities appear to vary from the formula. The formula is used only as rule of thumb, since capacities can also vary according to the health of the bladder. For example, following surgical procedures on the bladder or after recurrent infections, smaller capacities are documented.

A posterior and both posterior oblique images are obtained at a high-intensity setting, which demonstrates background activity throughout the field of view (Figure 18-11). In this manner minimal amounts of VUR are adequately demonstrated. Images are recorded for a total of 300,000 counts. Rarely, a fleeting minimal VUR occurs, which might not be demonstrated on permanent images. The technologist should note any other unusual occurrences to aid in the correct interpretation of the study. Then, a 2-min posterior image, including the entire bladder and upper urinary tract, is obtained. Total counts of the 2-min image are recorded for use in calculating the residual volume. This image is acquired at a lower intensity setting to visualize any abnormalities of the bladder. The patient is then seated to void into a bedpan or a urinal, and the gamma camera is positioned against the patient's back. As the balloon of the catheter is deflated, the patient is encouraged to void. As the patient begins to void, the catheter should slide out of the bladder. A voiding image is obtained as the patient empties the bladder. The same high-intensity setting as used for the prevoid images is set for the voiding image to demonstrate the minimal reflux that can occur only during the higher pressures of voiding. Finally, a 2-min postvoid image, including the bladder and the upper urinary tract, is obtained at a high-intensity setting. The residual volume, total volume at maximum capacity, and the reflux bladder volume for each kidney can be determined according to formulas reported by Weiss and colleagues.[49] Remember, none of the calculated volumes is accurate if urine is lost during the procedure.

The addition of simultaneous recording of bladder pressures during direct radionuclide cystography allows dysfunctional bladder abnormalities to be recognized.[30] A physiologic pressure transducer measures intravesical pressure through the drainage port of the Foley catheter. The use of this method—the radionu-

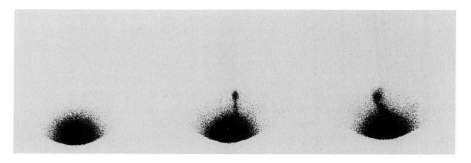

Figure 18-11 Posterior, LPO, and RPO images of the bladder and upper urinary tract demonstrate vesicoureteral reflux on the right.

clide cystometrogram—has enabled the characterization of four pressure patterns, including the normal, spastic-reflex, flaccid-paralytic, and uninhibited bladder contraction patterns. Patients with neurologic bladder disorders exhibit the spastic-reflex or flaccid-paralytic patterns. Children with voiding dysfunctions often have evidence of an uninhibited bladder contraction pattern.

Scrotal scintigraphic imaging. Scintigraphic imaging of the painful scrotum provides a useful screening study in determining the need for surgical exploration.[4,5] Torsion of the testis appears as a photopenic (cold) lesion because blood flow to the testicle is impaired due to the torsion (Figure 18-12). Inflammatory lesions usually have increased activity in the painful scrotum. In general, ischemic lesions (torsion, abscess, tumor) are managed surgically, whereas hyperemic lesions (epididymitis, orchitis, torsion of the appendix testes) are managed nonsurgically.

Scintigraphy should be performed with a magnification technique such as converging or pinhole collimation. A lead apron shield is placed around and beneath the scrotum and over the thighs. U-shaped cutouts of an old lead apron are suitable for the variable sizes of the scrotum at different ages. The penis is gently taped upward on the abdomen with nonallergenic tape. About 5-15 mCi of ^{99m}Tc pertechnetate (50 μCi/kg) is injected as a bolus to obtain a radionuclide angiogram of the scrotum to evaluate arterial perfusion. Angiographic images are obtained at 4 to 5 sec/image for 60

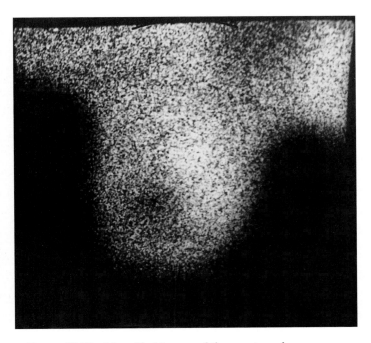

Figure 18-12 Magnified image of the scrotum demonstrates a photopenic lesion consistent with testicular torsion.

sec. Static scintigraphy for a minimum of 1 million counts/view is obtained immediately after the angiogram and 10 min after injection. Finally, it is useful to obtain a static scintigram with a lead strip marker on the median raphe of the scrotum, since edema often distorts the size of the side of the scrotum involved, making comparison with the normal side difficult.

Gastrointestinal System

Radionuclide studies of the gastrointestinal tract in children have been a boon to pediatric gastroenterologists in the difficult diagnosis of such entities as biliary atresia[31] and Meckel's diverticulum.[41,42] Other entities such as gastroesophageal reflux and gastrointestinal bleeding are investigated with radionuclide techniques. Technical considerations for the performance of these studies are different from those for the adult population, depending on the clinical entity in question.

Hepatobiliary scintigraphy. The primary indication for hepatobiliary scintigraphy in the pediatric patient is for the differentiation of the various causes of neonatal jaundice. Patients with biliary atresia present with hyperbilirubinemia and jaundice, which persists or increases in the neonatal period. Untreated, biliary atresia is a lethal condition at an early age. It is often possible to differentiate an inflammatory liver disease such as neonatal hepatitis from obstructive biliary tract disease such as biliary atresia using a ^{99m}Tc iminodiacetic acid (IDA) derivative radiopharmaceutical. The ^{99m}Tc IDA radiopharmaceuticals provide diagnostic images even in jaundiced patients with elevated direct serum bilirubin levels. There is a good hepatocyte extraction efficiency and short parenchymal transit time with these radiopharmaceuticals. We prefer to use ^{99m}Tc mebrofenin because of its rapid clearance and limited renal excretion. Normal transit times are not established for children but seem to be less than the normal $t_{1/2}$ for the adult.[24]

Other causes of neonatal jaundice, including neonatal hepatitis, are usually self-limiting conditions not associated with permanent interruption of the biliary drainage system. The differentiation of biliary atresia from other forms of obstruction or inflammatory disease is difficult based only on clinical laboratory tests and other radiologic imaging tests such as ultrasonography. Invasive procedures such as percutaneous transhepatic cholangiography are difficult to perform in children and have associated risks.

The biliary excretion of conjugated bilirubin is stimulated with the use of phenobarbital. Five mg/kg/day divided into two equal doses 3 to 7 days before the hepatobiliary imaging increases the sensitivity of diagnosis to 90% or greater in distinguishing biliary atresia from other causes of jaundice.[31]

Oral intake is restricted for 2 hr before injection of the radiopharmaceutical. Usually 100 μCi/kg of ^{99m}Tc disofenin is administered intravenously; 140 μCi/kg is administered to patients with a direct bilirubin greater than 5 mg/dl. Scintigraphy is begun immediately, with the patient in a supine position and with the appropriate magnification factor to obtain images that include only the xiphoid to the symphysis pubis within the field of view. Static images are obtained every 5 min for 45 to 60 min. Lateral images of the abdomen are obtained immediately thereafter. The key image is the left lateral projection. Any activity between the liver edge and the bladder within the abdomen anteriorly is evidence of gastrointestinal activity, which excludes the diagnosis of biliary atresia. Depending on the magnification factor as well as the collimation, images are obtained from 500,000 to 1 million counts/image. Additional images are obtained at various intervals, typically 3, 6, and 24 hr, or until radioactivity is demonstrated in the gastrointestinal tract.

Meckel diverticulum imaging. The most common gastrointestinal malformation is Meckel diverticulum. It occurs in approximately 1% to 3% of the population. Complications develop in about 25% of these individuals. Meckel diverticulum is the vestigial remnant of the omphalomesenteric duct and is usually found along the antimesenteric border of the distal ileum. Meckel diverticula often contain gastric mucosa, which leads to complications such as peptic ulceration and hemorrhage. Such complications occur most frequently in children and young adults and require surgery for correction.

Routine roentgenographic studies are usually considered of little value. Radionuclide imaging of Meckel diverticulum is based on the fact that ^{99m}Tc pertechnetate concentrates in gastric mucosa via active transport by the mucous surface cells. Nearly 60% of all Meckel diverticula contain gastric mucosa and thus are able to be imaged. Radionuclide imaging has an accuracy of 90% to 98%, making it the optimum examination for the identification of Meckel diverticulum. The clinical presentation is varied. The Meckel diverticulum is most often detected as an incidental finding at the time of surgery for other reasons. The patient may develop rectal bleeding as hematochezia (fresh blood tainting the stool), melena, or bright red symptomless bleeding.

The radionuclide detection of Meckel diverticulum is technique dependent. False-positives due to migration of secreted ^{99m}Tc pertechnetate from the stomach into the distal bowel have been reported. The following scintigraphic technique has been found to enhance the detectability of the Meckel diverticulum.[13]

Radionuclide imaging should be performed before barium sulfate studies or colonoscopy of the bowel. Such procedures can stimulate radionuclide localization due to irritation of the mucosa and cause false-positive interpretation. Barium sulfate attenuates photons and thus theoretically can mask localization of the radionuclide within the diverticulum, causing a false-negative interpretation. Because potassium perchlorate inhibits localization of pertechnetate within ectopic gastric mucosa, this drug should not be given before imaging. Potassium perchlorate should be administered following the radionuclide study to decrease the radiation dose to the thyroid gland. The patient should fast for at least 2 hr before imaging to reduce secretion and migration of ^{99m}Tc pertechnetate from the stomach into the bowel. Occasionally, in the presence of generalized bowel inflammation or irritable bowel, there is a rapid transit time of radionuclide throughout the bowel, resulting in difficult interpretation. The use of nasogastric suction to decrease transit of secreted nuclide may be helpful during a repeat examination. Premedication with cimetidine, which inhibits the secretion of pertechnetate from the cells into the lumen of the bowel, has been used as well. Because a Meckel diverticulum can be located close to the urinary bladder, the patient should void before and at intervals during the examination to prevent the ^{99m}Tc pertechnetate excreted by the kidneys into the bladder from masking a small diverticulum located adjacent to the bladder.

^{99m}Tc pertechnetate is administered intravenously, and imaging is begun immediately after injection. The usual amount of activity administered is 100 μCi/lb body weight. Anterior gamma-camera images are obtained every 5 min for 350,000-500,000 counts/view for a period of 1 hr. Oblique and lateral views can help isolate the Meckel diverticulum.

Scintigraphic interpretation criteria. Usually the Meckel diverticulum appears along with the gastric mucosa 10 to 20 min after injection. There might be a delayed appearance, but it rarely occurs after the 1-hr interval. The localization is usually prominent, rounded in appearance, and within a small focus. The majority of diverticula are found in the right lower quadrant of the abdomen but can be located anywhere within the abdomen and may be observed to move during the study. The activity should persist on multiple images during the study; however, the potential exists for emptying of the radioactive secretions within a Meckel lumen or dilution of the radioactivity by blood passing distally into the colon. This is a likely cause for the uncommonly reported false-negative studies. The diverticulum is generally intraabdominal and thus can be distinguished from activity within the retroperitoneal genitourinary tract, particularly on a lateral projection[13] (Figure 18-13).

Gastroesophageal reflux. One of the most common problems facing the pediatric practitioner is the infant

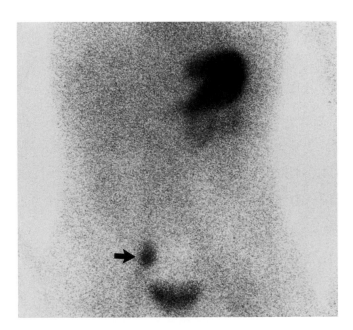

Figure 18-13 Meckel diverticulum is identified by localization in the prominent small, round focus of activity in the lower abdomen *(arrow).*

or child who constantly "spits up" or vomits. Such findings are a sign of gastroesophageal reflux (GER). It is not unusual for a child to occasionally regurgitate following feedings, but frequent regurgitation indicates a significant pathologic cause. In addition to anatomic abnormalities, such as esophageal stricture, tracheoesophageal fistula, and hiatal hernia, GER is associated with brain tumors, mental retardation, recurrent pneumonias, asthma, and sudden infant death syndrome (SIDS). Pediatricians are particularly concerned about the relationship of GER to unexplained recurrent pneumonias.

Clinical indications. Because of the incidence of the aforementioned disorders, a nuclear medicine practice with a busy pediatric component could, if it wanted to, perform many GER studies daily, both as a screening tool and as a confirmatory diagnostic tool. As a screening tool radionuclide GER studies lack the ability to identify significant abnormalities of the swallowing mechanism, nasopharyngeal reflux, and significant anatomic abnormalities of the esophagus. Therefore it is recommended that in most circumstances the x-ray esophagram be performed before the radionuclide GER study. If GER is present on the x-ray study, then the radionuclide GER study is unnecessary. The radionuclide GER study is indicated if the x-ray study is normal, since it is a more sensitive technique, primarily because it examines the process of GER over a longer interval than is possible with the x-ray study. In addition, the clinician is interested in determining the frequency of reflux and the magnitude of reflux. These factors

help determine the necessity of surgical intervention, such as the technique of a Nissen fundoplication. The radionuclide study therefore assists in determining the significance of GER. There are no criteria established for defining the significance of GER, but it would seem logical that more than three episodes during the examination, reflux that reaches the upper levels of the esophagus or regurgitates into the mouth, and evidence of pulmonary aspiration would most likely have clinical significance.

Factors affecting GER. It is well documented that a number of factors increase the incidence of GER.
1. *Position.* GER is detected most frequently in the supine position.[38] The incidence of reflux in other positions such as prone or decubitus is significantly smaller. If reflux or vomiting occurs with the child in the supine position, the technologist must be prepared to turn the child's face to the side to prevent aspiration of the refluxed gastric contents. This is rare, but it can occur in obtunded or severely retarded children unless preventive measures are taken. The vast majority of incidents of aspiration into the lungs occur during feeding and are due to abnormal swallowing mechanisms.
2. *Volume.* There is a direct relationship between the volume of the stomach contents and GER. An overdistended stomach is more likely to exhibit GER. Minimal reflux, which can occur when the stomach is fullest at the initiation of the examination, might be less significant than that which occurs later during the study.
3. *Consistency of stomach contents.* Liquids are more likely to reflux than solids. We prefer to mix the radiopharmaceutical with the patient's normal meal. Milk or milk with cereal assumes a semisolid consistency in the stomach as the milk curdles with stomach acids. To ensure uniformity of mixing, the radiopharmaceutical is placed into the milk or formula before ingestion. A small amount of nonradioactive milk or formula is given last to wash radioactivity out of the mouth and esophagus. If the child is a poor feeder, then the radiopharmaceutical should be instilled as an initial bolus to ensure adequate count rates for imaging in the presence of small stomach volumes.

   If the radiopharmaceutical is instilled into the stomach via an orogastric or nasogastric tube, it is important to ensure that the tip of the tubing is in the fundus of the stomach. Frequently gastric tubes are inserted too far, often into the duodenum or even jejunum. This results in a failed study. We prefer to insert the gastric tubes ourselves. It is seldom that tubing longer than the first marker is necessary when using a feeding tube. In addition, we instill a small portion of the radiopharmaceutical dose along with some saline to ensure that the tubing has been inserted into the stomach. If the child is crying lustily, it is unlikely that the tubing is within the trachea. However, in an obtunded or severely retarded child the placement of the tubing may be difficult to assess without instilling a small amount of isotope with saline. The patient's formula or milk should not be used as the bolus in such circumstances.

4. *Abdominal pressure.* The adult technique for studying GER includes the application of varying degrees of abdominal pressure with an abdominal band similar to a tourniquet. The GER appears according to the varying degrees of applied abdominal pressure. One should be cautious in attempting the same manipulation with a child and particularly with an infant, since the abdominal muscles play an important part in pediatric respiration. The abdominal venous return is also compromised by the application of tourniquets around the abdomen.

5. *Aspiration of saliva.* Recent studies have demonstrated aspiration of normal saliva in some patients. For that reason we frequently perform a "salivagram" before instilling radioactivity into the stomach or as a separate study. A drop of the radiopharmaceutical is placed on the patient's tongue, and the patient is monitored during normal swallowing of saliva before starting the GER study. Data is acquired in dynamic mode. Aspiration is readily recognized as activity in the trachea and bifurcation of the main bronchi (Figure 18-14). Time-activity curves are derived from ROIs over the lungs.[25]

Significance of GER. It is difficult to define the significance of GER. Taking into consideration all of the influencing factors, it would seem that up to three episodes of GER during an examination, especially if they are minimal and occur at the beginning of the examination, would be of little significance clinically. Multiple episodes of a large volume throughout that reaches the level of the patient's mouth, particularly late in the study, would be significant because the contents are potentially aspirable. Be that as it may, the potential for aspiration exists with any episode of GER, and findings should be correlated with the clinical situation, such as failure to thrive and multiple episodes of recurrent pneumonia.

Technical considerations. The radionuclide technique for GER involves the instillation of ^{99m}Tc sulfur colloid into the stomach, along with sufficient nonradioactive liquid to fill the stomach. About 150 μCi of ^{99m}Tc sulfur colloid is instilled into the stomach either by inges-

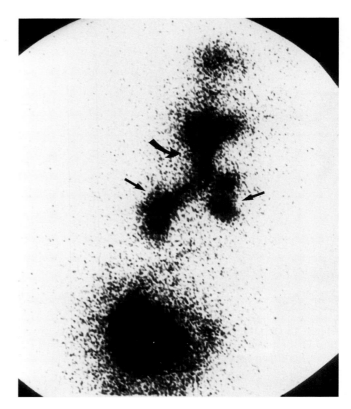

Figure 18-14 Salivagram image demonstrates activity in the trachea *(curved arrow)* and bronchi *(straight arrows).*

tion orally or via an orogastric or nasogastric tube, along with the infant's normal volume of formula, milk, juice, or glucose water. The patient should have fasted for a minimum of 2 hr before the procedure; when oral administration of the radiopharmaceutical is performed, the child usually accepts the radioactive feeding quickly. If the radionuclide is administered via orogastric or nasogastric tube, adequate placement of the tube in the fundus can be ensured by administering half of the radiopharmaceutical and, if necessary, repositioning the tube before instillation of the remainder of the feeding and the radiopharmaceutical. The technologist should wear gloves and use absorbent disposable pads around the child's shoulders to protect the clothing and skin from contamination. If contamination occurs, the absorbent pad can be quickly removed even during the examination. The gastric tube is removed immediately following administration of the radionuclide and feeding.

Occasionally an examination is performed on a child who has a gastrostomy tube in place. In such instances the tube should be clamped, with its free end secured to the lower abdomen so that any residual radioactivity in the tube will not be confused with reflux or aspirated activity on delayed images. The child is placed supine or in a left lateral decubitus position on top of the gamma camera. A low-energy collimator is used; magnification imaging is also used, depending on the size of the child. The upper abdomen and thorax should be included in the field of view. A radioactive marker is placed at the level of the upper end of the esophagus or the mouth. Analog images for 25,000 counts are acquired every 5 min for 1 hr or intentionally when reflux is recognized on the persistence scope. Digital images are obtained on the computer using 64×64 byte mode matrix at one frame/15 sec for the 60-min interval. Following the 60-min interval, 25,000 count anterior and left lateral images of the entire stomach and bowel are acquired for calculation of emptying percentage at 1 hr. In infants the gastric emptying rate at 1 hr varies considerably (10% to 90%), and standard values have not been defined.

Computer analysis of the data is performed by placing a region of interest (ROI) over the esophagus and a background region. A time-activity curve is generated from the background-subtracted esophagus area. Reflux episodes appear as spikes of increased activity above the background. Calculation of emptying percentage is accomplished by placing ROI over the stomach and the bowel for both the anterior and left lateral static images to obtain counts for each area. At a delayed interval of at least 3 hr an anterior image of the chest for 25,000 counts is obtained with markers at the shoulders and xiphoid to seek any evidence of reflux aspiration.

Cardiovascular System

The most common radionuclide studies of the heart in children are those used to detect and quantify cardiac shunts, either left-to-right through a septal defect or patent ductus arteriosus or right-to-left. The evaluation of surgically produced shunts is also frequently performed. All of the techniques involve the use of a radioactive tracer such as ^{99m}Tc pertechnetate or macroaggregated albumin to document the transit of the radionuclide through the cardiovascular system. The major advantages of these techniques are their noninvasive nature, rapidity, and low radiation dose compared with alternative procedures such as cardiac catheterization and contrast angiography.

Left-to-right shunt quantification involves the injection of a compact bolus of ^{99m}Tc pertechnetate, preferably through the jugular vein, and digital acquisition of 0.5-sec frames to document the transit through the cardiopulmonary circuit. Analog images are also acquired simultaneously. Following acquisition the pulmonary time-activity curve is generated and analyzed via the gamma variate analysis to determine the pulmonary-to-systemic flow ratio (QP/QS ratio). This method provides precise quantification of left-to-right shunts with a pulmonary-to-systemic ratio of 1.2 to 3.0, devised by Maltz and Treves.[32]

The detection of right-to-left cardiac shunts is accomplished by the administration of 25 μCi/lb of ^{99m}Tc macroaggregated albumin.[22] After injection of the radioactive particles, the distribution of activity between the systemic circulation and the lungs is determined. If no right-to-left shunt is present, more than 95% of the injected activity is trapped in the pulmonary vascular bed. Activity seen throughout the systemic circulation, including the kidneys, brain, and other organs, is evidence of a right-to-left shunt and can be quantified by acquisition of whole-body images and placement of ROI over the lungs and the rest of the body. Calculation of the magnitude of the right-to-left shunt is according to the following formula:

Percent right-to-left shunt =
$$\frac{\text{Total body count} - \text{Total lung count}}{\text{Total body count}}$$

The examination must be performed immediately after constitution of the radiopharmaceutical to avoid the possibility of radiopharmaceutical breakdown and increased counts from free pertechnetate in the kidneys or the bladder.

REFERENCES

1. Ami TB et al: Stress fractures after surgery for osteosarcoma: scintigraphic assessment, *Radiology* 163:157-162, 1987.
2. Berger RM et al: Bladder capacity (ounces) equals age (years) plus 2 predicts normal bladder capacity and aids in diagnosis of abnormal voiding patterns, *J Urol* 129:347-349, 1983.
3. Bressler EL, Conway JJ, Weiss SC: Neonatal osteomyelitis examined by bone scintigraphy, *Radiology* 152:685-688, 1984.
4. Chen DCP, Holder LE, Melloul M: Radionuclide scrotal imaging: further experience with 210 patients: part 1: anatomy, pathophysiology, and methods, *J Nucl Med* 24:735-742, 1983.
5. Chen DCP, Holder LE, Melloul M: Radionuclide scrotal imaging: further experience with 210 patients: part 2: results and discussion, *J Nucl Med* 24:841-853, 1983.
6. Cohen MD, Wood BP, Hodgman CH: The presence of parents with their children during imaging procedures, *Am J Roentgenol Rad Ther Nucl Med* 146:639-641, 1986.
7. Committee on Drugs: Guidelines for monitoring and management of pediatric patients during and after sedation for diagnostic and therapeutic procedures, *Pediatrics* 89:1110-1115, 1992.
8. Conway JJ: Avascular necrosis in septic arthritis of the hip (unpublished work).
9. Conway JJ: Communicating risk information in medical practice, *Radiographics* 12:207-214, 1992.

10. Conway JJ: *Musculoskeletal scintigraphy in children:* Audiovisual program CEL 226, New York, 1992, Society of Nuclear Medicine.

11. Conway JJ: Practical considerations in radionuclide imaging of pediatric patients. In Freeman LM, ed: *Freeman and Johnson's clinical radionuclide imaging,* ed 3, New York, 1984, Grune & Stratton.

12. Conway JJ: Radionuclide bone scintigraphy in pediatric orthopedics, *Pediatr Clin North Am* 33:1313-1334, 1986.

13. Conway JJ: Radionuclide diagnosis of Meckel's diverticulum, *Gastrointest Radiol* 5:209-213, 1980.

14. Conway JJ: Sedation, injection, and handling techniques in pediatric nuclear medicine. In James AE Jr, Wagner HN Jr, Cooke RE, eds: *Pediatric nuclear medicine,* Philadelphia, 1974, Saunders.

15. Conway JJ: *SPECT imaging in children: categorical course in nuclear radiology,* Weston, Virginia, 1989, American College of Radiology.

16. Conway JJ: The principles and technical aspects of diuresis renography, *J Nucl Med Technol* 17:208-214, 1989.

17. Conway JJ: "Well-tempered" diuresis renography: its historical development, physiological and technical pitfalls and standardized technique protocol, *Semin Nucl Med* 22:74-84, 1992.

18. Conway JJ et al: Detection of vesicoureteral reflux with radionuclide cystography: a comparison study with roentgenographic cystography, *Am J Roentgenol Rad Ther Nucl Med* 115:720-727, 1972.

19. Conway JJ, Filmer RB: Kidney: *Nuclear medicine in clinical pediatrics,* New York, 1975, Society of Nuclear Medicine.

20. Dodge EA: Vesicoureteral reflux: diagnosis with iodine-131 sodium orthoiodohippurate, *Lancet* 1:303-304, 1963.

21. Furosemide (Lasix). In *Physician's desk reference (PDR),* ed 43, Oradell, New Jersey, 1989, Medical Economics.

22. Gates GF, Orme HW, Dore EK: Cardiac shunt assessment in children with macroaggregated albumin technetium-99m, *Radiology* 112:649-653, 1974.

23. Gelfand MJ, Strife JL, Kereiakes JG: Radionuclide bone imaging in spondylolysis of the lumbar spine in children, *Radiology* 140:191-195, 1981.

24. Gilbert SA, Brown PH, Krishnamurthy GT: Quantitative nuclear hepatology, *J Nucl Med Technol* 15:38-47, 1987.

25. Heyman S, Respondek M: Detection of pulmonary aspiration in children by radionuclide "salivagram," *J Nucl Med* 30:697-699, 1989.

26. Holder LE, Cole LA, Myerson MS: Reflex sympathetic dystrophy in the foot: clinical and scintigraphic criteria, *Radiology* 184:531-535, 1984.

27. Howie DW et al: The technetium phosphate bone scan in the diagnosis of osteomyelitis in childhood, *J Bone Joint Surg* 65:431-437, 1983.

28. Keeter S et al: Sedation in pediatric CT: national survey of current practice, *Radiology* 175:745-752, 1990.

29. Ljung B, Andreásson S: Comparison of midazolam nasal spray to nasal drops for the sedation of children, *J Nucl Med Technol* 24:32-34, 1996.

30. Maizels M et al: The cystometric nuclear cystogram, *J Urol* 121:203-205, 1979.

31. Majd M, Reba RC, Altman RP: Effect of phenobarbital on ^{99m}Tc-IDA scintigraphy in the evaluation of neonatal jaundice, *Semin Nucl Med* 9:194-204, 1981.

32. Maltz DL, Treves S: Quantitative radionuclide angiocardiography: determination of Qp:Qs in children, *Circulation* 47:1049-1056, 1973.

33. McKay RJ Jr: Diagnosis and treatment: risks of obtaining samples of venous blood in infants, *Pediatrics* 38:906-908, 1968.

34. Nasrallah PF et al: The quantitative nuclear cystogram: an aid in determining the spontaneous resolution of vesicoureteral reflux, *Urology* 12:645-658, 1978.

35. Orzel JA, Rudd TG: Heterotopic bone formation: clinical, laboratory, and imaging correlation, *J Nucl Med* 26:125-132, 1985.

36. Papanicolaou N et al: Bone scintigraphy and radiography in young athletes with low back pain, *Am J Roentgenol Rad Ther Nucl Med* 145:1039-1044, 1985.

37. Paul DJ et al: A better method of imaging the abnormal hips, *Radiology* 113:466-467, 1974.

38. Piepsez A et al: Gastroesophageal scintiscanning in children, *J Nucl Med* 23:631-632, 1982.

39. Rosen PR, Micheli LJ, Treves S: Early scintigraphic diagnosis of bone stress and fractures in athletic adolescents, *Pediatrics* 70:11-15, 1982.

40. Roub LW et al: Bone stress: a radionuclide imaging perspective, *Radiology* 132:431-438, 1979.

41. Sfakianakis GN, Conway JJ: Detection of ectopic gastric mucosa in Meckel's diverticulum and in other aberrations by scintigraphy: I: pathophysiology and 10-year clinical experience, *J Nucl Med* 22:647-654, 1981.

42. Sfakianakis GN, Conway JJ: Detection of ectopic gastric mucosa in Meckel's diverticulum and in other aberrations by scintigraphy: II: indications and methods—a 10-year experience, *J Nucl Med* 22:732-738, 1981.

43. Smergel EM et al: Use of bone scintigraphy in the management of slipped capital femoral epiphysis (SCFE), *Clin Nucl Med* 12:349-353, 1987.

44. Starshak RJ, Simons GW, Sty JR: Occult fracture of the calcaneus—another toddler's fracture, *Pediatr Radiol* 14:37-40, 1984.

45. Strain JD et al: Intravenously administered pentobarbital sodium for sedation in pediatric CT, *Radiology* 161:105-108, 1986.

46. Strauss BS, Blaufox MD: Estimation of residual urine and urine flow rates without urethral catheterization, *J Nucl Med* 11:81-84, 1970.

47. Sty JR, Starshak RJ: The role of bone scintigraphy in the evaluation of the suspected abused child, *Radiology* 146:369-375, 1983.

48. Weiss S, Conway JJ: Radionuclide cystography, *J Nucl Med Technol* 15:66-74, 1987.

49. Weiss S, Conway JJ: The technique of direct radionuclide cystography, *Appl Radiology* 4:133-137, 1975.

50. Weiss SC, Conway JJ: An injection technique artifact, *J Nucl Med Technol* 12:10-12, 1984.

51. Whitfield HN et al: The distinction between obstructive uropathy and nephropathy by radioisotope transit times, *Br J Urol* 39:433-436, 1978.

52. Wilcox JR, Moniot AL, Green JP: Bone scanning in the evaluation of exercise-related stress injuries, *Radiology* 123:699-703, 1977.

53. Willi U, Treves S: Radionuclide voiding cystography, *Urol Radiol* 5:161-173, 1983.

54. Winter CC: A new test for vesicoureteral reflux: an external technique using radioisotopes, *J Urol* 81:105-111, 1959.

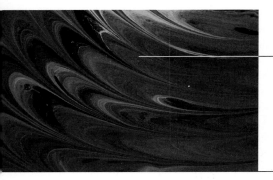

Glossary

A number   See *atomic mass.*

ablation   (1) Separation or detachment. (2) Destruction, that is, by radiation.

abscess   Localized collection of pus within tissue.

abscissa   The x, or horizontal, axis in a cartesian graph plot.

absorption (μ) coefficient   Constant representing the fraction of ionizing radiation absorbed per centimeter thickness of absorbing material.

accelerator   Device imparting high kinetic energy to a charged particle, causing it to undergo nuclear or particle reaction.

access time   The time required for a computer to locate and retrieve information from a specified location. In the case of memory, this is related to the electronic speed of the address register and read/write circuits. In the case of disks, the access time is the sum of the time taken for the read/write head to locate a particular track plus the time required for information to rotate into the read/write position.

accumulator   Register or data buffer used for temporary storage of data.

accuracy   Refers to whether a given measurement or set of measurements reflects a true or exact value.

ACE   Angiotensin converting enzyme.

achalasia   (1) Failure to relax; referring especially to pylorus, cardia, or any other sphincter muscles. (2) Obstruction of the terminal esophagus just proximal to the cardioesophageal junction.

acid   Any chemical compound that can either donate a proton or accept a pair of electrons in a chemical reaction.

acidophilic   (1) Stains easily with acid dyes. (2) Grows best in acid media.

acinus   Smallest lobule of a gland; secretes the product of the gland.

acquisition   Intake of data to the computer.

ACTH   See *adrenocorticotropin.*

activation analysis   Analytical procedure detecting and measuring trace quantities of elements after exposure to a flux of neutrons.

ADC   See *analog-digital converters.*

A/D converter   See *analog-digital converters.*

address   Label, name, or number that designates a location where information is stored.

adduct   An addition product, or complex, or one part of the same.

adenohypophysis   Anterior lobe of the pituitary.

adenoma   Epithelial tumor composed of glandular tissue.

adenosine   An endogenously produced nucleoside that causes coronary and systemic vasodilation.

adenylate cyclase   Enzyme found in the liver and muscle cell membranes.

adjuvant   That which aids or assists.

adrenal cortex   Outer portion of the adrenal gland; it produces cortisone.

adrenal medulla   Central portion of the adrenal gland; it produces adrenalin.

adrenergic   Relating to nerve fibers of the autonomic nervous system that liberate norepinephrine.

adrenocorticotropin   Compound isolated from the anterior pituitary having a stimulating effect on the adrenal cortex.

afferent   Carrying or conveying toward a center.

affinity   (1) Attraction of a specific reactor substance for a ligand. (2) An inherent attraction for substances to undergo reactions with one another.

affinity chromatography   Separation of compounds based on differences in their affinities for a given species.

agonist   A drug capable of combining with receptors to initiate drug action.

akinesia   Abnormal reduction of muscle movement.

ALARA   NRC operating philosophy for maintaining occupational radiation exposures "as low as is reasonably achievable."

albumin   Class of simple proteins; found in most tissues.

alcohol   Organic molecule containing the functional —OH group.

aldehyde   Organic molecule containing the

$$\overset{\displaystyle O}{\underset{\displaystyle \quad}{\|}}$$
—C—H group.

aldosterone   Sodium-retaining hormone of the adrenal cortex.

ALGOL (ALGOrithmic Language) High-level compiler language particularly well suited to arithmetic and string manipulations.

algorithm Prescribed set of well-defined rules or processes for the solution of a problem in a finite number of steps.

aliquot Specific measured amount of liquid.

alimentary canal Food tract starting with the mouth and ending with the rectum and anus.

alkane Hydrocarbon with a general formula of $C_nH_{2n + 2}$.

alkene Hydrocarbon that has one double bond and a general formula of C_nH_{2n}.

alkyl Alkane with one hydrogen atom removed.

alkyne Hydrocarbon that contains a triple bond and a general formula of $C_2H_{2n - 2}$.

alpha cells Cells in pancreatic islets containing large granules.

alpha particle (α) Nucleus of a helium atom emitted by certain radioisotopes upon disintegration.

ALU See *arithmetic unit.*

alveoli Terminal air pockets in the lungs.

amelioration Improvement of a disease.

amide Organic molecule with the functional group

$$\overset{\displaystyle O}{\underset{\displaystyle |}{\overset{\displaystyle \|}{-C}}} -NH_2.$$

amine Organic molecule containing the functional group $-NH_2$.

amino acid Organic acid containing an NH_2 and a COOH group, thus having both basic and acidic properties.

aminophylline A vasodilator and cardiac stimulant.

AMP Adenosine monophosphate; nucleotide containing adenine, a pentose sugar, and one phosphoric acid; product of metabolism.

amphoteric Having two opposite characteristics, especially having the capacity of reacting as either acid or base.

amplifier A device used to linearly increase pulse size.

amplitude The height of a waveform.

ampulla of Vater Dilation of ducts from the liver and pancreas where they enter the small intestine.

AMU See *atomic mass unit.*

amyloidosis A disease characterized by extracellular accumulation of amyloid in various organs and tissues.

analog (1) Representation of a parameter by a signal the magnitude of which voltage, current, or length is proportional to the parameter. (2) Structure with a similar function.

analog computer Computer that parameterizes data in terms of the magnitude of the incoming signals.

analog-digital converters (ADC) Electronic module used to convert an analog signal such as a pulse height into digital information recognizable by a computer.

anastomose To unite an end to another end; to bridge two vessels with a section of a vessel.

androgenic hormone Hormone stimulating male characteristics.

anemia Deficiency of red blood cells.

aneurysm Dilation of part of the wall of an artery.

Anger camera Type of gamma ray scintillation camera, named for its inventor Hal O. Anger.

angiography X-ray photography of the blood vessels with use of a radiopaque substance.

angiotensin Vasoconstrictor substance present in blood.

angstrom A measurement of wavelength (10^{-8} cm).

anion Negatively charged ion.

annihilation Reaction between a pair of particles resulting in their disintegration and the production of an equivalent amount of energy in the form of photons.

anode Positive electrode.

anoxia Deficiency of oxygen.

antecubital Area in front of the elbow.

antibiotics Drugs used to destroy bacteria; extracted from living organisms.

antibody Substance capable of producing specific immunity to a bacterium or virus; found in the blood.

anticholinergic Drugs blocking passage of impulses through the autonomic nerves.

antigen Molecule or particle capable of eliciting an immune response.

antineutrino Neutral nuclear particle emitted in either positron decay or electron capture.

antiserum Serum containing antibodies.

aorta Large artery stemming from the left ventricle.

apatite Crystalline phosphate of lime.

aplasia Failure of an organ to develop.

aplastic anemia Anemia characterized by absence of red blood cell regeneration.

application program Program that performs a task specific to a particular user's needs.

aqueous Referring to anything dissolved in water.

arachnoid Membrane covering the brain and spinal cord.

arene Hydrocarbon compound that contains an aromatic portion.

arithmetic and logic unit (ALU) See *arithmetic unit.*

arithmetic unit Unit within the computer architecture that performs all mathematical and logical operations. Sometimes called arithmetic and logic unit (ALU).

aromatic compound Chemical compound containing a ring system that has $(4n + 2)\pi$ electrons.

array processor A specially devised high-speed computer that performs computations on image array elements in a parallel fashion.

Arrhenius concept Concept stating that an acid is a compound that acts as a proton donor.

arrhythmia Variation of the heartbeat.

arterial thrombus Blood clot formed in an artery.

arthrography Radiography after the introduction of opaque contrast material into a joint.

ASCII Abbreviation for American Standard Code for Information Interchange, consisting of 128 seven-bit binary codes for uppercase and lowercase letters, numbers, punctuation, and special communication control characters.

ascites An accumulation of serous fluid in the peritoneal cavity.

ascorbic acid Vitamin C.

asepsis Sterile state.

assembler Programs that assemble symbolic programs into binary form.

assembly language Commands for the minicomputer system written in symbolic or mnemonic form. Typically, three-letter abbreviations, called mnemonics, are used to represent each instruction, and each mnemonic can usually be equaled to one machine-code or binary instruction. An assembly language program is translated to binary code by an assembler.

astrocytoma Central nervous system tumor composed of star-shaped cells.

asynchronous Mode of operation in which an operation is started by a signal that the operation on which it depends is completed. When referring to hardware devices, it is the method in which each character is sent with its own synchronizing information. The hardware operations are scheduled by "ready" and "done" signals rather than by time intervals. In addition, it implies that a second operation can begin before the first operation is complete.

asynchronous transfer Any sequential computer-operational signal that starts an operation when a necessary previous operation is completed.

ataxia Disorder of the neuromuscular system; lacking muscle coordination.

atherosclerosis Arterial hardening.

ATN Acute tubular necrosis.

atom Smallest unit of an element that can exist and still maintain the properties of the element.

atomic mass Mass of a neutral atom usually expressed in atomic mass units.

atomic mass unit Exactly one twelfth the mass of carbon 12; 1.661×10^{-24} g.

atomic number Number of protons in an atom, the symbol of which is Z.

atomic weight Average weight of the neutral atoms of an element.

ATP Adenosine triphosphate.

atrium Cavity of the heart receiving blood.

attenuation Any condition that results in a decrease of radiation intensity.

Auger electrons Electrons that participate in the production of x rays; pronounced o-zháy.

autofluoroscope A scintillation camera developed by M. Bender and M. Blau.

AV block Impairment of the normal conduction between the atria and the ventricles.

Avogadro's number Number of atoms in the gram atomic weight of a given element or the number of molecules in the gram molecular weight of a given substance: 6.022×10^{23} per gram mole.

avidity (1) Tendency of a specific reactor substance to hold its ligands. (2) The firmness of a combination of substances in reactions in terms of their dissociation.

axion The conducting portion of a nerve fiber.

axis of rotation In SPECT, an imaginary line passing through the center of the gantry about which the camera rotates.

background Detected disintegration events not emanating from the sample.

back-projection A computer manipulation of acquired image data back-projected into space.

backscattering Scattering of particulate radiation by more than 90 degrees.

bar phantom See *phantom.*

barn Area unit expressing the area of nuclear cross section; 1 barn = 10^{-24} cm^2.

Barrett esophagus Chronic peptic ulcer of the lower esophagus.

basal ganglia An aggregation of nerve cell bodies of the telencephalon.

base Any compound that either acts as a proton acceptor or an electron pair donor in a chemical process.

baseline Normal evaluation; evaluation before administration of a substance.

BASIC (Beginner's All-purpose Symbolic Instruction Code) High-level interactive, interpreter language for mathematical and string-variable manipulations.

batch mode Automatic computer mode that does not require specific programming instruction.

batch operation Computer operation that runs consecutively without operator intervention.

baud A unit of measurement of transmission speed; bits per second.

bequerel (Bq) The Système Internationale unit of activity, equal to one disintegration per second, 1 Bq = 1 dps.

beta cells Pancreatic cells in the islets of Langerhans.

beta (β^-) particle Electron whose point of origin is the nucleus; electron originating in the nucleus by way of decay of a neutron into a proton and electron (beta particle).

biconcave Having two concave surfaces.

bifunctional chelates Complexing agent with two sites for complexation.

bifunctional drug Drug with ability to attack two types of symptoms or disease.

biliary atresia A congenital absence of bile ducts.

biliary system System including the liver serving both a digestive and an excretory function.

binary Pertaining to the number system with a radix of two.

binary code A code that uses two distinct characters, usually the numbers 0 and 1.

binary digit One of the symbols 1 or 0; called a *bit*.

binder See *specific reactor substance*.

binding constant The equilibrium constant for a reaction between an antibody or binding protein and its antigen or ligand.

binding energy Energy released when a chemical bond is formed; amount of stabilization energy holding a nucleon in the nucleus.

binding sites Sites on a protein where they bind to radionuclides.

bioassay Determination of chemical strength by tests of living tissues.

biochemical Referring to the chemistry of living organisms.

biochemical analogs Chemicals of the living system that resemble one another in function but not in structure.

bioeffects Effects on the biologic system.

biologic distribution Normal distribution of a substance within the living system.

biologic half-life The elapsed time for the biologic elimination of 50% of a material from the body.

biologic matrix Basic materials of living systems.

biopsy Examination of tissue taken from the living body, usually without entirely removing the organ.

BIOS Basic input/output system.

biosynthesis Formation of a compound from other compounds by living organisms.

bisacodyl tablets Drugs used as a laxative.

bit An individual binary digit, either 1 or 0; acronyn for *bi*nary digi*t*.

bleomycin An antibody substance having antineoplastic properties.

block A group of bytes on a disk or magnetic tape used for data storage.

blood pool Vascular cavity.

bolus Rounded mass or lump quantity; a concentrated radiopharmaceutical given intravenously.

bombardment Exposure of a target to any ionizing radiation.

bootstrap loader Routine whose first instructions are sufficient to load the remainder of itself into memory from an input device and normally start a complex system of programs.

Bowman capsule Sac at the end of uriniferous tubules in the kidneys.

Bragg curve Curve showing specific ionization as a function of distance or energy.

bremsstrahlung x rays Photonic emissions caused by the slowing down of beta particles in matter.

briggsian logarithmic system System of logarithms based on the decimal system, using the base 10.

bromination Chemical addition of bromine to a compound.

bromocryptine A dopamine receptor agonist.

bronchiectasis Dilation of the small bronchial tubes.

bronchioles Small bronchial tubes leading to air cells.

bronchus Large passage carrying air within the lungs.

Brönsted-Lowry concept Concept stating that an acid is a proton donor and a base is a proton acceptor in a chemical process.

brownian movement Motion of minute particles suspended in liquid.

BSP Body substance precautions.

BTU British thermal unit; measurement of heat.

buffer (1) Storage area used to temporarily hold information being transferred between two devices or between a device and memory; often a special register or a designated area of memory. (2) A solution of a weak acid and one of its salts that resists change in pH; usually used to maintain a constant pH for a reaction in solution.

buffer solution Solution that has a specific pH value and is resistant to pH change by addition of acids or bases.

bug Error in a program.

bullous Referring to a bubble or a bladder.

bundle branch block Interventricular block due to interruption of one of the two main branches of the bundle of His.

bus A flat, flexible cable consisting of many transmission lines or wires; it interconnects computer system components to provide communication paths for addresses, data, and control information.

by-product material Radioactive material arising from controlled fission.

byte Group of binary digits usually operated upon as a unit and usually 8 bits long; in ASCII code one character occupies one byte of memory, and the maximum decimal integer that can be stored in an 8-bit byte is 255.

C Programming language for computer.

cache memory A high-speed memory, usually part of the CPU.

calyx (*pl.* calyces) Cuplike structure in the kidney that receives urine.

canaliculus Small canal or channel.

carbohydrate Compound consisting of carbon, hydrogen, and oxygen, such as sugars and starches.

carboxylic acids Organic molecules with the

$$-\overset{\overset{\displaystyle O}{\displaystyle \|}}{C}-OH$$

functional group, which have acidic properties because of this functional group.

carcinogen Substance stimulating the formation of cancer.

carcinoma Malignant tumor consisting of connective tissue enclosing epithelial cells.

cardiac ejection fraction That fraction of the total volume of blood of the left ventricle ejected per contraction.

cardiac output The quantity of blood ejected by the heart over a 1-min interval.

cardiomyopathy Subacute or chronic disorder of the heart muscle.

carrier Quantity of an element mixed with radioactive isotopes of that element to facilitate chemical operations.

carrier free Adjective describing a nuclide that is free of its stable isotopes.

carrier proteins Macroscopic amounts of nonlabeled proteins present with trace amounts of radiolabeled proteins.

cartesian coordinate system Utilization of numbers to locate a point in relation to two intersecting straight lines.

catabolism The breaking down within the body of complex chemical compounds into simpler ones.

cathode Negative electrode.

cathode ray tube (CRT) Electronic vacuum tube with a display screen where information is displayed.

cation Positively charged ion.

cauda equina End of the spinal cord containing the nerves that supply the rectal area.

CBG Cortisol-binding globulin.

CDC Centers for Disease Control and Prevention.

CEA Carcinoma embryonic antigen.

Celsius (1) Swedish astronomer and inventor. (2) Centigrade, the temperature scale in which there are 100 degrees between ice and boiling water at sea level.

central nervous system That part of the nervous system containing the brain, spinal cord, and nerves.

central processor unit (CPU) Unit of a computing system that includes the circuits controlling the interpretation and execution of instructions—the computer proper, excluding I/O and other peripheral devices.

centrifuge (1) To rotate or spin at high speed for separation. (2) Instrument for rotating or spinning samples at high speed.

cerebral radionuclide angiogram, cerebral radioangiogram Rapid sequential scintiphotos of the blood vessels of the brain.

cerebrospinal fluid (CSF) Fluid found in the cavities of the brain, brainstem, spinal cord, and meninges.

Chagas disease South American trypanosomiasis.

character A single letter, numeral, or symbol used to represent information.

charged-particle accelerators Device used to electronically accelerate any charged particle. See also *cyclotron* and *electron accelerator*.

chelate Ligand that has two or more potential bonding sites.

chemical equation Symbolic statement describing a process and showing the stoichiometric relationships among the individual species involved in the process.

chemical equilibrium State of lowest energy for a chemical system undergoing a chemical reaction.

chemical reaction Processes that result in chemical change of the participant molecules.

chemistry Study of matter and the changes that matter undergoes.

chi-square test A mathematical procedure applied to a series of observations to determine their amount of variability.

chloramine-T *N*-chloro-4-methylbenzenesulfonamide sodium salt; an oxidizing agent used in radioiodination of proteins.

chlormerodrin Diuretic containing mercury.

cholecystitis Inflammation of the gallbladder.

cholecystokinin Hormone secreted by the small intestine; stimulates contraction of the gallbladder.

choroid plexus Membrane lining the ventricles of the brain, concerned with formation of cerebrospinal fluid.

chromatography Method of chemical analysis where the solution to be analyzed separates into component parts; some types are gel permeation chromatography, paper chromatography, and affinity chromatography.

cistern Fluid reservoir; enclosed space.

CLIA 88 Clinical Laboratories Improvement Act of 1988.

clock A device within a computer system that keeps time, counts pulses, measures frequency, or generates periodic signals for synchronization.

cloud chamber Chamber where the paths of ionizing radiation can be observed.

COBOL (commercial and business oriented language) High-level incremental compiler language primarily suited to business applications.

cocktail A liquid scintillator.

code A system of symbols representing data or instructions executed by a computer.

coding The writing of instructions for a computer, using a system of symbols meaningful to a computer, an assembler, a compiler, or a language processor.

coefficient Constant by which a variable or other quantity is multiplied in an equation.

coefficient of variation A statistical measurement of the validity of serial observations on a changing parameter.

coincidence counting A means of detecting radiation by two detectors placed in opposition to one another; an event is recorded only when seen by both detectors simultaneously.

coincidence lines Events recorded by detectors placed in opposition.

collagen Protein found in bone and cartilage.

collimators Shielding device used to limit the angle of entry of radiation.

colloid Molecules in a continuous medium that measure between 1 and 100 nm in diameter.

colorimetry Measurement of color.

colostomy Artificial opening in the colon.

column generator Column device using a parent radionuclide absorbed to a support in a column; the daughter radionuclide is usually obtained by elution of the column with a solution that interacts with the daughter but not with the parent.

command A word, mnemonic, or character that, by virtue of its syntax is an input line, causes a computer system to perform a predefined operation.

competitive protein binding Type of competitive binding radioassay in which the specific reactor substance is a native nonimmunologic protein.

compile To produce a binary code program from a program written in source (symbolic) language, by selection of appropriate subroutines from a subroutine library, as directed by the instructions or other symbols of the source program; the linkage is supplied for combining the subroutines into a workable program, and the subroutines and linkage are translated into binary code.

compiler Program used to compile assembly code or source code.

complement A substance normally present in serum that is destructive to certain bacteria and other cells that have been sensitized by specific complement antibody.

complex ions The product resulting from the actions of neutral molecules with either a cation or an anion.

compound Distinct substance formed by a union of two or more elements in definite proportions by weight.

Compton edge See *Compton scatter.*

Compton plateau See *Compton scatter.*

Compton scatter One process by which a photon loses energy through collisions with electrons.

computer Programable electronic device that can store, retrieve, and process data.

computer program A plan or routine for solving a problem on a computer.

computer system A data processing system consisting of hardware devices, software programs, and documentation that describes the operation of the system.

concentration Strength of substance in a solution.

congener One of two or more things of the same kind.

congenital Existing at birth.

conjugate acid Remainder of a basic compound after it has either accepted a proton or donated an electron pair in a chemical process.

conjugate base Remainder of an acidic compound after it has either donated its acidic proton or accepted an electron pair in a chemical process.

constant A value that remains the same throughout a distinct operation.

conversion electron Orbital electron that has been excited (ionized) by internal conversion of an excited atom.

coordinate covalent bond Covalent bond formed by two atoms in which one atom donates both electrons for the bond.

core memory Main memory storage used by the central processing unit, in which binary data are represented by the switching polarity of magnetic cores.

coronal plane Plane that takes its name from the coronal suture of the skull dividing the body into the front and back portions.

corticosterone Compound isolated from the adrenal cortex.

cortisol Adrenocortical hormone.

Coulomb's law Basic law of electrostatics, which states that:

$$F = \frac{q_1 q_2}{4\pi\epsilon r^2} \quad \text{or} \quad F = \frac{qq'}{r^2}$$

covalent bond Chemical bond formed by sharing a pair of electrons by two nuclei.

covalent compound Compound held together by covalent bonds.

CPB See *competitive protein binding.*

CPR Cardiopulmonary resuscitation.

CPU See *central processor unit.*

crash *Hardware crash* is the complete failure of a particular device, sometimes affecting the operation of an entire computer system; *software crash* is the complete failure of an operating system characterized by some failure in the system's protection mechanisms.

CRFS Comprehensive renal function study.

critical organ (1) Organ of interest. (2) Organ most affected by a technique.

cross-reactivity Reaction of a molecule with an immunoglobulin directed toward another substance.

CRT See *cathode ray tube.*

crystallography Study of the crystal structure of a molecule.

CSF See cerebrospinal fluid.

CT Computerized tomography.

CU Control unit, a component of a computer's central processing unit.

curie Standard measure of rate of radioactive decay; based on the disintegration of 1 g of radium of 3.7×10^{-10} disintegrations per second.

cutie pie A type of ionization chamber.

CVA Cerebrovascular accident.

cyanocobalamine Vitamin B_{12}.

cyclotron Device for accelerating charged particles to high energies using magnetic and oscillating electrostatic fields, causing the particle to move in a spiral path with increasing energy.

data Facts, numbers, letters, and symbols; data are the basic elements of information that can be processed by a computer.

database A computer's compilation of information.

daughter radionuclide Decay product produced by a radionuclide. The element from which the daughter was produced is called the *parent.*

debug Detect, locate, and correct coding or logic errors in a computer program.

debugger Program to assist in tracking down and eliminating errors that occurs in the normal course of program development.

debusser Device used to erase material from a computer or recording tape.

decay Radioactive disintegration of a nucleus of an unstable nuclide.

decay constant Decay rate of a radionuclide based on its half-life.

decay factor Fraction of radionuclei that have decayed in a specified period, according to the following formula:

$$\lambda = \frac{0.693}{t_{1/2}}$$

decay schemes Diagram showing the decay mode or modes of a radionuclide.

dee A component of a cyclotron in which particle acceleration takes place.

deiodinate Removal of iodine from a compound.

delayed neutrons Neutrons that are emitted in a radioactive process at an appreciable time after fission.

dementia Mental deterioration from disease of the brain.

denaturation Change in chemical and physical properties from the normal state, usually irreversible.

dendrite One of the branching protoplasmic processes of the nerve cell.

densitometry A method of determining bone mineral content from single or dual gamma ray or x ray absorption measurements.

deuterons Nucleus of a deuterium atom ($^2_1$H) containing one proton and one neutron.

device A hardware unit such as an I/O peripheral, magnetic tape drive, or line printer.

device control unit A hardware unit that electronically supervises one or more of the same type of devices; it acts as a link between the computer and the I/O devices.

diabetes mellitus Pathologic condition with an absolute or relative insulin deficiency accompanied by elevated levels of glucose in the blood and urine.

diagnostic (1) Referring to determination of the disease; analysis of symptoms. (2) Pertaining to the detection and isolation of a malfunction (hardware) or mistake (software).

dialysis Process for separating crystalloids and colloids in solution by the difference in their rates of diffusion through a semipermeable membrane.

diastole Relaxation and dilation of the heart.

diethylenetriaminepentaacetic acid (pentetic acid, DTPA) Chelating agent that can be labeled with ^{99m}Tc and used for scintigraphy.

digit Character used to express one of the positive integers.

digital computer Device that operates on discrete data, performing sequences or arithmetic and logical operations in these data.

digitalis Cardiotonic agent from the *Digitalis* plant leaf.

dimer A compound produced by the combination of two like molecules; in the strictest sense, without loss of atoms, usually by elimination of water or similar small molecule between the two, but often by simple covalent bonding.

diphosphonate Organic phosphate compound that can be labeled with ^{99m}Tc and used for scintigraphy.

dipyridamole A potent coronary vasodilator.

direct-memory access Access to data in any location independent of sequential prohibitions.

directory A file in the form of a table containing the names of and pointers to files on a mass storage volume.

DIS Decay in storage.

discriminator An electronic barrier used to eliminate low-amplitude noise pulses.

disintegration General process of radioactive decay, usually measured per unit time; *dps* is disintegrations per second, and *dpm* disintegrations per minute; *dps* is equal to counts per second *(cps)* divided by the efficiency of the detector; *dpm* is equal to counts per minute divided by the efficiency of the detector.

disk Form of rotating memory consisting of a platter of aluminum coated with ferrous oxide that can be magnetized or read by a read/write head in proximity to the surface; most common form of bulk memory device.

display A peripheral device used to represent data graphically; normally refers to some type of cathode ray tube system.

diuretic Substance that promotes the secretion of urine.

diverticulum Blind pouch; usually in the intestine.

DLIS Digoxin-like immunoreactive substance.

DMA See *direct memory access.*

DMSA 2,3-Dimercaptosuccinic acid; a chelating agent that can be labeled with ^{99m}Tc for renal imaging.

DNA Deoxyribonucleic acid.

dopamine An intermediate in tyrosine metabolism and the precursor of norepinephrine and epinephrine; it is present in the central nervous system.

DOS Disk operating system.

dose Amount of ionizing radiation absorbed by a specific area or volume or by the whole body.

dose calibrator An ionization chamber designed to measure radionuclide doses.

dose response curve The graphic relationship between counts bound and amount of standard added in a radioimmunoassay; a standard curve.

dosimetry The accurate determination or calculation of dosage.

DOT Department of Transportation.

DPA (dual photon absorptiometry) A bone mineral content measurement technique using gamma or x-ray absorption with a dual energy photon-emitting source; the dual photons allow for accurate correction of soft tissue interference.

DST Dexamethasone suppression test.

DTPA See *diethylenetriaminepentaacetic acid.*

DVT Deep vein thrombosis.

dynode One of several metal plates with a positive voltage that attracts and accelerates electrons within a photomultiplier tube. There are 8-14 dynodes in a photomultiplier tube, each multiplying the number of electrons by a factor of 3 to 6 times.

dysplasia Abnormality of development.

dyspnea Difficulty in breathing.

ECAT Emission computerized axial tomography.

ECG See *electrocardiogram.*

ECT Emission computed tomography.

ED End diastole.

edema Excess fluid in the body.

edetic acid (ethylenediaminetetraacetic acid, EDTA) Chelating agent.

edge packing An area of increased brightness around the edge of a scintillation camera image.

editor Program to permit data or instructions to be manipulated and displayed. Most commonly used in the preparation of new programs or in the revision and correction of old programs.

EDTA See *edetic acid.*

EEG Electroencephalogram.

EF See *cardiac ejection fraction.*

effective half-life The elapsed time to eliminate a radioactive material from the body by a combination of biologic elimination and radioactive decay; determined from physical and biologic half-lives as $1/t_e = 1/t_p + 1/t_b$.

EI Excretion index.

ejection fraction See *cardiac ejection fraction.*

EKG See *electrocardiogram.*

elastic scattering Scattering caused by elastic collisions between nuclei that result in a conversion of the system's kinetic energy.

electrocardiogram A graphic record of the electrical currents that traverse the heart and initiate its contraction.

electrochemical process Chemical process involving oxidation and reduction of the reaction constituents.

electrolyte Substance that forms ions when dissolved in water.

electrolytic reactions Oxidation-reduction reactions.

electrometer Electrostatic instrument for measuring difference in potential.

electron Elementary particle of an atom with a charge of negative one and a mass of 9.1×10^{-28} g.

electron accelerators Machine used to accelerate electrons using potential differences.

electron capture Method of radioactive decay in which the nucleus captures an orbital electron, which then interacts with a proton, effectively negating the proton and transmuting the nucleus to that of another element.

electron configuration Refers to the space relationships of electrons in an atom.

electronegativity Tendency of a neutral atom to acquire electrons, measured relative to that of fluorine.

electronic structure Structure of the orbital electrons in an atom that satisfies the quantum mechanical Schrödinger equation.

electron microscope Microscope that uses an electron beam to form an image on a fluorescent screen.

electron spin resonance (ESR) Spectroscopic technique that determines structural features of a molecule based on electron resonance in a magnetic field.

electron volt (eV) Kinetic energy gained by an electron passing through a potential difference of 1 V.

electrophoresis Liquid paper chromatography carried out under the influence of an electric field.

element Pure substance consisting of atoms of the same atomic number that cannot be decomposed by ordinary chemical means.

eluate The material washed out of a chromatographic column.

elution Separation by solvent extraction.

embolism Matter that blocks a blood vessel.

emission computed tomography See *SPECT.*

empiric, empirical Referring to practical experience.

empirical formula Chemical formula that reflects only the simplest molar ratio of the elements in the compounds, not the actual molar ratio.

EMS Emergency medical system.

emulsion (1) Mixture of two liquids, one suspended within another; colloid system. (2) Suspended mixture in which one of the components is gelatin-like.

endocrine Pertaining to a gland that secretes internally.

endocrinology Study of hormonal secretion and of the endocrine glands.

endogenous Originating or produced within the organism or its parts.

endogonic Intake of energy.

endoscope Instrument, tubular in nature, carrying an

illumination source, inserted into a body cavity to permit visual inspection.

endosteum   Membrane lining of a hollow bone.

endotoxin   Poison from dead bacterial cells; formed while cells are living.

energy levels   Quantum levels of an atom satisfying the Schrödinger equation that are allowed levels for electron location.

enzyme   Protein catalyzing specific transformation of material.

eosinophil   (1) Cell stained readily by eosin. (2) White blood cell characterized by a two- or three-lobed nucleus and cytoplasms containing large granules.

EPA   Environmental Protection Agency.

epidemiology   Study of disease and its rate of occurrence, manner of spread, and prevalence.

epigastrium   Space in the abdomen just below the ribs.

epiphysis   (1) Portion of bone between the shaft and the cartilage. (2) Pineal gland.

epithelium   Cells of skin and mucous membrane.

equilibrium   State of equality between two opposing substances.

equilibrium constant   True constant that relates the concentration of products and reactants in a reversible chemical system where no further net change is occurring in those concentrations.

equivalent   Weight of chemical species that contains either 1 mol of electrons and 1 mol of replaceable hydrogen, or combines with exactly 8 g of oxygen.

erg   A unit of work in the gram-centimeter-second system equal to the amount of work of 1 dyne acting through the distance of 1 cm.

ergometer   Instrument used for measuring energy expended.

ERPF   Effective renal plasma flow.

error   Any discrepancy between a computed, observed, or measured quantity and the specific value or condition.

erythrocyte   Red blood cell.

erythrocytosis   Increase in red blood cells from a known stimulant.

erythroid   Reddish in color.

erythropoiesis   Formation of erythrocytes.

ES   End systole.

esters   Organic compound formed by the action of an acid with an alcohol; contains the functional group:

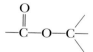

estradiol   The most potent, naturally occurring estrogen in mammals.

estrogenic hormone   Hormone producing female characteristics.

ether   Organic compound containing a C—O—C linkage.

ethylenediaminetetraacetic acid (EDTA)   See *edetic acid.*

etiology   Study of the causes of disease.

Euler's number   The base number (2.718) used in logarithmic calculations named after Leonhard Euler (1701-1783), a Swiss mathematician.

evagination   The protrusion of some part or organ from its usual position.

execute   To perform an instruction or run a program on a computer.

exergonic   Release of energy.

exogenous   Originating or produced outside the subject of reference.

exposure rate   Rate of exposure to radioactivity usually measured in units of rad per hour.

extirpation   Complete removal.

extractor   Device that removes something; liquid that removes another substance with it.

extranuclear   Referring to the space in an atom outside of the nucleus.

extrinsic testing   Scintillation camera uniformity testing done with the collimator in place.

families   Sets of elements that have the same valence-shell electronic configurations.

fast neutron   Neutron that has a minimum energy of 100 keV.

FDA   The U.S. Food and Drug Administration.

FDG   2 fluoro-2 deoxy-D-glucose

ferrokinetics   Study of iron within the body.

fibrinolysis   Dissolution or splitting of fibrin.

file   A logical collection of data that is treated as a unit, occupies one or more blocks on a mass storage volume, and has an associated file name and type.

film badge   Photographic film shielded from light; worn by an individual to measure radiation exposure.

filer   A computer algorithm applied to projections obtained from an imaging system to eliminate noise and artifacts.

fission   Splitting of a nucleus accompanied by a release of energy and neutrons.

flat-field collimator   See *collimator.*

flood phantom   See *phantom.*

flood-field uniformity   The ability of a scintillation camera to depict a uniform distribution of activity as uniform.

flow chart   A graphic representation for the definition, analysis, or solution of a problem in which symbols are used to represent operations, data flow, and equipment.

fluid thioglycollate   Medium that provides conditions for growth of aerobic and anaerobic bacteria; used in microbiologic sterility testing of radiopharmaceuticals.

fluor   A liquid scintillation medium.

fluorescence   Emission of light by an activated chemical complex.

FOCAL (formula calculation) High-level, conversational, interpreter language for mathematical and string variable manipulations developed for Digital Equipment Corporation (Maynard, Mass.) computers.

folate Salt of folic acid.

follicle Sac or pouchlike depression; cavity.

follicle-stimulating hormone (FSH) Anterior pituitary hormone that stimulates follicle growth in the ovaries and spermatogenesis in the testes.

foramen magnum Large opening in the occipital bone between the cranial cavity and the vertebral canal.

FORTRAN (formula translator) High-level compiler language for mathematical and scientific applications.

Fourier transform A mathematical process that converts matrix information into frequency space.

frame mode A method of computer data collection where x and y positional signals are stored in a single matrix.

free radicals Chemical complexes containing an unpaired electron.

frequency Number of cycles per unit time; normal unit is hertz, or cycles per second.

FSH See *follicle-stimulating hormone.*

F-test A statistical test of the null hypothesis.

FTI Free thyroxine index.

function An algorithm, accessible by name and contained in the system software, that performs commonly used operations; an example is the square root calculation function.

functional group Portion of a molecule responsible for its specific chemical properties.

fundus Base of an organ.

fusion Nuclear process in which two discrete nuclei collide and join together, forming a larger nuclide.

FWHM (full width at half maximum) A measurement of curve peak characteristics by comparing the curve width at half the peak height with the value at which the peak occurs. Used for a variety of applications, it is commonly used to express energy or spatial resolution. Results are expressed as a percentage: energy FWHM (%) = $(\Delta E/E) \times 100\%$.

GABA Gamma-aminobutyric acid.

gamma camera See *Anger camera.*

gamma decay See *gamma emission.*

gamma emission Nuclear process in which an excited nuclide deexcites by emission of a nuclear photon.

gamma globulin Globulins in plasma having the slowest mobility using electrophoresis in neutral or alkaline solutions.

gastrin Hormone stimulating secretion by the gastric glands.

gastroenteropathy Disease of the stomach and intestine.

gastroparesis A slight degree of stomach paralysis.

gate Electronic device capable of performing logic operations within a digital circuit. In nuclear medicine it implies a device that can provide a timing signal to the computer. This signal is usually associated with the QRS complex of the electrocardiograph.

gauss Unit for measuring magnetic field strength; 10,000 gauss = 1 tesla.

Geiger-Müller tube Ionization chamber measuring radiation in the region where the charge produced per ionizing event is independent of the number of primary ions produced by the initial ionizing event.

gel permeation chromatography Separation of compounds because of differences in their rates of permeation of a gel, especially useful for separation of large biomolecules such as proteins.

generator Device using a parent radionuclide to obtain its product, the daughter radionuclide, usually by addition of a solution that interacts only with the daughter.

genetic effects Dominant or recessive effects on progeny.

genitourinary tract Urinary system and the sex organs.

geometry A term used to denote the relationship of a radioactive source's position in terms of a detector's sensitive surface area.

GER Gastroesophageal reflux.

GFR Glomerular filtration rate.

g force Centrifugal force.

GH, GHA, glucoheptonate A ^{99m}Tc-labeled carbohydrate used for imaging the renal cortex and collecting system, which may also be used for brain imaging.

globulin Simple protein found in serum and tissue.

glomerulus Small cluster of blood vessels or nerve fibers.

glucagon Pancreatic secretion that increases concentration of the blood sugars.

glucocorticoid Hormone secreted by the adrenal cortex, stimulating the conversion of proteins to carbohydrates.

glucoheptonate Chelating molecule that can bind ^{99m}Tc and be used as an imaging agent.

glycogen Form in which carbohydrates are stored in animal tissue.

glycoprotein Protein and a carbohydrate that does not contain phosphoric acid, purine, or pyrimidine.

glycoside Compound formed between a sugar and another organic substance.

G-M tube See *Geiger-Müller tube.*

gonad Ovary or testicle; the sex gland.

graafian follicle Ovarian follicle where the ovum matures.

gram atomic weight Weight in grams of 1 mol of an element.

gram molecular weight Weight in grams of 1 mol of a chemical compound.

granulocyte White blood cell.

granuloma Tumor or neoplasm consisting of newly formed tissue induced by the presence of a foreign body or of bacteria.

Graves disease Diffuse toxic goiter.

gray (Gy) A unit of absorbed dose equal to 1 joule per kilogram in any medium.

growth hormone (GH) Hormone secreted by the anterior pituitary; stimulates growth.

GTT Glucose tolerance test.

half-life ($t_{1/2}$) A term used to describe the time elapsed until some physical quantity has decreased to half of its original value.

half-reaction Term used in an electrochemical reaction to describe either the oxidation process or the reduction process as a separate entity.

half-value layer (HVL) Thickness of absorbing material necessary to reduce the intensity of radiation by half; synonymous with half-thickness.

halide Compound containing a halogen.

halogens Family of chemical elements of similar electron structure (i.e., the valence shell is completely filled except for one electron)—fluorine, chlorine, bromine, iodine, and astatine.

HAMA Human antimouse antibodies.

H and D curve A logarithmic plot that describes a photographic film's response to a given amount of exposure; after Huerter and Deerfield.

hapten Molecule that cannot elicit immunoglobulin response by itself but can when bound to a larger carrier molecule.

hardware Physical equipment, such as mechanical, electrical, or electronic devices.

Hashimoto disease Infiltration of the thyroid gland with lymphocytes resulting in progressive destruction of the parenchyma and hypothyroidism.

haversian system System of canals in the bones where the blood vessels branch out.

HBV Hepatitis B virus

HCFA Health Care Financing Administration.

HCG Human chorionic gonadotropin.

HDP Hydroxymethylene diphosphonate, a ^{99m}Tc-labeled phosphate complex used in bone imaging.

heat-sensitive printer Type of printer that imprints characters on special sensitized paper by use of heat, without the use of an ink ribbon.

helium-3 (^{3}He) Isotope of helium with an atomic weight of three unified mass units.

hemangioma Tumor of blood vessels that is nonmalignant.

hematocrit Relative percentage of erythrocytes in whole blood.

hematology Study of blood and blood-forming organs.

hematopoietic system The blood system.

hemocytometer Instrument used to count blood cells.

hemoglobin Pigment of the blood that carries oxygen.

hemolysis Red blood cell destruction; escape of hemoglobin within the bloodstream.

hemorrhage Bleeding.

HEPA High-efficiency particulate air (filter).

heparin Mucopolysaccharide acid that occurs in tissues, mainly the liver; used in prevention and treatment of thrombosis, bacterial endocarditis, postoperative pulmonary embolism, repair of vascular injury, and to prevent clotting of blood.

hepatoblastoma Tumor of the liver.

hepatoma Tumor of the liver.

heptasulfide Technetium heptasulfide: ^{99m}Tc$_2$S$_7$; co-precipitates with colloidal sulfur particles stabilized with gelatin in ^{99m}Tc–sulfur-colloid preparation.

hertz Basic unit of frequency; 1 hertz (Hz) = 1 cycle per second.

hexadecimal Pertaining to the number system with a radix of 16.

hexane Alkane with the molecular formula C_6H_{14}.

HIDA N,N′-(2,6-dimethylphenyl) carbomolymethyl iminodiacetic acid; can be labeled with ^{99m}Tc and used as an imaging agent.

high-level language A programming language whose statements are translated into more than one machine language instruction; examples are BASIC and FORTRAN.

histochemical Referring to the deposit of chemical components in cells.

histogram A graph.

histology Study of the form and structure of tissues.

histopathology The science or study of diseased tissue.

HIV Human immunodeficiency virus.

HMO Health maintenance organization.

HMPAO Hexamethyl propylene animal oxime.

homeostasis The state of equilibrium in the body with respect to various functions and to the chemical compositions of the fluids and tissues.

hormone Chemical having a specific effect on the activity of a specific organ.

HVL See *half-value layer.*

hydrocarbon Compound containing carbon and hydrogen exclusively.

hydrolysis Processes of decomposition by the addition of water.

hydroxide The ion OH$^-$

hydroxyapatite Compound $Ca_{10}(PO_4)_6(OH)_2$; inorganic constituent of bone and teeth.

8-hydroxyquinoline (oxine) Compound that can form a complex with indium and gallium and be used to label blood cells.

hygroscopic Having an affinity for water.

hyperemia Excess blood in an organ or part of the body.

hyperglycemia Excessive sugar (glucose) in the blood.

hyperplasia An increase in the number of cells in a tissue or organ, excluding tumor formation.

hyperthyroidism Overactive thyroid gland.

hypoglycemia Not enough sugar (glucose) in the blood.

hypokinesia Diminished motor function.

hypopituitarism Insufficient secretion of the pituitary.

hypothalamus Part of the forebrain below the cerebrum.

hypothyroidism Insufficient activity of the thyroid.

ICRP International Commission on Radiation Protection.

IDA Iminodiacetic acid, a family of ^{99m}Tc-labeled radiopharmaceuticals used to evaluate the hepatobiliary system.

IF See *intrinsic factor.*

iminodiacetic acid Chelating group capable of binding technetium so that it can be attached to biologically active molecules, such as HIDA.

immunoactive Immunity produced by stimulation of antibody-producing mechanisms.

immunoglobulin Type of protein, isolated from the globulin fraction of serum having a characteristic shape and the ability to bind to molecules that are not endogenous to the species producing the immunoglobulin.

immunology Study of resistance to disease or disease agents.

immunoreaction Reaction taking place between an antigen and its antibody.

IMP Iodoamphetamine.

incubate To provide proper conditions for growth or a reaction to occur.

inelastic collision Interaction between two particles resulting in a net loss of kinetic energy in the system.

infarct Area deprived of its blood supply because of an obstruction.

infundibular pulmonic stenosis Obstruction in the outer passage from the right ventricle, restricting blood flow.

inhibition Prevention or interference of a chemical reaction.

inhibitor Substance preventing or interfering with a chemical reaction.

innominate vein Vein receiving blood from the head and neck region.

inoculate To protect against disease by injection of pathogenic microorganisms to stimulate production of antibodies.

inorganic Branch of chemistry having to do with compounds and processes that do not involve carbon.

input Transferal of data from auxiliary or external storage into the internal storage of a computer.

instruction A coded command that tells the computer what to do and where to find the values it is to work with; symbolic instructions must be changed into machine instructions before they can be executed by the computer.

insulin Hormone produced in cells of the pancreas essential for metabolism of carbohydrates.

interface Connection between two systems, such as a scintillation camera and a computer.

internal conversion Nuclear deexcitation process in which the radionuclide deexcites by transferring energy to an orbital electron.

interpreter Computer program that translates and executes each source-language statement before translating and executing the next statement.

interrupts Signals that, when activated, cause a transfer of control to a specific location in memory, thereby breaking the normal flow of control of the routine being executed. An interrupt is normally caused by an external event such as a condition in a peripheral.

interstices Small gaps between tissues or structures.

intrinsic factor (IF) Substance produced by the gastric mucosa and found in the terminal ileum that is necessary for absorption of vitamin B_{12}.

intrinsic testing Scintillation camera uniformity testing with the collimator removed.

intussusception The infolding of one segment of the intestine within another.

inulin Polysaccharide that on hydrolysis yields levulose, which can be used to test kidney function.

inulin clearance test Test of renal function.

inverse square law The radiation intensity of any source decreases inversely as the square of the distance between the source and the detector.

in vitro Outside a living organism.

in vivo Within a living organism.

I/O (input/output) device Computer device that either accepts input or prints out results.

iodination Addition of iodine to a compound.

iodohippuran Agent used for renal imaging.

ion Atom or group of atoms with a net electronic charge.

ion exchange Process involving reversible exchange of ions in a solution and in a solid.

ionic compound Compound held together by purely electrostatic forces.

ionic strength Half the sum of the terms obtained by multiplying the molarity of each ion by the square of its valence.

ionization Process of removing electrons from an atom to create an ion.

ionization chamber A gas-filled radiation detector.

IRMA Immunoradiometric assay.

irradiation Application of radiant energy for therapy or diagnosis.

ischemia Insufficient blood supply because of a spasm or constriction of the artery in an organ or part of the body.

ischemic damage Damage from a constriction of the blood vessel.

islets of Langerhans Pancreatic cells secreting insulin.

isobar Nuclides that have the same total number of neutrons and protons but are different elements.

isoelectric Having uniform electric potential; thus no current is given off.

isometric transition Change in the extranuclear portion of an atom from a high-energy level to a lower energy level accompanied by the release of electromagnetic radiation.

isomers Two compounds with the same molecular formulas and different structural formulas.

isopleth Graph showing frequency of an event as a function of two variables.

isotones Nuclides having the same number of neutrons but a different number of protons.

isotonic Physiologic; compatible with body tissues.

isotopes Nuclides of the same element with the same number of protons but different number of neutrons.

ITLC Instant thin layer chromatography.

ITP Idiopathic thrombocytopenia.

IUPAC International Union of Pure and Applied Chemistry.

JCAHO Joint Commission on Accreditation of Healthcare Organizations.

joystick An electronic pointing device for computers.

ketone Organic molecule with a carbon-oxygen double bond separating two alkyl portions

$$O$$
$$\|$$
$$(R—C—R)$$

kinetic energy That energy of a body due to its motion.

Kupffer cells Part of the reticuloendothelial system; star-shaped cells attached to the wall of the sinusoids of the liver.

lacuna Small hollow cavity.

LAL See *limulus amebocyte lysate.*

lambda Greek letter denoting the decay constant of radioactive species.

language Set of representations, conventions, and rules used to convey information.

Larmor frequency The characteristic frequency at which the resonance of the nucleus is excited in magnetic resonance imaging.

law of constant composition If two (or more) elements combine chemically to form a compound, the relative weights of the constituent elements will always be in a constant proportion to each other.

law of definite proportions If two (or more) elements chemically combine to form a compound, the relative number of moles of each constituent element will be in a proportion of simple whole numbers with each other.

law of mass action The velocity of the chemical reaction is proportional to the masses of the reactants.

law of multiple proportions If two elements form more than one compound, the number of moles of one element in the first compound is proportional to the number of moles of the same element in the second compound.

law of reciprocal proportions Two chemical elements unite with a third element in proportions that are multiples of the union of the first two elements.

Le Châtelier's principle If a system is initially at equilibrium and is forced away from equilibrium when a parameter is changed, the system will spontaneously return to a new equilibrium.

LET See *linear energy transfer.*

leukocyte White blood cell, either granular or nongranular.

leukopenia Less than the normal number of white blood cells.

leukotaxine Crystalline nitrogen substance appearing when tissue is injured.

Lewis concept An acid is an electron-pair accceptor and a base is an electron-pair donor.

LH Luteinizing hormone.

ligand (1) Molecule attached to a central atom using coordinate covalent bonds. (2) In radioimmunoassay an antigen or small molecule that binds to a native carrier protein.

light pen A device resembling a pencil or stylus that is used to input information to a CRT display system.

limulus amoebocyte lysate (LAL) In vitro test for pyrogens; it reacts with gram-negative bacterial endotoxins in nanogram or greater concentrations to form an opaque gel.

line spread function The profile of counts along a line running perpendicular to a line source.

linear attenuation coefficient That quantity by which radiation is decreased per unit path length through matter.

linear energy transfer Amount of energy lost by ionizing radiation by way of interaction with matter per centimeter of path length through the absorbing material.

linear regression A calculation generally performed to show a linear relationship between two variables to predict some y variable based on measurement of some x variable.

lingula Small tonguelike structure.

linker A program that combines many relocatable object modules into an executable module; it satisfies global references and combines program sections.

lipid Fat and fatlike substances.

lipophilic Capable of dissolving, of being dissolved in, or of absorbing lipids.

lipoproteins Combination of a lipid and a protein.

liquid-drop model Theoretical model of the nucleus

that assumes a simple continuous nuclear potential and spheroid shape.

liquid scintillation counter A system for detecting beta-emitting radionuclides using a liquid scintillator in which the radioactive source is dissolved.

list mode A method of computer data collection where x and y positional signals are stored sequentially in memory in the form of a list.

listing The printed copy generated by a line printer or terminal.

load To store a program or data in memory; to mount a tape on a device such that the read point is at the beginning of the tape; to place a removable disk in a disk drive and start the drive.

location An address in storage or memory where a unit of data or an instruction can be stored.

logarithm Exponent of the power of a base that equals a given number.

logit Mathematical relationship defined as $\ln \dfrac{y}{1-y}$.

loop A sequence of instructions executed repeatedly until a terminal condition prevails.

Lugol solution An iodine solution.

LV Left ventricle.

LVEF Left ventricular ejection fraction; see also *cardiac ejection fraction*.

lymphangiography Radiography of the lymph channels.

lymphocyte White blood cell with a single rounded nucleus.

lymphoma Tumor composed of lymph node tissue.

lyophilize To rapidly freeze and dehydrate a substance.

lysis (1) Separation of adhesions binding different structures. (2) Destruction of a cell by a specific agent. (3) Abatement of disease symptoms.

MAA Macroaggregated albumin.

machine code See *object code*.

machine language See *language*.

macro (1) Directions for expanding abbreviated text; a boilerplate that generates a known set of instructions, data, or symbols; a macro is used to eliminate the need to write a set of instructions that are used repeatedly. (2) Prefix meaning huge or of large scale.

macroglobulin Protein of high molecular weight.

macrophage Large white blood cell; active in bacterial destruction.

MAG3 Mercaptoacetyltriglycine.

magnetic field Field induced by moving electrical charges.

magnetic quantum number Quantum number (m, m_i, *or* M) that defines the orientation of an orbital in space.

magnetic tape A plastic-base tape in which data is imprinted magnetically.

malabsorption Inadequate absorption of nutrients in the gastrointestinal tract.

manometer Device used to measure the pressure of liquids.

mass Basic parameter of matter referring to the quantity of matter present. It is independent of the object's weight.

mass attenuation coefficient The quotient of the linear attenuation coefficient divided by the density of the matter through which it passes.

mass defect The difference in mass of an atom's constituent particles and its total mass.

mass storage A device that can store large amounts of data readily accessible to the computer.

matrix A rectangular array of elements; any matrix can be considered an array.

maximum permissible dose (MPD) Dose limitations, in rem, placed on each individual as specified by the Nuclear Regulatory Commission.

MDA Minimum detectable amount.

MDP Methylene diphosphonate, a ^{99m}Tc-labeled phosphate complex used in bone imaging.

mean Average of two or more quantities.

Meckel diverticulum Saclike pouch on the small intestine.

mediastinum Space behind the breastbone containing the heart.

medulloblastoma Tumor of the brain.

megakaryocyte A cell found in the bone marrow developing into blood platelets.

MEK Methyl ethyl ketone.

melanoma Tumor characterized by dark pigmentation.

memory Any form of data storage including main memory and mass storage in which data can be read and written; memory usually refers to the main memory.

mesenchyme Primitive tissue of the embryo.

metabolism Process for transforming foods into compounds used by the body.

metastable state Excited state of a nucleus or atom that has a measurable lifetime; also known as an isometric state.

metastasis Spreading of a disease process from one part of the body to another.

metathesis Chemical process in which two compounds exchange constituents.

microbiologic testing Any test for bacteria, virus, or other microorganism.

microlysis Destruction of a substance into microscopic size.

micrometer (μm) One millionth of a meter; formerly micron.

microprocessor A silicon chip containing many circuits.

microsphere Round mass of a small size, visible only with a microscope.

microvilli Projections of cell membranes greatly increasing the surface area of the cell.

migrating solvent Chromatographic solvent; used to differentially carry the unknown solute to be separated.

MIPS Million instructions per second.

mitral stenosis Deformity of the mitral valve of the heart.

mnemonic Aiding the memory; use of an acronym or other pattern to aid the memory.

mobile phase Phase in chromatography that differentially carries the unknown solutes.

modem From *mo*dulate and *dem*odulate. A device used to transmit computer data over telephone lines.

modulation transfer function A curve depicting the image to object contrast ratio as a function of spatial frequency.

molality Unit of solution concentration defined as the number of moles of solute per weight (kg) of solvent.

molal Unit of concentration associated with molality equal to the number of moles of solute per kilogram of solvent.

molar Concentration unit equal to number of moles of solute per liter of solution.

molarity Measure of solution concentration defined as the number of moles of solute per volume (liter) of solution.

mole See *gram molecular weight.*

molecular formula Chemical formula that states the actual number of atoms of each constituent per molecule of the compound.

molecular weight Weight in unified mass units of one molecule of a particular chemical compound.

molecule Basic unit of a chemical compound.

molybdate Compound containing a MoO_4^{-2} group.

monatomic One atom per molecule, usually referring to elements (such as the noble gases) in their native state.

monitor The master control program that observes, supervises, controls, or verifies the operation of a computer system; the collection of routines that controls the operation of user and system programs, schedules, operations, allocates resources, and performs I/O.

monoclonal antibodies Immunoglobulins, chemically identical in structure, produced by a group of cells that are genetically identical.

monocyte White blood cell having one rounded nucleus that increases in number during certain types of infections.

monoenergetic Having a single energy.

MOPS Manually operated pipetter/samplers.

morphology Study of the structure of tissues.

motility The power of spontaneous movement.

mouse An electronic pointing device for computers.

MPD See *Maximum permissible dose.*

MPST Mean platelet survival time.

MRI (magnetic resonance imaging) Body imaging technique to observe chemical makeup of tissue using magnetic fields and radiofrequency electromagnetic waves.

MTF See *modulation transfer function.*

mucoid (1) Mucuslike substance. (2) An animal conjugated protein.

mucosal biopsy Removal and examination of some of the tissue of the mucous membrane.

MUGA Multiple-gated acquisition.

multiformatter A photographic system designed to produce images from a cathode ray tube in various positions and sizes.

multiple-gated acquisition Composite heart-imaging technique performed by synchronizing a patient's heartbeat by means of an electrocardiograph to a scintillation camera/computer.

myeloblast A cell in the bone marrow that develops into a white blood cell.

myelofibrosis Replacement of the bone marrow by fibrous tissue.

myeloid (1) Referring to bone marrow. (2) Referring to the spinal cord. (3) Cell resembling a red bone marrow cell that did not originate in the bone marrow.

myocardial infarct Heart muscle damage secondary to loss of its blood supply.

myocardial ischemia Obstruction or constriction in the coronary arteries resulting in a deficiency of blood to the heart muscle.

myocardium Heart muscle.

N See *Neutron number.*

naperian logarithmic system Logarithmic system using the base *e,* which is a mathematical constant ($e = 2.71$).

nasopharyngeal Referring to that part of the pharynx above the soft palate.

natural logarithm See *naperian logarithmic system.*

NCRP National Council on Radiation Protection and Measurement.

negatron Negative electron.

NEMA National Electrical Manufacturers Association.

neonate Newborn to 4-week-old infant.

neoplasia Condition characterized by new tumors or growths.

nephrology Study of the kidney.

nephron Part of the kidney that secretes urine.

nephrosis Degeneration of the kidney.

neurinoma Enlargement of a node or tumor on a peripheral nerve.

neuroglia Nonnervous cellular elements of nervous tissue.

neurohormone Hormone stimulating the mechanism of the nerves.

neurohumeral Referring to a chemical secreted by a neutron.

neurohypophysis Main part of the posterior pituitary (hypophysis cerebri).

neuron Nerve.

neuropathology Study of nervous system diseases by examination of those tissues.

neutralization Chemical reaction in which an acid and a base react to form a salt and water.

neutrino Nuclear particle emitted during positron decay.

neutron Nuclear particle that is found in the nucleus, is electrically neutral, and has a mass of one mass unit.

neutron activation Nuclear process in which a nucleus absorbs a thermal neutron and deexcites by way of gamma-ray emission.

neutron flux Measure of neutron intensity defined as the number of neutrons passing through one square centimeter of area per second.

neutron number Number of neutrons in a nucleus (symbol for neutron number is N).

neutrophil White blood cell with three to five lobes connected by chromatin and cytoplasm containing five granules.

nidus (1) Focus of infection. (2) Depression in the brain surface.

NIST National Institute of Standards and Technology. Formerly National Bureau of Standards (NBS).

NMR (nuclear magnetic resonance) See *magnetic resonance imaging (MRI)*.

noble gas Any chemical element that has a completely filled valence-shell configuration in its neutral state—helium, neon, argon, krypton, xenon, and radon.

noise Extraneous interference in an electronic circuit of statistical manipulation.

nomogram Conversion scale.

nonpolar bond Chemical bond in which a pair of electrons is equally shared by two nuclei.

nonspecific binding (NSB) Binding of the radioligand to substances or surfaces other than the specific reactor substance.

normal Concentration unit defined as the number of equivalent weights of solute per liter of solution.

normality Method of expressing concentration defined as the number of equivalent weights of solute per volume of solution.

normalize A term used in association with computer-defined regions of interest to indicate that counts contained in the regions have been converted to the same size region.

NRC See *Nuclear Regulatory Commission*.

NSB See nonspecific binding.

nuclear charge Charge of the nucleus of an atom equal to the number of protons multiplied by the charge of a proton.

nuclear fission Nuclear process in which a nucleus splits into two pieces accompanied by neutron emission and energy release.

nuclear reactor Device that under controlled conditions is used for supporting a self-sustained nuclear reaction.

Nuclear Regulatory Commission (NRC) United States government agency regulating by-product material.

nuclear stability Condition to describe a nucleus that is stable with respect to radioactive decay.

nucleons Any particle commonly contained in the nucleus of an atom.

nucleus (1) Portion of an atom containing the neutrons and the protons. (2) Spheric body that is the core of a cell. (3) Mass of gray matter in the central nervous system.

NUTRAN High-level computer language.

object code Relocatable machine language code.

obtund To dull or blunt, especially to blunt sensation or deaden pain.

occipital Referring to the back of the head or occiput.

Occupational Safety and Health Administration (OSHA) United States government agency regulating health standards in the workplace.

octal The number system with a radix of 8; for example, octal 100 is decimal 64.

OIH See *ortho-iodohippurate*.

oleic acid (octadecanoic acid) Straight-chained organic acid with the molecular formula $C_{18}H_{36}O_2$.

oncocytoma Granular cell adenoma of the parotid gland.

optic chiasma The point of crossing of the fibers of the optic nerve.

orbital Energy sublevels occupied by electrons in an atom.

ordinate The y, or perpendicular, axis in a cartesian graph or plot.

organic chemistry Branch of chemistry dealing with the study of compounds of carbon.

organic compounds Any of the class of chemical compounds that contain carbon.

organomegaly Abnormal enlargement of an organ.

op code See *operation code*.

operand That which is affected, manipulated, or operated upon.

operating systems Collection of programs, including a monitor or executive and system programs, that organizes a central processor and peripheral devices into a working unit for the development and execution of application programs.

operation code Code used to start the operation of a program.

ortho-iodohippurate (OIH) Iodinated renal imaging agent.

OSHA See *Occupational Safety and Health Administration*.

osmoreceptor Specialized sensory nerve ending that (1) gives rise to sense of smell and (2) is stimulated by changes in osmotic pressures of the surrounding medium.

osseous Composed of bone.

osteoblast Immature bone-producing cell.

osteoclast Large multinuclear cell associated with destruction of bone.

osteocyte Cell lodged in flat oval cavities of the bone.

osteogenesis Bone development.

osteomyelitis Infection of the bone.

output Information transferred from the internal storage of a computer to output devices or external storage.

ovary Female reproductive gland.

oxidation Process by which a substance loses electrons in an oxidation-reduction reaction.

oxidation-reduction Chemical reaction in which electrons are transferred from one substance to another substance.

oxidizing agent Substance in an oxidation-reduction reaction that causes another substance to lose electrons.

oxine See *8-hydroxyquinoline.*

Paget's disease Osteitis deformans.

PAH Paraaminohippuric acid.

pair production Photonic deexcitation process in which a photon disintegrates into an electron-positron pair, each of which gains an equal amount of kinetic energy.

pancreas Large gland secreting enzymes into the intestines for digestion and manufacturing and secreting insulin.

papilla of Vater Prominent tissue in the duodenum where the bile duct enters the intestine.

parathormone Hormone secreted by the parathyroid gland.

parathyroid glands Four small endocrine glands on the lateral lobe of the thyroid that control calcium and phosphorus metabolism.

parenchyma Essential elements of an organ as distinguished from its framework.

parent radionuclide Radionuclide that decays to a specific daughter nuclide either directly or as a member of a radioactive series.

parotid gland Salivary gland.

Pascal A computer programming language.

PAS Paraaminosalicylic acid.

pathology Study of disease based on examination of diseased tissue.

pathophysiology Study of disordered function of organs.

Pauli exclusion principle Two electrons in the same atom cannot have the exact same set of quantum numbers.

Pauling scale A measure of electronegativity with fluorine arbitrarily assigned a value of 4.

pedicle Stemlike part of attaching structure.

PEG Poyethylene glycol.

pellet (1) Small pill. (2) A granule.

pentetic acid (diethylenetriaminepentaacetic acid,

DTPA) Chelating agent that can be labeled with ^{99m}Tc and used for scintigraphy.

peptide Low molecular weight compound containing two or more amino acids.

peptide hormone Hormones excreted by the pituitary, parathyroid, and pancreas.

percent trace binding The amount of radioactivity bound by a specific reactor substance in a solution containing the substance of interest, divided by the amount of radioactivity bound by a solution where the substance of interest is undetectable, times 100.

perchlorate Any chemical compound that contains the CIO_4 group.

perfusion Passage of a fluid into an organ to thoroughly permeate it.

pericardium Tissue sheath encasing the heart.

perineal region Floor of the pelvis.

period (1) In wave motion phenomena it is the time required to complete one cyclic motion, equalizing the reciprocal of the frequency. (2) Elements in a horizontal line on the periodic chart.

periodic chart Chart of the elements depicting the interrelationships among them based on their electronic configurations.

periosteal bone Bone that develops directly from and beneath the periosteum.

periosteum Thin tissue encasing bones that possesses bone-forming potential.

peripheral (1) Near the surface, distant; distal, opposite of proximal. (2) Any device distinct from the central processor that can provide input or accept output from the computer.

peripheral blood Blood that circulates in the vessels remote from the heart.

peripheral vessels Blood vessels that are remote from the heart.

pernicious anemia Anemia from lack of secretion by the gastric mucosa of intrinsic factor, which is important to blood formation.

pertechnetate Any chemical compound containing the TcO_4^- group.

PET Positron emission tomography.

PGA Pteroyglutamic (folic) acid.

pH Measure of the hydrogen ion concentration in a solution; equals the negative logarithm of the hydrogen ion concentration.

pH meter Device used to measure the pH of a solution based on the potential difference between the solution and a standard calomel electrode.

phagocyte Cell that destroys bacteria or other foreign bodies.

phagocytize To ingest cells or microorganisms by a cell (a phagocyte).

phagocytosis Destruction of bacteria or other foreign bodies by phagocytes.

phantom (1) Model of some part of the body in which radioactive material can be placed to simulate conditions in vivo. (2) A device that yields information concerning the performance of a medical imaging system.

pharmacokinetics Study of the activity of drugs and medicines.

pharmacology Study of drugs and medicine.

pharynx Back of the nasal passages and mouth; the throat.

phase The time relationship between two events.

phenols Organic compounds with the functional group OH^- attached to an aromatic ring.

phosphor Chemical compound that upon photonic absorption will deexcite slowly by emitting light.

phosphorylation Chemical process in which a molecule acquires a PO_4^{-3} group.

photocathode Negative electrode of a photomultiplier tube.

photodisintegration Disintegration event triggered by photonic interactions.

photoelectric effect Process by which photons deexcite through absorption by electrons, resulting in ionization phenomena.

photomultiplication Multiplication of the signal given off by the interaction of a photon in a scintillation detector.

photomultiplier tube An electronic tube that converts light photons to electric pulses.

photon Discrete packet of electromagnetic energy.

photopeak A peak or increase in a graphic representation of a radioactive spectrum characteristic of the radionuclide under study.

phrenic artery Artery in the diaphragm.

phylogenetic, phylogenic Referring to the developmental history of an organism or race.

physical half-life The elapsed time to reach half of the original quantity of radioactivity by decay.

physiology Study of the function of tissues or organs.

pipeline processing Computer instructions carried out in an assembly line fashion.

pipet (or pipette) (1) Device used to deliver a precise amount of a liquid. (2) The act of using such a device.

pituitary Endocrine gland located at the base of the brain; regulates growth and secretions of other endocrine glands.

pixel From *pic*ture *el*ement; a single image element.

PL/1 (programming language 1) High-level computer language.

placenta Organ attaching the embryo to the uterus; the afterbirth.

placental barrier Term used to describe the semipermeable barrier interposed between the maternal and fetal blood by the placental membrane.

Planck's constant 6.626186×10^{-27} erg-seconds.

planimetry Measurement of plane surfaces.

plasma Fluid of the blood not including the red and white blood cells.

platelet, blood platelet, thrombocyte Small, colorless disks that aid in blood clotting found in circulating blood.

plethysmography Measurement of changes in volume using a plethysmograph.

pleura Membrane lining of the chest cavity and lungs.

pleural effusion Fluid in the space that contains the lungs and the thoracic cavity.

PnAO Propylene amine oxime, a ^{99m}Tc-labeled complex that crosses the blood-brain barrier and is used to image regional cerebral perfusion.

point spread function The profile of counts along a line through a point source of radioactivity.

Poisson distribution A statistical distribution of events.

polar covalent bond Covalent bond formed by the unequal sharing of a pair of electrons between two atoms.

polarization The development of differences in potential between two points in living tissues.

polyatomic ion Ion composed of more than one atom.

polycythemia Disease characterized by an overabundance of red blood cells.

polycythemia vera (p. vera) Inherited disease characterized by increase of red blood cells and total blood volume accompanied by splenomegaly, leukocytosis, thrombocytosis, and bone marrow hyperactivity.

polymer Compound formed of simpler molecules, usually of high molecular weight.

polymerization Formation of a polymer.

polypeptide Compound containing two or more amino acids linked by a peptide bond.

polyphosphate Any molecule containing the $(PO_3)_n$ group.

pons (1) Slip of tissue connecting two parts of an organ. (2) Part of the base of the brain.

popliteal fossa Depression at the back of the knee.

porcine From a pig.

porta hepatis Part of the liver receiving the major blood vessels.

positron (β^+) Transitory nuclear particle with a mass equal to that of an electron and a charge equal to that of a proton.

potentiometer See *voltmeter*.

preamplifier A device placed between a detector and an amplifier used to shape and increase pulse size.

precipitate Solid compound that is produced in a chemical reaction between two soluble compounds in a solution.

precision Refers to the variations of individual measurements.

precordium Upper abdominal region.

pressure Force per unit area.

primary fluor A liquid scintillator.

primordial Formed early in the course of development.

principal quantum number (n or n_i) Relative distance from the nucleus at which the electron will be found and also its relative energy.

processor See *central processor unit*.

proerythroblast Primitive erythrocyte.

progesterone Hormone secreted by the ovaries.

program Complete sequence of instructions and routines necessary to solve a problem.

program development Process of writing, entering, translating, and debugging source programs.

prolactin Hormone secreted by the anterior pituitary.

promonocyte Intermediate cell between the monoblast and monocyte.

prompt neutrons Neutrons from a fission event that are emitted immediately after or during the event.

proportional counter A gas-filled radiation detector.

proprioception Process of receiving stimulation within the tissue.

prostaglandins Substance causing strong contractions of smooth muscle and dilation of the vascular bed.

prostatic hypertrophy Enlargement of the prostate because of an increase in the size of its cells.

protease Enzyme that digests protein.

protein High molecular weight compound of many amino acids linked by peptide bonds.

proteinuria Protein in the urine.

prothrombin Protein combining with other proteins to form thrombin, a clotting agent.

proton Nuclear particle with a mass of one unified mass unit and a charge of $+1.6 \times 10^{-9}$ coulomb.

psi Pounds per square inch; unit of pressure.

PTH Parathyroid hormone; parathyrin.

PTHrP Parathyroid hormone-related peptide.

ptosis Denotes a falling or downward displacement of an organ.

pulmonary Referring to the lungs.

pulmonic stenosis Obstruction from the right ventricle, restricting the outflow of blood.

pulse height analysis See *pulse height analyzer (PHA)*.

pulse height analyzer (PHA) Instrument that accepts input from a detector and categorizes the pulses on the basis of signal strength.

pulse height window See *window*.

PVC Premature ventricular contraction.

P wave The first complex of the electrocardiogram representing depolarization of the atria.

pyelonephritis Inflammation of the kidney and the pelvis of the kidney.

pylorus Part of the stomach just before the duodenum.

pyogenic Pus forming; bacterial.

pyrogen Fever-inducing substance.

pyrophosphate Chemical compound containing a $P_2O_7^{-4}$.

QF See *quality factor*.

QMP Quality management program.

QRS complex The principal deflection in the electrocardiogram representing ventricular depolarization.

qualitative chemical analysis Determination of the identity of each constituent in a chemical system.

quality control serum A serum sample that is analyzed many times to yield data about the statistical reproducibility of a radioassay.

quality factor (QF) Linear energy transfer–dependent factor by which absorbed doses are to be multiplied to account for the varying effectiveness of different radiations.

quantitative chemical analysis Branch of chemical analysis dealing with the determination of how much of a constituent there is in a chemical compound.

quantum mechanics Branch of physics dealing with the mathematical description of the wave properties of atomic and nuclear particles.

quantum number Value describing the location of an electron in the electron configuration of an atom.

quenching (1) Action of a gas added to a Geiger-Müller detector, allowing it to resolve. (2) An undesirable reduction of light output from a liquid scintillator.

R wave A portion of the QRS electrocardiographic signal denoting ventricular contraction and relaxation.

rad See *radiation absorbed dose*.

radial immunodiffusion Immunochemical method used for the determination of serum concentrations of physiologically important substances.

radiation absorbed dose (rad) Quantity of radiation that deposits 100 ergs of energy per gram of absorbing material.

radiation dose Quantity of radiation absorbed by some material.

radiation exposure Exposure to ionizing radiation.

radiation safety Methods of protecting workers and the general population from the deleterious effects of radiation.

radiochemistry Study of the chemistry of radioactive elements.

radiochromatography Chromatography using NaI crystal for detection of substances labeled with a radioisotope.

radiocolloids Colloid of a solid in a liquid where the solid phase contains a radioisotope.

radiograph Image of the internal structure of objects by exposure of film to x rays; roentgenogram.

radioimmunoassay Assay by immunologic procedures using radioactive antigens.

radionuclide Unstable nucleus that transmutes by way of nuclear decay.

radionuclidic purity Amount of total radioactive species in a sample that is the desired radionuclide.

radiopharmaceutical Radioactive drug used for therapy or diagnosis.

radiopharmacology Study of radioactive drugs and their therapeutic and diagnostic uses.

radiopharmacy Laboratory producing and dispensing

solutions labeled with radioisotopes for therapeutic and diagnostic purposes.

radioreceptor Sensory nerve terminal stimulated by radiant energy.

RAM (random access memory) Memory accessed in such a way that the next location from which data are obtained is not dependent on the location of the previously obtained data.

raphe A seam; the line of union of two contiguous and similar structures.

RAS Renal artery stenosis.

RAST Radioallergosorbent test.

rate meter Device, used in conjunction with a detector, that measures the rate of activity of a radioisotope; usually in units of counts per minute or counts per second.

RBE See *relative biologic effectiveness.*

reaction Any process resulting in a net change to the constituents of the system.

reactor See *nuclear reactor.*

read-only input (ROI) Input only from the memory or from an internal source. (Contrast *regions of interest [ROI].*)

read-only memory Internal acquisition of data from the memory in computers.

reagent Any chemical used in a process.

real time In computer terminology the actual time elapsed during the program.

real-time system System in which the computation is performed while a related physical activity is occurring; the program results are used in guiding the physical process.

receptor Sensory nerve terminal responding to stimulation by transmission of impulses to the central nervous system.

rectilinear scanner An imaging device that passes over the area of interest in a rectilinear fashion.

red blood cells (RBC) Any blood cells containing hemoglobin.

redox Abbreviation for an oxidation-reduction reaction.

reducing agent Substance that donates electrons in an oxidation-reduction reaction.

reduction In an oxidation-reducing reaction it is the process by which one substance gains electrons.

reflex A reaction or involuntary movement.

regions of interest (ROI) Portion of the data field that is to be studied. (Contrast *read-only input [ROI].*)

register A device capable of storing a specified amount of data such as a word. See also *accumulator.*

regression analysis See *linear regression.*

relative biologic effectiveness (RBE) Ratio of the biologic response derived from a particular radiation as compared with another radiation exposure.

rem See *roentgen equivalent man.*

renal cortex Smooth outer layer of the kidney.

replacement reaction Chemical process in which an ion is replaced by another species in a compound.

resolution The ability of a counting or imaging system to accurately depict two separate events in space, time, or energy as separate.

resolving time The length of time taken by a detector to sense and process a nuclear event.

resorption A loss of substance by lysis.

rest mass Mass that is not in motion.

reticuloendothelial cells Phagocytes.

RFQ Radiofrequency quadripole accelerator.

RIA See *radioimmunoassay.*

RISC Reduced instruction set computer.

RNA Ribonucleic acid; responsible for transmission of inherited traits.

RNC Radionuclide cystography.

ROC curve Receiver operating characteristic curve: a graphic representation of sensitivity and specificity.

roentgen (R) Quantity of x or gamma radiation per cubic centimeter of air that produces one electrostatic unit of charge.

roentgen equivalent man (rem) unit of radiation dose defined as the product of rad and RBE.

ROI See *read-only input* and *regions of interest.*

ROM See *read-only memory.*

RSO Radiation safety office(r).

run A single continuous execution of a program.

Rutherford scattering See *elastic scattering.*

RV Right ventricle.

RVG Radionuclide ventriculogram.

saccule Small sac or pouch.

sagittal (1) Plane or section parallel to the long axis of the body. (2) Arrowlike shape.

saline Sodium chloride in water.

saline solution, physiologic Salt solution compatible with body tissues.

salivary glands Glands secreting saliva, connected to the mouth by ducts; the three glands are the parotids, submaxillaries, and sublinguals.

saturation analysis A type of competitive binding assay where the specific reactor substance-binding sites are all occupied (saturated) by ligand; RIA is a type of saturation analysis.

scaler An electronic pulse counter.

Schilling test Test for primary pernicious anemia.

scientific notation A system of utilizing signs or numbers to represent numbers of greater and lesser magnitudes.

scintigraphic agent Substance injected to produce images of internal organs; usually a radioactive solution.

scintigraphy Imaging the distribution of a radionuclide with scintillation detection.

scintillation Flash of light produced in a phosphor by radiation.

scleroderma (1) Thickening of the skin by swelling. (2) Thickening of the fibrous tissue.

secondary fluor (waveshifter) A liquid scintillator.

secretin Hormone-stimulating secretion of pancreatic

juice and bile secreted by the duodenal mucous membrane.

secular equilibrium Parent-daughter radioisotope pair in which the parent has a much longer half-life than does the daughter radionuclide.

semiconductor Substance whose conductivity is enhanced by the addition of another substance or through the application of heat, light, or voltage.

senescent Growing old; characteristic of old age.

sensitivity (1) Pertains to the ability of a given test to determine what fraction or percentage of ill patients will have a positive test result. (2) Efficiency of a given detector system.

septal Referring to a wall or partition.

septum A wall or partition.

serous Referring to serum.

serum Liquid remaining after blood has clotted.

shells Energy levels in electronic configuration.

shielding Absorbing material used to attenuate ionizing radiation.

shunt Bypass; an alternate course.

SI Serum iron, see also *specific ionization*.

SIDS Sudden infant death syndrome.

sievert (Sv) Unit for dose equivalent. For a quality factor (QA) = 1, one sievert is the dose equivalent of one gray (100 rad); 1 Sv = 100 rem.

signal-to-noise ratio A ratio describing the relationship between desired and unwanted information.

sinogram The tracing of a sine wave.

sinusoid Beginning of the venous system in the spleen, liver, bone marrow, and so on, that has an irregularly shaped, thin-walled space.

sinusoidal (1) Referring to a recess or cavity. (2) Referring to an abnormal channel that permits the escape of pus.

Sjögren syndrome An aggregate of signs and symptoms including dryness of mucous membranes, purpuric spots on the face, and bilateral parotid enlargement.

SNR Signal-to-noise ratio.

software Collection of programs and routines associated with a computer.

software bootstrap A bootstrap activated by loading the instructions and specifying the appropriate load and start address.

sol Liquid colloid solution.

solid phase antibody An antibody chemically linked to a solid surface.

solute Material dissolved into a solution.

solution Physical system consisting of one or more substances dissolved in another substance.

solvent Substance that acts as the dissolving agent in a solution.

solvent extraction Use of a second solvent to preferentially dissolve a compound out of another solution.

sorption Adsorption or absorption.

SPA (single photon absorptiometry) Bone mineral content measurement technique using gamma-ray or x-ray absorption with a single energy photon-emitting source.

spallation To chip or flake off.

specific activity Unit pertaining to the disintegrations per gram of a radioisotope.

specific ionization (SI) Linear rate of energy attenuation of ionizing radiation measured in terms of the number of ion pairs produced per unit distance traveled.

specificity The ability of a given test to determine what fraction or percentage of well patients will have a negative test result. Ability of a substance to recognize and bind to only one other molecule.

specific reactor substance Material capable of specifically and reversibly reacting with another molecule.

SPECT (single photon emission computed tomography) An imaging technique associated with single gamma-ray–emitting radiopharmaceuticals obtained using a scintillation camera that moves around the patient to obtain images from multiple angles for tomographic image reconstruction.

spectrometer Device measuring electromagnetic radiation characteristics in a spectrum.

spectrophotometry Use of an instrument that measures light or color by photonic transmission.

spermatogenesis Process of forming sperm.

sphincter Muscle controlling a body opening.

splanchnic Pertaining to the interior organs in any of the four great body cavities.

splenic hilum Fissure where vessels and nerves enter the spleen.

spondylolysis Breaking down or dissolution of the body of the vertebra.

SRS See *specific reactor substance*.

SSKI Saturated solution of potassium iodide.

stable electron configuration Configuration of electrons about an atom in the atom's lowest energy state.

standard A solution of pure substance of known concentration to which unknown substances may be compared.

standard deviation The square root of the average of the squares of the deviation of the value of a set of measurements from each of the individual measurements.

stannous ion Ion of tin in the +2 valence state.

stationary phase Chromatographic phase that does not move with the solvent front.

steatorrhea Excess fat in the feces.

stellate Star shaped.

stenosis A narrowing of a canal or vessel.

Stenson ducts Canals that empty the parotid gland.

steroid Complex molecular structure containing four interlocking rings—three contain six carbon atoms each and the fourth contains five carbon atoms.

stoichiometry Study of numeric interrelationships between chemical elements and compounds and the mathematical laws governing such relationships.

storage Device into which data can be entered and held and from which it can be retrieved.

stroke volume The quantity of blood ejected by the heart in a single beat.

student's *t*-test A test of statistical significance of a deviation.

subarachnoid Below the membrane between the dura mater and the pia mater.

subendocardial Below the endocardium.

subphrenic Below the diaphragm.

subprogram A program or a sequence of instructions that can be called to perform the same task (although perhaps on different data) at different points in a program or in different programs.

sulcus Any of the grooves or furrows on the surface of the brain.

supernatant, supernate Liquid lying above or floating on a precipitated material.

survey meter Meter that measures rate of radioactive exposure, usually in units of milliroentgens per hour.

SVC Superior vena cava.

synapse The place where a nerve impulse is transmitted from one neuron to another.

synarthrosis Immovable joint, where bones lock within one another.

synchronous Performance of a sequence of operations controlled by an external clocking device; implies that no operation can take place until the previous operation is complete.

synchronous transfer Sequenced computer program operated by an external clock that does not permit a step to proceed until the previous step is completed.

syncope Fainting.

synovia Transparent fluid found in joint cavities.

synovitis Inflammation of joint-lining membrane.

Système Internationale (SI) International system of units used to replace traditional units as a result of U.S. metrication laws PL 93-380 and PL 94-168.

systole Contraction and expelling of blood from the heart.

T$_3$ Triiodothyronine.

T$_4$ Tetraiodothyronine; thyroxine.

target Object to be bombarded by ionizing radiation, usually in an accelerator or cyclotron.

TBG See *thyroid-binding globulin.*

TBPA Thyroxine-binding prealbumin.

terminal An I/O device such as an LA120 terminal that includes a keyboard and a display mechanism; in PDP11 systems a terminal is the primary communication device between a computer and a user.

tesla Unit for measuring magnetic field strength; 1 tesla = 10,000 gauss.

tentorium Fibrous tissue shelf separating the cerebrum from the cerebellum.

testosterone Hormone produced by the testes, influencing the male characteristics.

tetrahedron Molecular geometry in which the central atom is attached to four other atoms and the bond axes are directed along the diagonals of a cube.

tetralogy of Fallot Birth defect involving deformities of the blood vessels and walls of the heart chamber.

therapeutic Referring to the treatment of disease.

therapeutic window Range of dosage of a pharmaceutical that produces a beneficial effect.

thermal neutrons Neutrons with a maximum kinetic energy of 100 keV.

thermionic emission Electrons freed from an atom by heat.

thermodynamics Study of processes based on energy changes in the system.

thermoluminescent detector (TLD) Type of crystal used to monitor radiation exposure by emitting light; used in a film badge or ring badge.

thiols Family of organic compounds containing the functional group —SH.

thoracic cage Chest cavity.

thrombin Enzyme used as a clotting agent.

thrombocyte See *platelet.*

thrombosis Formation of a blood clot.

thyroid-binding globulin (TBG) Serum protein that is the primary agent for transport for thyroid hormone.

thyroid gland Endocrine gland that regulates metabolism.

thyrotropin (TSH) Hormone stimulating the thyroid secreted by the anterior pituitary.

thyroxine Hormone of the thyroid gland; 3,5,3′,5′-tetraiodothyronine.

time constant The speed of response of a rate meter.

time sharing Method of allocating central processor time and other computer services to multiple uses so that the computer, in effect, processes a number of programs simultaneously.

titer (1) Aliquot of titrant (solution of known concentration). (2) The quantity of a substance required to produce a reaction with a given amount of another substance.

Title 10 of the Code of the Federal Regulations, Part 20 (10 CFR, Part 20) *United States Nuclear Regulatory Commission Rules and Regulations, Standards for Protection against Radiation;* Title 10 of the CFR pertains to atomic energy.

titration Method of quantitative analysis in which one substance is volumetrically added to another substance with which it quantitatively reacts.

titrimetric procedures Chemical laboratory procedure for quantitative analysis by addition of solution of a known concentration to a solution of unknown concentration.

TLD See *thermoluminescent detectors.*

torcula Hollow, expanded area.

tomograph Any image representing three-dimensional information.

total count tube A tube in an RIA to which an aliquot of labeled ligand only has been added to serve as a check on the delivery of that material.

TQM Total quality management.

trabeculae Fibrous tissue supporting the structure of an organ.

tracer study Examination either in vivo or in vitro using a small amount of radionuclide-labeled substance to follow its path.

trackball An electronic pointing device for a computer.

transcobalamin Derivative of the cobalt-containing complex common to all members of the vitamin B_{12} group.

transferrin Serum globulin binding and transporting iron.

transient equilibrium Equilibrium reached by a parent-daughter radioisotope pair in which the half-life of the parent is longer than the half-life of the daughter.

transmittance The fraction of light that passes through photographic film.

transmutation Nuclear process by which one element is changed into another element.

transudate Term given to solvents and solutes that pass through a membrane.

transverse tomography Transverse scanning of a cross section of an organ, done from multiple directions, and then superimposed in a specific manner.

trauma Injury; wound.

TRH Thyrotropin-releasing hormone.

tritium Isotope of hydrogen with a mass of three unified mass units, consisting of one proton and two neutrons.

TSH Thyroid-stimulating hormone; See *thyrotropin.*

turnkey Computer system sold in a ready-to-use state.

T wave The next deflection in the electrocardiogram following the QRS complex; it represents ventricular repolarization.

Tyndall effect Light reflected or dispersed by particles suspended in a gas or liquid.

tyrosine Amino acid present in proteins that are susceptible to radioiodination.

UIBC See *unsaturated iron-binding capacity.*

ultrasonic nebulizer Device used for dispersing liquids in a fine mist through the use of sound waves.

ultrasonography Use of sound waves to image an internal structure of the body.

United States Pharmacopeia (USP) Official listing of all drugs and medications.

UNIX A computer operating system.

unsaturated iron-binding capacity (UIBC) Amount of serum transferrin that is not saturated with iron.

USP See *United States Pharmacopeia.*

vaccine Dead bacteria given to build specific immunity against disease.

valence electrons Electrons in the outermost energy level.

valence state Ionization state of an element in an ionic compound.

van der Waals bond Attraction between the charged portions of two molecules, known as dipoles.

variable The symbolic representation of a logical storage location that can contain a value which changes during a processing operation.

variance Degree of change.

vascular Referring to the vessels.

vascular bed Entire blood supply of an organ or structure.

vascular lesion Lesion that affects the vessels.

vasculature (1) Supply of vessels to a region. (2) Vascular system.

vasculitis Inflammation of a vessel.

vasoconstrictor Something that causes the constriction of blood vessels.

vasodilator Something that causes the dilation of blood vessels.

VDT Video display terminal.

venipuncture Placement of a needle within a vein.

venography Radiography of the veins using a contrast medium; phlebography.

venous thrombi Blood clots within the veins.

ventilation Process of supplying air.

ventilation-perfusion ratio (V/Q) Comparison of functioning ventilatory space and perfused tissue within the lung; ratio of minute flow of air through alveoli to minute flow of blood through pulmonary capillaries.

ventricular Referring to a small cavity or chamber.

ventriculography Radiography of the ventricles of the brain

vesicoureteral reflux Backward flow of urine through the bladder and into a ureter.

vitamin Organic compound necessary to maintain normal growth or function; found in some amounts in plants and animals.

volt Basic unit of electrical potential equal to one joule per coulomb.

voltmeter Device used to measure potential difference in electric circuits; potentiometer.

volume (1) Amount of space occupied in three dimensions. (2) A mass storage medium that can be treated as file-structured data storage.

volume dilution Dilution of a solution by addition of pure liquid solvent.

V/Q See *ventilation-perfusion ratio.*

VUR See *vesicoureteral reflux.*

wavelength Length per cycle in wave-motion mechanics.

well counter A thallium-activated sodium iodide crystal scintillation detector with a hole in the crystal to accommodate a sample vial.

white blood cell (WBC) Blood cell whose nucleus determines the type of cell: lymphocyte, monocyte, neutrophil, eosinophil, basophil.

window (1) Region of interest. (2) Limits of energy radiation accepted by a pulse-height analyzer.

wipe test Testing for removable contamination.

word Unit of data that may be stored in one addressable location (most microcomputers use 16-bit words).

WORM A type of optical disk drive; *write once read many.*

xerostomia Dryness of the mouth.

x-pulse In an Anger scintillation camera those pulses emanating from the resistor/capacitor network positioned in a horizontal manner.

x ray Photonic radiation originating from electronic deexcitation.

x-ray diffraction Spectroscopic method for determining crystal structure by the interaction of x rays with the atoms involved in the crystalline structure.

xiphisternum Inferior tip of the sternum.

y pulse In an Anger scintillation camera those pulses emanating from the resistor/capacitor network positioned in a vertical manner.

zipper effect Overlap of two or more images.

Z number See *atomic number.*

Zollinger-Ellison syndrome Familial polyendocrine adenomatosis.

z pulse In an Anger scintillation camera it represents the sum of the x and y pulses.

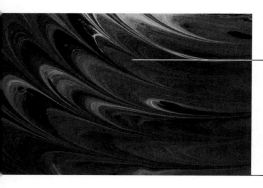

Index